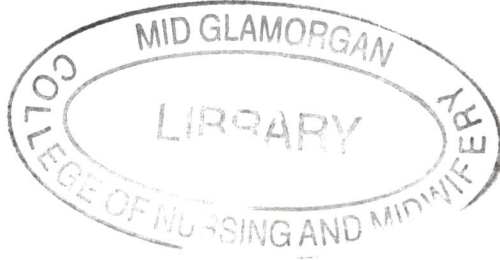
STANDARD LOAN

Renew Books on PHONE-it: 01443 654456

Books are to be returned on or before the last date below

Glyntaff Learning Resources Centre
University of Glamorgan CF37 4BD

POSTOPERATIVE MANAGEMENT

of the

CARDIAC SURGICAL PATIENT

Edited by

John P. Williams, M.D.

Associate Professor
Department of Anesthesiology
University of California, Los Angeles
UCLA School of Medicine
Director
Division of Cardiothoracic Anesthesiology
Department of Anesthesiology
Co-Director
Surgical Intensive Care Medicine
UCLA Medical Center
Los Angeles, California

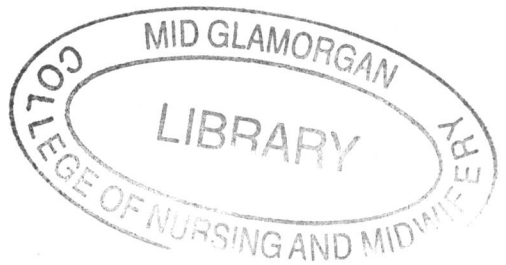

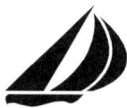

CHURCHILL LIVINGSTONE

New York, Edinburgh, London, Madrid, Melbourne, San Francisco, Tokyo

Library of Congress Cataloging-in-Publication Data

Postoperative management of the cardiac surgical patient / edited by
    John P. Williams.
        p.   cm.
    Includes bibliographical references and index.
    ISBN 0–443–08932–9
    1. Heart—Surgery. 2. Postoperative care. 3. Heart—
Pathophysiology.   I. Williams, John P. (John Phillip), date
    [DNLM: 1. Heart Surgery. 2. Postoperative Care. 3. Heart
Diseases—physiopathology. WG 169 P858 1996]
    RD598.P585 1996
    617.4`12059—dc20
    DNLM/DLC
    for Library of Congress   96–4759
                                                                            CIP

Distributed in the United Kingdom by Churchill Livingstone, Robert Stevenson
House, 1–3 Baxter's Place, Leith Walk, Edinburgh EH1 3AF, and by associated
companies, branches, and representatives throughout the world.

Accurate indications, adverse reactions, and dosage schedules for drugs are provided in this book, but it is possible that they may change. The reader is urged to
review the package information data of the manufacturers of the medications
mentioned.

The Publishers have made every effort to trace the copyright holders for bor-
rowed material. If they have inadvertently overlooked any, they will be pleased to
make the necessary arrangements at the first opportunity.

Acquisitions Editor: *Michael J. Houston*
Production Editor: *David Terry*
Production Supervisor: *Laura Mosberg Cohen*
Cover Design: *Jeannette Jacobs*

Printed in the United States of America

First published in 1996   7   6   5   4   3   2   1

To intensive care practitioners throughout the world

A group of physicians brought together through a common concern for the most gravely ill members of our society; a group without borders, nationality, creed, or religion

To Erin Sullivan

Without whom none of this would be possible (or worthwhile)

To Brynna

Here is at least one of the reasons your father was not in Houston

To UCLA

An institution that has taught me more about the necessity for vigilance, persistence, and thoroughness than any other

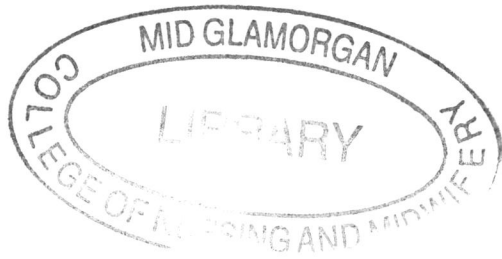

Contributors

Catherine Amrein, M.D.
Associate Clinical Professor, Department of Anesthesiology, Paris University Faculty of Medicine, Paris, France

S. Beloucif, M.D.
Assistant Professor, Lariboisière University Faculty of Medicine; Attending Physician, Department of Anesthesiology and Critical Care, Lariboisière Hospital, Paris, France

James Berry, M.D.
Assistant Professor, Department of Anesthesiology, University of Texas-Houston Medical School, Houston, Texas

Sture G. I. Blomberg, M.D., Ph.D.
Visiting Professor, Department of Anesthesiology, University of California, Los Angeles, UCLA School of Medicine; Attending Anesthesiologist, Department of Anesthesiology, UCLA Medical Center, Los Angeles, California

Howard I. Chait, M.D.
Associate Clinical Professor, Department of Anesthesiology, University of California, Los Angeles, UCLA School of Medicine, Los Angeles, California

Gordon A. Cohen, M.D.
Chief Resident, Department of Surgery, University of California, Los Angeles, UCLA School of Medicine, Los Angeles, California

John R. Cooper, Jr., M.D.
Clinical Associate Professor, Department of Anesthesiology, University of Texas-Houston Medical School; Associate Chief, Department of Cardiovascular Anesthesiology, Texas Heart Institute; Medical Director, Cardiovascular Recovery Room, St. Luke's Episcopal Hospital; Consultant in Cardiovascular Anesthesiology, Texas Children's Hospital, Houston, Texas

Nicholas Deutsch, M.D.
Attending Anesthesiologist, Department of Anesthesiology, Kaiser Permanente Medical Group, Sunset Medical Center, Los Angeles, California

Dominique Farge, M.D., Ph.D.
Professor, Department of Internal Medicine, Lariboisière University Faculty of Medicine, Saint Louis Hospital, Paris, France

Carin Hagberg, M.D.
Assistant Professor, Department of Anesthesiology, University of Texas-Houston Medical School; Associate Medical Director, Operative Services, Department of Anesthesiology, Hermann Hospital, Houston, Texas

Darryl T. Hiyama, M.D.
Assistant Professor, Division of General Surgery, Department of Surgery, University of California, Los Angeles, UCLA School of Medicine; Director, Surgical Nutritional Support Service, UCLA Medical Center, Los Angeles, California

Ron M. Jones, M.B., M.D., F.R.C.A.
Professor and Director, Department of Anaesthetics, Imperial College School of Medicine, London, England

Norman S. Kato, M.D.
Assistant Professor, Division of Cardiothoracic Surgery, Department of Surgery, University of California, Los Angeles, UCLA School of Medicine, Los Angeles, California

Jeffrey Katz, M.D.
Professor and Chairman, Department of Anesthesiology, University of Texas-Houston Medical School, Houston, Texas

Gregory Kerr, M.D.
Assistant Professor, Department of Anesthesiology, Cornell University Medical College; Associate Attending Physician, Department of Anesthesiology, The New York Hospital–Cornell Medical Center, New York, New York

Tiong H. Liem, M.D., Ph.D.
Anesthesiologist, Department of Anesthesiology, University of Nijmegen Faculty of Medicine; Director of Cardiac Anesthesiology, Department of Anesthesiology, University Hospital of Nijmegen, Nijmegen, the Netherlands

B. V. Murthy, M.V., B. S., F.R.C.A.
Registrar, Department of Anaesthetics, St. Mary's Hospital, London, England

Gerald V. Naccarelli, M.D.
Professor, Department of Medicine, and Chief, Division of Cardiology, Pennsylvania State University College of Medicine; Director, Penn State Cardiovascular Center, The Milton S. Hershey Medical Center, Hershey, Pennsylvania

Peter Nicolazzo, M.D.
Assistant Clinical Professor, Department of Anesthesiology, University of California, Los Angeles, UCLA School of Medicine; Staff Anesthesiologist, Department of Anesthesiology, West Los Angeles Veterans Affairs Medical Center, Los Angeles, California

D. Payen, M.D., Ph.D.
Professor, Lariboisière University Faculty of Medicine; Chairman, Department of Anesthesiology and Critical Care, and Head, Surgical Intensive Care Unit, Lariboisière Hospital, Paris, France

David T. Porembka, M.D., F.C.C.M., F.C.C.P.
Associate Professor, Departments of Anesthesia and Surgery, University of Cincinnati College of Medicine; Associate Director, Department of Surgical Intensive Care, and Director, Department of Transesophageal Echocardiography, University Hospital, Cincinnati, Ohio

Bruce D. Spiess, M.D.
Associate Professor, Department of Anesthesiology, and Chief, Division of Cardiothoracic Anesthesia, University of Washington School of Medicine, Seattle, Washington

Erin A. Sullivan, M.D.
Assistant Professor, Department of Anesthesiology, Director, Anesthesiology Residency Program, and Director, Anesthesiology Fellowship Program, University of California, Los Angeles, UCLA School of Medicine, Los Angeles, California

Stephen J. Thomas, M.D.
Professor, Department of Anesthesiology, Cornell University Medical College; Vice Chairman, Department of Anesthesiology, The New York Hospital–Cornell Medical Center, New York, New York

John P. Williams, M.D.
Associate Professor, Department of Anesthesiology, University of California, Los Angeles, UCLA School of Medicine; Director, Division of Cardiothoracic Anesthesiology, Department of Anesthesiology, and Co-Director, Surgical Intensive Care Medicine, UCLA Medical Center, Los Angeles, California

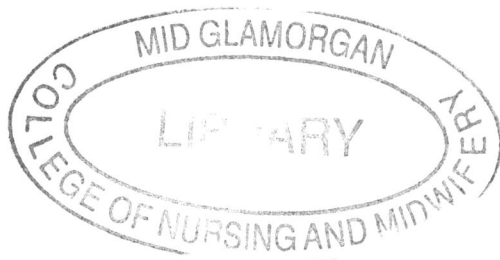

Preface

This book describes the management of the postoperative cardiac surgical patient, and provides ready access to clinical problems encountered by such patients. The book's tripartite organization permits the reader to explore recent research into the pathophysiologic mechanisms of cardiac illness, to understand the effects of cardiopulmonary bypass upon such mechanisms, and to anticipate specific postoperative problems. The book also serves as a valuable preoperative reference.

Authors from France, England, Sweden, and the Netherlands provide a global perspective for clinical management, offering their considerable expertise in the areas of hemodynamic and pharmacologic, renal, and pain management in the postoperative period. Authors from throughout the United States also offer perspectives on the management of pulmonary, cerebral, dysrhythmic, and hematologic disturbances. The authors are all recognized experts in their respective fields and bring a large body of knowledge and peer-reviewed publications to this book.

Special sections are included that describe the application of echocardiography and mechanical circulatory support to the field of cardiac intensive care. These areas are rapidly developing and are increasingly incorporated as integral aspects of complete postoperative intensive care.

As noted previously, the book is divided into three sections. This arrangement allows the authors in the clinical management section to concentrate on postoperative management, thus avoiding repetitive descriptions of pathophysiology.

The first section describes the pathophysiologic changes that result in the need for surgical intervention in the cardiac patient population. The pathophysiologic consequences of valvular heart disease and cardiomyopathic disorders are described in this section, as are the basics of transplantation immunology.

In the second section, the interaction of these pathophysiologic changes with cardiopulmonary bypass are considered with special emphasis on how these changes affect the postoperative management of the patient. The reader is encouraged to follow each section in a stepwise fashion; however, cross references have been provided for finding relevant topics throughout the book.

The third and largest section is dedicated to the actual systems-level management of the postoperative patient. Each of the systems is covered in detail and management of specific complications are discussed in each chapter. While many of the pathophysiologic consequences following cardiopulmonary bypass surgery may overlap, the reader is referred to specific chapters when this occurs.

This is the first clinical book available that covers the postoperative management of the cardiac surgical patient. This book is unique in its niche. The focus of moving a patient from pathophysiology through surgery and into the postoperative period allows the reader to explore cogently the reasons for choosing specific management techniques.

Day-to-day management of specific problems is easily examined by using a systems-level approach. For example, the reader interested in the management of renal insufficiency can move directly to the chapter on renal dysfunction to discover the latest in intraoperative management as well as post-operative care of the patient following cardiac surgery.

The intended audience is any critical care professional who is involved in the care of postoperative cardiac patients. Both the consultant-level practitioner as well as the general intensivist will find the book useful in the daily management of the postoperative cardiac surgical patient.

John P. Williams, M.D.

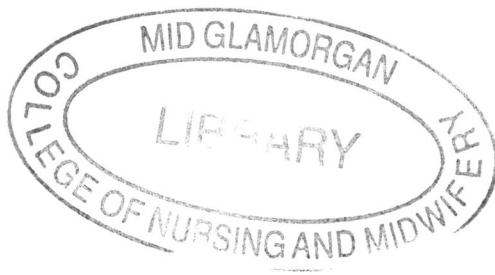

Acknowledgments

I wish to acknowledge the work of the following people:

The chapter authors, for their dedication and timely submission of their manuscripts; Barbara J. Carter, for her unflagging and dedicated efforts to unscramble my mysterious and often cryptic editing marks; and Churchill Livingstone, for offering me the opportunity to publish a work in my chosen field of critical care medicine.

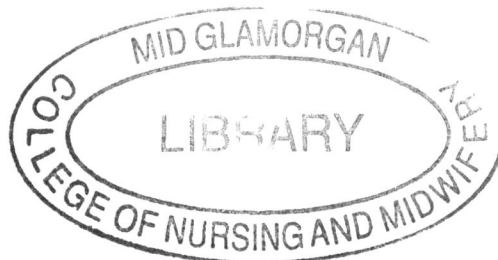

Contents

Color plates appear after pp. 258 and 268.

1

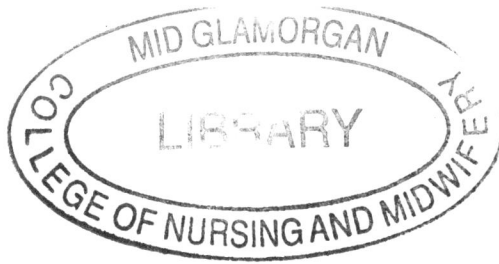

Regurgitant Valvular Disorders

John P. Williams

This chapter comprises three parts. The first section describes in brief the etiology of valvular regurgitation. There is no intent to contrast the various causes unless the description is clinically relevant (i.e., the difference between acute and chronic regurgitation). Similarly, the second section, pathophysiology, dwells not on differences between various causes of regurgitation, but rather on their hemodynamic similarities. As such, the second section is divided into two subsections on atrial and ventricular changes accompanying valvular regurgitation. The third and final section of this chapter deals with the special concerns presented by groups of patients with either right- or left-sided regurgitant lesions. Specifically, this section covers those concerns related to pre-existing organ dysfunction and the implication this carries for care in the postoperative period.

Unlike stenotic lesions, regurgitant lesions may be subdivided into acute and chronic types. This distinction is important on both morphologic and functional bases. While the physiologic adaptive mechanisms are similar in both regurgitant subtypes, they differ in their relative success (as measured by sur-

vival of the patient). Further distinction relates to the number of possible causes of regurgitant versus stenotic lesions. There are a large number of possible causes of regurgitant lesions (Table 1-1), while causes of stenotic lesions are comparatively few.

A final, but important, difference involves the timing of surgery. Those patients with stenotic lesions are often symptomatic for many years before surgical intervention is required. Patients with regurgitant lesions may remain asymptomatic even after the onset of irreversible left ventricular dysfunction. This complicates both the timing of surgical intervention as well as the postoperative care.

ETIOLOGY AND HISTORY

Etiology

CHRONIC REGURGITANT LESIONS

The common causes of valvular regurgitation are broadly divided into six classes: congenital, inflammatory, ischemic, infective, vascular, and traumatic (Table 1-1). The relative predominance of one class of lesions is relatively unimportant. Isolated, purely regurgi-

Table 1-1. Etiology and Classification of Valvular Heart Disease

Valve Involved	Class	Etiology
Mitral	Congenital	Marfan syndrome Anatomic aberrancy ("floppy")
	Inflammatory	Rheumatoid arthritis Carcinoid
	Ischemic	Papillary dysfunction or rupture
	Infectious	Rheumatic fever Endocarditis
	Traumatic	Penetrating
Aortic	Congenital	Anatomic aberration Marfan syndrome
	Inflammatory	SLE Ankylosing spondylitis
	Infectious	Syphilitic Endocarditis Rheumatic fever
	Vascular	Aortic dissection
	Traumatic	Penetrating Blunt
Tricuspid	Congenital	Ebstein's anomaly Anatomic aberrancy
	Inflammatory	Carcinoid
	Infectious	Endocarditis Rheumatic fever
	Ischemic	Papillary muscle dysfunction
	Vascular	Pulmonary hypertension
	Traumatic	Penetrating Radiation
Pulmonary	Congenital	Anatomic aberrancy
	Inflammatory	Carcinoid
	Infectious	Endocarditis Rheumatic Fever
	Vascular	Pulmonary hypertension
	Traumatic	Catheter induced

Abbreviation: SLE, systemic lupus erythematosus.

tant lesions are uncommonly rheumatic (as compared to stenotic lesions); however, if more than one valve is involved, the cause is almost always rheumatic.[1,2] The overall incidence of regurgitant lesions in operative valvular candidates is approximately 19 percent.[3] The mitral valve is the most frequently involved (59 percent), followed by the aortic valve (40 percent), and the tricuspid valve (1 percent). When combined multivalvular dis-

ease is involved, only 4 percent of valves excised at the time of surgery are found to be regurgitant; thus the predominant modifying physiologic influence in multivalvular disease is stenosis (see Ch. 2).

These numbers compare well with a series of patients with fatal valvular diseases. Twenty-six percent of necropsy specimens were purely regurgitant. The relative percentages of involvement were aortic valve (12 percent), mitral valve (10 percent), and multi-valvular (4 percent).[3] Purely regurgitant mitral valves are rarely associated with commiseral fusion, calcific deposits, or chordal alterations. In a recent cohort of 97 patients following operative intervention for mitral regurgitation (MR), the overwhelming cause (62 percent) was morphologic alteration (prolapse) of valves, with only 2 percent demonstrating rheumatic involvement.[1]

Aortic involvement is most commonly associated with rheumatic disease, accounting for variously 26 to 49 percent of valves excised surgically.[4,5] The disease process usually results in diffuse fibrosis and thickening of each cusp with retraction of one or more cusps. Only small amounts of calcific deposits are typically present.

Very little time and space is used here to discuss etiologic agents for right-sided valvular lesions, as they rarely account for more than 1 percent of all valves excised surgically. Table 1-1 covers the most common causes of right-sided valvular dysfunction.

ACUTE REGURGITANT LESIONS
Acute MR is a common complication following myocardial infarction. The incidence varies with anatomic location of the infarct (15 percent of anterior and up to 40 percent of posterior infarcts).[5] However, most of these episodes of MR resolve spontaneously, with less than 1 percent of all anterior acute ischemic MR requiring emergent surgical intervention.[6] Acute MR secondary to endocarditis frequently occurs in association with aortic valvular disease and is commonly associated with pre-existing aortic involvement (45 percent of cases).[7]

Aortic regurgitation (AR) is most commonly a result of endocarditis, dissection (Marfan syndrome, hypertension, etc.), or trauma.[8]

Natural History
CHRONIC REGURGITANT LESIONS
The capacitance of the left atrium is the single most important determinant of the symptomatic course of MR. A large-capacity atrium is able to "absorb" a large volume of regurgitant flow from the left ventricle; this will limit the onset of symptomology. The slow insidious nature of chronic MR allows the left atrium to gradually enlarge and adapt to the increasing end-systolic volume.

Most patients remain asymptomatic for many years or even decades before evincing the first overt symptoms: fatigue and dyspnea.[9] Fatigue is generally indicative of a failure of cardiac output to rise with increases in demand, while dyspnea generally represents increased alveolar fluid content. Moderate to severe pulmonary hypertension follows if surgical intervention is not forthcoming.[10] A group of patients treated medically demonstrated a 40 percent mortality at 10 years without surgical intervention.[11]

Similarly, AR cloaks its insidious nature by allowing normal (at times even vigorous) physical activities without symptomatology.[12,13] This asymptomatic period will last from 10 to 15 years before the onset of symptoms: exertional dyspnea or prominent neck pulsations. If surgical intervention is withheld, an ineluctable progress toward left ventricular decompensation, failure, and death typically ensues over an 8- to 10-year period.[13] In a cohort of 35 patients treated medically, only 63 percent survived 10 or more years after diagnosis.

ACUTE REGURGITANT LESIONS
Acute MR or AR is uniformly fatal if not treated surgically.[3,5,7,8] Although surgical mortality is high with either disorder, AR is generally associated with lower mortality than MR.

Risk Stratification
MITRAL REGURGITATION
The patient with chronic regurgitation often presents a clinical dilemma. Although the determinants of poor outcome following valvular surgery have not changed, the type of surgery is rapidly changing. The factors that are traditionally associated with poor survival are

Table 1-2. Predictions of Poor Outcome After Mitral Valve Replacement

Age (>60 yrs)
NYHA class (3 or 4)
Associated CAD
Cardiac Index <2.0 L·min^{-1}·m^{-2}
LVEDP >12 mmHg
Pulmonary hypertension
End-systolic volume index (ESVI) >90 ml·m^{-2}
Ejection fraction <50% (cath data)
ESWS/ESVI ratio (≤2.4)

Abbreviations: NYHA, New York Heart Association; CAD, coronary artery disease; LVEDP, left ventricular end-diastolic pressure; ESWS, end-systolic wall stress.

listed in Table 1-2.[14–20] The reliability of these predictors is under review because the advent and ascendency of mitral repairs[21–25] and aggressive vasodilator therapy[26] may have altered these traditional risk modifiers.

It is increasingly common for patients with lesser degrees of ventricular impairment to present for mitral repair. Operative mortality is reported as the same or lower than that experienced by patients undergoing valve replacement.[27–29] Further, the morbidity from subsequent thromboembolism, endocarditis, and anticoagulation is substantially reduced with repair.[27,29,30]

Unfortunately, the results following valvular repair are generally surgeon specific (at least with regard to experience), and other factors that are patient specific (i.e., mitral calcification, under-reporting of symptoms, patient reliability and compliance) are often as important as the predictors for poor outcome listed in Table 1-2.

Patients with symptomatic MR are uniformly recommended for surgery. Unfortunately, symptomatic patients all exhibit some degree of ventricular dysfunction.[31] The presence of symptomatology severe enough to result in a New York Heart Association (NYHA) classification of III or IV is associated with a poor outcome, although load-independent measures of ventricular function (end-systolic volume index [ESVI] or the ratio of end-systolic wall stress [ESWS] to ESVI) are better discriminators.

In brief, the systolic unloading characteristics of MR (see next section) render many ejection phase estimates of left ventricular function useless. This not only makes judgments of when to send a patient for surgery difficult, but also obfuscates expectations regarding postoperative function. In general, patients with ejection fractions of less than 50 percent or ESVI greater than 90 ml·M^{-2}, and especially those with symptoms, should be considered higher-risk candidates.

AORTIC REGURGITATION

The situation with AR is significantly different. Although the lowered diastolic pressure does diminish workload during early systolic ejection (see following sections), this is insufficient to significantly alter ejection phase indices of performance. As the occurrence of symptoms in AR is generally concomitant with decrements in ventricular performance, general recommendations for surgery hinge on ventricular function regardless of symptomatology.[8,18,32] A list of findings and demographic data that offer predictive value for survival is found in Table 1-3.[20,33–39] Not all of these are predictors in all studies, however, and most are long-term and not strictly postoperative in their focus. In those studies that focus on postoperative outcome, elevated left ventricular end diastolic pressure (LVEDP) and pulmonary pressure are common predictors, as are the end-systolic volume index, left ventricular dilation (greater

Table 1-3. Suggested Predictors of Poor Outcome After Aortic Valve Replacement

Age (>65 yrs)
Male sex
NYHA class (3 or 4)
Exercise capacity (<22.5 min)
Cardiothoracic ratio (>0.60)
Cardiac index (<2.5 L·min^{-1}·m^{-2})
Pulmonary hypertension
Ejection fraction (<50% on cath or 60% on echo)
End-systolic diameter (>55 mm)
End-systolic volume index (>90 ml·m^{-2})

Abbreviation: NYHA, New York Heart Association.

than 5.5 cm), and reduced fractional shortening or ejection fraction.

Similar to acute MR, AR occurring suddenly is a surgical emergency.[8,31,32] This does not imply that attempts to ameliorate the symptoms of massive left ventricular volume overload are unnecessary. In fact, most of these patients require emergent medical management prior to operative intervention. However, operative repair in the emergent setting is associated with a higher mortality (10 to 27 percent).[8,40]

PATHOPHYSIOLOGIC ALTERATIONS

Functional Alterations

The classic finding in the heart with chronic volume overload is eccentric hypertrophy (i.e., an increase in both chamber size and wall thickness).[41] While this description is generally true of all regurgitant lesions, the loading conditions experienced by the ventricle in these disorders vary greatly (Table 1-4).

MITRAL REGURGITATION

MR represents a relatively pure form of volume loading. The ventricle progressively dilates in response to the increase in volume; however, in chronic MR the atrium acts as a high-capacity, low-impedance reservoir for the excess volume. This progressively lowers both peak and instantaneous wall stress on the ventricle. The result is a reduction in both ventricular afterload and maintenance of cardiac output, but with an augmentation of stroke volume.[42] All ejection phase measures of function are preserved until late in the course of this disorder.

In a sense, the ventricle is being "trained" to work as a high-volume, low-pressure pump. Volume work in the setting of low pressure requires the myocardial fibrils to perform work in shortening rather than tension development. It is in effect similar to skeletal muscle training for an endurance event (e.g., marathon running) rather than a power event (e.g., weightlifting). This also has the unfortunate side effect of "deconditioning" the ventricle for power events (i.e.,

Table 1-4. Typical Functional Changes Associated With Regurgitant Lesions

Disorder	Ventricle	Atrium
Chronic AR	Augmentation of preload Ejection phase indices increased initially, then decreased Cardiac output maintained	Few changes until late in the disease Gradual dilation following increases in left-ventricular end-diastolic pressure
Chronic MR	Dilation of ventricle Cardiac output maintained Ejection phase indices increased or normal Deconditioning of ventricle for tension development	Progressive dilation Atrial fibrillation Low left atrial pressure Little pulmonary hypertension (until late in the disease)
Acute AR	Rapid increase in end-diastolic pressure Ejection phase indices fall immediately Dilated, hypocontractile ventricle	Left atrial pressure rises concomitantly with end-diastolic pressure Pulmonary edema and congestion
Acute MR	Immediate increase in end-diastolic pressure and volume but less than AR No change or decrease in wall tension Enhanced early diastolic filling Marked reduction of stroke volume	Marked reduction of left atrial pressure Pulmonary congestion and right heart failure Sinus rhythm the norm Little change in chamber size

Abbreviations: AR, aortic regurgitation; MR, mitral regurgitation.

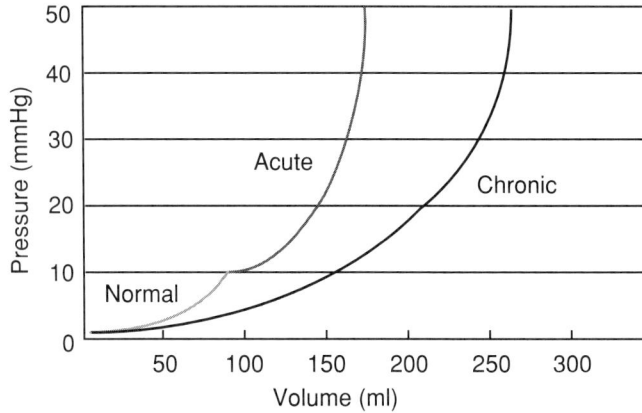

Fig. 1-1. Changes in ventricular complicance occur over time with the onset of aortic valvular regurgitation. If the onset of regurgitation is acute, the ventricular pressures rise rapidly, moving from the "normal" range into the "acute" range. If the degree of regurgitation increases slowly, the ventricular morphology will change to adapt to the volume increase and move to the "chronic" curve.

tension development) following mitral repair or replacement.

This functional disparity between shortening and tension work is the basis for the diagnostic versus prognostic discrepancy describing the typical patient undergoing mitral valve surgery. Diagnostic ejection phase indices in the low "normal" range are not reliably prognostic of a good surgical outcome because the ventricle is not exposed to "normal" (i.e., postsurgical) afterload. This also ensures that these ventricles are exquisitely afterload-sensitive in the immediate postoperative period.

Alternative strategies for surgical decision-making might include the following: sequential biopsy of the left ventricle to determine when sufficient fibril alteration occurs to represent an increased surgical risk; the use of materials for annuloplasty that gradually constrict the mitral annulus (ameroid, magnetic, etc.); and balloon "challenges" of the left ventricle to assess tension resiliency (i.e., short periods of systolic mitral occlusion with simultaneous measurement of ejection indices measured once every year or two). Each of these approaches offers a more direct assessment of morphologic and functional changes than current practice. The use of a slowly progressive annuloplasty implies that the ventricle can be retrained for tension development if sufficient time is available.

ACUTE MITRAL REGURGITATION

Acute MR is dramatically different in both presentation and functional alterations from chronic MR (Fig. 1-1). If the degree of MR is severe, such as occurs following papillary muscle rupture after myocardial infarction, the result is rapidly fatal.[43] However, acute MR is generally better tolerated than similar degrees of AR.[44,45] This is primarily related to the decrease in late systolic wall tension (afterload) in MR, which increases fractional shortening.[46,47] The changes of acute MR rarely result in a large increase in myocardial oxygen consumption; however, if acute regurgitation persists, end-diastolic pressure rises, which gradually increases wall tension.[48,49] This increase in wall tension will increase myocardial oxygen consumption and may ultimately result in myocardial ischemia.[50]

AORTIC REGURGITATION

The principal functional difference between AR and MR is afterload. As noted previously, the regurgitant volume in MR is ejected into a low-impedance system. In AR, the regurgitant fraction is ejected into a high-impedance system (the systemic circulation). This difference in impedance results in significant changes in function. While the reduction in afterload offers the majority of compensation in MR, preload dependent forces (i.e., increases in ventricular end-diastolic volume) offer the most compensation in AR. Patients with AR as a group have the largest increases in end-diastolic volume of all valvular lesions. This results in *cor bovinum* (literally "cow heart"). Volume overload is the most common stimulus for eccentric hypertrophy.[41] Interestingly, however, these morphologic alterations rarely decrease ventricular compliance, which results in little or no increase in end-diastolic pressure.

As in MR, ejection phase indices remain normal until late in the course of the disease. Unlike MR, however, ejection indices are a reliable if slightly late measure of ventricular decompensation in AR.[51–53] The gradual rise in ventricular end-diastolic volume eventually leads to afterload mismatch (chamber size increase outstripping wall thickness increase), which in turn leads to decrements in contractility and an increase in end-systolic volume.[54,55] Most, if not all, of these changes will precede the onset of symptoms. Finally, the large increase in muscle mass combined with a decrease in diastolic pressure leads to marked reductions in coronary flow reserve.[56]

ACUTE AORTIC REGURGITATION

Unlike the scenario in chronic AR, acute onset of AR results in immediate ventricular decompensation. In experimental animals, this is experienced as a rise in preload, wall tension, and myocardial oxygen consumption.[57,58] This limits the ability of the ventricle to augment stroke volume, which leads to a rapid increase in ventricular end-diastolic pressure (Fig. 1-2). Thus, the patient with acute AR will have a much narrower pulse pressure than one with chronic AR for similar degrees of regurgitation.[59]

Morphologic Alterations

VENTRICULAR ALTERATIONS

Eccentric hypertrophy refers to enlargement of chamber size (dilation) and wall thickness such that the ratio between the two remains constant.[60] This is presumably a physiologic response of the myocardium to maintain wall tension constant.

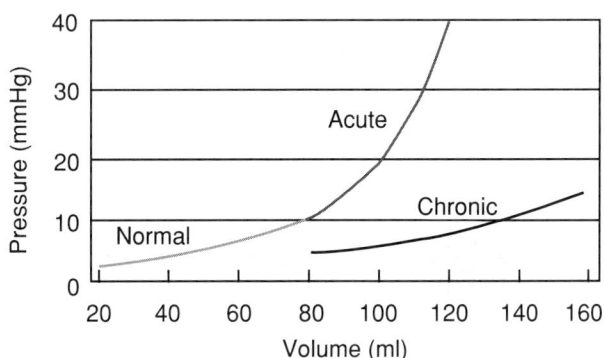

Fig. 1-2. Similar to the changes related to aortic regurgitation, atrial level responses to acute and chronic mitral regurgitation define two compliance curves. If the degree of regurgitation increases rapidly, then atrial pressures will rise steeply, moving from the "normal" area to the "acute" region. If the degree of regurgitation increases over many years, the atrium will dilate and atrial pressure will change very little, although volume will increase dramatically.

Wall tension is related to wall thickness and chamber size through Laplace's equation:

$$T = \frac{PR}{2} \qquad (1)$$

where T = tension, P = pressure, and R is the radius.

However, volume overload also increases end-diastolic wall stress, determined as follows:

$$S = \frac{PR}{2h} \qquad (2)$$

where S = stress and h = wall thickness.

The increase in end-diastolic wall stress causes the sarcomeres to replicate in series rather than in parallel (parallel replication occurs with pressure overload). This allows the ventricle to accommodate large increases in volume while simultaneously maintaining a low end-diastolic pressure (compliance increases) and effective forward stroke volume (fractional shortening remains constant).

Left ventricular mass increases concomitant with the degree of hypertrophy. The imposition of any additional restrictions on coronary blood flow (i.e., superimposed coronary artery disease), however, results in a reduced response to the volume overload stimulus. This implies that the diagnosis of coronary atherosclerosis associated with ventricular dysfunction results in an increase in surgical risk; both of which are true (Table 1-3).

If, however, no change occurs in coronary flow, the insidious increase in end-diastolic volume continues until no further morphologic changes occur. Once this stage of the disease is reached, progressive decreases in myocyte shortening, ejection fraction, diastolic compliance, and cardiac output result[61] with simultaneous increases in end-diastolic pressure and symptomatology.[61,62] In the patient with longstanding MR, the accompanying ventricular dilation will increase mitral annular size, thereby increasing regurgitation and actually accelerating the development of ventricular decompensation.[42]

The degree of ventricular hypertrophy in MR is significantly less than that in AR, however.[62] The ratio of chamber size to wall thickness is higher in MR,[41,62] indicating an elevated level of wall stress (see equation 2). Only the presence of a low-afterload outlet (the regurgitant valve and compliant left atrium) serves to reduce wall stress to near normal levels (Fig. 1-3).

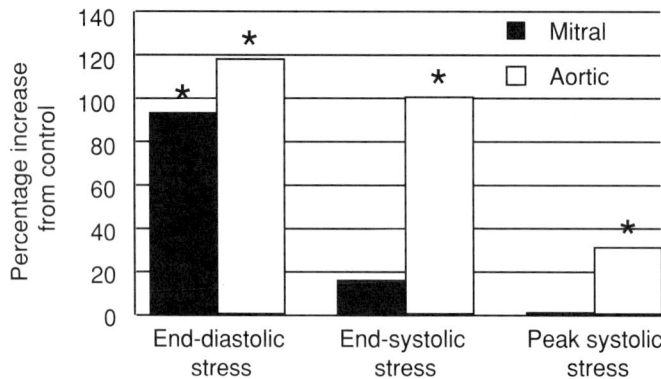

Fig. 1-3. Effect of regurgitation on ventricular stress. There is similar increase in end-diastolic stress in both aortic and mitral regurgitation. However, increases in peak systolic and end-systolic stress only occur with aortic regurgitation. This explains in part the difference in responses following surgical correction of similar degrees of regurgitation. Asterisks (*) indicate $P < 0.05$ versus control.

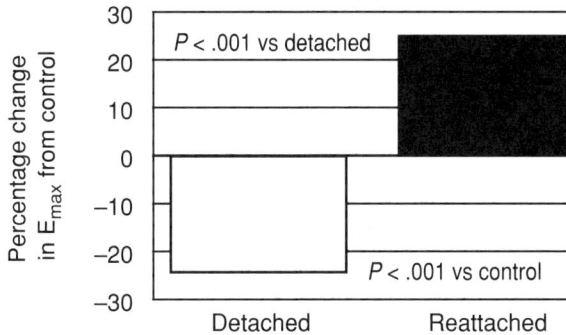

Fig. 1-4. Another possible cause for the decline in ventricular function following mitral valve replacement is removal of the chordal attachments. If the mitral apparatus is removed in dogs, there is a 25 percent decline in ventricular function (E_{max}). If the apparatus is then reattached in those same animals, it is associated with a 22 percent rise in ventricular function.

Further degradation in ventricular structure and function occurs if the mitral valve apparatus is removed[63–65] (Fig. 1-4). This in large part accounts for the improvement in outcome with mitral repair compared to replacement. The attachments of the mitral valve to the papillary muscles cause the long axis of the ventricle to shorten and the short axis to lengthen during early isovolemic systole. This early systolic increase in short axis length enhances late systolic function through the Frank-Starling mechanism.[64,66]

An additional problem encountered in this group of patients is the increase in diastolic stiffness associated with the slow decline in ejection fraction.[67] This decrease in diastolic compliance may be related to excessive hypertrophy[68–70] or fibrosis,[71–73] but not to chamber geometry.[67] Further, the increase in ventricular stiffness does not appear to be related to a decrease in coronary reserve blood supply.[74]

Others have noted that there are no changes in interstitial volume in animals following 3 months of chordal disruption and MR[75] (Fig. 1-5). However, this model did result in a lengthening of cardiac myocytes and decreases in the sarcomere shortening and relaxation velocities. These results imply that the contractile and relaxation defects in an acute model of MR are intrinsic to the myo-

cyte and not the milieu in which the myocyte is immersed.[76] Further, the myofibrils constituted a statistically smaller portion of each myocyte in those dogs with the greatest degree of global contractile dysfunction. There were no changes in mitochondrial density. These changes are typical of those seen in acute MR[77] and myocardial failure[78]; they are *not* as characteristic of chronic, *compensated* MR.[77]

ATRIAL ALTERATIONS

The morphologic response of the atrium in MR is entirely dependent upon the level of distention and the time course of the disease. Thus, with acute MR, there is little time for morphologic alteration and the atrium is a stiff, noncompliant reservoir. If the increase in distension is gradual, the atrium responds in a manner qualitatively similar to the ventricle but quantitatively to a lesser degree. A singularly problematic event accompanying the increase in left atrial compliance occurs secondary to left atrial dilation: atrial fibrillation. Further, the increase in size and decrease in atrial function associated with atrial fibrillation creates large areas of stagnant or eddying flow. This stagnation predisposes the atrium to thrombus formation.

The associated morphologic changes accompanying atrial dilation are thin fibrotic

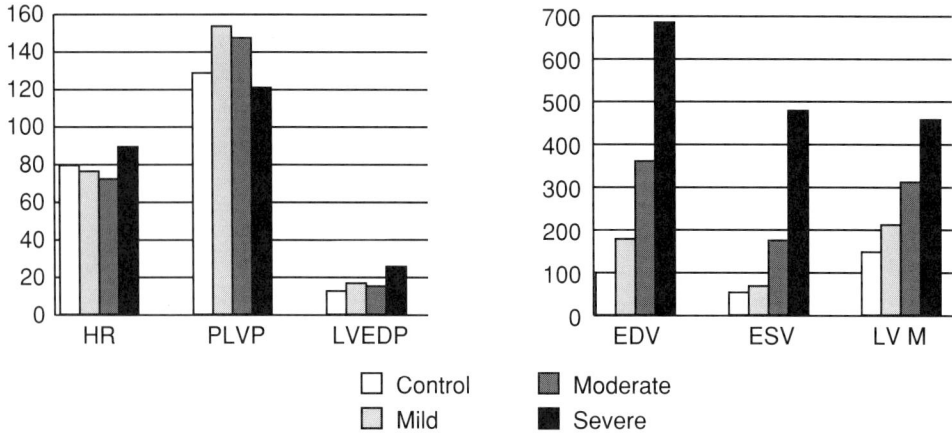

Fig. 1-5. Degree of ventricular dysfunction (i.e., *mild, moderate,* or *severe*) as assessed by the relationship of wall stress to ejection fraction and time-varying elastance (E_{max}). *Control* (11 patients) represents no departure from normal for either measure; *Mild* (12 patients) an abnormality in stress-ejection relationships only; *moderate* (16 patients), an abnormal E_{max}; and *severe* (4 patients), both an abnormal E_{max} and stress-ejection relationship. There is little difference between patients in their hemodynamic characteristics (PLVP, HR, or LVEDP). However, there are marked differences between groups based on their ventricular volumes and mass (EDV, ESV, and LVM). Thus, knowledge of these parameters is of greater value than isolated hemodynamic measurements (including ejection fraction) for predicting difficulty in the postoperative period. PLVP, peak left ventricular pressure (in mmHg); HR, heart rate (in beats·min^{-1}); LVEDP, left ventricular end-diastolic pressure (in mmHg); EDV, end-diastolic pressure (in ml); ESV, end-systolic pressure (in ml); LV Mass, left ventricular mass (in g). (From Starling et al.,[75] with permission.)

walls and disorganization of the myocardial cells. It is interesting to speculate that similar genetic processes are stimulated in the atrium and ventricle that result in a thin-walled fibrotic response. Conversely, atrial walls that are thick, muscular, and poorly dilated are often associated with a stiff, noncompliant response in the ventricle. It may be that the oft reported relationship of a poor surgical outcome associated with the latter ventricular morphology may not occur purely as a result of the lack of a high-compliance outlet.[42] Rather, the genetically determined response to volume overload in the patient with a poorly compliant ventricle may predispose them to a poor surgical result. Further, the lack of atrial dilation may not be the cause of this aberrant compliance but rather a marker for an excessive hypertrophic response. More research into the genetic response to volume overload is required.

When compared to MR, the atrial response to AR is less dramatic regardless of whether the lesion is acute or chronic. In acute AR the rapid rise in LVEDP results in a matched, although lesser, rise in atrial pressure. The typical relationship wherein a rise in atrial pressure is less than a rise in ventricular end-diastolic pressure is preserved as long as the mitral valve remains competent and the rhythm is sinus. With increasing degrees of ventricular hypertrophy and dilation, the mitral annulus dilates and may result in MR in addition to AR. Also, the previously described decrease in left ventricular compliance associated with AR results in a relentless rise in left atrial pressure. The gradual dilation of the left atrium in response to the increase in left atrial wall tension in turn leads to atrial fibrillation. The onset of atrial fibrillation often heralds the appearance of symptoms in AR.[3] Although many of the atrial morphologic changes associated with chronic AR resemble the early changes of MR, they rarely occur to the same degree as in MR.

Genetic Alterations

There is a relative paucity of information specifically regarding atrial genetic activation during valvular regurgitation; thus, this section focuses on various aspects of ventricular hypertrophy in response to volume overload. However, the reader is encouraged to explore Chapter 2, as there seems to be some concordance in the genetic response to hypertrophy regardless of etiology.[79,80]

A general description of the genetic response to volume overload may be divided into two broad categories: hypertrophy and function. The "function" category includes changes in the number or size of cells as well as alterations in subcellular organelles (e.g., mitochondria and the sarcoplasmic reticulum) and protein isoforms (e.g., altered forms of contractile proteins such as actin, myosin, and tropomyosin).[81] As expected, this implies that a variety of different systems are responsible for cellular signaling; however, there is no general agreement as to which system is subservient or dominant.

Broadly, these systems are divided into three areas (Table 1-5): growth factors (peptides that regulate cell proliferation and differentiation), stress proteins (proteins expressed in response to any type of myocardial stress), and proto-oncogene expression (proto-oncogenes are myocardial gene sequences that match oncogenes normally expressed by acute transforming viruses.[79] There is general agreement that the release of atrial naturetic peptides (ANP) in one of two forms, an atrial (aANP) or a brain (bANP) version, is correlated with the activation of proto-onocogene sequences.[79,82] Further, several investigators note that increases in both atrial and ventricular stretch alone result in activation of the mRNA sequence coding for bANP.[83] In animals, the expression of ANP is directly proportional to both the degree and duration of physical distension.[82] However, hypertrophy did not appear in these studies until well after increases in ANP were noted.

Protein isoform switches involving the heavy chain of myosin are also common occurrences in both volume and pressure hypertrophy.[79,80,82,83] Heavy chain units exist in two isoforms, α and β (located on the same chromosome, the α-site about 4,000 base pairs downstream).[84] The V_1 isozyme consists of two α chains, V_2 one α and one β chain, and V_3 two β subunits. Although both animals and humans demonstrate the isoform switch, the human ventricle is composed primarily (more than 90 percent) of the V_3 isozyme (structurally identical to the

Table 1-5.   Listing of Various Genetic Triggers for Myocardial Growth and Modification

Growth Factors	Stress Proteins	Proto-oncogenes
Transforming growth factor-β (TGF-β)	Heat shock proteins	c-*myc*
	70	c-*raf*
Insulinlike growth factor (IGF)	71	c-*erb*-A
Nerve growth factor (NGF)	110	c-*ras*-H
	90-α	c-*ski*
acidic fibroblast growth factor (aFGF)	90-β	c-*cis*
basic fibroblast growth factor (bFGF)	60	c-*fos*
	47	c-Ha-*ras*
Endothelial cell growth supplement (ECGS)	27	c-*jun*
Epidermal growth factor (EGF)	$\alpha\beta$-Crystalline	Egr-1
	Ubiquitin	
Growth hormone (GH)	Heme-oxygenase	
	Glucose-regulated proteins	

"slow" form of skeletal muscle).[85,86] These heavy chain subunits contain the ATPase site necessary for interaction with the actin subunit. There are similar isoform switches in the atria, where two further isozymes, A_1 and A_2, are located. These chains consist of α-type isoforms linked to an atrial-type light chain. Chronic MR results in displacement of the α by the β isoform. Functionally, this results in a switch to the ventricular version of the isozyme and is correlated with the degree of atrial enlargement (Fig. 1-6).[87]

Actin myofilaments are highly conserved (less than 1 percent base-pair divergence versus about 20 percent for myosin); however, two isoforms of actins exist.[79,80] Both isogenes are expressed in humans (α-skeletal and α-cardiac mRNA); however, the proportional representation clearly favors the α-skeletal mRNA (greater than 60 percent). There is evidence that this ratio is not altered with advanced stages of heart failure.[88] Further, these ratios are very different from those reported in animals.[80,88] The reason for this differential behavior of expression of myosin heavy chains (MHC) and actin isoforms is not known; however, substitution of a single amino acid in insect muscle results in an altered frequency of wing motion.[89] This suggests that actin myofilaments are more highly developed from an evolutionary perspective. Small changes in structure lead to dramatic alterations in function (and rarely in a positive direction), which may be a teleologic explanation for the divergent genetic expression.

The role that heat shock proteins play in the hypertrophic response to volume overload is less clear.[90] These proteins do play a role in conditioning the ventricle to recover from ischemic insults.[91] The release of heat shock proteins occurs in all organisms and is best described as an acute response by the cell to a variety of noxious stimuli. The proteins produced are members of a family of stress proteins, such as glucose-regulated proteins, ubiquitin, $\alpha\beta$-crystallin, and heme-oxygenase. This protein family can be subdivided into three groups according to molecular mass: high (HMM), medium (MMM), and low (LMM).

The HMM group contains three members, 110, 90-α, and 90-β, of which the latter two appear to regulate steroid receptors. The MMM group is the most abundant of the three groups and includes the 70 series (three to four members) and 60 series. While small amounts of the 70 series proteins are

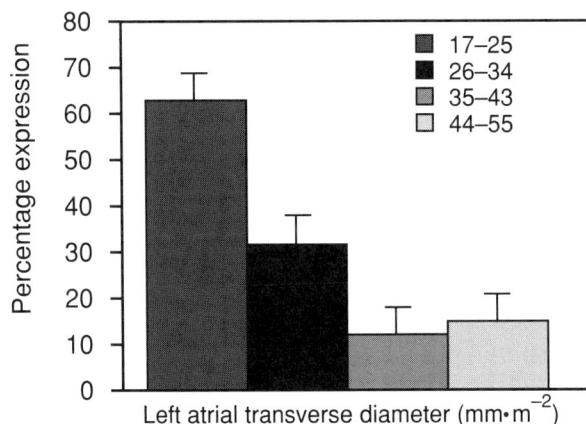

Fig. 1-6. Effect of atrial size on α-myosin heavy chain expression. As atrial dilation increases, expression of the α-myosin subunit decreases. $P < 0.05$ for all comparisons except 35 to 43 versus 44 to 55 mm·m^{-2}.

expressed in primates at all times, their response to oxidative stress of any sort is dramatic. The 60 series protein is expressed by the nucleus but resides in mitochondria, where it may assist in the assembly of macromolecules.

The LMM group contains 47,27, $\alpha\beta$-crystallin, heme-oxygenase, and ubiquitin. Protein 47 resides in the endoplasmic reticulum and presents a high binding affinity for collagen. Protein 27 appears to be a target for phosphorylation following exposure to mitogens or tumor promoters. Although $\alpha\beta$-crystallin is abundant in cardiac muscle cells, its role is unclear. Ubiquitin plays an important role in protein degradation.[92]

A theoretical model for the role of HSP 70 is available. Normally HSP 70 is bound to a genetic activating protein (heat shock factor, HSF). When the concentration of denatured proteins (which commonly occur after all forms of stress) in the cytoplasm increases, HSP 70 binds to them. This allows HSF proteins to aggregate into a trimer (instead of their usual monomer) form, which subsequently activates transcription of more HSP 70.

HSP 70 exists in mammalian cardiac cells in two forms. The first is a constitutive form and the second an inducible form. Following an oxidative stress, inducible HSP levels rise rapidly and confer protective effects during subsequent ischemic events. The degree of myocardial protection afforded is directly related to the amount of HSP 70 present.[93,94] What role, if any, these proteins play in the hypertrophic response remains an area of active investigation.

The role for peptide growth factors is equally uncertain. The action of these chemicals is typically carried out through cell surface receptor activation and secondary messenger signaling (G-proteins, protein kinases, and inositol phosphates). Both platelet-derived growth factor and fibroblast growth factor are associated with the activation of certain oncogenes mentioned later in this section.[95,96] Thus, a chicken-and-egg hypothesis is set up for these growth factors. Are they the result of oncogene activation or do they result in oncogene activation, both, or neither? Much work remains.

There are also associated changes in the isozyme systems of the sarcoplasmic reticulum. The well-described decrease in relaxation (negative lusitropy) noted in the discussion of functional alterations earlier in this chapter may be related to these isozyme changes.[80] A reduction in the rate of calcium transport by the sarcoplasmic enzyme systems and an absolute decrease in the number of functional Ca^{++}-ATPase molecules are described in pressure overload hypertrophy.[97] Decreases in the concentration of Ca^{++}-ATPase mRNA of 30 percent in animals and 48 percent in humans are recorded.[80,98] What these investigators did not find, however, was a switch in the isoform expressed.

This reduction in active enzyme systems is not only quantitatively and qualitatively different from the regulation of expression noted with the MHC, but may also contribute to rapid onset of myocardial failure seen in the terminal stages of chronic volume overload. If the switch in isoforms and the absolute concentration of myosin increases with hypertrophy while the rate of calcium uptake continuously declines, there is likely to be a point at which ancillary compensatory mechanisms for the regulation of cytoplasmic calcium are exhausted. This would lead to an accelerated pace for depletion of all available energy stores in response to low-level continuous activation of the troponin-tropomyosin contractile apparatus. Further, this interaction may explain the relatively rapid downhill course many patients experience at the end of the natural history of valvular regurgitation.

Finally, although both growth hormone and insulin growth factor I (IGF-I) (Table 1-5) are associated with the hypertrophic response to volume overload, their up-regulation is not required for hypertrophy to occur.[99]

The cellular signaling mechanism for the

eccentric hypertrophic response also remains elusive. While the induction of ANP is
a marker for hypertrophy, the exact transduction mechanism is unclear. The H-*ras* proto-
oncogene is a low-molecular-weight guanosine triphosphate (GTP) binding protein. Injection of this proto-oncogene into the cytoplasm results in expression of the ANP gene
as well as the c-*fos* gene, both of which are
linked to the hypertrophic response.[100] Additionally, protein kinases A, C, mitogene activated, and calmodulin dependent are involved in the proximal signaling mechanism.
These kinases in turn phosphorylate cytoplasmic transcriptional factors (i.e., agents
such as the cAMP response element binding
protein, or CREB) that subsequently control
nuclear level (i.e., expression of the hypertrophic response) events. All of the foregoing
notwithstanding, there is *no* direct evidence
linking any of the proto-oncogenes listed in
Table 1-5 with activation of a target gene during hypertrophy.[100] However, a close temporal relationship does exist between stretch
activation of cultured myocytes and c-*fos* and
c-*myc* expression. Although c-*fos* levels
peaked at 30 minutes and c-*myc* at 60 minutes
following the stretch stimulus, both were un-
detectable at 240 minutes following the stimulus.[101]

Similarly in isolated heart preparations, increases in left ventricular wall stress increased levels of c-*fos* and c-*jun* mRNA levels
three- to fourfold.[102] Norepinephrine infusions will also result in transient rises in both
c-*fos* and c-*myc,* peaking within 30 minutes
(fivefold increase) and 90 minutes (3.8-fold
increase), respectively, and declining to control ranges by 90 and 120 minutes, respectively.[103] Acute volume overload demonstrated a qualitatively similar, although
markedly reduced, result (a 1.8- and a 2.8-
fold increase, respectively). This latter result
is similar to that of other studies in dogs,
where pressure overload resulted in a 30 percent increase in myosin heavy chain synthesis compared to either control or acutely volume overloaded animals.[104]

SPECIAL CONCERNS

Thromboembolism

The incidence of embolic phenomena in
patients with increases in left atrial size is increased (the incidence is 10 to 15 percent
in patients with severe MR).[105] When these
patients undergo valvular resection, every
effort is made to remove the thrombotic
source simultaneously. In the postoperative
period, the timing of restarting anticoagulation for prosthetic valves is critical. It is best
to delay the use of any anticoagulants for 24
hours after surgery or return of normal coagulation as measured by the prothrombin
time/partial thromboplastin time (PT/PTT).
Although some centers prefer initiating anticoagulation with heparin, most begin warfarin at 48 hours.[18] The aim is to attain a PT of
1.5 to 2 times the normal range. If the patient
is considered high risk, dipyridamole is
added.[106]

Similarly, patients with either bioprosthetic valves (those made from glutaralde-
hyde-fixed tissue) or postvalvular repair may
require warfarin for 8 to 12 weeks following
surgery (required principally for placement
of the sewing ring). After that time, continued
use of anticoagulants is necessary only in
those patients with a prior history of systemic
embolization or where left atrial thrombi are
remnant. Patients who undergo mitral repair
without placement of an annular prosthetic
ring may require even shorter periods of anticoagulation.

Pre-existing Organ Dysfunction

Those patients with longstanding MR and
AR may present with varying degrees of ancillary organ insufficiency. These organs may
be affected as a result of chronic ischemia
secondary to poor cardiac output (renal and
mesenteric beds) or chronic venous congestion (pulmonary and hepatic).

Severe valvular regurgitation and high left
atrial pressures often result in increased lung
weight.[107] This in turn increases the work of

breathing concomitant with the decrease in pulmonary compliance. This increase in lung weight also removes most if not all of the normal safety factors preventing the onset of pulmonary edema.[108] Thus, these patients are at particularly high risk for perioperative pulmonary insufficiency.

Right ventricular failure is a secondary complication of a longstanding increase in left atrial and pulmonary venous pressure. As the pulmonary venous bed slowly hypertrophies, the increase in intravascular pressure is gradually transmitted to the pulmonary arterial bed, resulting in pulmonary hypertension. Pulmonary hypertension in turn acts as a pressure overload on the right ventricle, ultimately leading to hypertrophy. Hypertrophy is accompanied by a decrease in diastolic compliance and a gradual but ineluctable rise in right ventricular end-diastolic pressure and subsequently right atrial pressure.

As right ventricular pressures rise, symptoms of venous congestion in the systemic bed occur. This often leads to hepatic congestion with subsequent decrease in both synthetic and excretory functions. Patients with congestive hepatic dysfunction will present a variety of problems from coagulation to drug metabolism. If signs or symptoms of right ventricular failure are present, the intensive care clinician must anticipate an increased incidence of bleeding problems in the immediate postoperative period. Additionally, all of the pharmacokinetic and pharmacodynamic alterations discussed in Chapter 16 are expected.

Similarly, chronic ischemia of the mesenteric or renal beds (secondary to low cardiac output) will result in malnutrition (poor absorption and decreased appetite) and renal insufficiency. These changes are at least additive and may be synergistic with the previously discussed hepatic and pulmonary impairment. The clinician must be alert to these patients and may insist on preoperative hyperalimentation (see Ch. 8) as one mechanism to decrease postoperative complications.

Other Problems

Postoperative management of bleeding, endocarditis, isotropic support, and arrhythmia management are covered in their respective chapters.

REFERENCES

1. Waller BF, Morrow AG, Maron BJ et al: Etiology of clinically isolated, severe, chronic, pure mitral regurgitation: analyses of 97 patients over 30 years of age having mitral valve replacement. Am Heart J 104:288, 1982
2. Roberts WC: Morphologic features of the normal and abnormal mitral valve. Am J Cardiol 51:1005, 1983
3. Brest AN: Valvular heart disease: comprehensive evaluation and management. pp. 4–104. In Frankl WS, Brest AN (eds): Cardiovascular Clinics. FA Davis, Philadelphia, 1986
4. Roberts WC, Morrow AG, McIntosh CL et al: Congenitally bicuspid aortic valve causing severe pure aortic regurgitation without superimposed ineffective endocarditis. Am J Cardiol 47:206, 1981
5. Davies JJ: Pathology of Cardiac Valves. Butterworth, London, 1980
6. Roberts WC, Cohen LS: Left ventricular papillary muscles: description of the normal and a survey of conditions causing them to be abnormal. Circulation 46:138, 1972
7. Arnett FN, Roberts WC: Active infective endocarditis: a clinicopathologic analysis of 137 necropsy patients. Curr Probl Cardiol 1:2–76, 1976
8. Benotti JR, Dalen JE: Aortic valvular regurgitation: natural history and medical treatment. pp. 1–54. In Cohn LH, DiSesa VJ (eds): Aortic Regurgitation, Medical and Surgical Management. Marcel Dekker, New York, 1986
9. Stapleton JF: Natural history of chronic valvular disease. pp. 105–47. In Frankl WS, Brest AN (eds): Cardiovascular Clinics. FA Davis, Philadelphia, 1986
10. Braunwald E: Mitral regurgitation: physiologic, clinical and surgical considerations. N Engl J Med 281:425–33, 1969
11. Rapaport E: Natural history of aortic and mitral valve disease. Am J Cardiol 35:221–7, 1975

12. Spagnuolo M, Kloth H, Taranta A et al: Natural history of rheumatic aortic regurgitation: criteria predictive of death, congestive heart failure, and angina in young patients. Circulation 44:368, 1971

13. Segal J, Harvey WP, Hufnagel C: A clinical study of one hundred cases of severe aortic insufficiency. Am J Med 21:200, 1956

14. Phillips HR, Levine FH, Carter JE et al: Mitral valve replacement for isolated mitral regurgitation: analysis of clinical course and late postoperative left ventricular ejection fraction. Am J Cardiol 48:647, 1981

15. Hammermeister KE, Fischer L, Kennedy JW et al: Predictors of late survival in patients with mitral valve disease from clinical, hemodynamic, and quantitative angiographic variables. Circulation 57:341, 1978

16. Salomon NW, Stinson EB, Griepp RB et al: Patient-related risk factors as predictors of results following isolated mitral valve replacement. Ann Thorac Surg 24:519, 1977

17. Chaffin JS, Daggett WM: Mitral valve replacement: a nine-year follow-up of risks and survivals. Ann Thorac Surg 27:312, 1979

18. Brest AN, Frankl WS: Valvular heart disease: comprehensive evaluation and treatment. pp. 58–291. In Brest AN, Frankl WS (eds): Cardiovascular Clinics. FA Davis, Philadelphia, 1986

19. Carabello BA, Stanton SP, McGuire LB: Assessment of preoperative left ventricular function in patients with mitral regurgitation: value of the end-systolic wall stress–end-systolic volume ratio. Circulation 64:1212, 1981

20. Borow KM, Green LH, Mann T et al: End-systolic volume as a predictor of postoperative left ventricular performance in volume overload from valvular regurgitation. JAMA 68:655–63, 1980

21. Duran CG, Revuelta JM, Gaite L et al: Stability of mitral reconstructive surgery at 10–12 years for predominantly rheumatic valvular disease. Circulation 78:I91–6, 1988

22. Carpentier A, Chauvaud S, Fabiani JN et al: Reconstructive surgery of mitral valve incompetence: ten year appraisal. J Thorac Cardiovasc Surg 79:338–48, 1980

23. Duran CG, Revuelta JM et al: Stability of mitral reconstructive surgery at 10–12 years for predominantly rheumatic valvular disease. Circulation 78(suppl. I):I-91–6, 1988

24. Rankin JS, Feneley MP et al: A clinical comparison of mitral valve repair versus valve replacement in ischemic mitral regurgitation. J Thorac Cardiovasc Surg 95:165–77, 1988

25. Pitarys CJ, Forman MB et al: Long-term effects of excision of the mitral apparatus on global and regional ventricular function in humans. J Am Coll Cardiol 15:557–63, 1990

26. Duran CG, Pomar JL, Revuelta JM et al: Conservative operation for mitral insufficiency. J Thorac Cardiovasc Surg 79:326, 1980

27. Kay GL, Kay JH, Zubiate P et al: Mitral valve repair for mitral regurgitation secondary to coronary artery disease. Circulation 74:188, 1986

28. Sand ME, Naftel DC, Blackstone EH et al: A comparison of repair and replacement for mitral valve incompetence. J Thorac Cardiovasc Surg 94:208, 1987

29. Cohn LH, Kowalker W, Bhatia S et al: Comparative morbidity of mitral valve repair versus replacement for mitral regurgitation with and without coronary artery disease. Ann Thorac Surg 45:284, 1988

30. Orszulak TA, Schaff HV, Danielson GK et al: Mitral regurgitation due to ruptured chordae tendinae. J Thorac Cardiovasc Surg 89:491, 1985

31. Levine HJ: Is valve surgery indicated in patients with severe mitral regurgitation even if they are asymptomatic? Dilemmas in clinical cardiology. pp. 161–213. In Brest AN (ed): Cardiovascular Clinics. FA Davis, Philadelphia, 1990

32. Zaibad MA, Halim MA: Mitral valve regurgitation. pp. 187–260. In Zaibag MA, Duran C (eds): Valvular Heart Disease. Marcel Dekker, New York, 1994

33. Hirshfeld JW, Epstein SE, Roberts AJ et al: Indices predicting long-term survival after valve replacement in patients with aortic regurgitation and patients with aortic stenosis. Circulation 50:1190, 1974

34. Copeland JB, Griepp RB, Stinson EB et al: Long-term follow-up after isolated aortic valve replacement. J Thorac Cardiovasc Surg 74:875, 1977

35. Bonow RO, Borer JS, Rosing DR et al: Preoperative exercise capacity in symptomatic patients with aortic regurgitation as a predictor of postoperative left ventricular function and

long-term prognosis. Circulation 62:1280, 1980

36. Stone PH, Goldschlager N, Selzer A et al: Determinants of prognosis of patients with aortic insufficiency undergoing aortic valve replacement. Circulation 60(suppl II):II-38, 1979
37. Forman R, Firth BG, Barnard MS: Prognostic significance of preoperative left ventricular ejection fraction and valve lesion in patients with aortic valve replacement. Am J Cardiol 45:1120, 1980
38. Henry WL, Bonow RO, Rosing DR et al: Observations on the optimum time for operative intervention for aortic regurgitation. II. Serial echocardiographic evaluation of asymptomatic patients. Circulation 61:484, 1980
39. Cunha CLP, Giuliani ER, Fuster V et al: Preoperative M-mode echocardiography as a predictor of surgical results in chronic aortic insufficiency. J Thorac Cardiovasc Surg 79: 256, 1980
40. Carabello BA: Aortic regurgitation: hemodynamic determinants of prognosis. pp. 87–106. In Cohn LH, DiSesa VJ (eds): Aortic Regurgitation, Medical and Surgical Management. Marcel Dekker, New York, 1986
41. Grossman W, Jones D, McLaurin LP: Wall stress and patterns of hypertrophy in the human left ventricle. J Clin Invest 56:56–64, 1975
42. Ionescu MI, Cohn LH: Mitral Valve Disease; Diagnosis and Treatment. Butterworths, Stoneham, MA, 1985
43. Morrow AG, Cohen LS, Roberts WC et al: Severe mitral regurgitation following acute myocardial infarction and ruptured papillary muscle: hemodynamic findings and results of operative treatment in four patients. Circulation 37(suppl II):124, 1968
44. Urschel CW, Covell JW, Sonnenblick EH et al: Myocardial mechanics in aortic and mitral valvular regurgitation: the concept of instantaneous impedance as a determinant of the performance of the intact heart. J Clin Invest 47:867, 1968
45. Braunweld E: Mitral regurgitation: physiological, clinical and surgical considerations. N Engl J Med 281:425, 1969
46. Corin WJ, Monrad ES, Murakami T et al: The relationship of afterload to ejection performance in chronic mitral regurgitation. Circulation 76:59, 1987
47. Hwasokwa O, Camesas A, Weg I, Bodenheimer MM: Differences in left ventricular adaptation to chronic mitral and aortic regurgitation. Chest 95:106, 1989
48. Katayama K, Tajimi T, Guth BD et al: Early diastolic filling dynamics during experimental mitral regurgitation in the conscious dog. Circulation 78:390, 1988
49. Knotos GJ Jr, Schaff HV, Gersh BJ, Bove AA: Left ventricular function in subacute and chronic mitral regurgitation: effect on function early postoperatively. J Thorac Cardiovasc Surg 98:163, 1989
50. Keren G, Katz S, Strom J et al: Dynamic mitral regurgitation: an important determinant of the hemodynamic response to load alterations and inotropic therapy in severe heart failure. Circulation 89:306, 1989
51. Mehmel HC, Olshausen KV, Schuler G et al: Estimation of left ventricular myocardial function by the ejection fraction in isolated chronic, pure aortic regurgitation. Am J Cardiol 54:610, 1984
52. Iskandrian AS, Hakki AH, Kane-Marsch S: Left ventricular pressure/volume relationship in aortic regurgitation. Am Heart J 110: 1026, 1985
53. Shen WF, Roubin GS, Choong CY-P et al: Evaluation of relationship between myocardial contractile state and left ventricular function in patients with aortic regurgitation. Circulation 71:31, 1985
54. Schon HR: Hemodynamic and morphologic changes after long-term angiotensin converting enzyme inhibition in patients with chronic valvular regurgitation. J Hypertension 12(suppl 4):S95–S104, 1994
55. Scognamiglio R, Fasoli G, Ponchia A, Dalla-Volta S: Long-term nifedipine unloading therapy in asymptomatic patients with chronic severe aortic regurgitation. J Am Coll Cardiol 16:424, 1990
56. Nitenburg A, Foult J-M, Antony I et al: Coronary flow and resistance reserve in patients with chronic aortic regurgitation, angina pectoris, and normal coronary arteries. J Am Coll Cardiol 11:478, 1988
57. Urschel CW, Covell JW, Graham TP et al: Effects of acute valvular regurgitation on the

oxygen consumption of the canine heart. Circ Res 23:33–43, 1968

58. Pelenkie I, Rademaker A: Acute and chronic changes after aortic valve damage in the intact dog. Am J Physiol 241:H95, 1981

59. Downes TR, Nomeir A-M, Hackshaw BT et al: Diastolic mitral regurgitation in acute but not chronic aortic regurgitation: implications regarding the mechanism of mitral closure. Am Heart J 117:1106, 1989

60. Dodge HT, Kennedy JW, Petersen JL: Quantitative angiocardiographic methods in the evaluation of valvular heart disease. Prog Cardiovasc Dis 16:1–23, 1973

61. Kleaveland JP, Kussmaul WG, Vinciguerra T et al: Volume overload hypertrophy in a closed-chest model of mitral regurgitation. Am J Physiol 254(Heart Circ Physiol 23): H1034–41, 1988

62. Wisenbaugh T, Spann JF, Carabello BA: Differences in myocardial performance and load between patients with similar amounts of chronic aortic versus chronic mitral regurgitation. J Am Coll Cardiol 3:916–23, 1984

63. Wong CYH, Spotnitz HM: Systolic and diastolic properties of the human left ventricle during valve replacement for chronic mitral regurgitation. Am J Cardiol 47:40–50, 1981

64. Rozich J, Carabello B, Usher B et al: A mechanism by which ejection performance is preserved following mitral valve repair but not replacement for chronic mitral regurgitation, abstract. Circulation 84(suppl 2):578, 1991

65. David TE, Uden DE, Strauss HD: The importance of the mitral apparatus in left ventricular function after correction of mitral regurgitation. Circulation 68(suppl 2):76–82, 1983

66. Carabello BA: The changing unnatural history of valvular regurgitation. Ann Thorac Surg 53:191–9, 1992

67. Corin WJ, Murakami T, Monrad ES et al: Left ventricular passive diastolic properties in chronic mitral regurgitation. Circulation 83: 797–807, 1991

68. Peterson K, Tsui J, Johnson A et al: Diastolic left ventricular pressure-volume and stress-strain relations in patients with valvular aortic stenosis and left ventricular hypertrophy. Circulation 58:77–89, 1978

69. Taniguchi K, Nakano S, Kawashima Y et al: Left ventricular ejection performance, wall stress, and contractile state in aortic regurgitation before and after aortic valve replacement. Circulation 82:798–807, 1990

70. Glantz SA, Parmley WW: Factors which affect the diastolic pressure-volume curve. Circ Res 42:171–80, 1979

71. Hess OM, Ritter M, Schneider J et al: Diastolic stiffness and myocardial structure in aortic valve disease before and after valve replacement. Circulation 69:855–65, 1984

72. Fuster V, Danielson MA, Robb RA et al: Quantification of left ventricular myocardial fiber hypertrophy and interstitial tissue in human hearts with chronically increased volume and pressure overload. Circulation 55: 504–8, 1977

73. Villari B, Campbell S, Hess OM et al: Influence of collagen network on left ventricular systolic and diastolic function in aortic valve disease. J Am Coll Cardiol 22:1477–84, 1993

74. Carabello BA, Nakano K, Ishihara K et al. Coronary blood flow in dogs with contractile dysfunction due to experimental volume overload. Circulation 83:1063–75, 1991

75. Starling MR, Kirsh MM, Montgomery DG et al: Mechanisms for left ventricular systolic dysfunction in aortic regurgitation: importance for predicting the functional response to aortic valve replacement. J Am Coll Cardiol 17:887–97, 1991

76. Urabe Y, Mann DL et al: Cellular and ventricular contractile dysfunction in experimental canine mitral regurgitation. Circulation Res 70:131–147, 1992

77. Marino TA, Kent RL, Uboh CE et al: Structural analysis of pressure versus volume overload hypertrophy of cat right ventricle. Am J Physiol 249:H371–9, 1985

78. Ferrans VJ: Human cardiac hypertrophy: Structural aspects. Eur Heart J 3(suppl A): 15–27, 1982

79. Bugaisky LB, Gupto M, Gupto MP et al: Cellular and molecular mechanisms of cardiac hypertrophy. pp. 162–70. In Fozzard et al (eds). Raven Press, New York, 1992

80. Schwartz K, Boheler KR, de la Bastie D et al: Switches in cardiac muscle gene expression as a result of pressure and volume overload. Am J Physiol 262:R364–9, 1992

81. Buckingham ME, Minty AJ: Contractile protein genes. Essays Biochem 20:77–109, 1985

82. Gu J, D'Andrea M, Seethapathy M et al: Physical overdistension converts ventricular

cardiomyocytes to acquire endocrine property and regulate ventricular atriala natriuretic peptide production. Angiology 42: 173–86, 1991

83. Mantymaa P, Vuolteenaho O, Marttila M et al: Atrial stretch induces rapid increase in brain natriuretic peptide but not in atrial natriuretic peptide gene expression in vitro. Endocrinology 133:1470–3, 1993

84. Mahdavi V, Chambers A, Nadal-Ginard B: Cardiac α and β-myosin heavy chain genes are organized in tandem. Proc Natl Acad Sci USA 81:2626–30, 1984

85. Gorza L, Mercadier J, Schwartz K et al: Myosin types in the human heart: an immunofluorescence study of normal and hypertrophied atrial and ventricular myocardium. Circ Res 54:694–702, 1984

86. Mercadier JJ, Bouveret P, Gorza L et al: Myosin isoenzymes in normal and hypertrophied human ventricular myocardium. Circ Res 53:52–62, 1983

87. Mercadier JJ, de la Bastie D, Menasche P et al: Alpha-myosin heavy chain isoform and atrial size in patients with various types of mitral valve dysfunction: a quantitative study. J Am Coll Cardiol 9:1024–30, 1987

88. Schwartz K, Carrier L, Lompre LM et al: Contractile proteins and sarcoplasmic reticulum calcium-ATPase gene expression in the hypertrophied and failing heart. Basic Res in Cardiol 87(suppl 1):285–90, 1992

89. Drummond DR, Peckham M, Sparrow JC, White DCS: Alteration in crossbridge kinetics caused by mutations in actin. Nature (London) 348:440–2, 1990

90. Delcayre C, Samuel J-L, Marotte F et al: Synthesis of stress proteins in rat cardiac myocytes 2–4 days after imposition of hemodynamic overload. J Clin Invest 82:460–8, 1988

91. Currie RW, Karmazyn M, Kloc M, Mailer K: Heat-shock response is associated with enhanced postischemic ventricular recovery. Circ Res 63:543–9, 1988

92. Mestril R, Dillmann WH: Heat shock proteins and protection against myocardial ischemia. J Mol Cell Cardiol 27:45–52, 1995

93. Hutter MM, Sievers RE, Barbosa V, Wolfe CL: Heat shock protein induction in rat hearts: a direct correlation between the amount of heat shock protein induced and the degree of myocardial protection. Circulation 89:355–60, 1994

94. Marber MS, Walker JM, Latchman DS, Yellon DM: Myocardial protection after whole body heat stress in the rabbit is dependent on metabolic substrate and is related to the amount of the inducible 70 kD heat stress protein. J Clin Invest 93:1087–94, 1994

95. Delli Bovi P, Curatola AM, Kern FG et al: An oncogene isolated by transfection of Kaposis sarcoma DNA encodes a growth factor that is a member of the FGF family. Cell 50:729–37, 1987

96. Yarden T, Escobedo JA, Kuang WJ et al: Structure of the receptor for platelet-derived growth factor helps define a family of closely related growth factor receptors. Nature 323: 226–32, 1986

97. de la Bastie D, Levitsky L, Rappaport L et al: Function of the sarcoplasmic reticulum and expression of its Ca2+-ATPase gene in pressure overload-induced cardiac hypertrophy on the rat. Circ Res 66:554–64, 1990

98. Mercadier JJ, Lompre AM, Duc P et al: Altered sarcoplasmic reticulum Ca2+-ATPase gene expression in the human ventricle during end-stage heart failure. J Clin Invest 85: 305–9, 1990

99. Isgaard J, Wahlander H, Adams MA et al: Increased expression of growth hormone receptor mRNA and insulin-like growth factor-I mRNA in volume-overloaded hearts. Hypertension 23(part 2):884–8, 1994

100. Chien R: Signaling mechanisms for the activation of an embryonic gene program during the hypertrophy of cardiac ventricular muscle. Basic Res Cardiol 87(suppl 2):49–58, 1992

101. Sadoshimi J, Jahn L, Takahashi T et al: Molecular characterization of the stretch-induced adaptation of cultured cardiac cells. J Biol Chem 267:10551–60, 1992

102. Schunkert H, Jahn L, Izumo S et al: Localization and regulation of c-fos and c-jun proto-oncogene induction by systolic wall stress in normal and hypertrophied rat hearts. Proc Natl Acad Sci USA 88:11480–4, 1991

103. Kolbeck-Ruhmkorff C, Horban A, Zimmer H-G: Effect of pressure and volume overload on proto-oncogene expression in the isolated working rat heart. Cardiovasc Res 27: 1998–2004, 1993

104. Imamura T, McDermott PJ, Kent RL: Acute changes in myosin heavy chain synthesis rate in pressure versus volume overload. Circ Res 75:418–25, 1994

105. Komuro I, Kaida T, Shibazaki Y et al: Stretching cardiac myocytes stimulates proto-oncogene expression. J Biol Chem 265:3595–8, 1990

106. Stein PD, Kantrowitz A: Antithrombotic therapy in mechanical and biological prosthetic heart valves and saphenous vein bypass grafts. Chest 95(suppl):107S, 1989

107. Ota T, Tsukube T, Matsuda H et al: Effect of mitral valve surgery on severely impaired pulmonary function. Thoracic and Cardiovascular Surgeon 42:94–9, 1994; discussion, 99–102

108. Allen SJ, Drake RE, Williams JP et al: Recent advances in pulmonary edema. Crit Care Med 15:963–70, 1987

2

Stenotic Valvular Disorders: Adaptive Strategies to Chronic Pressure Overload

Peter Nicolazzo

LEFT VENTRICULAR PRESSURE OVERLOAD

Adult myocytes are unable to undergo mitosis[1]; enlargement of the ventricle of the heart in response to hemodynamic overload occurs by the growth of existing cells (hypertrophy, rather than hyperplasia). The hallmark of ventricular hypertrophy due to chronic pressure overload is concentric myocardial hypertrophy. This morphologic change is accompanied by an alteration in genetic expression, resulting in a ventricle that is not simply an enlarged version of the previous structure, but one that has a modified composition and function. The human ventricle adapts to chronic pressure overload by developing a slower and more economic force of contraction. Although there are detrimental consequences, myocardial hypertrophy can be considered an adaptive process that the heart undertakes to normalize mechanical wall stress in response to hemodynamic overload.

It is often technically difficult or impractical to determine hemodynamic indices such as pressure, volume, and wall thickness in the clinical setting that describe the functional consequences of ventricular hypertrophy. Much of the current understanding of the functional, morphologic, and molecular changes associated with ventricular hypertrophy is derived from experimental models in which acute increases in afterload are produced by surgical banding of the great arteries. Although pressure overload hypertrophy can be reliably produced in such banded animal models, the resulting alterations do not necessarily resemble pressure overload hypertrophy in humans; and important distinctions have been described.[2]

Pathologic left ventricular hypertrophy (LVH) confers a grave prognosis.[3,4] Results from the Framingham Study demonstrate an eightfold increased risk of cardiovascular mortality in persons having electrocardiographic (ECG) evidence of LVH, with 5-year

21

mortality rates approximating 30 percent.[5] When myocardial hypertrophy is diagnosed by echocardiography, a more sensitive method, it is a significant independent predictor of morbidity and mortality.[6]

AORTIC STENOSIS

Aortic outflow tract obstruction can occur at supravalvular, valvular, and subvalvular levels. Subvalvular aortic stenosis may be due to a discrete lesion or myocardial thickening as seen in hypertrophic cardiomyopathy (HCM). Aortic stenosis (AS) at the valvular level can be due to degenerative (senile) changes involving fibrosis, calcification, and fusion of aortic valve cusps, sometimes in a congenitally malformed aortic valve. About 1 percent of live births have a congenitally bicuspid aortic valve.[7] Although a bicuspid valve can function normally over a lifetime, it can pose an increased risk of stenosis by inducing turbulent flow, accelerated fibrosis, and calcification. A congenitally unicuspid valve is rare but can result in symptomatic AS during infancy. Rheumatic AS is almost always accompanied by mitral valve (MV) involvement leading to mitral stenosis (MS) due to fusion of the cusps at their commissures. Diabetes and hypercholesterolemia are associated risk factors for the development of AS.[8]

Objective quantification of the degree of stenosis involves the calculation or measurement of the systolic pressure gradient across the aortic valve and a calculation of the aortic valve area (AVA). Both values can be determined invasively (cardiac catheterization) or noninvasively (echocardiography with Doppler ultrasound). Generally accepted values for "critical" AS are a systolic pressure gradient greater than 50 mmHg and AVA less than 0.5 cm^2. In assessing the severity of AS, the transvalvular systolic pressure gradient can be misleading in advanced disease with LV failure. Low cardiac output across the severe stenosis can cause the gradient to be paradoxically low. For determination of AVA

from catheterization data, the Gorlin equation[9] is used:

$$\text{AVA (cm}^2) = \frac{\text{cardiac output/systolic ejection period} \times \text{HR}}{44.5 \times \sqrt{\text{mean aortic pressure gradient}}}$$

If normal heart rate is assumed, the following simplified formula is used:

$$\text{AVA (cm}^2) = \frac{\text{cardiac output}}{\sqrt{\text{mean aortic pressure gradient}}}$$

Echocardiographically guided Doppler ultrasonography provides a convenient noninvasive means for measuring both the transvalvular systolic pressure gradient and the AVA. For the former, a modification of the Bernoulli equation is used with good correlation cardiac catheterization data.[10] For the latter, the continuity equation is used with close correlation to catheterization data,[10] especially when the true AVA is less than 1.0 cm^2. Since the Gorlin equation relies on flow and systolic pressure gradient, either of which can be depressed in advanced disease, the continuity equation can be more useful for assessment of AVA for patients with severe AS.[11]

Clinical Manifestations of Aortic Stenosis

Patients with AS are usually asymptomatic until late in their disease process. Increased LV filling pressures secondary to impaired diastolic relaxation associated with concentric LVH are responsible for congestive symptoms such as shortness of breath and dyspnea on exertion. The occurrence of syncope is more related to the systolic transaortic pressure gradient.[12] Shortness of breath is the most common presenting symptom.[13] Once the symptoms of angina, syncope, and congestive heart failure (CHF) appear, the patient has a very poor prognosis without therapeutic intervention. A paradoxic decline in the intensity of the systolic murmur in advanced AS may occur similar to the decline in the systolic pressure gradient. Classically, the time period between symptom manifestation and death is 5 years for patients with angina, 3 years for those with syncope, and 2 years for patients with CHF due to AS.[14,15] Orthopnea and paroxysmal nocturnal dyspnea (PND) due to pulmonary hypertension are often late findings.

Angina is a frequent symptom in patients with AS and may not correlate with the existence of significant coronary artery disease (CAD).[16,17] In one series of patients with severe AS, two-thirds of patients presented with angina, and of this group, one-third of patients had no CAD on catheterization.[17] Identifying coexisting CAD in patients with AS is essential, since patients with CAD have an increased mortality rate after aortic valve replacement (AVR); however, concurrent coronary artery bypass grafting (CABG) improves survival.[18,19]

Electrocardiography of Patients with Aortic Stenosis

LVH criteria is met in about 85 percent of ECGs of patients with AS.[20] ST-segment depression and T-wave inversion (strain pattern) are commonly present. Occasionally a "pseudoinfarct pattern" develops with loss of the R-wave in the right-sided precordial leads and a T-wave inversion. Left atrial enlargement, identified by a biphasic a-wave in lead V1, is frequently observed.[21] Occasionally, the ECG reveals a delayed conduction or heart block due to the extension of aortic calcification into the conduction system.[22]

Ventricular Response to Pressure Overload: A Hemodynamic Perspective

The stimulus for myocardial hypertrophy is an increase in force per unit area of myocardium, referred to as wall "stress."[23] Both experimental[24] and human data[24] suggest that volume overload (diastolic wall stress) as seen in mitral regurgitation (MR) stimulates less of a hypertrophic response than the pressure overload (systolic wall stress), as seen in AS.

The distribution of wall stress is nonhomogeneous in normal and hypertrophied ventricles. This inhomogeneity is represented by both regional (higher wall stress in the equator of the ventricle than in the apex[25]) and global (higher wall stress in the endocardial than in the epicardial regions) alterations. This phenomenon is represented by the greater sarcomere length in the endocardial than in the epicardial regions.[26] During pressure overload and in conditions of depressed contractility, recruitment of sarcomeres from the epicardial and apical regions takes place, resulting in a more homogeneous distribution of wall stress.

Increased end-diastolic fiber stretch (preload) and increased wall tension result in the augmentation of contractile force (the Frank-Starling mechanism).[27] Preload becomes less of a determinant of ejection performance as diastolic filling pressures increase and the Frank-Starling mechanism is exhausted.[25] Increasing end-diastolic volume with further in-

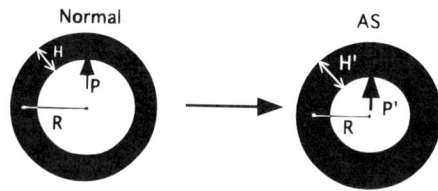

$$\text{WALL TENSION (STRESS)} = \frac{(P)(R)}{2(H)} = \frac{(P')(R)}{2(H')}$$

Fig. 2-1. Calculation of left ventricular wall tension (stress) based on the law of Laplace. The ventricle, schematically represented as a sphere in cross section, will strive to maintain a normal wall stress under chronic hemodynamic overload. Pressure overload is represented by P', with an increased ventricular wall thickness represented by H'. A chronic increase in P (pressure overload, concentric hypertrophy) or R (volume overload, eccentric hypertrophic [not illustrated]) will be compensated by an increase in wall thickness. P, mean left ventricular cavity pressure during systole; R, mean left ventricular radius during systole; H, mean myocardial wall thickness during systole; AS, aortic stenosis.

creases in diastolic pressure results in a minimal gain in stroke volume (SV).[28]

The initial stress of pressure overload (stenotic valve lesions) will cause replication of sarcomeres in parallel, as opposed to serial replication as seen in volume overload (regurgitant valve lesions). Parallel sarcomere replication produces concentric hypertrophy. With this increase in LV wall thickness, the myocardial wall stress returns toward normal in accordance with the law of Laplace[29,30] (Figs. 2-1 to 2-3).

As evident on the pressure-volume loop for AS (Figs. 2-2A and 2-4), the indices of systolic function, as represented by ejection fraction

(EF) and SV, are usually preserved in AS. This is accomplished by an "adequate" LVH response—enough concentric hypertrophy to maintain a normal LV wall stress.

The result of a lack of hypertrophic response to pressure overload has been described by the term *afterload mismatch*.[27,31,32] An inadequate ventricular hypertrophic response will not accomplish a normalization of wall stress and result in a decreased systolic function (lower EF) with limited preload reserve.[31] Elevated diastolic filling pressures are a frequent hallmark.[33]

For those patients who had evidence of inadequate hypertrophy (afterload mismatch),

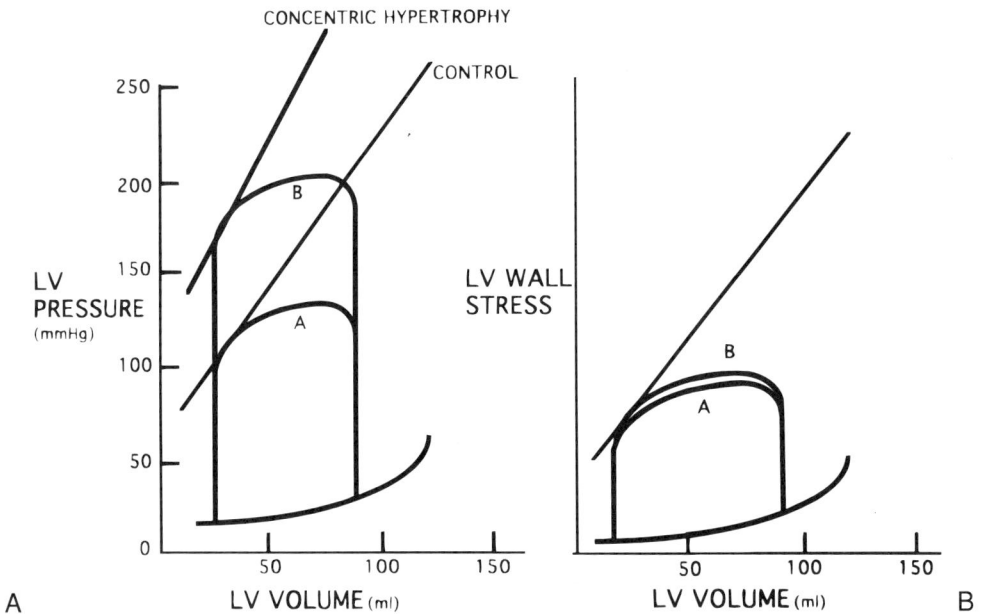

Fig. 2-2. Adaptation of the left ventricle to chronic pressure overload. **(A)** Left ventricular (LV) pressure-volume relations with the curvilinear diastolic pressure-volume curve and the linear end-systolic pressure-volume relation. Loop A of left ventricular contraction occurs before the development of concentric hypertrophy. Loop B shows the response under conditions of chronic concentric hypertrophy when the left ventricular end-diastolic and end-systolic volumes are normal but the left ventricular systolic pressure is markedly elevated. As shown experimentally, there is a shift of the end-systolic pressure-volume relation upward and to the left, indicating hemodynamic hyperfunction of the ventricle under these conditions. **(B)** Same contractions shown in Fig. A plotted as wall-stress volume loops. Loop A before concentric hypertrophy and loop B after concentric hypertrophy are essentially superimposable (wall thickening results in normal wall stress), and they reach the same linear end-systolic left ventricular wall stress-volume relation. Thus, concentric hypertrophy, considered within the wall stress-volume framework, appears to occur without a change in myocardial contractility. (From Ross,[32] with permission.)

aortic stenosis

↓

left ventricular pressure overload

↓

wall stress

↓

mechanotransducers,
second messengers

↓

altered genetic expression

enhanced protein synthesis   altered calcium handling

↓   ↓

myocardial hypertrophy   decreased Vmax

↓   ↓

normalization of wall stress   greater economy

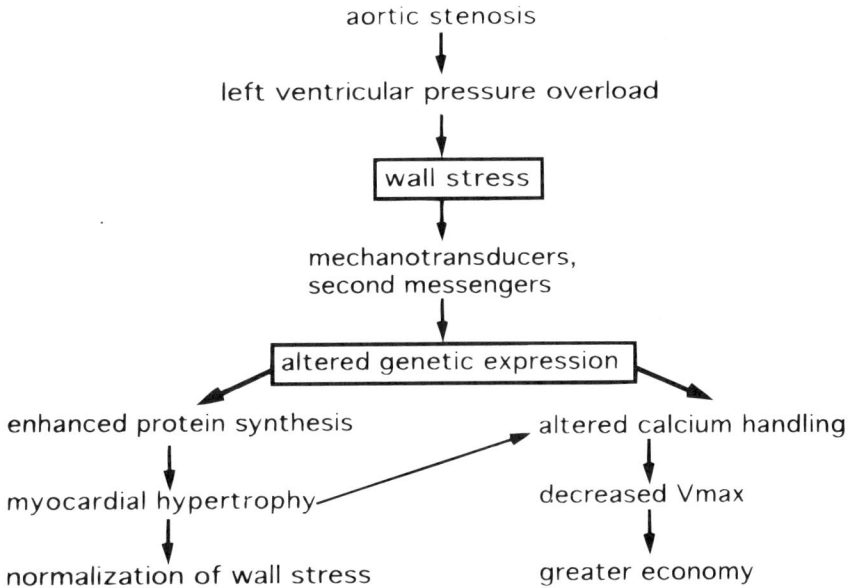

Fig. 2-3. Schematic representation of the adaptive strategy of the left ventricle in response to pressure overload. Mechanical adaptation is met by concentric hypertrophy of myocardial cells, with replication of sarcomeres in parallel, normalizing wall stress. Functional adaptation occurs through altered calcium handling and a slower maximal velocity of shortening (V_{max}), improving the economy of the system. The initial signal for transformation is increased wall stress, which activates mechanotransducers, humoral mediators, and second messenger pathways. For the human ventricle, the alteration in calcium handling appears to be secondary to a decreased density of sarcoplasmic reticulum calcium "pumps," as the cell hypertrophies, resulting in less calcium cycled per beat.

as measured by a decreased LV wall thickness-to-LV cavity radius ratio, a higher wall stress was correlated with a lower EF.[34] This decreased EF due to afterload mismatch presents an increased risk of CHF.[35] The origin of poor hypertrophic response leading to afterload mismatch may be due to a lack of the necessary triggering mechanism. In addition, myocardial ischemia, either from coexisting coronary disease or from subendocardial ischemia in the presence of normal coronaries (a frequent finding in patients with aortic stenosis,[34]) may contribute to poor hypertrophic response as well.

Atrial Contribution in Aortic Stenosis

As a result of the decreased LV diastolic compliance and prolongation of isovolumic relaxation period, early diastolic (passive) flow across the mitral valve is decreased. As a result, atrial contraction has a greater contribution to LV stroke volume in patients with AS. For example, in one study it was found that in patients with AS, atrial contraction contributes 45 percent of LV end-diastolic volume and 39 percent of LV stroke volume, compared to only 20 percent of LV end-diastolic volume and 26 percent of LV stroke volume in normal subjects.[36] Atrial contraction will elevate left ventricular end-diastolic pressure (LVEDP) with only a transient rise in left atrial pressure (LAP), so that mean LAP and hence pulmonary venous pressure is lower in the presence of sinus rhythm.[37] In severe AS, the atrial contribution to stroke volume may be critical, and junctional rhythm or atrial fibrillation may in some instances precipitate severe hypotension requiring immediate cardioversion. Mitral

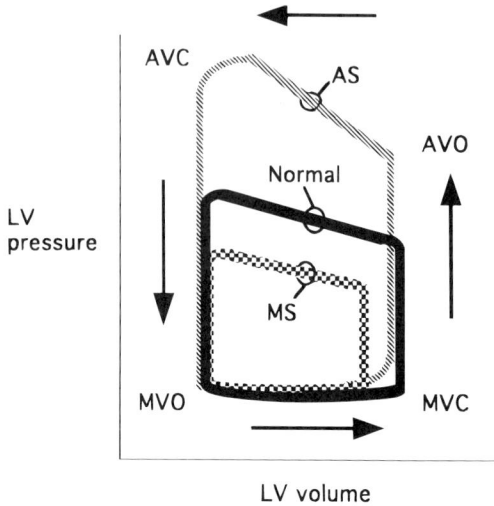

Fig. 2-4. Idealized schematic of the left ventricular pressure-volume relationship during the cardiac cycle in patients with chronic stenotic valve lesions of the left heart. In compensated aortic stenosis (AS) with concentric hypertrophy, systolic function (as represented by the volume axis) is usually preserved under increased interventricular pressures. The higher end-diastolic pressure reflects the noncompliant thick-walled ventricle. The ventricle in mitral valve stenosis (MS) is both pressure and volume underloaded. MVO, mitral valve opening; MVC, mitral valve closure; AVO, aortic valve opening; AVC, aortic valve closure.

regurgitation (MR), impairing atrial contribution, can be a coexisting finding in patients with severe AS. However, MR usually improves following AVR.[38]

Changes in Contractility

The use of positron emission tomography (PET) confirms that hypertrophied ventricles have less oxygen consumption than that of normal ventricles at any comparable work load (per weight of tissue with corrections made for rate-pressure product and afterload/gradient). This is consistent with deceased contractile states for these patients.[39] In a study that measured afterload (wall stress) and contractility in 76 patients with aortic stenosis, advanced myocardial hyper-

trophy was associated with depressed contractility, independent of afterload.[40] Until the field of molecular biology provided answers, hemodynamic data concerning the decreased contractility of pressure-overloaded ventricles were abundant; however, an explanation was lacking.

GENETIC ALTERATIONS

Recent findings in molecular biology have established that pressure-overloaded ventricles undergo a genetic conversion to an altered contractile state (Fig. 2-3). The type of ultrastructural transformation that takes place has been shown to be species-specific.[41,42] Myosin structure and calcium handling are the major determinants of contractility. The human ventricle adapts to chronic pressure overload by developing a slower and more economic force of contraction by a genetic change in proteins responsible for calcium transport, whereas myocytes in the human atrium undergo an ultrastructural change that involves a change in myosin isoform.

The thick filaments of the sarcomere are composed primarily of myosin, while the thin filaments contain actin, tropomyosin, and the troponin apparatus. There are three primary isoforms of myosin in mammalian ventricular muscle, designated V_1, V_2, and V_3. They differ in their rate of ATP hydrolysis, with V_1 having a rate three to five times faster than V_3.[43] The V_3 isoenzyme allows more mechanical work per ATP. Myosin ATPase activity is closely correlated with the initial speed of myocardial shortening at zero load (V_{max}).

Contractile proteins studied in rodent models of pressure overload hypertrophy are modified to produce more V_3-type myosin, creating slow, economic force development represented by a lower V_{max}.[41,43–45] In the human ventricle, the initial myosin isoform is almost completely of the V_3 type; there appear to be no isoenzyme shifts in either myosin or actin.[46] The lower V_{max} in human ventricular pressure overload hypertrophy is related to altered calcium handling with less calcium cycled per beat.[41,43,47] The adaptive strategy of the human ventricle to chronic pressure overload thus involves an altered state of calcium handling to achieve greater economy. A correlation between increased aortic valve gradient and economical energy utilization (increased respiratory chain capacity) was demonstrated to exist in patients with pressure overload LVH undergoing aortic valve replacement.[48]

Atrial Modification in Pressure Overload

The expression of oncogenes in response to aortic banding is more pronounced initially in the atria.[49] The myosin composition of the atria gives it a two to three times faster maximum velocity of shortening, V_{max}, than that of the ventricle.[50] As described previously, V_{max} is an intrinsic property of the cardiac muscle determined by myosin ATPase activity and calcium transient.[51] In the normal human atrium, the composition of myosin is that of the fast isoform, V_1, compared to the normal human ventricle, which is composed of the slower V_3 isoform. Several laboratories have demonstrated a shift in human atrial myosin isoform from the V_1 type to the V_3 form, after chronic hemodynamic overload due to either aortic or mitral stenosis.[43,51,52] Clinically, the transverse diameter of the atrium correlates with its V_3 content.[53] Thus, the adaptive strategy of the human atrial myocardium involves an altered myosin isoform, a change similar to that of the ventricular myocardium of some species used in laboratory investigations of pressure overload hypertrophy.[41,42]

Altered Calcium Handling in the Pressure-Overloaded Ventricle

Careful measurements of systolic and diastolic function in patients with hemodynamic overload due to aortic valvular disease, using simultaneous left ventriculography and LV pressure measurements, indicate that diastolic relaxation abnormalities precede systolic dysfunction.[54] Myocardial relaxation is an active process that occurs early in diastole. Delayed relaxation is due to residual crossbridges among contractile elements. Delayed removal of calcium from the contractile apparatus contributes to intracellular calcium overload in diastole and results in impaired diastolic filling.

Troponin-C has four binding sites for free calcium ions, and myocardial relaxation proceeds with the release of calcium from troponin-C. Relaxation thus depends on the ability of the cell to closely regulate and expel intracellular calcium. Two processes are primarily involved here: the calcium ATPase on the sarcoplasmic reticulum, which stores free calcium ions for myocardial contraction, and the sodium calcium exchanger of the cellular membrane.

Reuptake of calcium by the sarcoplasmic reticulum (SR), specifically by the sarcoplasmic calcium ATPase (SR-ATPase) enzyme, is largely responsible for the speed of relaxation. A reduction in calcium transport by the SR is observed in investigational chronic pressure overload[43] and in biopsied myocardium of patients with chronic pressure overload.[55] The genes encoding this sarcoplasmic calcium transport protein are not induced by the hypertrophic process; thus, as the muscle cell hypertrophies, there is a resulting decrease in density of these SR-ATPase pumps.[43,45,47,52,53,56–58] This produces an SR that stores less calcium and releases less calcium. The slower rate of calcium uptake appears to be a result of a decreased density of these pumps, rather than a qualitative change (phenotypic shift).[43]

Mechanotransducers

On the molecular level a chain of events links the mechanical signal of hemodynamic overload to a change in genetic expression. Hemodynamic load on the myocyte, simply

described as cellular *stretch,* can act as an initial signal for the altered genetic expression leading to hypertrophy.[42,59–61] Several studies have employed in vitro mechanical loads placed by stretching adherent cells in myocardial cell cultures isolated from neural or hormonal influences. These stretched myocytes rapidly produce increased amounts of mRNA, new protein products, and an increased capacity for protein synthesis (i.e., increased ribosome content and DNA transcriptional activity) (Fig. 2-5). This activation is enhanced when the myocytes are stimulated to contract.[62] Furthermore, a preferential accumulation of new myosin protein can be demonstrated in the areas of the heart subjected to the stretch.[43]

Sadoshima and Izumo[63] reviewed possible mechanisms by which this "mechanotranscription" coupling process might be initiated: stretch applied to the cell surface may directly cause a conformational change in certain membrane molecules, which in turn are responsible for activating second messenger pathways.[64] These stretch-activated ion channels (SACs) may be modulated by growth factors and may require sodium influx through deformation-dependent channels.[59,62] Another possibility is that mechanical stretch may release growth factors that subsequently activate second messenger cascades. When nonstretched cardiocytes are exposed to media from stretched cells, nonstretched cells behave as if they were stretched with

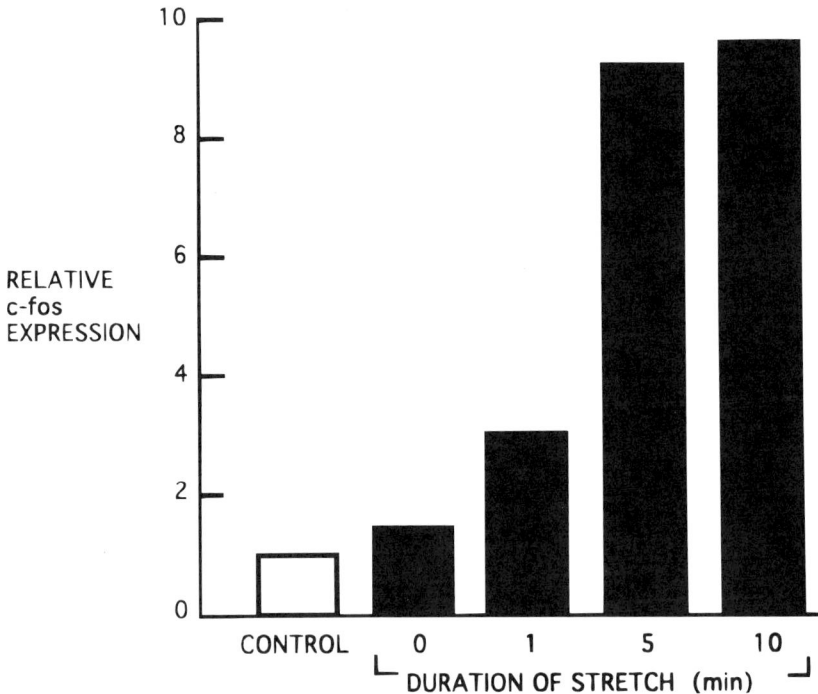

Fig. 2-5. Effects of "stretch-conditioned" media on c-*fos* expression in nonstretched cardiocytes. Cardiocytes were stretched for the times indicated. The culture medium of the stretched cells was transferred to nonstretched cardiocytes. The cells were incubated in the stretch-conditioned medium for 30 minutes and c-*fos* expression was examined by Northern blot analysis. Hybridization was assessed as relative to the value obtained from nontreated cells. Zero minute stretch indicates the medium transfer from nonstretched cardiocytes. Data are from a representative experiment. Similar results were obtained from four additional experiments. (From Sadoshima and Izumo,[63] with permission.)

activated second messenger pathways and altered genetic expression.[63]

Adrenergic Agents

Catecholamines have been implicated as causative agents in the pathogenesis of myocardial hypertrophy, reviewed by Long et al.[65] A correlation between LV mass and plasma norepinephrine levels has been demonstrated in humans.[66] Initial investigations in animal models also suggested a "hormonal" effect of norepinephrine in this respect. Chronic subhypertensive doses of norepinephrine were demonstrated to cause significant ventricular hypertrophy in canine models.[67] It must be emphasized that dogs remained normotensive in this study, eliminating increased afterload as a cause of LVH.

Recent investigations using cell cultures have linked the α_1-adrenergic receptor to specific changes in genetic expression leading to hypertrophic growth of a similar pattern to that of pressure overload hypertrophy in vivo.[68] Cardiocytes under α_1-adrenergic stimulation produced mRNA sequences and increased amounts of protein products associated with hypertrophy. This effect was blocked by α_1-adrenergic antagonism and not significantly modified by α_2-adrenergic effects.[69,70] Evidence thus far supports a role for both the α_1- and β-cardiac receptors, with differences in resulting genetic expression detected between the two remaining to be defined.[65,71]

Renin-Angiotensin System

The classic endocrine renin-angiotensin (RA) system involves the cascade of renin, acting on the hepatically produced substrate angiotensinogen to produce angiotensin I, converted by angiotensin-converting enzyme (ACE) to the active compound angiotensin II (AGT II). There are also separate "local" RA systems located in individual organs; these local RA systems can include all the protein and genetic components of the classical cascade. Such a local RA systems exists in the myocardium and is independently regulated.[72–74]

AGT II can induce myocardial hypertrophy phenotypically similar to that produced by pressure overload. AGT II appears to induce hypertrophy via the same second messengers and genetic activation as mechanical loading, including a role for calcium.[75,76] Whether the hypertrophic action of AGT II is mediated by systemic or locally produced hormone, or both, remains to be defined. One study found no correlation between plasma AGT II and cardiac hypertrophy.[77]

Intracardiac ACE activity is enhanced[78] and LV angiotensinogen mRNA is increased[79] in animal models of pressure overload hypertrophy. Ventricular AGT II receptors are up-regulated in animal models of LVH and, when treated with a specific receptor antagonist, LVH can be completely reversed.[73] It still is unclear whether RAS activity induces LVH or is associated with its maintenance.[80] Although a distinct mechanism remains to be proved, ACE inhibitors can cause the regression of ventricular hypertrophy in doses which do not alter afterload.[72,77,79–82]

Intracellular Calcium

Cyclic fluctuations in the concentration of intracellular calcium, or calcium transients, can be demonstrated for each cardiac cycle. Although the calcium transient is closely regulated, an increase in intracellular free calcium in the myocardium has been demonstrated to occur in the acute response to stretch of myocardial cells[83] and elevated aortic pressure.[84] Indeed, evidence exists for elevated coronary perfusion pressure,[85] acute afterload increase,[84] α_1-adrenergic stimulation,[86] and angiotensin II[87] to all increase intracellular calcium concentration. An increase in intracellular calcium concentration is linked to activation of proto-oncogene DNA sequences known to be activated in hypertrophy.[84,88] Marban and Koretsune[84] reviewed the abundant evidence that links increased intracellular calcium concentrations to the increased protein synthesis seen in ventricular hypertrophy. These investigators demonstrated a significant increase in intracellular calcium to increased perfusion pressure.

Calcium signaling is ubiquitous in cellular processes and is often mediated through calcium receptor proteins; therefore, the concept that a change in intracellular calcium concentration in response to an acute rise in pressure load coincidentally acts as a signal for genetic adaptation for the cell is appealing. The precise mechanism for this acute increase in calcium concentration to elevated perfusion pressures is unknown. The existence of stretch-sensitive ion channels permeable to calcium has been identified in chick myocyte culture. The inward calcium flux from these stretch-sensitive ion channels may contribute to the Frank-Starling mechanism and also serve as a signal for hypertrophic response to stretch.[89] Similar data exist in other cell systems; for example, calcium flux in depolarized neural cells induces genetic transcription.[90]

Growth Factors

Mechanical load induces the accumulation of peptide growth factors.[43,65,91–93] Culture media exposed to stretched myocytes for as short as 1 minute will accumulate undefined trophic factors that can induce c-*fos* proto-oncogene expression (a genetic marker seen in models of ventricular hypertrophy) in nonstretched myocytes.[63]

Second Messengers

Convincing evidence for receptors in the etiology of LVH exists (i.e., the α_1-receptor); these receptors must exert an influence at the nuclear level to alter the observed changes in genetic transcription, presumably through second messengers. Cell stretch is known to activate numerous second messenger transduction pathways, including tyrosine kinase, mitogen-activated protein (MAP)

kinases, protein kinase C (PKC), phospholipase D, and phospholipase A2.[63] PKC may serve as a second messenger in response to stretch,[60,61] possibly initiated by the α_1-adrenergic receptor.[65,94] Phosphoinositol (PI) cycle is activated in stretched myocyte cultures.[60,61] Pressure-induced hypertrophy involves a cAMP-dependent mechanism[95]; cAMP levels appear to mediate the increase in ribosome content in the pressure-overloaded myocyte.[96] New experimental evidence suggests that a specific second messenger, a PKC isoform, specifically activates the myosin type of gene seen in pressure overload hypertrophy.[65]

Enhanced Protein Synthesis

The machinery for protein synthesis appears to respond rapidly to elevated aortic pressures, specifically at the ribosomal level, where mRNA sequences are translated into protein products. An in vitro heart muscle model clearly demonstrates a preferential increase in the synthesis of new ribosomes within 1 to 2 hours of an increased aortic pressure from 60 to 120 mmHg.[97] Thus, a greater capacity for protein synthesis is initiated very early in the hypertrophic process.

In experimental pulmonary artery banding, both the capacity of protein synthesis (total number of ribosomes available) and the efficiency of protein synthesis (total number of peptide bonds formed per unit time) are increased at days 2 and 4, respectively.[98] Mechanical stretching has been shown to stimulate MAP kinase, which increases the efficiency of ribosome protein synthesis.[61] Increased intraventricular pressure from 0 to 25 mmHg or aortic pressure from 60 to 120 mmHg in an arrested heart preparation will still accelerate protein synthesis by more than 40 percent.[99]

Oncogenes: Transiently Induced Genes Regulating Growth

Oncogenes were first discovered as the DNA sequences transmitted by retroviruses to host cells causing neoplastic transformation. Retroviruses causing malignancy are believed to have incorporated host oncogenes (c-*onc*) into their viral genomes (v-*onc*), transforming normal genetic effects in the process.[100] Subsequently, these genes have been identified as normal-occurring sequences in all eukaryotic genomes and are called proto-oncogenes. Proto-oncogenes code for specific protein products necessary for normal cell growth and regulation. Proto-oncogenes mapped to the human genome, for example, code for growth factors, membrane receptors, protein kinases, and DNA binding proteins. In the pressure-overloaded myocyte, mRNA sequences coding for oncogenes can be identified by using c-DNA probes. For example, the c-*myc* and c-*fos* oncogenes are involved in the mitosis of nonmuscular cells, whose expression is documented in stretched myocyte cultures.[49,60,69] The process of mechanogenetic transduction occurs rapidly (Fig. 2-5). The c-*fos* proto-oncogene can be detected after 1 minute of stretch to cardiocyte culture[63] and, within 30 minutes, after acute aortic banding (with the c-*myc* oncogene detected within 2 hours).[101]

Heat-shock proteins (HSP) are another group of transiently induced genes expressed in response to pressure overload; their role may be to protect mRNA.[102] Genetic transformation initially involves proto-oncogenes and HSP genes, followed by activation of genes normally expressed during the fetal period, such as atrial natriuretic factor and fetal-type isomyosin proteins.[103]

Increased Connective Tissue: Role of Collagen

Experimental cardiac hypertrophy produced by banding in animal models results in excess hyperplasia of nonmuscular elements, marked fibrosis, necrosis, and resultant artifactual changes that do not resemble findings in hypertrophied human hearts.[2] In one such model of the papillary muscle from a pressure-overloaded ventricle induced to grow by

50 percent, there was a 48 percent hyperplasia of endothelial cells and a 35 percent increase in the number of connective tissue cells, with no increase in the number of myocytes. For the different tissue types, cell volumes increased by 35 percent, 64 percent, and 53 percent, respectively.[104]

An increased concentration of collagen has been shown in experimental chronic pressure overload[105,106] as well as the biopsied myocardium of patients with aortic stenosis.[48,107] Decreased ventricular diastolic compliance is correlated with an increased collagen content[108,109] as well as the orientation and location of collagen fibers.[51,110] A reversal of relaxation abnormalities can be achieved by inhibitors of collagen synthesis.[111]

Increased collagen content is the result of a proliferation of active fibroblasts and possibly due to a decreased amount of collagenolysis.[112] On the molecular level, it is known that transforming growth factor (TGF) is an important stimulant of collagen synthesis in cardiac fibroblasts. Increased levels of mRNA coding for TGF have been detected in models of ventricular hypertrophy.[113] Norepinephrine also enhances levels of TGF through mechanisms that remain to be defined. Furthermore, aldosterone levels can modify the degree of fibrosis.[51] In experimental infrarenal aortic stenosis, in which aldosterone levels are normal, LVH develops without fibrosis, while significant fibrosis develops in LVH due to renovascular hypertension or under continuous infusion of aldosterone. A cardiac mineralocorticoid receptor has been identified that does not exist in other organ systems.

Although the increased amount of connective tissue is detrimental to the contractile performance of the pressure-overloaded ventricle, the degree of fibrosis present does not completely correlate with the depressed systolic function seen in patients with pressure overload hypertrophy.[114] This lends support to the altered intrinsic properties of the myocardium itself as a cause of depressed contractile function.[114]

Dysrhythmias

Dysrhythmias occur more often in echocardiographically diagnosed ventricular hypertrophy and are linked to an increased incidence of sudden death among these patients. Ischemia, altered metabolism, mechanical wall stress, sympathetic activity, and fibrosis all contribute to this dysrhythmogenic potential. Myocyte stretching can make the cell more vulnerable to spontaneous ectopic impulse formation.[3,4,51] The proximity of the atrioventricular (AV) node and bundle of His to degenerative calcific deposits may lead to AV block or to a left or right bundle branch block,[115] or these conditions may develop after AVR due to surgical trauma.[22]

By prolonging the duration of local action potentials and refractory periods, and by causing fragmentation of conduction, fibrosis can lead to reentrant dysrhythmias. Supraventricular dysrhythmias, when present, may also be related to coexisting disease[115] (e.g., metabolic disease, alcoholism) or coexisting cardiac pathology, such as enlarged left atrium or mitral regurgitation. Such supraventricular disturbances could be threatening for the AS patient who is dependent on sinus rhythm for LV filling.[115]

A reduction in LVH diminishes the incidence of dysrhythmias.[3,4,36] Whether this translates into a reduction in cardiovascular morbidity and mortality remains to be determined.[4]

Calcium homeostasis contributes to the increased dysrhythmogenicity often seen in hypertrophied hearts.[52] Both the channels responsible for calcium release from the SR and those responsible for uptake are diminished.[52,116,117] Thus, any agent or intervention that can modify intracellular calcium is of potential significance to the hypertrophied myocardium, including digitalis, hypokalemia, ischemia, sympathetic stimulation, and temperature (recovery from hypothermic cardioplegia).[52,115]

Impaired Response to Inotropes

The total number of β_1-adrenergic receptors remains unchanged during myocardial hypertrophy in animal models, resulting in a 30 to 50 percent decrease in their density. The consequence is a decreased response to catecholamine inotropes (i.e., isoproterenol).[57,118] Since β_1-adrenergic receptors in the heart are linked to adenylate cyclase by the G-protein, a decreased inotropic response of failing hypertrophied hearts to phosphodiesterase inhibitors may be a consequence as well.[119] The ratio of β-adrenergic receptors to muscarinic receptors is unchanged.[41]

Myocardial Oxygen Supply and Demand in Pressure Overload Hypertrophy

The ventricle under pressure overload is exquisitely sensitive to ischemia. Increased systolic pressure in AS leads to increased myocardial wall tension, especially in an inadequately hypertrophied ventricle. Basal myocardial oxygen demand is increased due to increased muscle mass. In addition, patients with AS can have a relatively prolonged ejection phase, increasing myocardial oxygen demand.[120]

On the supply side, total blood flow to the ventricle with concentric hypertrophy is increased; however, blood flow per unit mass of myocardial tissue is reduced, even with disease-free coronary arteries.[121] The prolonged systolic ejection time and delayed relaxation lead to a relatively decreased time available for coronary perfusion during diastole. Myocardial perfusion is also decreased by a higher interventricular end-diastolic pressure in a poorly compliant ventricle.

Epicardial coronary vessels do not enlarge in proportion to the degree of LVH.[122,123] In addition, the number of capillaries in LVH is not increased in proportion to the degree of hypertrophy. As myocardial cells hypertrophy, capillary growth fails to maintain normal density per unit tissue,[121,122,124–127] resulting in increased intercapillary distance.[104,128]

As reviewed by Schwartzkopff et al.,[112] there is an important distinction between coronary vascular changes in LVH due to aortic stenosis and that in LVH due to systemic hypertension. In the former, subendocardial coronary perfusion pressure is exceeded by LV systolic wall tension; in the latter, coronary perfusion pressure can equal or exceed LV wall tension.[129] Most experimental models of LVH employ aortic banding in which supravalvular aortic pressures and therefore coronary perfusion pressures are much higher than in true valvular stenosis. In such models, evidence of medial wall thickening of the coronary vasculature can be seen.[130] In experimental hypertension and in postmortem hearts of hypertensive patients, hypertrophy of the medial layer and increased perivascular fibrosis are responsible for reduced luminal diameter of coronary arterioles. This type of medial wall thickening is apparently absent on coronary arterioles in patients with aortic stenosis.[112]

Studies on coronary flow dynamics have shown that flow rates are cyclical, according to the cardiac cycle in both normal and hypertrophied ventricles. However, in models of aortic stenosis with LVH, the decrease in coronary flow during systole can be dramatic, even reaching negative flow rates (reversal of forward flow) during systole.[131] In addition to increased transmural pressures causing this reversal, a fluid mechanics model of AS suggests that a negative pressure gradient can develop during systole near the coronary sinuses, especially at more rapid heart rates.[132] Clinically, retrograde flow of contrast in coronary arteries in AS patients has been documented.[133] This reversal of coronary flow, at least at the beginning of systole, disappears following aortic valve replacement.[134]

Coronary Reserve in Patients With Pressure Overload Hypertrophy

Blood flow to vital organs is autoregulated to maintain an adequate energy/oxygen supply. Local metabolic environment and demand is a major determinant of regional blood flow. *Coronary reserve* is the difference between autoregulated and maximally vasodilated blood flows through the coronary circulation (Fig. 2-6). Under pathologic changes in organ structure and function, autoregulatory mechanisms are less efficient and can even become detrimental when "steal" perfusion exists (vasodilation causing decreased perfusion of an already jeopardized area). Compromised blood flow to the hypertrophied heart and compromised autoregulatory mechanisms create an organ that is susceptible to ischemia from a decreased autoregulatory reserve, or coronary reserve[135] (Figs. 2-6 and 2-7).

As reviewed by Guyton et al.,[129] there are regional differences in coronary reserve. Coronary arterioles in the subendocardial regions have a lower resistance due to a greater degree of dilation than subepicardial regions. This baseline dilated state translates into a decreased coronary reserve for the inner layers of the heart. In experimental conditions, coronary hypotension leads to subendocardial ischemia.[130,136] A steal phenomenon can develop as the subepicardial regions, with greater dilatory reserve capacity, receive greater blood flow.

Patients with impaired coronary reserve are at increased risk of ischemia when diastolic blood pressures are decreased.[137] A plot of diastolic blood pressure versus cardiac morbidity and mortality forms a characteristic J-shape, or *J-curve*. This curve correlates the risk of lowered diastolic blood pressure to the incidence of myocardial infarction (MI) in hypertensive patients. A recent review of the literature on this subject in the hypertensive population suggests a therapeutic threshold of 85 mmHg diastolic pressure.[138] One-half of patients with hyper-

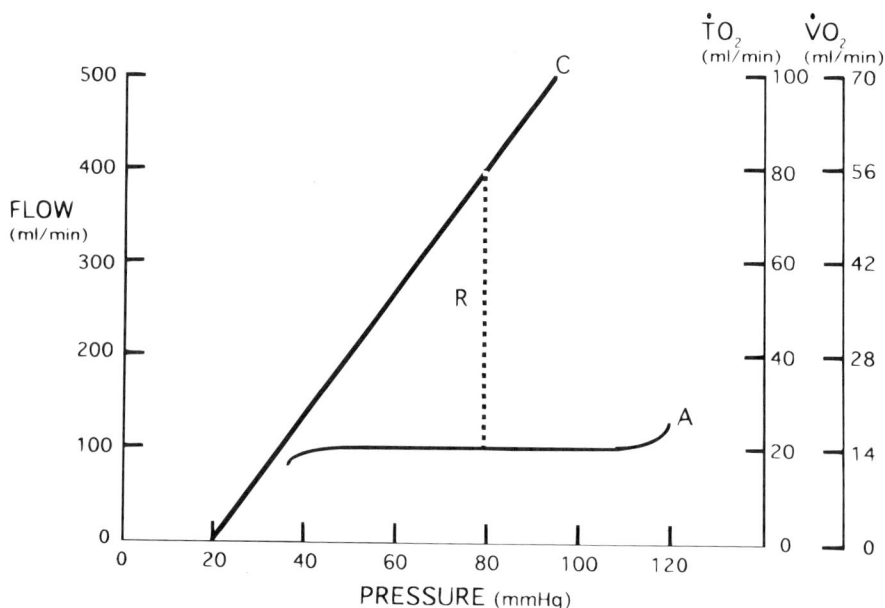

Fig. 2-6. Coronary pressure-flow relations in a normal left ventricle during autoregulation (A) and maximal vasodilation (C). The dashed vertical line indicates the coronary flow reserve at that perfusing pressure. Right-hand scales show the values of coronary oxygen transport ($\dot{T}O_2$) and myocardial oxygen consumption ($\dot{V}O_2$) that correspond to the flows on the left-hand scale. (From Hoffman et al.,[177] with permission.)

tension and LVH who had diastolic pressures rapidly lowered to between 85 and 90 mmHg showed ischemic changes on ECG.[139] This risk is significantly exacerbated by CAD and LVH.[137] In patients with coexisting coronary artery disease, flow reserve is reduced by approximately one-half with an 80 percent narrowing.[140] Further clinical evidence is illustrated in hypertensive human subjects with LVH and with normal coronaries who experienced angina with exercise in response to lowering of systemic diastolic blood pressure with nitrates.[141] This same study demonstrated that in patients with concentric LVH, a significant decrease in coronary blood flow (26 percent lower compared to normal ventricles) and an increase in myocardial oxygen extraction occurs at coronary perfusion pressures lowered beyond 85 mmHg.

When coronary perfusion pressure is decreased in a patient with AS, as during periods of decreased afterload (hypotension),

myocardial ischemia will lead to a decreased active ventricular relaxation and increased chamber stiffness (less available ATP for calcium reuptake). The result will be a vicious cycle of decreased LV compliance and decreased coronary perfusion, leading to myocardial ischemia and acute cardiac failure. Thus, maintaining an adequate afterload is one of the primary concerns in the treatment of patients with uncorrected AS, paradoxically requiring the use of a vasopressor, rather than a vasodilator, for treatment of acute myocardial ischemia.

Reversibility of Hypertrophic Changes Following Aortic Valve Replacement

Patients with isolated AS can be expected to experience reversal of LV dysfunction and improvement in functional capacity following AVR, even when preoperative heart failure is

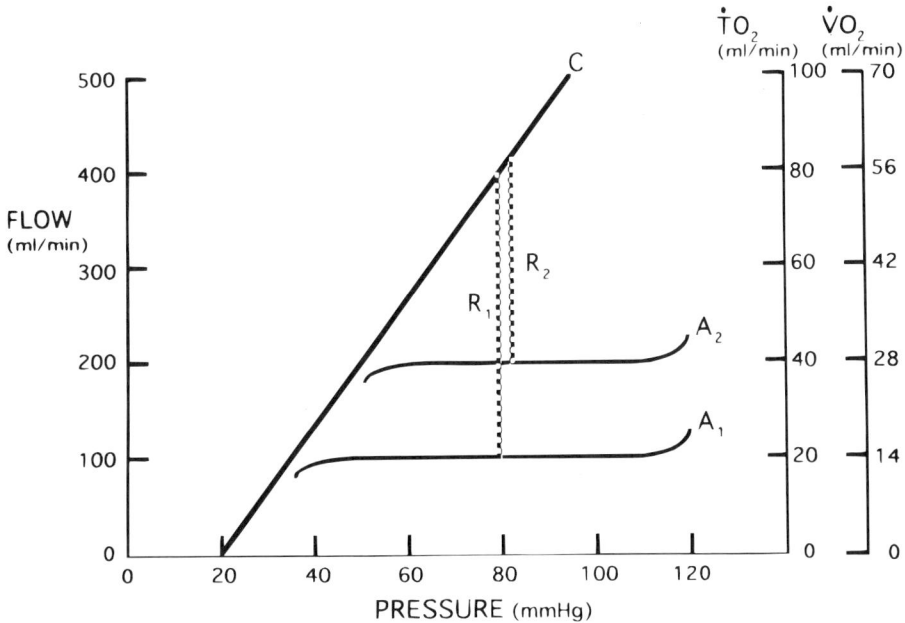

Fig. 2-7. Coronary pressure-flow relations during maximal vasodilation (C) and autoregulation in normal (A_1) and hypertrophied (A_2) left ventricles. The coronary flow reserve is shown by the vertical dashed lines. R_1 normal ventricle; R_2, hypertrophied ventricle. Right-hand scales are as in Fig. 2-6. (From Hoffman et al.,[177] with permission.)

severe.[142] LV mass typically regresses following successful AVR[142-144] with ventricular hemodynamics at rest returning to normal on 6-month follow-up of AVR patients.[114,145,146] Theoretically, the development of fibrosis may preclude complete regression of myocardial distensibility following AVR; however, reversibility of elevated stiffness has been documented even in patients with markedly elevated calculated wall stiffness.[33] There is persistent diastolic dysfunction during the immediate postoperative period; patients remain vulnerable to ischemia, especially in the presence of tachycardia. This persistent diastolic dysfunction is more pronounced in patients with concentric hypertrophy compared to patients with eccentric hypertrophy.[12] The improvement in clinical cardiac function suggests that many of the ultrastructural changes in the hypertrophied myocardium are reversible, although data on the molecular biology of this reversal remain to be described.

Pulmonary Hypertension in Patients With Aortic Stenosis

Severe pulmonary hypertension (SPAP greater than 50 mmHg) is an infrequent finding in patients with isolated AS. When present, pulmonary hypertension is related to LV diastolic dysfunction with a significant correlation to elevated LVEDP[147] and a poor correlation with aortic valve area and EF.[148] A decrease in pulmonary hypertension can be expected during the first few days following AVR, even in patients with severe pulmonary hypertension.[147] The operative mortality for isolated AVR in these patients does not appear to be increased.[148,149]

MITRAL STENOSIS

Rheumatic heart disease is the etiology of mitral stenosis (MS) in more than 99 percent of patients.[150] Commissural fusion, calcific deposits, and shortened fibrotic chordae tendineae are a common finding.[150,151] The leading cause of heart disease in the developing countries and with a reported resurgence in the 1980s in the United States, acute rheumatic fever (RF) develops several weeks after an upper respiratory tract infection with group A β-hemolytic streptococcus. The degree of immune response by the host is positively associated with the development of RF.[152] The precise mechanism of mitral valve involvement is not clear, but much investigation has centered on the autoimmune response induced by streptococcal antigens.[152]

Clinical manifestations of MS include symptoms related to hemodynamic overload proximal to the mitral valve. Dyspnea on exertion, pulmonary edema, hemoptysis, atrial fibrillation, and recurrent systemic emboli can be presenting symptoms for MS.[153]

Electrocardiogram in Mitral Stenosis

The ECG is not a sensitive diagnostic tool in patients with MS. However, findings may include left atrial enlargement, as demonstrated by tall P-waves in lead II and biphasic or inverted P-wave in lead V1.[54]

Measurement of Mitral Valve Area

The normal adult mitral valve has an orifice measuring approximately 4.0 cm², with no transvalvular gradient.[155] The "critical" mitral valve area (MVA) (stenosis likely to produce advanced symptoms) in patients with MS is approximately 1 to 1.2 cm².[156]

Echocardiography provides a noninvasive means of measuring MVA. A continuous-wave Doppler provides a velocity profile of transvalvular mitral blood flow when it is aligned along the axis of the stenotic jet. The more prolonged the deceleration curve of blood flow across the stenosis, the smaller the calculated MVA.[157] This method using Doppler ultrasound correlates well with data from cardiac catheterization (the Gorlin formula)[11,157–159] and is less influenced by mitral regurgitation or tachycardia.

As stated for AS, transvalvular pressure gradients alone are not a valid assessment for the degree of stenotic disease. In the case of severe AS, gradients can be paradoxically low. In the case of MS, the gradient is dynamic, as a modification of the Gorlin equation illustrates:

$$MVA\ (cm^2) = \frac{\text{transmitral flow rate}}{(\text{mitral orifice constant}) \times 44.5 \times \sqrt{\text{mean mitral pressure gradient}}}$$

If MVA is held constant

$$\begin{array}{l}\text{Mean mitral} \\ \text{pressure} \\ \text{gradient}\end{array} \cong (\text{transmitral flow rate})^2$$

$$\cong \frac{(\text{cardiac output})^2}{(\text{diastolic filling time})^2}$$

As the formula predicts, the transvalvular mitral gradient increases by the square of the cardiac output or reduction in diastolic filling time (which occurs at accelerated heart rates). A twofold increase on mitral flow produces a fourfold increase in mitral pressure gradient.[153] As reviewed by several investigators on the natural history of MS, an acutely increased mitral valve gradient manifesting in pulmonary edema may occur after any event that increases cardiac output (e.g., sympathetic stimulation, exercise) and/or causes tachycardia (e.g., metabolic derangements, anemia.)[160]

Dysrhythmias in Mitral Stenosis

As LAP increases and left atrial enlargement progresses, a patient with MS may demonstrate frequent premature atrial contractions and eventually develop atrial flutter or fibrillation. As reviewed by Horstkotte,[155] there is indeed a positive correlation between the frequency of atrial fibrillation (AF) and the severity of stenosis. The onset of these atrial dysrhythmias can be marked by an acute elevation of pulmonary vascular pressures with resultant pulmonary edema.[22] The atrial systolic contribution to LV end-diastolic volume is minimal in those patients with MS who maintain sinus rhythm.[36] This can be represented by the diminished or absent A-wave (transmitral flow due to atrial contraction) seen on Doppler examination of the mitral valve. Thus, the onset of congestive symptoms with the loss of sinus rhythm is due to the increased ventricular rate (increasing the transmitral pressure gradient), rather than the loss of atrial contribution.[155,161] Attempts to slow the rapid ventricular rate with digoxin or a β-blocker should be undertaken in such cases.

Restoration of sinus rhythm in patients who had AF at the time of mitral valve replacement (MVR) occurred in only 8 percent at 1-year follow-up and could be positively correlated with smaller left atrial size.[155] This same study, which involved follow-up in 842 patients, also revealed a low frequency of patients converting from SR to AF post-MVR that was positively correlated with a larger left atrial size.

Myocardial Modification in Mitral Stenosis

MS is unique among valve lesions of the left heart in that the LV is spared from both pressure and volume overload (Fig. 2-4). The demonstrated tendencies for these patients to have decreased LV ejection fractions and end-diastolic volumes is predictable due to the mechanical obstruction of the stenotic mitral valve. However, Gaasch and Folland[162] have reviewed the perhaps less obvious reasons for further mechanical impairment. These include abnormal LV wall motion observed in the posterobasal area due to a restricted mitral valve apparatus, and abnormal interventricular septal motion due to RV volume overload. Although a specific mechanism has not been established, this relative underloading of the LV may in some cases lead to a thin-walled ventricle susceptible to impaired systolic performance. This was suggested by results from a study by Gash and associates,[163] who found that MS patients with reduced LV ejection performance tended to have thinner LV wall thickness

compared to MS patients with normal LV ejection performance.

Under hemodynamic overload, the human atrial myosin isoform appears to change from the fast-inefficient V_1 type to the slow-efficient V_3 isoform.[43,51,52] Whether the human LV undergoes significant genetic alteration in the unloaded state remains to be elucidated.

Pulmonary Hypertension in Mitral Stenosis

In chronic MS, elevated pulmonary vascular pressures can develop and are associated with medial hypertrophy of medium-size branches of the pulmonary arteries.[164] Pulmonary hypertension is reversible following surgical replacement of the mitral valve.[165,166]

Chronically elevated pulmonary vascular pressure due to MS can be associated with airway narrowing and bronchial hyperreactivity.[167–169] Airway narrowing in MS patients demonstrates an obstructive pattern involving both large and small airways, with the average airway resistance of MS patients approximately doubled over that of controls.[170] Patients with MS who undergo a challenge with a bronchial inflammatory mediator (cholinergic agonist) demonstrate a five times greater sensitivity than displayed by normal subjects.[169] The mechanism for airway obstruction undoubtedly involves edema and vascular distension, with the mechanism for bronchial hyperresponsiveness remaining controversial.[167]

Right Ventricular Dysfunction in Mitral Stenosis

With progressive disease and the onset of pulmonary hypertension, the RV will experience pressure overload. Several clinical studies have indicated that the RV can sustain this hemodynamic load well. In patients with moderate pulmonary hypertension and elevated systolic RV pressures due to MS, the RV will tend to maintain a normal ejection fraction and size.[171] Furthermore, the RV seems to maintain a normal V_{max} (contractile force), even in patients with pulmonary hypertension due to MS in whom RV failure has developed.[172]

Systemic Embolism in Patients With Mitral Stenosis

At surgery, 43 percent of patients with significant MS were shown to have left atrial thrombi.[173] Approximately 20 percent of MS patients will have a systemic embolism during the course of their disease, with one-half of detected events occurring in the cerebral circulation.[153] The diagnosis of left atrial thrombus is most efficiently acclomplished with the use of a transesophageal (TEE) examination. Other methods, including transthoracic echocardiography, left atrial and coronary angiography, and magnetic resonance imaging (MRI), have a high specificity, but low sensitivity. This is due in part to the ten-

dency for one-half of all thrombi to be located in the left atrial appendage, which can be well visualized by TEE.[174] For patients with MS, there is a higher incidence of thromboembolic events in those with AF, and to a lesser extent in those with larger atrial diameters[155] (Fig. 2-8). In most cases, anticoagulation will reduce the incidence of thromboembolic events in patients with MS and AF.[175]

An excellent review by Agathos and Starr[151] summarizes how patients remain at risk of thromboembolic events related to the technique of insertion or to the mechanical prosthesis itself following MVR. Calcific emboli may result from inadequate scavenging of particles during intraoperative debridement of the diseased mitral valve. Alternatively, inadequate removal of calcific deposits or suture entrapment can cause prosthetic valve incompetency. Malplaced sutures can also cause a perivalvular leak (visualized on TEE) or potentially damage structures in

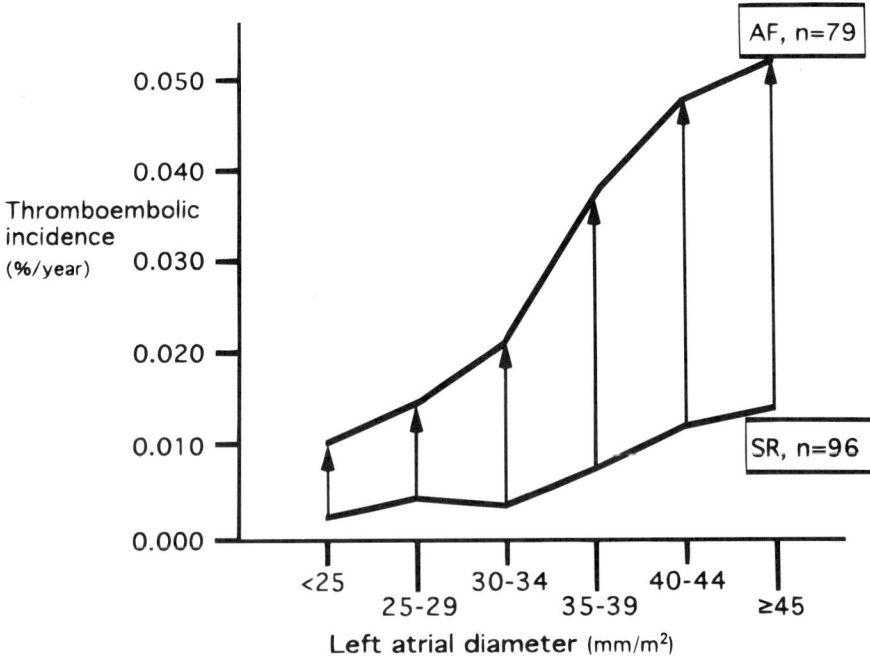

Fig. 2-8. Influence of rhythm and left atrial diameters on the thromboembolic incidence of nonanticoagulated patients with mitral stenosis (n = 879). AF, atrial fibrillation; SR, sinus rhythm. (From Horstkotte,[155] with permission.)

proximity to the repair, such as the circumflex coronary artery, coronary sinus, or noncoronary aortic cusp.[151]

Post-MVR, blood contact with the immobile elements of the tissue or mechanical valve prosthesis will initiate thrombus formation. Chronic anticoagulation with the vitamin K antagonist warfarin will reduce the risk of thromboembolism to 0.5 percent per year.[176]

REFERENCES

1. Zak R, Kizu A, Buaisky L: Cardiac hypertrophy: its characteristics as a growth process. Am J Cardiol 44:941–6, 1979
2. Bishop S, Melsen L: Myocardial necrosis, fibrosis, and DNA synthesis in experimental cardiac hypertrophy induced by sudden pressure overload. Circ Res 39:238, 1976
3. Messerli F: Left ventricular hypertrophy, arterial hypertension and sudden death. J Hypertens, suppl 7. 8:S181, 1990
4. Messerli F, Grodzicki T: Hypertension, left ventricular hypertrophy, ventricular arrhythmias and sudden death. Eur Heart J, suppl D, 13:66, 1992
5. Kannel W, Sorlie P: Left ventricular hypertrophy in hypertension: prognostic and pathogenic implications (the Framingham study). pp. 223–33. In Strauer B (ed): The Heart in Hypertension. Springer-Verlag, Berlin, 1981
6. Casale P, Devereux R, Milner M et al: Value of echocardiographic measurement of left ventricular mass in predicting cardiovascular morbid events in hypertensive men. Ann Intern Med 105:173, 1986
7. Roberts W: Valvular heart disease of congenital origin. In Frankl W, Brest A (eds): Valvular Heart Disease: Comprehensive Evaluation and Treatment. FA Davis, Philadelphia, 1993
8. Deutscher S, Rockette H, Krishnaswami V: Diabetes and hypercholesterolemia amoung patients with calcific AS. J Chron Dis 37:407, 1984
9. Gorlin R, Gorlin S: Hydrolic formula for calcuation of the area of the stenotic mitral valve, other cardiac valves, and central circulatory shunts. Am Heart J 41:1–29, 1951
10. Oh J, Taliercio C, Homes D et al: Prediction of the severity of aortic stenosis by Doppler aortic valve area determination: prospective Doppler-catheterization correlation in 100 patients. J Am Coll Cardiol 11:1127–34, 1988
11. Nitter-Hauge S: Does mitral stenosis need invasive investigation? Eur Heart J, suppl B, 12:81–3, 1991
12. Hess O, Ritter M, Schneider J et al: Diastolic stiffness and myocardial structure in aortic valve disease before and after valve replacement. Circulation 69:855, 1984
13. Kelly T, Rothbart R, Cooper M: Comparison of outcome of asymptomatic to symptomatic patients older than twenty years of age with valvular aortic stenosis. Am J Cardiol 61:123, 1988
14. Frank S, Johnson A, Ross J: Natural history of valvular aortic stenosis. Br Heart J 53:41, 1973
15. Ross J, Braunwald E: The influence of corrective operations on the natural history of AS. Circulation, suppl 5. 37:61, 1968
16. Lombard J, Selzer A: Valvular aortic stenosis: a clinical and hemodynamic profile of patients. Ann Intern Med 106:292–8, 1987
17. Hakki A, Kimbiris D, Iskandrian K et al: Angina pectoris and coronary disease in patients with severe aortic valvular disease. Am Heart J 100:441, 1980
18. Lund O, Nielsen T, Pilegaard H et al: The influence of coronary artery disease and bypass grafting on early and late survival after valve replacement for aortic stenosis. J Thorac Cardiovasc Surg 100:327–37, 1990
19. Czer L, Gray R, Stewart M et al: Reduction in sudden late death by concomitant revascularization with aortic valve replacement. J Thorac Cardiovasc Surg 95:390, 1988
20. Braunwald E: Valvular heart disease. p. 1040. In Braunwald E (ed): Heart Disease. Vol. 4th Ed. WB Saunders, Philadelphia, 1992
21. Gooch A, Calatawud J, Rogers P, Garman P: Analysis of the P wave in severe AS. Dis Chest 49:459, 1966
22. Dreifus L: Arrhythmias in valvular heart disease. In Frankl W, Brest A (eds): Valvular Heart Disease: Comprehensive Evaluation and Treatment. FA Davis, Philadelphia, 1993
23. Badeer H: Biological significance of cardiac hypertrophy. Am J Cardiol 14:133–8, 1964
24. Carabello B, Zile M, Tanaka R, Cooper G: Left ventricular hypertrophy due to volume

overload versus pressure overload. Am J Physiol 263:H1137, 1992

25. Buchi M, Hess O, Murakami T, Krayenbuehl H: Left ventricular wall stress distribution in chronic pressure and volume overload: effect of normal and depressed contractility on regional stress-velocity relations. Basic Res Cardiol 85:367, 1990

26. Yoran C, Covell J, Ross JJ: Structural basis for the ascending limb of left ventricular function. Circ Res 32:297, 1973

27. Jacob R, Brandle M, Dierberger B, Rupp H: Functional consequences of cardiac hypertrophy and dilation. Basic Res Cardiol suppl 1. 86:113, 1991

28. Jacob R, Dierberger B, Kissling G: Functional significance of the Frank-Starling mechanism under physiological and pathophysiological conditions. Eur Heart J, suppl E. 13:7, 1992

29. Yin F: Ventricular wall stress. Circ Res 49: 829, 1981

30. Grossman W, Jones D, McLaurin L: Wall stress and patterns of hypertrophy. J Clin Invest 56:56, 1975

31. Ross J: Afterload mismatch and preload reserve: a conceptual framework for the analysis of ventricular function. Prog Cardiovasc Dis 18:255, 1976

32. Ross J: Afterload mismatch in aortic and mitral valve disease: implications for surgical therapy. J Am Coll Cardiol 5:811–26, 1985

33. Peterson K, Tsuji J, Johnson A et al: Diastolic left ventricular pressure-volume and stress-strain relations in patients with valvular aortic stenosis and left ventricular hypertrophy. Circulation 58:77, 1978

34. Gunther S, Grossman W: Determinants of ventricular function in pressure-overload hypertrophy in man. Circulation 59:679, 1979

35. Grossman W: Cardiac hypertrophy: useful adaptation or pathologic process? Am J Med 69:576, 1980

36. Stott D, Marpole D, Bristow D et al: The role of left atrial transport in aortic and mitral stenosis. Circulation 41:1031–1041, 1970

37. Braunwald E, Frahm C: Studies on Starling's law of the heart. Observations on the hemodynamic function of the left atrium in man. Circulation 24:633, 1961

38. Tunick P, Gindea A, Kronzon I: Effect of aortic valve replacement for aortic stenosis on severity of mitral regurgitation. Am J Cardiol 65:1219–21, 1990

39. Hicks R, Savas V, Currie P et al: Assessment of myocardial oxidative metabolism in aortic valve disease using positron emission tomography with C-11 acetate. Am Heart J 123:653, 1992

40. Huber D, Grimm J, Koch R, Krayenbuehl H: Determinants of ejection performance in aortic stenosis. Circulation 64:126, 1981

41. Swynghedauw B: The biological limits of cardiac adaptation to chronic overload. Eur Heart J, suppl G. 11:87, 1990

42. Mann D, Urabe Y, Kent R et al: Cellular versus myocardial basis for the contractile dysfunction of hypertrophied myocardium. Circ Res 68:402, 1991

43. Schwartz K, Boheler K, De La Bastie D et al: Switches in cardiac muscle gene expression as a result of pressure and volume overload. Am J Physiol 262:R364, 1992

44. Alpert N, Mulierri L, Litten R: Functional significance of altered myosin adenosine triphosphate activity in enlarged hearts. Am J Cardiol 44:947, 1979

45. De La Bastie D, Levitsky D, Rappaport L et al: Function of the sarcoplasmic reticulum and expression of its Ca^{2+}-ATPase gene in pressure overload-induced cardiac hypertrophy in the rat. Circ Res 66:554, 1990

46. Schwartz K, Carrier L, Lompre A et al: Contractile proteins and sarcoplasmic reticulum calcium-ATPase gene expression in the hypertrophied and failing heart. Basic Res Cardiol, suppl 1. 87:285, 1992

47. Alpert N, Hasenfuss G, Mulieri L et al: The reorganization of the human and rabbit heart in response to haemodynamic overload. Eur Heart J 13:9, 1992

48. Maurer I, Zierz S: Positive correlation between aortic valve pressure gradient and mitochondrial respiratory chain capacity in hypertrophied human ventricle. Clin Invest 70: 896, 1992

49. Swynghedauw B: Biological adaptation of the myocardium to a permanent change in loading conditions. Basic Res Cardiol, suppl 2. 87:1, 1992

50. Urthaler F, Walker A, Hefner L, James T: Comparison of contractile performance of canine atrial and ventricular muscle. Circ Res 37:762, 1975

51. Klug D, Robert V, Swynghedauw B: Role of mechanical and hormonal factors in cardiac remodeling and the biologic limits of myocardial adaptation. Am J Cardiol 71:46A, 1993

52. Swynghedauw B, Carre F: The biological basis of modified myocardial function in hypertensive cardiopathy. Acta Cardiol 46:167, 1991

53. Mercadier J, Lompre A, Duc P et al: Altered sarcoplasmic reticulum Ca^{2+}-ATPase gene expression in the human ventricle during end-stage heart failure. J Clin Invest 85:305, 1990

54. Villari B, Hess O, Kaufmann P et al: Effect of aortic valve stenosis (pressure overload) and regurgitation (volume overload) on left ventricular systolic and diastolic function. Am J Cardiol 69:927, 1992

55. Cooper I, Fry C, Webb-Peploe M: Mechanical restitution of isolated human ventricular myocardium subjected to in vivo pressure and volume overload. Cardiovasc Res 26:978, 1992

56. Gwathmey J, Morgan J: Altered calcium handling in experimental pressure-overload hypertrophy in the ferret. Circ Res 57:836, 1985

57. Chevalier B, Charlemagne D, Callens-el Amrani F et al: The membrane proteins of the overloaded and senescent heart. Basic Res Cardiol, suppl 1. 87:187, 1992

58. Levitsky D, De La Bastie D, Schwartz K, Lompre A: Ca^{2+}-ATPase and function of sarcoplasmic reticulum during cardiac hypertrophy. Am J Physiol, suppl 4. 261:23, 1991

59. Cooper G IV, Kent R, Mann D: Load induction of cardiac hypertrophy. J Mol Cell Cardiol, suppl 5. 21:11, 1989

60. Komuro I, Katoh Y, Kaida T et al: Mechanical loading stimulates cell hypertrophy and specific gene expression in cultured rat cardiac myocytes. Possible role of protein kinase C activation. J Biol Chem 266:1265, 1991

61. Yazaki Y, Komuro I: Role of protein kinase system in the signal transduction of stretch-mediated myocyte growth. Basic Res Cardiol, suppl 2. 87:11, 1992

62. Kent R, Hoober J, Cooper G IV: Load responsiveness of protein synthesis in adult mammalian myocardium: role of cardiac deformation linked to sodium influx. Circ Res 64:74, 1989

63. Sadoshima J, Izumo S: Mechanical stretch rapidly activates multiple signal transduction pathways in cardiac myocytes: potential involvement of an autocrine/paracrine mechanism. EMBO J 12:1681, 1993

64. Watson P: Function follows form: generation of intracellular signals by cell deformation. FASEB J 5:2013, 1991

65. Long C, Kariya K, Karns L, Simpson P: Sympathetic modulation of the cardiac myocyte phenotype: studies with a cell-culture model of myocardial hypertrophy. Basic Res Cardiol, suppl 2. 87:19, 1992

66. DeQuattro V, Lee D, Shkhvatsabaya I et al: Primary hypertension: left ventricular mass and function, sympathetic nervous system activity, and therapy. Health Psychol, suppl. 7:165, 1988

67. Laks M: Noreponephrine—the myocardial hypertrophy hormone? Am Heart J 91:674, 1976

68. Long C, Kariya K, Karns L, Simpson P: Sympathetic activity: modulator of myocardial hypertrophy. J Cardiovasc Pharmacol, suppl 2. 17:S20, 1991

69. Starksen N, Simpson P, Bishopric N et al: Cardiac myocyte hypertrophy is associated with c-myc protooncogene expression. Proc Natl Acad Sci USA 83:8348, 1986

70. Meidell R, Sen A, Henderson S et al: Alpha 1-adrenergic stimulation of rat myocardial cells increases protein synthesis. Am J Physiol 251(5 pt 2):H1076, 1986

71. Simpson P, Kariya K, Karns L et al: Adrenergic hormones and control of cardiac myocyte growth. Mol Cell Biochem 104:35, 1991

72. Paul M, Ganten D: The molecular basis of cardiovascular hypertrophy: the role of the renin-angiotensin system. J Cardiovasc Pharmacol, suppl 5. 19:S51, 1992

73. Suzuki J, Matsubara H, Urakami M, Inada M: Rat angiotensin II (type 1A) receptor mRNA regulation and subtype expression in myocardial growth and hypertrophy. Circ Res 73:439, 1993

74. Lindpaintner K, Ganten D: The cardiac renin-angiotensin system: a synopsis of current experimental and clinical data. Acta Cardiol 46:385, 1991

75. Sadoshima J, Izumo S: Signal transduction pathways of angiotensin II-induced c-fos gene expression in cardiac myocytes in vitro.

Roles of phospholipid-derived second messengers. Circ Res 73:424, 1993

76. Moalic J, Bauters C, Himbert D et al: Phenylephrine, vasopressin and angiotensin II as determinants of proto-oncogene and heatshock protein gene expression in adult rat heart and aorta. J Hypertens 7:195, 1989

77. Linz W, Scholkens B, Ganten D: Converting enzyme inhibition specifically prevents the development of and induces regression of cardiac hypertrophy in rats. Clin Exp Hypertens A11:1325, 1989

78. Schunkert H, Dzau V, Tang S et al: Increased rat cardiac angiotensin converting enzyme activity and mRNA expression in pressure overload left ventricular hypertrophy. Effects on coronary resistance, contractility, and relaxation. J Clin Invest 86:1913, 1990

79. Baker K, Chernin M, Wixson S, Aceto J: Renin-angiotensin system involvement in pressure-overload cardiac hypertrophy in rats. Am J Physiol 259(2 pt 2):H324, 1990

80. Fernandez-Alfonso M, Ganten D, Paul M: Mechanisms of cardiac growth. The role of the renin-angiotensin system. Basic Res Cardiol, suppl 2. 87:173, 1992

81. Schelling P, Fischer H, Ganten D: Angiotensin and cell growth: a link to cardiovascular hypertrophy? J Hypertens 9:3, 1991

82. Lindpaintner K, Ganten D: Tissue renin-angiotensin systems and their modulation: the heart as a paradigm for new aspects of converting enzyme inhibition. Cardiology, suppl 1. 79:32, 1991

83. Allen D, Kurihara S: The effects of muscle length on intracellular calcium transients in mammalian cardiac muscle. J Physiol 327:79, 1982

84. Marban E, Koretsune Y: Cell calcium, oncogenes, and hypertrophy. Hypertension 15:652, 1990

85. Kitakaze M, Marban E: Cellular mechanism of the modulation of contractile function by coronary perfusion pressure in ferret hearts. J Physiol (Lond) 414:455, 1989

86. Simpson P: Role of proto-oncogenes in myocardial hypertrophy. Am J Cardiol 62:13G, 1988

87. Taubman M, Berk B, Izumo S: Angiotensin II induces c-*fos* mMRA in aortic smooth muscle. Role of Ca^{2+} mobilization and protein kinase C activation. J Biol Chem 264:526, 1989

88. Mommaerts W: Relationship between cardiac work and cardiac growth: some general thoughts on cardiac hypertrophy. pp. 52–65. In Ter Keurs H, Schipperheyn J (eds): Cardiac Left Ventricular Hypertrophy. Martinus Nijhoff, Boston, 1983

89. Ruknudin A, Sachs F, Bustamante J: Stretch-activated ion channels in tissue-cultured chick heart. Am J Physiol 264:H960, 1993

90. Morgan J, Curran T: Role of ion flux in the control of c-*fos* expression. Nature 322:552, 1986

91. Schneider M, McLellan W, Black F, Parker T: Growth factors, growth factor response elements, and the cardiac phenotype. Basic Res Cardiol, suppl 2. 87:33, 1992

92. Schneider M, Parker T: Cardiac growth factors. Prog Growth Factor Res 3:1, 1991

93. Black F, Packer S, Parker T et al: The vascular smooth muscle alpha-actin gene is reactivated during cardiac hypertrophy provoked by load. J Clin Invest 88:1581, 1991

94. Simpson P, Long C, Waspe L et al: Transcription of early developmental isogenes in cardiac myocyte hypertrophy. J Mol Cell Cardiol 21:79, 1989

95. Xenophontos X, Watson P, Chua B et al: Increased cyclic AMP content accelerates protein synthesis in rat heart. Circ Res 65:647, 1989

96. Watson P, Haneda T, Morgan H: Effect of higher aortic pressure on ribosome formation and cAMP contentin rat heart. Am J Physiol 256(6 pt 1):C1257, 1989

97. Chua B, Russo L, Gordon E et al: Faster ribosome synthesis induced by elevated aortic pressure in rat heart. Am J Physiol 252(3 pt 1):C323, 1987

98. Nagai R, Low R, Stirewalt W et al: Efficiency and capacity of protein synthesis are increased in pressure overload cardiac hypertrophy. Am J Physiol 255:H325, 1988

99. Xenophontos X, Gordon E, Morgan H: Effect of intraventricular pressure on protein synthesis in arrested rat hearts. Am J Physiol 251:C95, 1986

100. Gordon H: Oncogenes. Mayo Clin Proc 60:697, 1985

101. Komuro I, Kurabayashi M, Takaku F, Yazaki Y: Expression of cellular oncogenes in the

myocardium during the developmental stage and pressure-overloaded hypertrophy of the rat heart. Circ Res. 62:1075, 1988

102. Delcayre C, Samuel J, Marotte F et al: Synthesis of stress protein in rat cardiac myocytes 2–4 days after imposition of hemodynamic overload. J Clin Invest 82:460, 1988

103. Izumo S, Nadal-Ginard B, Mahdavi V: Protooncogene induction and reprogramming of cardiac gene expression produced by pressure overload. Proc Natl Acad Sci USA 85: 339, 1988

104. Anversa P, Olivetti G, Melissari M, Loud A: Stereological measurement of cellular and subcellular hypertrophy and hyperplasia in the papillary muscle of adult rat. J Mol Cell Cardiol 12:781, 1980

105. Weber K, Nanicki J, Schroff S et al: Collagen remodeling of the pressure overloaded, hypertrophied nonhuman primate myocardium. Circ Res 62:757, 1988

106. Chapman D, Weber K, Eghbali M: Regulation of fibrillar collagen type I and III and basement membrane type IV collagen gene expression in pressure overloaded rat myocardium. Circ Res 67:787, 1990

107. Krayenbuehl H, Hess O, Monrad E et al: Left ventricular myocardial structure in aortic valve disease before, intermediate, and late after aortic valve replacement. Circulation 79:744, 1989

108. Weber K, Brilla C: Pathological hypertrophy and cardiac interstitium. Fibrosis and the renin-angiotensin-aldosterone system. Circulation 83:1849, 1991

109. Weber K, Jalil J, Janicki J, Pick R: Myocardial collagen remodeling in pressure overload hypertrophy. A case for interstitial heart disease. Am J Hypertens 2:931, 1989

110. Swynghedauw B, Delcayre C, Cheav S et al: Biological basis of diastolic dysfunction of the hypertensive heart. Eur Heart J, suppl D, 13:2, 1992

111. Bing O, Fanburg B, Brooks W, Matsushita S: The effect of the lathyrogen β-amino proprionitrile (BAPN) on the mechanical properties of experimentally hypertrophied rat cardiac muscle. Circ Res 43:632, 1978

112. Schwartzkopff B, Frenzel H, Dieckerhoff J et al: Morphometric investigation of human myocardium in arterial hypertension and valvular aortic stenosis. Eur Heart J, suppl D. 13:17, 1992

113. Eghbali M: Cardiac fibroblast: function, regulation of gene expression, and phenotypic modulation. Basic Res Cardiol, suppl 2. 87: 183, 1992

114. Schwarz F, Flameng W, Schaper J et al: Myocardial structure and function in patients with aortic valve disease and their relation to postoperative results. Am J Cardiol 41:661, 1978

115. Kremer R: Arrhythmias in the natural history of aortic stenosis. Acta Cardiol 47:135–40, 1992

116. Moalic J, Charlemagne D, Mansier P et al: Cardiac hypertrophy and failure—a disease of adaptation. Modifications in membrane proteins provide a molecular basis for arrhythmogenicity. Circulation, suppl 5. IV 87: 21, 1993

117. Chevalier B, Callens F, Charlemagne D et al: Signal and adaptational changes in gene expression during cardiac overload. J Mol Cell Cardiol, suppl 5. 21:71, 1989

118. Chevalier B, Mansier P, Callens-El Amrani F, Swynghedauw B: The beta adrenergic system is modified in compensatory pressure cardiac overload in rats. Physiological biochemical evidence. J Cardiovasc Pharmacol 13:412, 1989

119. Swynghedauw B: Remodeling of the heart in chronic pressure overload. Basic Res Cardiol, suppl 1. 86:99, 1991

120. Smucker M, Tedesco C, Manning S: Demonstration of an imbalance between coronary perfusion and excessive load as a mechanism of ischemia during stress in patients with AS. Circulation 78:573, 1988

121. Johnson L, Sciacca R, Ellis K et al: Reduced left ventricular myocardial blood flow per unit mass in aortic stenosis. Circulation 57: 582, 1978

122. Stack R, Schirmer B, Greenfield J: Coronary artery luminal diameters in normal and hypertrophied canine ventricles. Circulation, suppl 3. 62:64, 1980

123. Alyono D, Anderson R, Parrish D: Alterations of myocardial bllod flow associated with experimental canine LVH secondary to valvular aortic stenosis. Circ Res 58:47, 1988

124. Shipley R, Shipley L, Wearn J: The capillary supply in normal and hypertrophied hearts of rabbits. J Exp Med 65:29, 1937

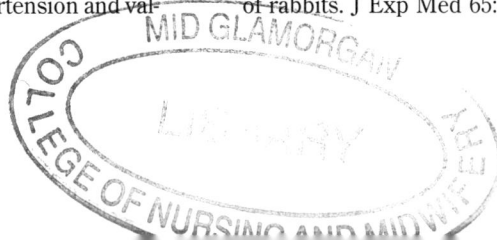

125. Roberts J, Wearn J: Quantitative changes in the capillary-muscle relationship in human hearts during normal growth and hypertrophy. Am Heart J 21:617, 1941

126. Hinquell L, Odoroff C, Honig C: Intercapillary distance and capillary reserve in hypertrophied rat hearts beating in situ. Circ Res 41:400, 1979

127. Rakusan K: Quantitative morphology of capillaries of the heart. Number of capillaries in animal and human hearts under normal and pathologic conditions. Methods Arch Exp Pathol 5:272, 1971

128. Linzbach A: Heart failure from the point of view of quantitative anatomy. Am J Cardiol 5:370, 1960

129. Guyton R, McClenathan J, Newman G, Michealis L: Significance of subendocardial S-T segment elevation caused by coronary stenosis in the dog. Am J Cardiol 40:373, 1977

130. O'Keefe D, Hoffman J, Cheitlin R et al: Coronary blood flow in experimental canine left ventricular hypertrophy. Circ Res 43:43, 1978

131. Pyle R, Lowensohn H, Khouri E et al: Left circumflex coronary artery hemodynamics in conscious dogs with congenital subaortic stenosis. Circ Res 33:34, 1973

132. Bellhouse B, Bellhouse F: Fluid mechanics of model normal and stenosed aortic valves. Circ Res 25:693, 1969

133. Carroll R, Falsetti H: Retrograde coronary artery flow in aortic valve disease. Circulation 54:494, 1976

134. Fujiwara T, Nogami A, Masaki H et al: Coronary flow velocity waveforms in aortic stenosis and the effects of valve replacement. Ann Thorac Surg 48:518, 1989

135. Wicker P, Tarazi R: Coronary blood flow in left ventricular hypertrophy: a review of experimental data. Eur Heart J, suppl A. 3: 111–18, 1982

136. Rouleau J, Boerboom L, Surjadhana A, Hoffman J: The role of autoregulation and tissue diastolic pressures in the transmural distribution of left ventricular blood flow in anesthetized dogs. Circ Res 45:804, 1979

137. Cruickshank J: The role of coronary perfusion pressure. Eur Heart J suppl D. 13:39, 1992

138. Farnett L, Mulrow C, Linn W et al: The J-curve phenomenon and the treatment of hypertension. JAMA 265:489, 1991

139. Pepi M, Alimento M, Maltagliati A, Guazzi M: Cardiac hypertrophy in hypertension. Repolarization abnormalities elicited by rapid lowering of pressure. Hypertension 11:84, 1988

140. Klocke F: Measurements of coronary flow reserve: defining pathophysiology versus making decisions about patient care. Circulation 76:1183, 1987

141. Polese A, De Cesare N, Montosorsi P et al: Upward shift of the lower range of coronary flow autoregulation in hypertensive patients with hypertrophy of the left ventricle. Circulation 83:845, 1991

142. Krayenbuehl H, Hess O, Monrad E et al: Function and structure of the failing left ventricular myocardium in aortic valve disease before and after valve replacement. Basic Res Cardiol, suppl 3. 86:175–85, 1991

143. Kennedy J, Doces J, Stewart D: Left ventricular function before and following aortic valve replacement. Circulation 56:944, 1977

144. Monrad E, Hess O, Murakami T et al: Time course of regression of left ventricular hypertrophy after aortic valve replacement. Circulation 77:1345, 1988

145. Croke R, Pifarre R, Sullivan H et al: Reversal of advanced left ventricular dysfunction following aortic valve replacement for aortic stenosis. Ann Thorac Surg 24:38, 1977

146. Smith N, McAnulty J, Rahimtoola S: Severe aortic stenosis with impaired left ventricular function and clinical heart failure; results of valve replacement. Circulation 58:255, 1978

147. Tracy G, Proctor M, Hizny C: Reversibility of pulmonary artery hypertension in aortic stenosis after aortic valve replacement. Ann Thorac Surg 50:89–93, 1990

148. Aragam J, Folland E, Lapsley D et al: Cause and impact of pulmonary hypertension in isolated aortic stenosis on operative mortality for aortic valve replacement in men. Am J Cardiol 69:1365, 1992

149. Johnson L, Hapanowicz M, Buananno C et al: Pulmonary hypertension in isolated artic stenosis. Hemodynamic correlations and follow-up. J Thorac Cardiovasc Surg 95:603, 1988

150. Waller B, Howard J, Fess S: Pathology of mitral valve stenosis and pure mitral regurgitation—Part I. Clin Cardiol 17:330–36, 1994

151. Agathos E, Starr A: Mitral valve replacement. Curr Probl Surg 30:482–592, 1993
152. Burge D, DeHoratius R: Acute rheumatic fever. In Frankl W, Brest A (eds): Valvular Heart Disease: Comprehensive Evaluation and Treatment. FA Davis, Philadelphia, 1993
153. Burckhardt D, Hoffmann A, Kiowski W: Treatment of mitral stenosis. Eur Heart J, suppl B. 12:95–8, 1991
154. Goldstein M, Michelson E, Dreifus L: The electrocardiogram in valvular heart disease. In Frankl W, Brest A (eds): Valvular Heart Disease: Comprehensive Evaluation and Treatment. FA Davis, Philadelphia, 1993
155. Horstkotte D: Arrhythmias in the natural history of mitral stenosis. Acta Cardiol 47:105–13, 1992
156. Carabello B, Grossman W: Calculation of stenotic valve orifice area. pp. 152–65. In Grossman W (ed): Cardiac Catheterization and Angiography. Lea & Febiger, Philadelphia, 1991
157. Hatle L, Angelsen B, Tromsdal A: Noninvasive assessment of atrioventricular pressure half-time by Doppler ultrasound. Circulation 60:1096–1104, 1979
158. Odemuyiwa O, Bourke J, Peart I et al: Valvular stenosis: a comparison of clinical assessment, echocardiography, Doppler ultrasound and catheterization. Int J Cardiol 26:59–66, 1990
159. Carabello B: Timing of surgery in mitral and aortic stenosis. pp. 229–38. In Carabello B (ed): Cardiology Clinics. Vol. 9. WB Saunders, Philadelphia, 1991
160. Jackson J, Thomas S: Valvular heart disease. p. 629. In Kaplan J (ed): Cardiac Anesthesia. 3rd Ed. WB Saunders, Philadelphia, 1993
161. Meisner J, Keren G, Pajaro O et al: Atrial contribution to ventricular filling in mitral stenosis. Circulation 84:1469–1480, 1991
162. Gaasch W, Folland E: Left ventricular function in rheumatic mitral stenosis. Eur Heart J, suppl B. 12:66–9, 1991
163. Gash A, Carabello B, Cepin D et al: Left ventricular ejection performance and systolic muscle function in patients with mitral stenosis. Circulation 67:148–54, 1983
164. Chopra P, Bhatia M: Chronic rheumatic heart disease in India: a reappraisal of pathologic changes. J Heart Valve Dis 1:92, 1992
165. Braunwald E, Braunwald N, Ross J: Effective mitral valve replacement with pulmonary vascular dynamics for patients with pulmonary hypertension. N Engl J Med 273:509, 1965
166. Dalen J, Matloff J, Evans G et al: Early reduction of pulmonary vascular resistance after mitral valve replacement. N Engl J Med 277:387–94, 1967
167. Snashall P, Chung K: Airway obstruction and bronchial hyperresponsiveness in left ventricular failure and mitral stenosis. Am Rev Respir Dis 144:945–56, 1991
168. Cabanes L, Weber S, Matran R et al: Bronchial hyperresponsiveness to methacholine in patients with impaired left ventricular function. N Engl J Med 320:1317–22, 1989
169. Rolla G, Bucca C, Caria E et al: Bronchial responsiveness in patients with mitral valve disease. Eur Respir J 3:127–31, 1990
170. Wood T, McLeod P, Anthonisen N, Macklem P: Mechanics of breathing in mitral stenosis. Am Rev Respir Dis 104:52–60, 1971
171. Wroblewski E, Spann J, Bove A: Right ventricular performance in mitral stenosis. Am J Cardiol 47:51–5, 1981
172. Stein P, Sabbah H, Anbe D et al: Performance of the failing and nonfailing right ventricle of patients with pulmonary hypertension. Am J Cardiol 44:1050–5, 1979
173. Hall R: Rheumatic mitral valve disease. In Julian D, Camm A, Fox K, Hall R (eds): Diseases of the Heart. Bailliere Tindall, London, 1989
174. Acar J, Cormier D, Grimberg D et al: Diagnosis of left atrial thrombi in mitral stenosis—usefulness of ultrasound techniques compared to other methods. Eur Heart J, suppl B. 12:70–6, 1991
175. Horstkotte D, Niehues R, Strauer B: Pathomorphological aspects, aetiology and natural history of acquired mitral valve stenosis. Eur Heart J, suppl B. 12:55–60, 1991
176. Vidne B, Erdman S, Levy M: Thromboembolism following heart valve replacement by prosthesis: survey among 365 consecutive patients. Chest 63:713–7, 1973
177. Hoffman JIE, Graftan MT, Hanley FL, Marina LM: Total and transmural perfusion of the hypertrophied heart. p. 129. In Ter Keurs HEDJ, Schipperheyn JJ (eds): Cardiac Left Ventricular Hypertrophy. Kluwer Academic, Dordrecht, 1983

3

Cardiomyopathies

Gordon A. Cohen
Norman S. Kato
Peter Nicolazzo

The definition and classification of cardiomyopathy are controversial. Many physicians treating cardiac disease would include any form of heart failure caused by myocardial insufficiency, including ischemic heart disease, nutritional deficiency, and myocarditis.[1] However, there exists a more generally accepted view that the cardiomyopathies specifically exclude entities developing secondary to ischemic heart disease, pulmonary and systemic hypertension, and valvular and congenital heart disease. Thus, there has been a great deal of objection to the term *ischemic cardiomyopathy*.

In 1980, the World Health Organization Task Force defined cardiomyopathies as "heart muscle diseases of unknown cause."[2] A second class of disorders known as "specific heart muscle disease" was developed. Thus, the classification of cardiomyopathy as just defined has been greatly simplified as follows: dilated or congestive cardiomyopathies; hypertrophic cardiomyopathies; and restrictive/obliterative cardiomyopathies. Those forms of myocardial dysfunction associated with a toxic etiology, such as metabolic disease, neuromuscular disease, storage disorder, or those that are infiltrative in origin, are all part of the larger category referred to as specific heart muscle diseases. Despite this specific definition, the specific heart muscle diseases are still commonly referred to as secondary cardiomyopathies.

As for the purpose of this chapter, the cardiomyopathies are classified on an etiologic basis. Two fundamental forms are recognized: a primary type consisting of heart muscle disease of unknown cause and a secondary type consisting of a myocardial disease of known cause that may or may not be associated with a disease involving other organ systems (Table 3-1). Specific heart muscle diseases often show a dilated restrictive or hypertrophic characteristic, making them hemodynamically similar to those that have primary myocardial involvement. Although it is important to understand the technical difference in terms of the definition of the cardiomyopathies, as opposed to the specific heart muscle diseases, for the purpose of this discussion, they are all referred to as primary and secondary cardiomyopathies. Most clini-

Table 3-1.   Classification of Cardiomyopathy

Disorder	Description	Hemodynamic Marker
Dilated cardiomyopathy	Biventricular dilation and hypertrophy	Pump failure
Hypertrophic cardiomyopathy	Severe ventricular hypertrophy especially of the intraventricular septum	Obstruction and poor ventricular compliance
Restrictive cardiomyopathy	Ventricular restriction similar to constrictive pericarditis	Poor ventricular compliance
Obliterative cardiomyopathy	Massive fibrosis of the endocardium with ventricular enlargement but cavity restriction	Poor ventricular compliance

cians still refer to these diseases as primary and secondary cardiomyopathy because physiologically there appears to be no difference in terms of their pathophysiology and management.

CLASSIFICATIONS

Since the cardiomyopathies represent a diverse group of diseases, they are best managed in terms of their hemodynamic characteristics. While there are four hemodynamic categories of cardiomyopathy[3] (Table 3-2), the physiologic consequences are easily sep-arated into two groups: diminished compliance (filling problems), and diminished contractile response (pump failure).

The restrictive and obliterative cardiomyopathies are often combined into a single category. For the purpose of this review, restrictive and obliterative are referred to as a single category. However, some investigators believe that separate categories for these conditions are still warranted, as the purely restrictive cardiomyopathies involve only the myocardium, whereas the obliterative cardiomyopathies have major endocardial anomalies as well. Despite the pathologic differ-

Table 3-2.   Secondary Cardiomyopathies

Metabolic disorders	Toxic	Connective tissue disorders
Thyroid dysfunction	Doxorubicin	Scleroderma
Abnormal serum potassium	(Adriamycin)	Rheumatoid arthritis
Nutritional deficiencies	Cyclophosphamide	Polyarteritis nodosa
Storage disorders	Alcohol	Systemic lupus
Fabry's disease	Catecholamines	erythematosus
Sandhoff's disease	Carbon monoxide	Dermatomyositis
Glycogen storage disease	Lithium	Peripartum heart disease
Hunter-Hurler syndrome	Hydrocarbons	Endocardial fibroelastosis
Infiltrative	Arsenic	
Hemachromatosis	Cobalt	
Emoidosis	Infective	
Sarcoidosis	Viral myocarditis	
Malignancy	Bacterial myocarditis	
Leukemia	Fungal myocarditis	
Neuromuscular disease	Protozoal myocarditis	
Muscular dystrophy	Metazoal myocarditis	
Myotonic dystrophy		
Friedreich's ataxia		
Refsum's disease		
Congenital atrophies		

ences, these two categories are essentially identical, from a hemodynamic perspective.

CLASSIFICATION OF CARDIOMYOPATHIES BASED ON ETIOLOGY

Of the known causes of cardiomyopathy, dilated cardiomyopathy associated with excessive alcohol intake is one of the more common forms. A great deal of evidence suggests that ethanol is able to suppress or depress cardiac function directly.[4] However, alcohol abuse is also associated with malnutrition, and this may be a contributing factor. Clinically, after stopping alcohol consumption, a recovery of function occurs in the absence of nutritional repletion. An example of an idiopathic form of cardiomyopathy is one that occasionally develops in women within the last month of pregnancy and may occur as far along as 4 months following parturition. This form of cardiomyopathy is known as *peripartum cardiomyopathy* and is idiopathic. It is most likely not due to underlying subclinical cardiomyopathy. In most cases, the disease occurs well after the period in which the mother has gone through the most physiologically stressful part of the pregnancy.[5]

In most cases, when a cardiomyopathy has a clearly definable etiology, the signs of that primary disease process are quite evident. There are rare situations in which the cardiac involvement precedes the other systemic manifestations of the underlying primary problem. This may be the case with some cardiomyopathies classified as idiopathic in nature. For example, viral cardiomyopathy may represent the late sequelae of an underlying or resolving viral infection. Coxsackie B virus has been commonly associated with cardiomyopathies.[6] There appears to be a significantly higher prevalence of HLA-B27 and HLA-DR4 in patients with dilated cardiomyopathy concurrent with, or after, a viral infection.[7] Other investigators have also demonstrated a reduced suppresser cell activity or autoimmune processes.[8] Patients who have a viral infection associated with cardiac dysfunction or who have just recovered from a viral infection have been shown on endomyocardial biopsy to have active myocarditis. Whether the viral infection is the sole cause of the myocarditis, or some other relationship between the viral infection and the cardiomyopathy exists, is unclear.

Chagas disease is primarily seen in parts of South America; it is caused by a parasitic infection. With the increased number of immigrants into the United States over the past decade, there has been a slight increase in the numbers of patients seen with dilated cardiomyopathy secondary to Chagas disease. This is a relatively rare form of cause of dilated cardiomypathies in the United States.

DILATED OR CONGESTIVE CARDIOMYOPATHIES

The characteristic finding associated with dilated or congestive cardiomyopathy is dilation of the left, right, or both ventricles. Although ventricular hypertrophy usually supervenes, ventricular function is reduced.[9] The hemodynamic and morphologic consequences of dilated cardiomyopathies include decreased cardiac output, decreased stroke volume (SV), increased filling pressures, increased chamber size, decreased ejection fraction, either a normal or decreased diastolic compliance, and associated mitral or tricuspid valve regurgitation.[3] Often, the end result is congestive heart failure (CHF). The underlying etiology of the ventricular dilation and poor hemodynamic performance is unclear. The dilated cardiomyopathies have many different origins and ultimately represent a common end result for a number of different forms of myocardial injury, including those associated with hypertension, valvular heart disease, congenital heart disease, or coronary artery disease. It is important to note that dilated or congestive cardiomyopathies caused by beri beri or thyrotoxicosis are associated with a high cardiac output, unlike the other cardiomyopathies of this category.[3] In patients who have a primary cardiomyopathy, treatment is usually limited to symptomatic improvement. In patients with a secondary cardiomyopathy, treatment should be directed at the primary disease process, as some of these conditions are reversible. If symptomatic treatment is refractory in either situation, the only choice is orthotopic cardiac transplantation.

Grossly, these hearts are increased in weight and may weigh as much as 1 kg. Dilated cardiomyopathies often have mural thrombi present, particularly in the left ventricular apex, due to poor cardiac contraction and stasis of blood in the cardiac chambers. The right ventricle, the right atrial appendage, and the left atrial appendage may also have thrombi due to blood stasis. Operative procedures on these hearts should involve minimal manipulation of the heart before application of the aortic cross-clamp to minimize the risk of embolization; they often require intraoperative echocardiology to identify thrombi. Grossly, the cardiac valves are usually normal, and most often the coronary arteries have minimal to moderate atherosclerosis as compared to other patients of the same age group, unless the cause of the cardiomyopathy is atherosclerosis.[9]

Histologic examination of the heart at necropsy or from endomyocardial biopsy usually demonstrates vague and nonspecific changes. Twenty-five percent of these hearts have are no significant alterations or atrophy of myocardial cells; some increase in interstitial fibrous tissue suggestive of a previous viral myocarditis is the most common change. Some cases exhibit mild to moderate endocardial thickening, usually localized to the ventricles. Small interstitial foci of mononuclear inflammatory cells are occasionally observed. Electron microscopy and histochemistry have been unable to identify specific biochemical or anatomic changes, demonstrating only regressive alterations.[9]

Clinically, patients with this condition usually present with symptoms of left- and right-sided CHF. Clinical manifestations of this include dyspnea on exertion, fatigue, orthopnea, paroxysmal nocturnal dyspnea, peripheral edema, and palpitations. Patients usually describe a progressive nature of the symptoms. Many patients have left ventricular dilation for months, or even years, before becoming symptomatic. Occasionally, patients complain of vague chest pain; however, typical angina pectoris is unusual and suggests the presence of concomitant coronary artery disease.

On physical examination, variable degrees of cardiac enlargement and findings of CHF are usually seen. As the disease progresses, a narrowed pulse pressure and jugular venous distension develop. An S_3 gallop and an S_4 can be identified, and murmurs consistent with mitral or tricuspid regurgitation are often present. Clinical findings such as diastolic murmurs and hypertension and valvular calcification and vascular changes in the optic fundi are suggestive of a process other than cardiomyopathy. Laboratory evaluation of the patient with dilated or congestive cardiomyopathy demonstrates a number of different changes. Chest radiography will show evidence of moderate to marked cardiac enlargement and pulmonary venous hypertension. The electrocardiogram (ECG) will show nonspecific ST- and T-wave abnormalities.

Echocardiograms display evidence of left ventricular dilation and marked dysfunction, and a pericardial effusion is often identified. More sophisticated studies, such as radionuclide studies and cardiac catheterization, will show evidence of left ventricular dilation and dysfunction. Endomyocardial biopsy may be useful and can be diagnostic in certain conditions such as myocardial infiltration by amyloid. In addition, biopsy evidence of myocardial inflammation can be suggestive of an inflammatory etiology such as viral myocarditis.[3]

The clinical course of patients with a dilated cardiomyopathy is usually one of progressive deterioration. Most patients with this condition, particularly those over 55 years of age, will die within 2 years from the onset of symptoms. Death is usually secondary to CHF or ventricular dysrhythmia. Sudden death of a dysrhythmic origin is a constant threat.[10] Because of the presence of intracardiac thrombi as well as low cardiac output states, systemic embolization and stroke are often seen. Consequently, patients with dilated or congestive cardiomyopathy usually undergo anticoagulant therapy. Since by definition the cause of primary dilated cardiomyopathy is unknown, it is not possible to administer specific therapy for the disease process.

Treatment of this disorder is usually palliative in nature. Some clinicians have advocated strict bed rest for up to 1 year or more. However, this form of therapy is controversial because its effectiveness appears limited, and in most cases compliance is extremely poor. Strenuous exertion should be avoided. Treatment of this form of cardiomyopathy is usually similar to that of congestive heart failure. Patients are placed on a salt-restricted diet; diuretics, digitalis, and vasodilators have proved of limited efficacy in terms of providing symptomatic improvement. Pharmacologic therapy with inotropic agents such as dopamine and milrinone has also demonstrated some clinical improvement but have not improved survival.[11] In those patients who have endomyocardial biopsy-proven myocardial inflammation, treatment is often directed toward reducing the inflammation. Pharmacologic agents that have been tried include corticosteroids, often in association with azathioprine. Other pharmacologic approaches to treating this disease entity have included gradual increasing dosages of β-adrenergic blocking agents, and various antidysrhythmic agents.[12]

Because most patients are resistant to pharmacologic amelioration, surgical therapy has gained favor because it demonstrates a more effective approach to treating these patients. The most common forms of surgical intervention for the dilated cardiomyopathies include surgical interruption of the dysrhythmic circuit or implantation of an automatic internal cardiodefibrillator (AICD). Patients with advanced disease refractory to medical therapy are referred for cardiac transplantation.

HYPERTROPHIC CARDIOMYOPATHY

Overview

Hypertrophic cardiomyopathy (HCM) is a pathologic hypertrophy of the myocardium in the absence of valvular stenosis. HCM has also been given other labels, such as asymmetric septal hypertrophy, idiopathic hypertrophic subaortic stenosis, and hypertrophic obstructive cardiomyopathy. Nonetheless, the name hypertrophic cardiomyopathy is preferable because the cardiac changes are not always obstructive and the hypertrophy is not always subaortic or asymmetric. Hypertrophy is the primary event in HCM, unlike aortic stenosis (AS), in which hypertrophy is a compensatory response to pressure overload. Although the obstructive mechanism and myocardial thickening in this setting would suggest alterations in hemodynamics similar to those seen in pressure overload left ventricular hypertrophy (LVH), important distinctions exist.

Demographics and Genetic Linkage of Hypertrophic Cardiomyopathy

The lesion is congenital in more than 50 percent of cases.[13] The incidence is approximately 3 per 10,000. Males are affected twice as often as females, although no X-linked inheritance is known, and some studies suggest an autosomal dominant mode of inheritance. There is evidence that in humans, chromosome 14 is involved in the etiology of HCM in some cases.[14] Although other studies demonstrate an increased prevalence of HLA-B12 in Caucasions and HLA-B5 in African Americans, both loci are located on chromosome 6.

Morphologic and hemodynamic characteristics of HCM include marked hypertrophy of the left and occasionally right ventricle, with disproportionate hypertrophy of the cardiac septum. Cardiac output is usually normal, while stroke volume is either normal or increased. Ventricular filling pressures are either normal or increased, chamber size is either normal or decreased, ejection fraction is increased, and end-diastolic compliance is decreased. Mitral regurgitation is often present, usually related to obstruction between the intraventricular septum and the septal leaflet of the mitral valve. In one-half of undiagnosed patients, sudden death may be the presenting symptom.[15]

The clinical course of HCM is quite variable. Many patients develop atrial fibrillation late in the course of the disease, and this usually leads to a marked increase in symptomatology. However, others demonstrate an improvement or plateau of their symptoms over time. If atrial fibrillation is sustained and uncontrolled, it can often lead to rapid cardiac deterioration and death due to a fall in coronary perfusion pressure and loss of the atrial contribution to cardiac output. Interestingly, patients in the younger age group who have minimal or no evidence of obstruction appear to be at particular risk.

However, clinical features of HCM are often subtle or absent. Often, these asymptomatic patients are close relatives of people with known disease. Unfortunately, because this disease is often clinically silent, the first obvious manifestation may be sudden death. As noted, in one-half of undiagnosed patients, sudden death may be the presenting symptom.[15] This frequently occurs in young adults and children, usually during or after some physical exercise. The most common complaints of symptomatic patients are shortness of breath (as a result of elevated left ventricular diastolic and left atrial pressure), followed by angina, syncope, palpitations, and overt CHF.[16] The annual mortality rate is up to 5 percent in patients with HCM.[14] In one study addressing the incidence of sudden death, more than 70 percent of deaths occurred in patients younger than 30 years of age.[17] In addition, level of activity, occurrence of dysrhythmias, and the use of β-blockers are not reliably predictive of mortality for these patients.[17–19]

Areas of Involvement

Approximately 90 percent of patients with HCM have a reduction in the volume of the ventricular cavities, while three-fourths demonstrate endocardial thickening or mural plaque formation in the left ventricular outflow tract. Mitral valve thickening is seen in three out of four patients, dilated atria are seen in virtually all patients, and abnormal intramural coronary arteries are seen in about one-half of patients. Traditionally, HCM was thought of as an obstructive disorder, with similarities to valvular stenotic lesions perpetuated by such descriptive terms as "subaortic stenosis" and "obstructive cardiomyopathy." Yet, hemodynamic studies suggest that HCM is also a filling disorder. One conclusion is that the pathology that describes HCM exists along a continuum from the obstructive theory to the filling disorder theory. The thickest portion of the septum in those patients who have developed obstructive symptoms is toward the base of the heart behind the mitral leaflet. In those patients without obstructive symptoms, the thickest portion of the septum is usually located more apically and therefore does not contribute to mitral valve dysfunction.[9]

The lesion is not necessarily "stenotic" due to this variability in location of the thickening (Fig. 3-1). The most common site of myocardial thickening is the ventricular septum, typically in the subaortic region; however, thickening may occur in the basal, mid, or apical areas of the septum, or be more concentric in nature. Microscopically, the myofibers are disarrayed so that they are no longer oriented in the usual parallel array within the ventricular septum and the free wall. There also appears to be intracellular

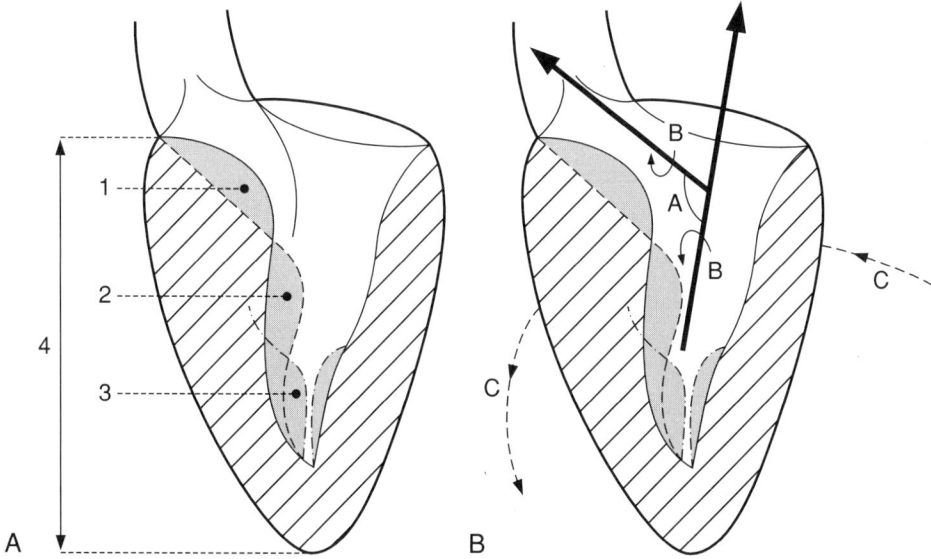

Fig. 3-1. Concept of cavity angulation. Depending on the site of the septal deformity, the major axis, and hence the left ventricular cavity, will be or will not be angulated. **(A)** Morphology. Basal septal *(1);* and septal *(2);* apical *(3);* total septal *(4).* **(B)** Geometry. Angulation of long axis *(A);* torsion of upper half with respect to lower half of LV cavity *(B);* spatial rotation *(C);* preferential flow toward mitral orifice *(arrow).* (From Van der Wall,[43] with permission.)

disarray of the myofibrils and myofilaments within individual myofibers. With obstructive manifestations, the myofiber disarray is more prominent in the septum than in the free wall. Although these changes can also be seen with ordinary or physiologic hypertrophy, the changes in this form of cardiomyopathy are much more striking.

Characteristic findings seen in the evaluation of hypertrophic cardiomyopathy are numerous. Chest radiographs usually demonstrate mild to moderate cardiac enlargement, whereas the ECG usually demonstrates nonspecific ST-segment and T-wave abnormalities. The ECG also demonstrates changes consistent with left ventricular hypertrophy, and often abnormal Q-waves. An echocardiogram may show evidence of asymmetric septal hypertrophy or systolic anterior motion of the mitral valve. Radionuclide studies may show evidence of vigorous systolic function or asymmetric septal hypertrophy. Cardiac

catheterization may demonstrate profound systolic dysfunction, dynamic ventricular outflow obstruction, or elevated left- and right-sided filling pressures.

The broad spectrum of lesions may involve the right side of the heart as well. HCM is not truly hypertrophic since the involved regions show a high percentage of disorganized myofibers and connective tissue elements, rather than hypertrophied myocytes. As previously noted, disorganized regions may not be limited to areas of gross wall thickening but may also occur in nonhypertrophied areas of the left ventricle, further contributing to impaired diastolic function.

Septal myotomy or partial myomectomy often results in significant reduction in subaortic gradient[20] and relief of impaired diastolic filling.[21] In a retrospective study, surgical repair of symptomatic patients demonstrated a significantly better survival than in medically treated patients,[22] although recurrence of the lesion following surgical myotomy is not uncommon. The perioperative mortality has improved in recent years but remains at about 5 percent.[23] Surgical complications can be related to the transaortic surgical approach, resulting in a damaged aortic valve or new-onset aortic regurgitation. Further complications are related to the need to obtain an adequate resection to prevent the recurrence of left ventricular outflow tract (LVOT) obstruction: that is, left bundle branch block, septal infarct, secondary ventricular septal defect, or cerebral emboli.

Hypertrophic Cardiomyopathy as an "Obstructive Disorder"

Most investigators agree that there is a true mechanical obstruction to flow by systolic anterior motion (SAM) of the mitral valve against the hypertrophied ventricular septum. When HCM is associated with a pressure gradient, there is an abnormal SAM of the anterior and sometimes posterior leaflets of the MV. The severity of SAM-septal contact and LVOT pressure gradients is related quantitatively.[24]

Hypertrophic Cardiomyopathy as a "Filling Disorder"

Van der Wall[21] and Goodwin[25] have reviewed the filling disorder theory for HCM. First, gradients across the LVOT are dynamic and without correlation to symp-

toms[26]; second, 90 percent of the left ventricular volume is rapidly expelled during the first half of systole before mechanical obstruction takes place[27,28]; and third, the ejection fractions in this disease tend to be normal or supranormal.

Atrial systole contributes approximately 15 to 20 percent of left ventricular end-diastolic volume in the normal ventricle. Poor ventricular compliance results in a greater dependence on sinus rhythm and "atrial kick" for adequate diastolic filling. In HCM, the atrial contribution is comparable to that in AS; typically occurs at a much higher resistance as compared to patients with AS[21] (Table 3-3). The atrial contribution to the final ventricular SV may approach 75 percent in some HCM patients.[29] Van der Wall[21] emphasizes the significant atrial contribution to left ventricular filling in HCM by the term *atrioventricle* (Fig. 3-2) and emphasizes the need to maintain sinus rhythm in patients with this disease.

The variable location of the septal hypertrophy can significantly alter the direction of the ejected ventricular volume away from the LVOT, described as "cavity angulation"[21] (Fig. 3-1). Cavity angulation during early systolic emptying creates a high-velocity flow through the narrowed LVOT, which enhances the characteristic mitral-septal contact or SAM as the mitral valve apparatus is "pulled along." This dynamic interaction also typically contributes to mitral valve insufficiency, which occurs in late systole.[30]

Table 3-3.   Atrial Contribution to Left Ventricular Filling in Hypertrophic Cardiomyopathy Compared to Aortic Stenosis and Normal Hearts

	Normal (n = 20) Mean ± SD	AS (n = 19) Mean ± SD	HCM (n = 23) Mean ± SD
ΔV-as (%)	20 ± 4	20 ± 6	23 ± 9
ΔP-as (mmHg)	2 ± 2[a]	7 ± 4[a]	17 ± 5[a]

Abbreviations: V-as, atrial contribution to left ventricular diastolic volume expressed as a percentage of the end-diastolic volume; P-as, atrial contribution to left ventricular end-diastolic pressure expressed as the change in pressure from pre-a wave to peak-a wave pressure ("atrial kick"); AS, aortic stenosis; HCM, hypertrophic cardiomyopathy; SD, standard deviation.
[a] $P = 0.0001$.
(From Van der Wall,[43] with permission.)

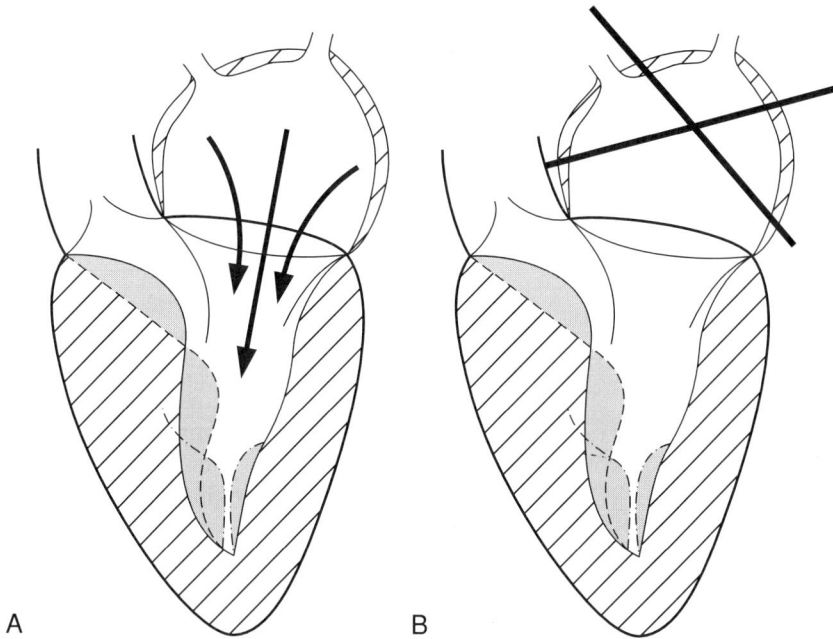

Fig. 3-2. The concept of "atrioventricle" in the heart with hypertrophic cardiomyopathy (HCM). An inseparable combination of a small thick-walled nondilated left ventricle with a normal-size or dilated left atrium. **(A)** The atrium in HCM is converted to a pressure pump from a booster pump. **(B)** The loss of atrial drive. (From Van der Wall,[43] with permission.)

Perioperative Management of Patients With Hypertrophic Cardiomyopathy

The strategy for hemodynamic management of patients with HCM traditionally centers on the reduction of the SAM and subsequent LVOT obstruction. Thus, maneuvers that increase contractility, reduce afterload, and decrease preload should be avoided. Perioperative pharmacologic treatment of hypertrophic cardiomyopathy usually includes negative inotropic agents such as β-adrenergic blocking agents or verapamil in an attempt to attenuate the degree of the angina pectoris and syncope that these patients experience. There is, however, no evidence that β-adrenergic blocking agents have any protective effect against the occurrence of sudden cardiac death (thought to be secondary to malignant ventricular dysrhythmias).[31]

Studies are available demonstrating that amiodarone reduces the frequency of occurrence of both supraventricular and ventricular dysrhythmias. Calcium channel blocking agents have been shown to reduce the stiffness of the ventricle and thus reduce the elevated diastolic pressures. As a result, patients taking calcium channel blocking agents often show improvement in exercise tolerance.[32] Attempts to reduce left ventricular contractility and the outflow gradient with disopyramide are of limited value.[33] It appears that surgical intervention results in the most lasting symptomatic improvement. During anesthesia and surgery, the administration of cardiodepressants (i.e., β-blockers or inhalation anesthetics during general anesthesia) will maintain or improve cardiac output. Vasodilators should be avoided and an adequate vascular resistance maintained, along with an adequate volume status and filling pressures.

In those patients with known LVOT pressure gradients, it is best to avoid diuretics, nitrates, and digitalis preparations.

Surgical myotomy or surgical myomectomy of the hypertrophied septum is often efficacious but carries a mortality of approximately 5 percent. These operations are reserved for those patients who are extremely symptomatic, who demonstrate a high-grade obstruction, or who are refractory to medical management.[34]

Mitral Regurgitation in Hypertrophic Cardiomyopathy

Mitral regurgitation (MR) commonly accompanies HCM. The severity of MR directly correlates with the magnitude of the LVOT gradient.[35] Surgical myotomy and relief of subaortic obstruction result in significant decrease in MR, so that mitral valve replacement is usually not required.[36] MR due to HCM has the opposite response to pharmacologic and hemodynamic manipulations as the classic MR. In HCM, a decreased afterload results in a smaller left ventricular chamber size in systole and a subsequent worsening of MR, whereas an increased afterload maintains a higher left ventricular end-systolic volume and decreases MR.

Diastolic Dysfunction in Hypertrophic Cardiomyopathy

Patients with HCM demonstrate some similar derangements in diastolic function as those with AS. The isovolumic relaxation time (time from AV closure to MV opening) is prolonged. Also, the time to peak rate of left ventricular filling is significantly prolonged in patients with HCM.[37] It has been hypothesized that derangements in calcium sequestration during diastole, similar to that proven in AS, can account for poor diastolic compliance.[23] Another consequence of impaired diastolic relaxation in HCM is that afterload re-

duction and vasodilation fail to improve ventricular function.[23]

Oxygen Supply and Demand in Hypertrophic Cardiomyopathy

Ischemia is less common in patients with HCM compared to those with AS; however, anginal chest pain can be a presenting symptom. Similar to AS, global myocardial oxygen demand is significantly increased due to the increased mass of the left ventricle and the increased pressure work. There is also a compromise on the supply side similar to AS: capillary density is decreased; an elevated left ventricular end-diastolic pressure (LVEDP) results in a decreased coronary perfusion pressure; and prolonged systolic ejection time compromises diastolic time available for coronary perfusion. There are also unique pathologies to HCM that compromise oxygen supply. These include extramural compression of septal perforators by the interventricular septum[38] and metabolic derangements in oxygen extraction.[39]

Dysrhythmias in Hypertrophic Cardiomyopathy

Sudden death is a significant risk for patients with HCM, particularly in the younger age groups. There have been many attempts to link ventricular dysrhythmias, which are frequently found in HCM, to the occurrence of sudden death. The results have not been conclusive. In one study, ventricular dysrhythmias were significantly associated with sudden death, whereas supraventricular dysrhythmias were not.[40] In this study, 24 of 86 patients had at least one attack of ventricular tachycardia on a 72-hour Holter-ECG monitor. Of the seven patients who died suddenly over a mean follow-up of 2.6 years, five patients had documented ventricular tachycardia on Holter.

By contrast, at least two other studies have failed to show a correlation between incidence of sudden death in HCM and the incidence of ventricular tachycardia, abnormal ECG, cardiac symptoms, or hemodynamic variables.[17,18] These two studies do not support aggressive long-term pharmacologic management of ventricular dysrhythmias in these patients. Surgical approaches to this condition consist of ablation of the atrioventricular nodal conduction system and placement of an atrioventricular sequential pacemaker.

RESTRICTIVE-OBLITERATIVE CARDIOMYOPATHY

Restrictive-obliterative cardiomyopathy is rare. The common feature of this disorder is restriction of ventricular filling. A number of different unrelated disease entities appear to induce this form of cardiomyopathy. Diseases such as cardiac amyloidosis, sarcoidosis, endocardiocardial fibroelastosis, endomyocardial fibrosis, and Loeffler's endocarditis all appear to induce this disorder. Other disease processes, such as hemachromatosis, glycogen deposition, and neoplastic infiltration, also cause a restrictive type pattern, but these usually have substantial concurrent systemic disease. Partial obliteration of the ventricular cavity occurs by fibrous tissue formation; mural thrombus contributes to the abnormally high resistance to ventricular filling. Cardiac amyloidosis can appear along with systemic amyloidosis, or it may affect only the heart. If this occurs in the elderly, it is often referred to as "senile isolated cardiac amyloidosis." Some studies have suggested that senile cardiac amyloidosis has been identified in more than 50 percent of individuals over the age of 70 years; however, this is often an incidental finding.[9]

Endomyocardial fibrosis and Loeffler's endocarditis are both very rare. Some investigators have suggested that the pathologic features of these two disease entities are so similar that they may in fact be a single disease at different stages of development. Endomyocardial fibrosis is principally a disease of children and young adults in Africa and is not commonly seen in the United States. Loeffler's endocarditis is also identified by endomyocaridal fibrosis. This disease is commonly seen in temperate climates but has also been reported in Africa, Scandinavia, and Europe.[41]

Endocardial fibroelastosis is also an uncommon heart disease of a relatively obscure etiology. This disease is characterized by focal or diffuse cartilagelike fiber elastic thickening of the mural endocardium involving the left side of the heart, but it may involve, far less commonly, the right side or both sides of the heart. Endocardial fibroelastosis is the final common outcome of a variety of forms of cardiac damage. This disease process is not limited to any specific age group; however, it is most commonly seen in children within the first 2 years of life and is often associated with congenital malformations in the heart or elsewhere in the body. The pattern of transmission of this disease is unclear; however, numerous cases have been reported in identical twins and siblings. Nonetheless, the vast majority of cases occur as isolated events. Some investigators have hypothesized that both an autosomal dominant inheritance with incomplete penetrance or an autosomal recessive inheritance form a genetic basis for the pathologic changes.[9]

The morphologic and hemodynamic characteristics of restrictive-obliterative cardiomyopathy are quite varied. Morphologically, patients may have reduced ventricular compliance, thickened endocardium or mural thrombi, infiltration of the myocardium by amyloid hemosideran or glycogen, or some other space-occupying type of lesion. These patients have normal or decreased cardiac output, normal or decreased stroke volume, increased ventricular filling pressures, a range of chamber sizes from increased to normal to decreased, a normal to decreased ejection fraction, and decreased diastolic compliance. Other findings associated with restrictive-obliterative cardiomyopathy include ventricular pressure tracings essentially identical to those seen in constrictive pericarditis. Grossly, patients with endomyo-cardial fibrosis have a ventricular endocardium that extends from the apex toward the inflow tract of the right or left ventricle, or both. Although largely subendocardial, there may be scarring that extends into the inner one-third of the myocardium. The fibrotic process may also involve the tricuspid and mitral valves, and occasionally the fibrous tissue will become calcified, leading to a fibrocalcific distortion of these valves. Ventricular mural thrombi may be present, and it has been suggested that this fibrous tissue will result in the organization of a mural thrombus. Microscopically, various degrees of inflammatory cells may be present, which include eosinophils often found at the junction between the scarring and the preserved myocardium.[3]

In patients with Loeffler's endocarditis, the pattern of marked endomyocardial fibrosis is very similar to that of the endomyocardial fibrosis. Large mural thrombi are almost always present in patient's with Loeffler's endocarditis. Microscopically, other organs may be involved, including eosinophilia in the peripheral blood smear and infiltration of various organs including the heart by eosinophils; in some cases, an eosinophilic leukemia may develop. However, in other cases, no peripheral eosinophilia may be present. The histologic development of Loeffler's endocarditis begins as foci of myocardial necrosis, followed by an eosinophilic infiltrate present in the inner third of the myocardium. This leads to scarring of the necrotic areas and to layering of the endocardium by thrombus.

Endomyocardial fibroelastosis usually appears as a patchy opaque thickening of the mural endocardium, usually localized to the left ventricle. However, the other chambers of the heart may be involved. Grossly, this thickening usually has a glossy whitish appearance and lines the mural endocardium to a depth 5 to 10 times normal. The fibroelastic blanket is usually itself covered by an intact endocardium. Aortic stenosis and mitral stenosis are often present; however, the valves on the right side of the heart are rarely if ever affected. Cardiac enlargement is usually present due to either left ventricular hypertrophy or dilation. Histologically, the endocardial thickening appears as an increase of collagenous and elastic fibers on the endocardial surface. Impairment of the vascular supply to the muscle fibers may result in cellular necrosis of the myocardium. Histologic evidence of myocarditis or myocardial scarring is seen in approximately one-third of cases.[33]

The hallmark of restrictive cardiomyopathies is abnormal diastolic function and increased resistance to ventricular filling. This results in persistently elevated venous pressure and dependent edema and an enlarged tender liver. As the jugular venous pressure is abnormally elevated, it does not fall within a normal pattern. A Kussmaul sign, a rise in the venous pressure with inspiration, is present. Heart sounds are usually distant and an S_3 and S_4 are usually present. The apical impulse is usually easy to palpate, a key factor in differentiating this disease from constrictive pericarditis, which this disease closely resembles in terms of clinical presentation. Diagnostic studies do not generally produce as much information for the restrictive type of cardiomyopathy as compared to the other two categories. Chest radiography reveals only mild cardiac enlargement, if any enlargement at all. ECG may reveal only low-voltage conduction defects. An echocardiogram will demonstrate normal systolic function but usually shows increased left ventricular wall thickness. Radionuclide studies and cardiac catheterization show normal systolic function but abnormal diastolic function with elevated left- and right-sided filling pressures. Cardiac catheterization may not be useful in differentiating this disease from constrictive pericarditis.[42]

One must always evaluate for constrictive pericarditis as an easily treatable form of restrictive cardiomyopathy. Although constrictive pericarditis can be due to viral or idiopathic etiologies, tuberculosis is a very common cause.

PREOPERATIVE MANAGEMENT

Medical Management of Heart Failure in the Preoperative Period

The vast majority of patients who undergo heart surgery do not suffer from serious hemodynamic complications. However, in patients presenting with pre-existing impaired ventricular function, the incidence of intraoperative hemodynamic dysfunction increases markedly. Marked hemodynamic deterioration results in low cardiac output syndrome or cardiogenic shock.

In the patient with a cardiomyopathy, the acute heart failure that develops is a result of an anatomic or functional abnormality of the heart. The failing heart is associated with a sudden and dramatic reduction in cardiac output, with symptomatology resulting from poor end-organ perfusion or acute congestion of the venous system proximal to the affected ventricle. In some cases of heart failure, both may occur simultaneously. In the cardiomyopathic patient who is otherwise stable with medical management and then suddenly develops acute heart failure, it is important to identify rapidly any coexisting problem that may be responsible for this sudden deterioration. Problems such as pulmonary or systemic infection, cardiac dysrhythmia, fluid overload, myocardial ischemia, changes in vascular resistance, as well as a host of other problems are potentially treatable and should be appropriately dealt with, if this is the case. However, it is important to recognize that the deterioration in the patient's cardiac function may be due to progression of the patient's underlying disease process and thus may not be treatable. When patients have progression of the underlying disease, this phenomenon is usually characterized by more gradual onset of the symp-tomatology rather than an acute onset. Nonetheless, any patient presenting with evidence of severe cardiac decompensation requires immediate therapy.

In the cardiomyopathic patient, initial therapy is accomplished with administration of a variety of pharmacologic agents. This involves the administration of diuretics to reduce total body water and the use of nitrates and peripheral vasodilators to reduce ventricular work by decreasing systemic and pulmonary vascular resistance and ventricular preload and afterload. Therapy is also directed at increasing myocardial contractility with the use of sympathomimetic amines. It is important to emphasize that the addition of sympathomimetic amines increases myocardial oxygen consumption; thus severe heart failure may require a mechanical assist device. Mechanical assist devices are the only means available to reduce myocardial oxygen consumption and increase cardiac output (see Ch. 17).

DIURETIC THERAPY

Numerous diuretics are employed in the treatment of heart failure. The primary objective of diuretic therapy is to reduce the circulating blood volume, thereby decreasing preload and causing movement to the left on the Starling curve. Aggressive diuretic therapy is often used with advancing heart failure, with relatively few side effects. However, electrolytes should be monitored to reduce the incidence of cardiac dysrhythmias. In addition, one must avoid reducing preload so excessively that an optimal cardiac output can no longer be maintained. On the other hand, in HCM, the left ventricle has a markedly decreased compliance and requires a higher left ventricular end-diastolic pressure. Vigorous diuresis in these patients often results in decreases in left ventricular end-diastolic pressure cardiac output. The use of a pulmonary artery or a bedside echocardiography catheter provides the ability to closely monitor the patient if central venous pressure and blood pressure are misleading.

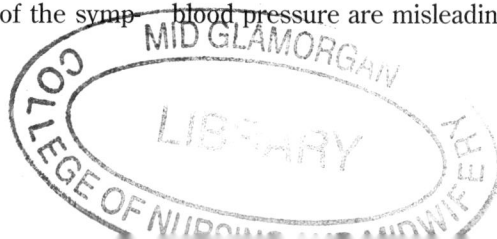

INOTROPIC THERAPY

Although reducing intravascular volume by diuresis is a key therapeutic maneuver in the treatment of heart failure, increasing myocardial contracility also serves a very important role. The use of positive inotropic agents plays a critical role in the management of severe or acute systolic dysfunction. Ever since William Withering first recognized the hemodynamic improvement in patients who chewed the leaf of the foxglove plant, the digitalis glycosides have become a mainstay in the management of chronic heart failure. However, because of the long onset of action for the digitalis glycosides, these are currently used primarily in patients with chronic heart failure, rather than in patients with acute heart failure. In order to treat an acute event, it is necessary to have a pharmachologic agent that has a rapid onset of action and a relatively short half-life. This allows for careful titration of the agent so as to maximize the patient's cardiac condition. Historically, inotropic drugs such as dobutamine, dopamine, epinephrine, and norepinephrine were used to treat acute heart failure because of their relatively short half-lives. This makes these drugs ideal agents for titrating to the desired inotropic response. More recently, the intravenous phosphodiesterase inhibitors such as amimone and milrinone are increasing in popularity because of their vasodilatory properties.

The therapeutic goal in patients with acute heart failure is to increase stroke output and decrease the ventricular filling pressure. Inotropic agents are ideal for this. Pharmacologic agents in this category have a positive inotropic effect on the myocardium; as a result, they increase stroke output directly. One important consideration when using these inotropic agents is the fact that none of these drugs is a truly selective agent. Therefore, although they may have a positive inotropic effect, their response may be either attenuated or augmented, depending on the peripheral effect of the agent. Specifically, the degree to which filling pressures decrease and stroke output increases is usually dependent in part by the effect of the agent on vascular resistance.

The phosodiesterase inhibitors increase cardiac output as well as decrease ventricular filling pressure. However, because of their mechanism of action, they also cause a systemic vasodilation. Thus, these drugs tend to have an enhanced cardiac effect as a result of their peripheral effects. Although dobutamine is considered to be a selective β-agonist, it does appear to have some mild α-agonist effect. Nonetheless, this does not appear to be clinically relevant and, as a result of the predominant β effect produced by dobutamine, it, like the phosphodiastase inhibitors, is able to increase cardiac output and decrese ventricular filling pressure. Since dobutamine has peripheral β-agonist qualities as well, it is able to produce systemic vasodilation, significantly enhancing the cardiac effects of dobutamine. By contrast, dopamine is not as selective an agent as dobutamine and has very dose-dependent effects. In moderate doses, dopamine has an effect very similar to that of dobutamine. However, as the dose increases, a predominant α effect is observed, resulting in increased peripheral vascular resistance. Thus, when using dopamine at higher doses, the peripheral α effects may cause an actual increase in left ventricular filling pressure as well as a decrease in stroke volume. Norepinephrine is relatively nonselective, although its agonistic effects on the various receptor subtypes differ in terms of their sensitivities to this agent. Nonetheless, because of its nonselective effects, norepinephrine is also capable of attenuating its cardiac effects as a result of its effect on systemic impedance. Finally, epinephrine is similar to dopamine in that it is a nonselective agent with dose-dependent effects. Because of its predominant β effects, it can be beneficial at low to mid-range doses, as it produces a peripheral vasodilation, thereby increasing stroke output and decreasing ventricular filling pressure. However, as the dose of epinephrine rises, its ability to stimulate peripheral α-receptors becomes a pharmacologic consideration, as it is also capable of causing a peripheral vasoconstriction, resulting in decreased stroke output and increased ventricular filling pressure. As a result of the varied actions of these various agents, the pharmacologic inotropes of choice in the management of acute heart failure are the phosphodiesterase inhibitors amrinone and milrinone, as well as the sympathomimetic amine dobutamine.

As mentioned earlier, digitalis glycoside preparations play an important role in the management of chronic heart failure. These preparations are reserved for the more chronic conditions because of their long half-life, as well as slow onset of action. Digitalis is successful as a therapeutic agent becuase of its ability to increase stroke volume by significantly increasing the force of myocardial contraction. Its efficacy in the failing heart is remarkable considering that it has a direct effect on constricting both veins and arterial resistance vessels. It is this ability that has kept the digitalis glycoside preparations as one of the primary agents in the treatment of chronic heart failure for nearly two centuries.

COMBINATION DRUG THERAPY

The contemporary management of acute and severe heart failure is to employ the beneficial effects of each of the agents previously discussed. Clearly, diuretics, the nitrates, vasodilators, and the inotropic agents all play a role in the management of the patient with the failing heart. However, the patient's condition can be optimized by using pharmacologic agents from each of these categories in combination with one another. The ultimate goal in the treatment of the failing heart is to increase cardiac performance while at the same time causing the minimal increase in myocardial oxygen demand. Often, combining inotropic and vasodilation drugs will increase coronary blood flow and maximize a patient's pulmonary capillary wedge pressure more than either drug alone.

The dose-dependent nonselective nature of dopamine can, in fact, be a beneficial property in terms of treating heart failure. However, if the other effects of dopamine are not taken into account at higher doses, dopamine will cause an unwanted increase in pulmonary capillary wedge pressure as a result of its α-adrenergic properties. Thus, in a patient with an otherwise reasonable pressure, dopamine should be used only at the lowest doses. However, in hypotensive cases, the α-adrenergic properties of dopamine may be particularly useful. Dopamine can be titrated upward so as to cause an increase in peripheral vascular resistance, thereby increasing blood pressure. Once a satisfactory blood pressure is obtained in the acute phase, the dopamine can be titrated downward, demonstrating a predominant β effect, and the addition of a nitrovasodilator may be useful in decreasing the pulmonary capillary wedge pressure and may decrease peripheral vascular resistance, thereby enhancing cardiac output.

In essentially all cases, low-dose dopamine can serve to provide a beneficial effect. It can be combined with any of the other agents used to treat heart failure. This is because of its ability to increase renal blood flow and cardiac output, resulting in improved diuresis, as long as lower doses of dopamine are used. It is not until the dose of dopamine is increased that its cardiovascular effects should be considered.

Likewise, dobutamine increases stroke output and causes a moderate decrease in pulmonary capillary wedge pressure. One downfall in the use of dobutamine is that it causes an increase in myocardial oxygen consumption by as much as 30 to 40 percent. However, when dobutamine is used in combination with a nitrovasodilator, an overall increase in cardiac output as well as a decrease in pulmonary capillary wedge pressure is observed with a moderate decrease in the myocardial oxygen consumption, as compared with dobutamine alone.

Diuretic therapy is also an important therapeutic intervention in the treatment of the failing heart. Diuretic therapy can be employed with any of the cardiovascular agents. Because of their ability to decrease intravascular volume, decrease pulmonary capillary wedge pressure, and in some cases even decrease peripheral vascular resistance, their effect is almost always beneficial. Nonetheless, because of their potent ability to cause electrolyte wasting, careful monitoring of a patient's serum electrolytes or empiric replacement therapy should always be considered. Finally, when administered intravenously, the phosphodiesterase inhibitors cause an increase in cardiac function similar to that seen with the use of dobutamine. In fact, the hemodynamic consequenses of the phosphodiesterase inhibitors are comparable to those seen when using a combination of dobutamine and a nitrovasodilator agent such as sodium nitroprusside. Essentially, phosphodiesterase inhibitors have a positive inotropic effect and a direct vasodilator effect combined within a single pharmacologic agent. One key to the success of phosphodiesterase inhibitor use in the treatment of the failing heart is that vasodilator actions balance the increase in myocardial oxygen consumption that would otherwise be required as a result their positive inotropic effect. Thus, phosphodiesterase leads to an increase in cardiac output with little change in myocardial oxygen consumption. Because of this property when amrinone and milrinone are used in combination with the sympathomimetic agents, a synergistic effect of the agents can be observed with a relatively small increase in myocardial oxygen consumption, thus maximizing cardiac performance with only a very small increase in the energy requirement.

The various pharmacologic actions of these different therapeutic agents should be considered when trying to maximize a patient's cardiac status during medically the pre- or perioperative period. If all these actions are considered and appropriately employed in combination, the patient's cardiac performance is easily optimized.

SUMMARY

All the cardiomyopathies demonstrate some variable form of pump failure. With the dilated or congestive cardiomyopathy, systolic pump function is impaired. In the case of HCM, the pathophysiologic abnormality is not systolic, but rather diastolic dysfunction. Two primary hemodynamic features of HCM are an elevated left ventricular diastolic pressure, due to diminished left ventricular compliance. Although it is diastolic dysfunction that occurs with HCM, decreased cardiac output will ultimately result. The mechanism responsible for this is due to a dynamic type of obstruction, rather than a mechanical obstruction. Because this disease has been associated with an increased left ventricular contractility, ventricular systolic volume is reduced and the ejection velocity of blood moving through the outflow tract is increased. Consequently, the anterior mitral valve is drawn against the septum as a result of the reduced filling pressure. Next, the decrease in ventricular volume results in a decreased preload. This leads to a further reduction in the size of the outflow tract. Finally, the reduction in aortic impedance and pressure results in a decreased afterload. This ultimately increases the velocity of flow through the subaortic area and reduces ventricular systolic volume, consequently reducing cardiac output. With the restrictive or obliterative type of cardiomyopathy, the characteristic feature is abnormal diastolic function; the ventricular walls are excessively rigid and there is slow ventricular filling. The abnormal diastolic function associated with the restrictive-obliterative type of cardiomyopathy results in persistently elevated venous pressures, which in turn lead to symptoms of congestion: pulmonary edema for the left ventricle and dependent edema and enlarged liver for the right ventricle. Ultimately, decreased cardiac output occurs.

It is the reduction in left ventricular function or systemic cardiac output that is the most difficult and most significant problem to manage in most, but not all, cases. The reduction in left ventricular function or systemic cardiac output makes patients very susceptible to the development of CHF and even cardiogenic shock. Once patients begin to demonstrate evidence of heart failure, if not dealt with appropriately, there is an ineluctable progression to cardiogenic shock and circulatory deterioration.

REFERENCES

1. Johnson RA, Palacios I: Dilated cardiomyopathies of the adult. N Engl J Med 307:1051, 1982
2. Dec GW, Fuster V: Idiopathic dilated cardiomyopathy. N Engl J Med 331:1564, 1994
3. DeSanctis RW: Cardiomyopathies. Sci Am Med 14:1989
4. Rubin E: Alcoholic myopathy in heart and skeletal muscle. N Engl J Med 5:28, 1979
5. Horrians DC: Peripartum cardiomyopathy. N Engl J Med 312:1432, 1985
6. Cambridge G, MacArthuur CGC, Waterson AP: Antibodies to Coxsackie B viruses in congestive cardiomyopathy. Br Heart J 41: 692, 1979
7. Anderson JL, Cariquist JF, Lutz JR: HLA, A, B and DR typing in idiopathic dilated cardiomyopathy: a search for immune response factors. Am J Cardiol 53:1325, 1984
8. Eckstein R, Mempel W, Bolte H: Reduced suppressor cell activity in congestive cardiomyopathy and in myocarditis. Circulation 65:1224, 1982
9. Robbins, Cotran, Kumar: Robbins, Cotran, Kumar (eds): Pathologic Basis of Disease. 3rd Ed. WB Saunders, Philadelphia, 1984 13, The Heart. p. 596–602.
10. Van Olshausen K, Schafer A, Mehmel HC: Ventricular arrhythmias in idiopathic dilated cardiomyopathy. Br Heart J 51:195, 1984
11. Packer M, Leter CV: Survival in congestive heart failure during treatment with drugs with positive inotropic actions. Circulation, suppl IV. 75:55, 1987
12. Swedberg K, Hjalmerson A, Waagstein F: Beneficial effects of long-term beta-blockade in congestive cardiomyopathy. Br Heart J 44: 117, 1980
13. Clark C, Henry W, Epstein S: Familial prevelence and genetic transmission of idiopathic hypertrophic subaortic stenosis. N Engl J Med 289:709, 1973
14. Elstein E, Liew C, Sole M: The genetic basis of hypertrophic cardiomyopathy. J Mol Cell Cardiol 24:1471, 1992
15. Maron B, Roberts W, Edwards J et al: Sudden death in patients with hypertrophic cardiomyopathy; characterization of 26 patients without functional limitation. Am J Cardiol 41:803, 1978
16. Wynne J: Cardiomyopathies and myocarditides. pp. 1394–1450. In Braunwald E (ed): Heart Disease. 4th Ed. WB Saunders, Philadelphia, 1992
17. Maron B, Roberts W, Epstein S: Sudden death in hypertrophic cardiomyopathy: a profile of 78 patients. Circulation 65:1388, 1982
18. Viersma J, Van Veldhuisen D, Hamer J et al: Arrhythmias in hypertrophic cardiomyopathy: prognostic significance and clinical relevance. pp. 21–32. In Van der Wall E, Lie K (eds): Recent Views on Hypertrophic Cardiomyopathy. Martinus Nijhoff, Dordrecht, 1985
19. Savage D, Seides S, Maron B et al: Prevalence of arrhythmias during 24-hour electrocardiographic monitoring and exercise testing in patients with obstructive and nonobstructive hypertrophic cardiomyopathy. Circulation 59: 866, 1979
20. Williams W, Wigle E, Rokowski H et al: Results of surgery for hypertrophic obstructive cardiomyopathy. Circulation 76:104, 1987
21. Van der Wall E: Recent views on hypertrophic cardiomyopathy: hemodynamic concepts and their clinical applications. pp. 71–100. In Van der Wall E, Lie K (eds): Recent Views on Hypertrophic Cardiomyopathy. Martinus Nijhoff, Dordrecht, 1985
22. Seiler C, Hess O, Schoenbeck M et al: Long term follow-up of medical versus surgical therapy for hypertrophic cardiomyopathy: a retrospective study. J Am Coll Cardiol 17:634, 1991
23. Jackson J, Thomas S: Valvular heart disease. p. 629. In Kaplan J (ed): Cardiac Anesthesia. 3rd Ed. WB Saunders, Philadelphia, 1993
24. Pollick C, Rakowski H, Wigle D: Muscular subaortic stenosis: the quantitative relation-

ship between systolic anterior motion and the pressure gradient. Circulation 69:43, 1984

25. Goodwin J: Recent views on hypertrophic cardiomyopathy. pp. 1–8. In Van der Wall E, Lie K (ed): Recent views on hypertrophic cardiomyopathy. Martinus Nijhoff, Dordrecht, 1985

26. Buda A, MacKenzie G, Wigle D: Effect of negative intrathoracic pressure on left ventricular outflow tract obstruction in muscular subaortic stenosis. Circulation 63:875, 1981

27. Murgo J, Alter B, Dorethy J et al: Dynamics of left ventricular ejection in obstructive and non-obstrucive hypertrophic cardiomyopathy. J Clin Invest 66:1369, 1980

28. Murgo J, Alter B, Dorethy J et al: The effects of intraventricular gradients on left ventricular ejection dynamics. Eur Heart J, suppl F. 4:23, 1983

29. Hanrath P, Mathey D, Kremer P et al: Effect of verapamil on left ventricular isovolumic relaxation time and regional left ventricular filling in hypertrophic cardiomyopathy. Am J Cardiol 45:1258, 1980

30. Blanksma P: Pressure-volume and stress-strain relationships in hypertrophic cardiomyopathy. pp. 53–70. In Van der Wall E, Lie K (eds): Recent Views on Hypertrophic Cardiomyopathy. Martinus Nijhoff, Dordrecht, 1985

31. Maron BJ, Bonow RO, Cannon RO: Hypertrophic cardiomyopathy: interrelations of clinical manifestations, pathophysiology, and therapy. N Engl J Med 316:844, 1987

32. Rosing DR, Kent KM, Maron BJ: Verapamil therapy: a new approach to the pharmacologic treatment of hypertrophic cardiomyopathy: ill effects on exercise capacity and symptomatic status. Circulation 60:1208, 1979

33. Pollick C: Muscular subaortic stenosis: hemodynamic and clinical improvement after disopyramide. N Engl J Med 307:997, 1982

34. Krajcer Z, Leachman RD, Cooley DA: Mitral valve replacement and septal myomectomy in hypertrophic cardiomyopathy: ten-year follow-up in 80 patients. Circulation, suppl. 78:1, 1988

35. Silver M, Buda A, MacKenzie G et al: The variable nature of mitral regurgitation in muscular subaortic stenosis. Circulation, suppl 3. 55:217, 1977

36. Leachman R, Krajcer Z, Azic T, Cooley D: Mitral valve replacement in hypertrophic cardiomypathy: ten year follow-up in 54 patients. Am J Cardiol 60:1416, 1987

37. Spirito P, Maron B, Chiarella F et al: Diastolic abnormalities in patients with hypertrophic cardiomyopathy: relation to magnitude of left ventricular hypertrophy. Circulation 72:310, 1985

38. Nishimura K, Nosaka H, Saito T et al: Another possible mechanism of angina in hypertrophic cardiomyopathy. Circulation 68:162, 1983

39. Grover-McKay M, Schwaiger M, Krivokapich J et al: Regional myocardial blood flow and metabolism at rest in mildly symptomtic patients with hypertrophic cardiomyopathy. J Am Coll Cardiol 13:317, 1989

40. McKenna W, England D, Doi Y et al: Arrhythmia in hypertrophic cardiomyopathy. I. Influence on prognosis. Br Heart J 46:168, 1981

41. Baandrup U: Loeffler's endocarditis and endomyocardial fibrosis—a nosologic entity. APMIS 85:869, 1977

42. Benotti JR, Grossman W, Cohn PF: Clinical profile of restrictive cardiomyopathy. Circulation 61:1206, 1980

43. Van der Wall E: Recent views on left ventricular function in hypertrophic cardiomyopathy: hemodynamic concepts and their clinical implications. p. 71. In Van der Wall E, Lie KI (eds): Recent Views on Hypertrophic Cardiomyopathy. Kluwer Academic, Dordrecht, 1985

4

Transplantation Immunology

Dominique Farge
Catherine Amrein

After organ transplantation, the donor's allogeneic cells are recognized as foreign by host lymphocytes, leading to graft rejection. The cellular differentiation and subsequent clonal expansion induced by the donor's allo-antigen is closely associated with lymphokine production by the recipient's CD4+ T-inducer/helper cells, especially interleukin 2 (IL2). These lymphokines enhance the immune response and induce proliferation of T- and B-effectors cells (Fig. 4-1). Autoimmune tolerance of the allograft is obtained with several immunosuppressive agents, each having a predominant action on one step of the immune response. The first chemical immunosuppressor, 6-mercaptopurine, was prescribed with steroids in basic conventional immunosuppression following organ transplantation in 1960. The use of polyclonal antilymphocyte globulins (1970), cyclosporine (1975), and monoclonal antibodies (1980) progressively changed the principles of immunosuppression.

As treatments became more specific and were directed against subpopulations of lymphocyte receptors against the lymphokines involved in the immune response, lower morbidity and mortality resulted (when compared to conventional immunosuppression) with a 15 percent increase in graft survival. The introduction of cyclosporine reduced the incidence of rejection by a further 10 to 15 percent, followed by significant progress in heart and heart-lung transplantation. The use of cyclosporine permitted a decrease in the very high doses of steroids with subsequent reductions in the incidence of infections. The third generation of immunosuppressive drugs (FK-506, deoxyspergualine) with selective and powerful actions on the immune response may help avoid several of the remaining adverse side effects. These agents will constitute an alternative therapeutic approach following transplantation in the next decade.

Immunosuppressive therapy for heart or heart-lung transplant recipients starts immediately before surgery and is continued thereafter in the intensive care unit (ICU) according to a variety of protocols, which differ not only according to the transplanted organ but also from one surgical team to another.

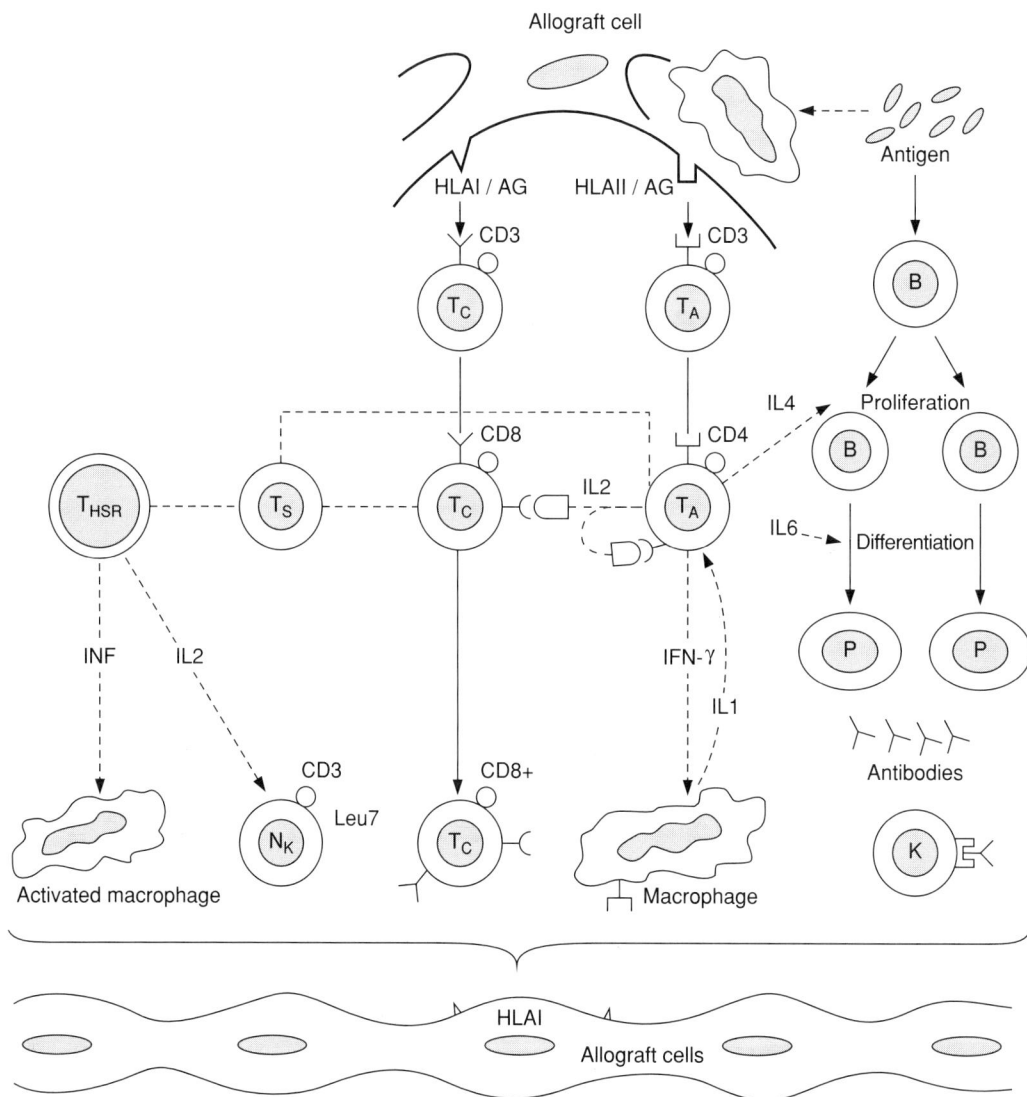

Fig. 4-1. Various steps of cellular activation, with the major sites of action for immunosuppressive drugs, during the process of allograft rejection. AG, antigen; HLAI/II, human lymphocyte antigen type I/II; T_c, cytotoxic T-cells; T_A, auxilliary T-cells; B, B-cells; P, plasmocytes; T_{HSR}, T-cell producers of lymphokines; T_S, suppressive T cells; N_K, natural killer cells; K, killer cell.

Therefore, this chapter focuses on the principles of immunosuppression and on the critical care required in the early postoperative transplant period, following the toxic side effects of immunosuppressive therapy or early failure of the transplanted organs due to acute rejection.

IMMUNOSUPPRESSIVE DRUGS

Azathioprine

STRUCTURE–ACTIVITY RELATIONSHIP

Azathioprine is a purine analogue, derived from 6-mercaptopurine. Its immunosuppressive action requires passage through the liver to become active via its metabolite (6-thio-inosinic acid), which inhibits DNA and RNA synthesis, the interconversion between purines and nucleotides and de novo purine synthesis.[1,2]

ACTION

In vitro, azathioprine has a predominant action on T-cells and inhibits mixed lymphocyte reaction (MLR). It also inhibits IL2 production and lowers the number of natural killer (NK) cells and monocytes. In vivo, azathioprine increases graft survival after organ transplantation with no change in lymphocyte subpopulations or in the levels of preexisting antibodies.

PHARMACOKINETICS

Hepatic transformation in 6-mercaptopurine occurs within a few minutes after either oral or intravenous administration. Azathioprine absorption is rapid and almost complete. Degradation of mercaptopurine occurs by direct oxidation via xanthine-oxidase or enzymatic methylation. Thiopurine nucleotides are active intracellular metabolites with homogeneous distribution. Inactive metabolites are eliminated in urine as thiouric acids. Renal insufficiency does not alter pharmacokinetics. Hepatic insufficiency reduces azathioprine biotransformation and its inhibitory action on T-cells in vitro.

CLINICAL TOXICITY

The major toxic effect of mercaptopurine is bone marrow suppression. This cytotoxicity is not reflected in the peripheral blood cell count before 7 days after starting therapy: granulocytopenia can be followed by thrombocytopenia, but rarely by decreased hematocrit with megaloblastic anemia and reticulocytopenia. There is little evidence of hepatic toxicity. Hyperuricemia with hyperuricosuria may occur during treatment. Allergic reactions as well as acute pancreatitis are rare.

DRUG-DRUG INTERACTIONS

Allopurinol is a powerful inhibitor of xanthine-oxidase; therefore, simultaneous prescription of azathioprine and allopurinol can lead to leukopenia and pancytopenia, with a risk of acute agranulocytosis and death. If this co-prescription is necessary, patients treated with both drugs should receive 50 percent of the usual dose of azathioprine.

THERAPEUTIC USES

Azathioprine is part of the early immunosuppressive strategy to prevent both acute and chronic rejection, but it has only moderate effects on the reversal of acute rejection. It can be administered intravenously and then orally without an alteration in dosage. Daily dosages vary from 1 to 3 mg $\cdot$ kg^{-1}, according to the hematologic tolerance. Azathioprine should be discontinued if the white blood cell count is below 3,500 $\cdot$ mm^{-3} or the platelet count is below 50,000 $\cdot$ mm^{-3}.

Corticosteriods

Natural steroids (cortisone) at pharmacologic doses have potent immunosuppressive actions. Synthetic steroids (prednisone and prednisolone) have a four to five times greater anti-inflammatory effect with less mineralocorticoid effect. These drugs form the basis of prophylactic and curative treatment of acute rejection (Table 4-1).

MECHANISM OF ACTION

Glucocorticoids react with a specific intracytoplasmic receptor-protein. The steroid-receptor complex migrates into the nucleus, where it binds to glucocorticoid-responsive elements (GRE) within the chromatin. These are specific DNA nucleotides that ultimately interfere with the synthesis of specific proteins. Glucocorticoids also act through calcium ionophore channels to modify transmembranous calcium flux. In vitro, they inhibit lymphocyte proliferation after stimulation of the CD3/Ti receptor.

ACUTE AND CHRONIC ANTI-INFLAMMATORY PROPERTIES

Acute and chronic anti-inflammatory properties are nonspecific. Steroids inhibit both the early and late process of inflammation. This

Table 4-1. Glucocorticoids Used After Heart and Lung Transplantation

Name	Trade Name	Dosage	Plasmatic Half-life (hr)	Biologic Half-life (hr)	Required Doses
Prednisone	Cortancyl Deltasone Prednicen Sterapred	5-, 10-mg pills	3	12–36	*Rejection prophylaxis:* 1.5 mg·kg^{-1}·day^{-1} × 10–15 days, progressively tapered
Prednisolone	Hydrocortancyl Deltacortef	5-mg pills 1-, 2-, 5-mg pills	3	12–36	Maintenance doses: 0.2–0.5 mg·kg^{-1}·day^{-1} *Rejection treatment:* 1 mg·kg^{-1}·day^{-1} × 8–10 days progressively tapered
Prednisolone sodium metasulfobenzoate	Solupred	5-, 20-mg pills	3–3.5	12–36	
Methylprednisolone	Solu-Medrol Depo-Medrol Medrol	20, 40, 120, 500 mg IV	2–3	12–36	*Rejection prophylaxis:* From day 0 to day 3 postgraft: 2.5–5 mg·kg^{-1}·day^{-1} *Rejection treatment:* 500–1,000 mg·day^{-1} IV × 3 days

68

inhibition generally decreases polymorpho-nuclear leukocyte and monocyte migration, monocyte-macrophage maturation and macrophage phagocytic activity, and delays cicatrization.

The corticosteroids act on various steps of the immune response. They inhibit T-lymphocyte proliferation. Cooperation between monocyte-macrophage and lymphocytes is decreased, as well as binding of complement factors, IgG and IgE, to lymphocyte receptors during the proliferative response. Corticosteroids inhibit IL1 production by the monocyte-macrophages and IL2 and interferon production by activated T-cells in the presence of the alloantigen. The T-cell proliferation reaction dependent on IL1 and IL2 is decreased. NK and T-cell cytotoxicity, dependent on interferon and IL2, is altered. Antigen presentation at the macrophage surface, dependent on HLA class II antigens, is also diminished. Glucocorticosteroids have no significant effect on the level of circulating antibodies in humans.

EFFECT ON CELLULAR SUBPOPULATIONS

Steroids induce significant granulocytosis due to their demargination from capillary endothelium and increased rate of entrance into the blood from bone marrow.[3] A transient decline of about 70 percent in circulating lymphocytes and of more than 90 percent in monocytes occurs within 4 to 6 hours after glucocorticoid administration, due to redistribution of cells (essentially a loss of T-lymphocytes) and decreased issue of monocytes from bone marrow. Eosinophil and basophil numbers decrease within a few hours after a single dose of glucocorticosteroids and remain low during treatment.

PHARMACOKINETICS

In the plasma, 80 percent of glucocorticosteroids are reversibly bound to transcortine, a cortisol binding globulin (CBG), and 10 percent to albumin. Only the free-fraction interacts with cytosolic receptors. Prednisone and

prednisolone have the same immuno-suppressive action, but prednisone becomes active only after hepatic transformation to prednisolone via the 11-β-hydroxydehydrogenase. Inactive metabolites are eliminated in the urine. Biologic half-life takes into account anti-inflammatory action and is more important in clinical practice than plasma half-life.

CLINICAL TOXICITY

Clinical toxicity is important (Table 4-2). In the early postoperative period, high-dose steroids may lead to life-threatening toxicity. Peptic ulceration should be prevented by use of appropriate anti-H_2-agonists or antacids to maintain gastric acidity greater than 4.5 (checked by direct pH measurement). Colonic perforation in the presence of diverticular disease is rare but requires immediate surgery. Pancreatitis was thought to be related to steroids but is probably related to excessive immunosuppression or a recrudescence of a viral infection. Psychiatric disturbances also occur: euphoria, depression, severe mood swings, and agitation and frank psychosis, including catatonia (which requires lowered doses of steroids and psychotropic drugs). Onset of diabetes may be related to steroids alone and requires insulin therapy. Hypertension can be severe, and diuretics are useful in counteracting water and sodium retention.

DRUG-DRUG INTERACTIONS

The drugs listed in Table 4-3 all alter steroid biodisposition and thus potentiate their adverse side effects.

THERAPEUTIC USES

Prednisone and prednisolone are the major drugs for prophylaxis and treatment of rejection in heart transplant recipients. Prophylaxis of rejection requires high doses of intravenous methylprednisolone (200 to 500 mg IV) before or at transplantation and for 3 days thereafter. Oral steroids are then tapered progressively from 1 mg $\cdot$ kg^{-1} in the first postoperative week to 0.2 mg $\cdot$ kg^{-1} $\cdot$ day^{-1} at

Table 4-2. Adverse Side Effects of Glucocorticoids

Side Effects	Prevention
Metabolic side effects	Diet
Water and salt: water and salt retention, edema, hypertension	Low-salt diet (3 g·day^{-1} NaCl)
K$^+$: hypokalemia, cramps	K$^+$ supplementation (2 g·day^{-1} K$^+$)
Ca$^+$, P$^+$: hypercalciuria, hyperphosphaturia	Vitamin D, Ca^{++} supplementation
Uric acid: hyperuraturia	(1–2 g·day^{-1} Ca^{++})
Glucoids: glucose intolerance	Lower glucoids
Lipids: ↑ cholesterol, ↑ triglycerides	<300 mg·day^{-1} cholesterol
Proteins: muscular atrophy, cushingoid faces, delayed cicatrization	High proteins
Organic side effects	
Digestive: ulceration, perforation	Anti-acids, anti-H$_2$-agonists
Infections: bacterial, viral, fungal, parasitic—all types	Antibioprophylaxis, hygienic rules
Ocular: glaucoma, keratitis, long-term cataract	
Psychiatric disturbances	

1 month. In lung transplant recipients, the introduction of steroids is delayed, after one perioperative course of intravenous steroids (200 to 500 mg methylprednisolone), up to day 7 or 10, in order to allow the cicatrization of tracheal and/or bronchial anastomoses.

Methylprednisolone (IV) is the major drug used for first-line treatment of acute rejection. It is administered alone or with other immunosuppressive drugs at a dose of 10 to 12 mg · kg^{-1} · day^{-1} (usually 1 g · day^{-1}) for 3 consecutive days, although longer therapeutic courses are occasionally required. In the early postoperative period, steroids can be abruptly discontinued when faced with life-threatening complications with little risk of adrenal insufficiency.

Cyclosporine

STRUCTURE AND ACTIVITY

Cyclosporine A (Sandimmune)[4–11] is a cyclic undecapeptide extracted from a Norwegian fungus (*Tolypocladium inflatum gams*).[4] This highly hydrophobic drug is soluble in lipids. After crossing the cell membrane, cyclosporine first binds to cyclophiline, a cytosolic enzyme from the rotamase family. The cyclophiline-cyclosporine complex then binds to calmodulin, a calcium phosphatase and a calcineurine-dependent target protein.[5] The protein-receptor complex migrates toward the chromosome, where it interferes with lymphokine synthesis and down-regulates the transcription of lymphokine RNA messengers (mainly IL2).

ACTION

Cyclosporine increases allograft survival in a dose-dependent fashion in animals and humans.[6] It inhibits mixed lymphocyte reaction

Table 4-3. Pharmaceutical Interactions of Glucocorticosteroids

Compete with steroid effects
  Antacids: ↓ steroid absorption
  Barbiturates, rifampin, antiepileptic: ↑ steroid hepatic metabolism

Synergistic with steroid effects
  Erythromycyn: ↓ steroid catabolism
  Hypoalbuminemia: ↓ steroid-free fraction

Caution when prescribed with steroids
  Oral anticoagulant: stable hypocoagulation difficult to obtain
  Cyclosporine: methylprednisolone → ↑ cyclosporine blood levels

Forbidden associations
  Attenuated live vaccine
  Non-steroidal anti-inflammatory drugs (↑ nephrotoxicity)

via direct inhibition of IL2 production by CD4 + activated T-lymphocytes. The production of cytotoxic T-cells depends on IL2 and is inhibited; but T-suppressor cell action, IL2-receptor expression and activated T-lymphocyte responses to various lymphokines are not blocked. Cyclosporine inhibits the production of IL1 by the macrophages and of interferon by the activated T-lymphocytes. It has little action on B-lymphocytes, but inhibition of lymphokine production indirectly affects B-cell activation.

PHARMACOKINETICS AND BLOOD LEVELS

Absorption of cyclosporine is incomplete (20 to 50 percent) with wide intra- and interindividual variability, which are further aggravated if administered simultaneously with other drugs.[4,7] Cyclosporine is rapidly distributed within all tissues except muscle and brain, with higher concentrations in liver, kidney, pancreas, and fatty tissues. Within the blood, 50 to 70 percent of cyclosporine is bound to erythrocytes; 20 percent appears in the plasma, mainly bound to lipoproteins. Hepatic metabolism occurs within the cytochrome P-450 microsomal system. More than 10 metabolites with very little pharmacologic activity are eliminated via an enterohepatic cycle. Biliary excretion (greater than 90 percent) is delayed in the presence of hepatic insufficiency. Renal insufficiency does not alter circulating blood levels, and cyclosporine is not dialyzable. Dose monitoring[7] in the early postoperative period should be performed often: daily for lung and twice weekly for heart transplant recipients, whether cyclosporine is used alone or with other drugs. Blood levels are usually measured by radioimmunoassay (RIA) or by polarized fluorescence technique (TDX, Abbott); high-performance liquid chromatography (HPLC) permits cyclosporine separation from its metabolites. Whole blood dosages should be performed on specimens drawn into tubes containing EDTA.

ADVERSE SIDE EFFECTS

Cyclosporine exerts direct and dose-dependent nephrotoxicity, potentiated by nephrotoxic drugs or the presence of renal dysfunction. This emphasizes the need for careful early monitoring of trough blood levels. Cyclosporine nephrotoxicity is responsible for acute renal failure characterized by a fall in renal blood flow and glomerular filtration rate and an increase in filtration fraction and proximal sodium reabsorption. It reverses rapidly after a reduction in, or cessation of, the drug. On very rare occasions, acute nephrotoxicity presents as a sudden arrest of both cortical and medullary perfusion with microarteriopathy.[8] The resulting signs and symptoms resemble closely those of the hemolytic/uremic syndrome. Hypertension, renal failure, microangiopathic and hemolytic anemia, schizocytosis, and thrombocytopenia are observed and are attributed to acute vascular lesions within the kidney, such as arteriolar fibrinoid necrosis and glomerular and arteriolar thrombosis.[9] Cyclosporine should be decreased or discontinued until resolution of the symptoms. Chronic nephrotoxicity with interstitial fibrosis and tubular degeneration appears within 3 to 6 months following initiation of therapy and is responsible for chronic renal insufficiency in most heart and heart-lung transplant recipients. Hypertension at this time is favored by water and salt retention following high doses of steroids. Although it is responsive to furosemide, therapy must be initiated slowly to avoid enhancing cyclosporine nephrotoxicity. Calcium channel blockers and converting enzyme inhibitors directly counteract stimulation of the renin-angiotensin system induced by cyclosporine[10] (see Ch. 9). Hepatotoxicity is uncommon. High-dose cyclosporine may lead to cholestasis with elevated conjugated bilirubin and/or cytolysis, which are always reversible with dose reduction.

Neurotoxicity

Generalized seizures are rare and are generally exacerbated by other factors: hypocholesterolemia, high steroid doses, water and electrolyte abnormalities, hypomagnesemia, aluminum overload, high cyclosporine blood levels, or viral encephalopathy (CMV). Computed tomography (CT) examination reveals demyelinating lesions in the white matter.[11]

Metabolic Effects

Hypomagnesemia due to increased renal clearance of Mg^{++} should be systematically prevented, especially in heart and heart–lung transplant recipients. Hyperuricemia due to lower renal excretion may occur. Nausea or vomiting may be observed when starting oral cyclosporine therapy.

DRUG–DRUG INTERACTIONS

Cyclosporine levels are affected by many different drugs and drug types. This necessitates careful monitoring of cyclosporine dosages when other drugs are introduced[7] (Table 4-4).

THERAPEUTIC USES

Cyclosporine is started in the early postoperative period. Particular attention to acute nephrotoxicity is necessary in patients with altered hemodynamics. In heart transplant recipients, cyclosporine is started orally at 3 to 4 $mg \cdot kg^{-1} \cdot day^{-1}$ on the third postoperative day, once stable cardiac output and renal function have been achieved (serum creatine below 2.5 to 3 $mg \cdot dl^{-1}$). If glucocorticoids are withheld for the first 10 days after lung transplantation, cyclosporine is routinely started on day 1 at an initial dose of 1 $mg \cdot kg^{-1} \cdot day^{-1}$ IV and increased according to daily blood level monitoring. The oral daily dose is about 4 to 5 $mg \cdot kg^{-1} \cdot daily^{-1}$ and can be given as an oily suspension or by pills. Modification of daily doses of cyclosporine require 5 days to stabilize because of the extended biologic half-life.

NEW IMMUNOSUPPRESSIVE DRUGS

FK-506

FK-506 (tacrolimus) was isolated in Japan in 1983 from *Streptomyces tsukubaensis.*[12] This highly lipophilic macrolide has a powerful immunosuppressive action in vivo. In vitro, FK-506 is a potent inhibitor of T-lymphocyte activation at doses 100 times lower than cyclosporine and also has antihumoral properties. FK-506 is similar to cyclosporine in that it blocks Ca^{++}-channel-dependent T-lymphocyte proliferation. Although the bioavailability of FK-506 is only 30 percent, its absorption is independent of biliary salts. Peak blood levels are obtained within 1 to 4 hours following oral administration with rapid clearance and a large volume of distribution. Detailed hepatic metabolism, which is dependent on cytochrome P-450, is still unknown. Less than 1 percent is eliminated in the urine. Adverse side effects and nephrotoxicity are as frequent and severe as with cyclosporine, although hypertension is much reduced. FK-506 has a significant diabetogenic effect.

FK-506 is administered intravenously at dosages of 0.06 to 0.15 $mg \cdot kg^{-1} \cdot day^{-1}$ then orally at 0.2 to 0.3 $mg \cdot kg^{-1} \cdot day^{-1}$. FK-506 is capable not only of reversing acute humoral cardiac allograft rejection, but also of providing effective prevention of recurrent humoral rejection episodes with long-term immunosuppression of antidonor immunoglobulin production.[13] According to the surgical team and treatment protocol, it is administered instead of cyclosporine for prophylaxis or treatment of rejection. This use is either as a first-line immunosuppressive agent in the early postoperative period or as a second-line drug in the event of cyclosporine intolerance or failure.[12,13]

RAPAMYCINE

Rapamycine is a macrolide, isolated from *Streptomyces hygroscopius,* with a structure close to that of FK-506.[14] Rapamycine nonselectively inhibits T-cell proliferation. In vitro, its action is synergistic with cyclosporine. This effect must still be demonstrated in animals before it can be administered to humans.

BREDININE

Bredinine (Brequinar) is an imidazolic nucleotide used widely in Japan since 1982. This compound inhibits nucleic acid synthesis as

Table 4-4. Pharmaceutical Interactions of Cyclosporine[a]

Increase cyclosporine blood levels	*Antibiotics*
Antibiotics	*Nafcillin*
Macrolides	*Platelet antiaggregant agents*
Erythromycin	*Sulfinpyrazone*
Josamycin	**Enhance cyclosporine nephrotoxicity**
Pristinamycin	Antifungal agents
Roxithromycin	Amphotericin B
Cephalosporins	Aminoglycosides
Antifungal agents	Gentamicin
Imidazoles	Tobramycin
Ketocanazole	Amykacin
Metronidazole	Anticarcinogens
Itraconazole	Melfalan
Calcium antagonists	Sulfonamides
Nicardipine	Cotrimoxazole PO
Diltiazem	*Nonsteroidal anti-inflammatory drugs*
Verapamil	*Diclofenac*
Corticosteroids	*Indometacin*
Prednisolone	*H_2-Receptor antagonists*
Methylprednisolone	*Ranitidine*
Oral contraceptives	**No interaction demonstrated**
Androgenic steroids	Vitamin K antagonists
Diuretics	Warfarin
Furosemide	Antibiotics
Acetazolamide	Macrolides
Decrease cyclosporine blood levels	Spiramycin
Antitubercular agents	Tetracyclines
Rifampicin	Doxycycline
Anticonvulsants	Anticonvulsants
Phenobarbital	Valproate
Phenytoin	Antifungal agents
Carbamazepine	Fluconazole
Primidone	H_2-Receptor antagonists
Sulfonamides	Cimetidine
Cotrimoxazole IV	Quinolones
Sulfametomidine	Ciprofloxacin
	Pefloxacin

[a] Drugs in italics are suspected but not proven to result in significant interaction.

does azathioprine. It is used as an azathioprine substitute in association with steroids and cyclosporine. It is currently being tested for immunosuppression following heart transplantation.

15-DEOXYSPERGUALINE

15-Deoxyspergualine (DSG) was isolated in 1981 from *Bacillus laterosporus*.[15] DSG inhibits T-cytotoxic lymphocyte production differently from cyclosporine: inhibition is not suppressed by exogenous IL2, but by interferon. Its beneficial effect in association with cyclosporine is under examination.[15]

BIOLOGIC AGENTS: ANTILYMPHOCYTE GLOBULINS

Polyclonal Antilymphoid Globulins

Since 1980, various heterologous polyclonal antibodies against human lymphocytes have become available as immunosuppressive agents for prophylaxis against and particularly the treatment of rejection.

STRUCTURE AND ACTIVITY

The composition, purity, and efficiency of heterologous globulins vary according to time and place of preparation.[16] They are usually prepared from horses or rabbits, but alternative species include sheep and goats. Their specificity is directed against various antigens, including purified human thymocytes (ATGAM, Upjohn), defined cultivated T-cell lines (ATG, Fresenius), and thoracic duct lymphocytes (ALG, Merieux). The immunosuppressive action is carried out almost exclusively by the IgG fraction of γ-globulins. The fraction is purified prior to injection in humans. The method by which allograft survival is increased remains debatable. Antilymphocyte globulins (ALG) are powerful immunosuppressive agents, which work partially by T-lymphocyte depletion and reduction of long-lived circulating lymphocytes. These ALGs may mask cell surface antigens with antibodies directed against T- and B-lymphocytes and macrophages: anti-CD2, -CD3, -CD4, -CD18, or anti-β-chain of LFA-1 molecules and anti-HLA-DR. Other antibodies against β_2-microglobulin and endothelial cells are responsible for adverse side effects. Early and significant lymphopenia can be observed after the first injections.

ADVERSE SIDE EFFECTS

Most side effects are dose dependent and reversible. Hypersensitivity reactions due to both specific and heterologous proteins can induce fever or chills (5 to 10 percent) and erythema and pruritus (1 percent). Thrombocytopenia occurs in up to 30 percent of patients due to cross-reactive antibodies. Treatment should be stopped if platelets fall below 50,000 per mm³. Thrombocytopenia generally develops within 7 to 10 days after starting therapy and is associated with serum sickness or hemolysis.[16] Anaphylactic reactions, shortness of breath, hives, and occasional hypotension or even shock are extremely rare.

INDICATIONS

Polyclonal antilymphocyte globulins (ALG and ATG) are part of the induction therapy for prophylaxis of rejection immediately after heart and heart-lung transplantation. On return from the operating room, they maintain strong immunosuppression, whereas cyclosporine introduction is often delayed. Further use of ALGs in the early postoperative period significantly enhances long-term survival.[17] They are also indicated in the treatment of allograft rejection when steroids may be undesirable or inefficient. In this setting, up to 80 percent of patients will respond.

TREATMENT MODALITIES AND INDICATIONS

ALGs are given by daily infusion through central intravenous lines for 3 to 5 days.[17] Dosing of the agent depends on the source of the preparation. Equine globulins are usually administered at 15 mg · kg^{-1} · day^{-1}, to a maximal dose of 1 g. Rabbit globulins are administered at dosages of 1 to 3 mg · kg^{-1} · day^{-1} for 3 to 5 days following heart and heart-lung transplantation. Initial administration of the agents should be concomitant with steroids, histamine agonists, and antipyretic agents. A complete blood cell count is checked daily during therapy. Effectiveness is monitored by FACS enumeration of various T-cell subtypes.

Monoclonal Antibodies: AntiCD-3 Monoclonal Antibody

Monoclonal-antibodies are immunoglobulins isolated from hybridomas and are produced in mice according to the technique described by Kohler and Milstein.[16,18] The unique specificity (class, subclass, antibody affinity) and purity of MAs have lead to their replacing ALGs in many instances.

STRUCTURE AND AFFINITY

OKT3 is a murine anti IgG, directed against the human CD3 receptor present on mature peripheral CD3+ T-cells. In vivo, OKT3 induces disappearance of CD3+ cells with coincident lymphopenia.[19] In vitro, OKT3 inhibits cytotoxic T-cell effector function via antigenic modulation of the CD3/Ti complex receptor.[20] OKT3 stimulates the Ti receptor with a capping phenomenon at one cellular pole; then, CD3 and Ti disappear by endocytosis or by dropping out. In vitro, OKT3 has a mitogenic action on mature T-cells with increased lymphokine production. This effect may be hazardous, as it could favor the onset of rejection with a rebound phenomenon following cessation of OKT3 therapy.[19,20]

PHARMACOKINETICS

After a 5-mg IV injection, OKT-3 peak serum level is obtained within 1 to 2 hours and trough serum levels within 24 hours. Circulating T-cells (CD3+, but also CD4+ and CD3+ CD8+) disappear 20 to 60 minutes after the first injection. Between day 2 and 5 of treatment, antigenic modulation leads to T-cells with CD3− phenotypes, able to express the CD3 molecule in vitro.[19] The appearance of circulating anti-OKT3 antibodies (of the IgM and/or IgG class) within 10 days of treatment is due to development of antimouse and/or anti-idiotypic antibodies that should be monitored.[21] Anti-isotypic antibodies (mouse anti-IgG2a) do not inhibit OKT3 fixation at the target cell; however, anti-idiotypic antibodies block the action of OKT3. Immunization against OKT3 is inversely related to the degree of immunosuppression obtained by azathioprine, steroids, and cyclosporine prescribed simultaneously and is a major impediment to the prolonged use of OKT3.[21]

ADVERSE SIDE EFFECTS

First dose effects are frequent and are thought to be secondary due to lymphokines released by T-cell destruction. The risk of acute respiratory distress syndrome with noncardiogenic pulmonary edema is important and, if possible, hemodynamic stability should be present prior to first injection. Fever, rigors, diarrhea, and/or vomiting are preventable with the administration of histamine antagonists and antipyretic drugs. Leukopenia, hypo- or hypertension, hypoglycemia, headaches, and/or aseptic meningitis are less frequent (8 percent) complications.

INDICATIONS AND TREATMENT MODALITIES

In the early postoperative period, OKT3 antibody (Ortho) can be used for prophylaxis of rejection, instead of polyclonal antilymphoid globulins, although there is no significant benefit to this use.[22] However, OKT3 offers an alternative therapy for patients made allergic to horse or goat serum (previous exposure) or when toxic side effects occur from ALGs. OKT3 is indicated as first-line treatment of severely or moderately acute rejection after heart and heart-lung transplantation with 85 percent efficacy.[23] OKT3 (5 mg · day^{-1} IV for 10 days) should be administered through a peripheral vein for a period of less than 2 minutes.

Other Monoclonal Antibodies

Several other monoclonal antibodies have been used on an experimental basis in humans for prophylaxis or treatment of renal allograft rejection.[24–31] Some of them are currently being tested after heart transplantation in the early postoperative period; the reader can refer to their characteristics in Table 4-5. Preliminary results suggest effectiveness in preventing rejection in highly sensitized patients, but the development of anti-idiotypic antibodies precludes any prolonged use. Since monoclonal antibodies tend to induce sensitization much earlier than do polyclonal antibodies (which recognize antigens by several epitopes), their use remains limited, especially when repeated administration is required.

MONITORING THE IMMUNE FUNCTION AND INFECTION IN THE EARLY POSTOPERATIVE PERIOD

Acute Rejection

Although onset of acute rejection is common within the first 3 months after heart or lung transplantation, its occurrence within

Table 4-5. Monoclonal Antibodies Used in Organ Transplantation

Monoclonal Antibody	Sub-class	Target Antigen	Target Cells	% Labeled Circulating Lymphocytes	Refer-ences
OKT3	IgG2a				24
WT32		CD3	T mature cells	65–85	31
CAMPATH 3	IgG2b				32
BMA 031	IgG2b				32
T10-B9-1A.31 A	IgMk	Ti receptor	T mature cells	65–85	27
33B31	IgG2a	II.2 receptor	IL2R ± T-cells		28
CAMPATH 6	IgG2b	(chain P55-TAC)			32
OKT4-LEU-3a	IgG1	CD4	CD4 + T-cells inducer/helper	40–60	
T12	IgM	CD6	T mature cells	65–75	
OKT8-Leu-2a	IgG1	CD8	CD8 + T-cells cytotoxic/ suppressor	20–40	
CAMPATH 1	IgM		Peripheral monocytes and lymphocytes	95	29
CHAL 1	IgM		Mononuclear cells	99	30
CBL 1			T- and B-cells, monocytes	<5	

the first 2 to 7 days after transplantation is very rare. Typically, hemodynamic adjustment of the graft to the recipient's circulation and recovery from ischemia are the two major problems (see Ch. 7). Intense immunosuppressive therapy usually allows early acceptance of the graft. Onset of hyperacute or of acute rejection is unpredictable; however, some patients, such as second graft recipients and/or patients with cytotoxic antibodies, are at high risk of such complications in the early postoperative period. Therefore, only careful follow-up in the early postoperative period (Table 4-6) will permit early diagnosis of rejection.

Routine endomyocardial biopsy is mandatory to diagnose graft rejection. The assessment of severity uses histologic criteria, as established by the International Society of Transplantation[32] (Table 4-7). Clinical (fever or cardiac failure) or electrocardiographic (ECG) signs (microwaves) are delayed, and their presence corresponds to severe degrees of acute or hyperacute rejection. Ultrasound examinations may reveal early signs of ventricular dysfunction, which remain nonspecific in the early postoperative period. Treatment is dictated by the histologic degree of rejection and local protocols.

Table 4-6. Daily Monitoring of Immune Function and Infections in Heart and/or Heart-Lung Transplant Recipients Within the First Week After Grafting

Clinical examination: daily
    Temperature, blood pressure
    Sternal wound
    Pulmonary and cardiac auscultation
    Weight/24-hr diuresis
    Complete clinical examination
    Tubes
Chest radiographs + ECG: daily
Biologic examinations: daily
    Blood cell count
    Sedimentation rate, C-reactive protein
    Urea + creatinine (blood + urine)
    Ca^+, P^+ (serum)
    24-hr urinary proteins
    Hepatic function, hemostasis
Cyclosporine blood levels: daily in lung, twice weekly in heart transplant recipients
Bacteriologic exmainations: daily
    Tubes, electrodes, sputums, urine (± blood)
Serum antibody levels: once a week
    CMV, Herpes, HBs, HVC, EBV, HIV1 and 2, *Toxoplasma, Candida, Aspergillus, Legionella*
Heart echodoppler ultrasonography: once a week
Endomyocardial biopsy: once a week
Bronchoalveolar lavage + lung biopsy at day 15 in lung recipients

Table 4-7. Various Stages of Acute Heart Rejection According to the Histologic Degree of Rejection[a]

Grade	Degree of Rejection
0	No rejection
1	A: Focal (perivascular or interstitial) infiltrate without necrosis
	B: Diffuse but sparse infiltrate without necrosis
2	One focus only with aggressive infiltration and/or focal myocyte damage
3	A: Mutlifocal aggressive infiltrates and/or myocyte damage
	B: Diffuse inflammatory process with necrosis
4	Diffuse aggressive polymorphous ± infiltrate ± edema, ± hemorrhage, ± vasculitis, with necrosis

[a] Resolving rejection denoted by a lesser grade; resolved rejection denoted by grade 0.

The diagnosis of acute lung rejection is difficult at this early postoperative stage and includes clinical signs, chest radiographic abnormalities, and histologic monitoring. However, none of the clinical symptoms (fever, dyspnea, wheezing, ronchi, or auscultation) or radiologic signs (diffuse alveolar infiltration with or without pleural effusion) is specific for rejection. Bronchoalveolar lavage is performed first to rule out potential infection, a more frequent occurrence than hyperacute or acute rejection in the early postoperative period. Infection is also associated with rejection but remains the primary concern. Only transbronchial lung biopsies Tableallow precise diagnosis. The treatment of acute rejection is dictated by the histologic degree of rejection[33] (Table 4-8).

Immunosuppressive Strategy in Case of Infection

All types of immunosuppressive therapy are deleterious to host-defense mechanisms. Overwhelming infection with superimposed allograft rejection is all too common. Empiric

misdiagnosis and treatment of rejection based on nonhistologic findings will further predispose to infection. Since rejection is the second most common cause of mortality in heart or heart-lung recipients, an individualized and judicious approach is warranted. Infections that are self-limited (urogenital tract sepsis, superficial wound infection) or easily

Table 4-8. Various Stages of Acute Lung Rejection According to Histologic Degree of Rejection

Acute rejection
  Grade 0—no significant abnormality
  Grade 1—minimal acute rejection
    With evidence of bronchiolar inflammation
    Without evidence of bronchiolar inflammation
    With large airway inflammation
    No bronchioles are present
  Grade 2—mild acute rejection
    With evidence of bronchiolar inflammation
    Without evidence of bronchiolar inflammation
    With large airway inflammation
    No bronchioles to evaluate
  Grade 3—moderate acute rejection
    With evidence of bronchiolar inflammation
    Without evidence of bronchiolar inflammation
    With large airway inflammation
    No bronchioles to evaluate
  Grade 4—severe acute rejection
    With evidence of bronchiolar inflammation
    Without evidence of bronchiolar inflammation
    With large airway inflammation
    No bronchioles to evaluate
Active airway damage without scarring
  Lymphocytic bronchitis
  Lymphocytic bronchiolitis
Chronic airway rejection
  Bronchiolitis obliterans—subtotal
    Active
    Inactive
  Bronchiolitis obliterans—total
    Active
    Inactive
Chronic vascular rejection
Vasculitis

treated do not necessitate a major reduction in immunosuppressive therapy. Leukopenia or neutropenia due to azathioprine may potentiate bacterial or fungal infections, and the dose is appropriately reduced. OKT3 is a strong potentiator of many opportunistic pathogens, including cytomegalovirus, *Legionella, Listeria, Cryptococcus,* and *Pneumocystis.* It should be avoided unless severe concomitant rejection is proved by histologic criteria. In the case of life-threatening infections or complications, immunosuppression is decreased.

REFERENCES

1. Walker RG, D'Apice AJF: Azathiprine and steroids. p. 319. In Morris PJ (ed): Kidney Transplantation: Principles and Practice. 3rd Ed. WB Saunders, Philadelphia, 1989
2. Flye MW: Immunosuppressive therapy. p. 155. In: Principles of Organ Transplantation. WB Saunders, Philadelphia, 1989
3. Fauci AS, Dale DC, Balon JE: Glucocorticosteroid therapy mechanisms of action and clinical considerations (NIH conference). Ann Intern Med 84:304–15, 1976
4. Borel JF, Di Pavoda F, Mason J et al: Pharmacology of cyclosporine (Sandimmune). Pharmacol Rev 41:239–434, 1989
5. Harding MW, Handschumacer ER: Cyclophilin, a primary molecular target for cyclosporine: structural and functional implications. Transplantation 46:29S–34S, 1988
6. Green CJ: Experimental transplantation and cyclosporine. Transplantation 46:3S–10S, 1988
7. Task Force on Cyclosporine Monitoring: Critical issues in cyclosporine monitoring. Clin Chem 33:1269–88, 1987
8. Myers BD: Cyclosporine nephrotoxicity. Nephrology forum. Kidney Int 30:964–74, 1986
9. Guillemain R, Farge D, Dreyfus G et al: Thrombotic microangiopathy with reversible acute renal failure in a cardiac transplant recipient under cyclosporine. Clin Nephrol 34:237–8, 1990
10. Julien J, Farge D, Kreft Jais C et al: Stimulation of the renin angitensin system in hypertensive cardiac and liver transplant recipients under cyclosporine. Transplantation 56:885–91, 1993
11. Scheinman SJ, Reinitz ER, Petro G et al: Cyclosporine central neurotoxicity following renal transplantation. Transplantation 49:215–6, 1990
12. Starzl TE, Todo S, Groth C, Fung JJ: FK 506, a potential breakthrough in immunosuppression: clinical implication. Transplant Proc 23:1–113, 1990
13. Woodle ES, Phelan DL, Saffitz JE et al: Reversal of humorally mediated cardiac allograft rejection in the presence of preformed class I antibody. Transplantation 56:1271–5, 1993
14. Ochiai T, Gunji Y, Nagat M et al: Effects of rapamycin in experimental organ allografting. Transplantation 56:15–9, 1993
15. Yuh DD, Morris RE: The immunopharmacology of immunosuppression by 15-deoxyspergualin. Transplantation 55:578–91, 1993
16. Cosimi AB: Antilymphocyte globulin and monoclonal antibodies. p. 343. In Morris JP (ed), Kidney Transplantation: Principles and Practice. 3rd Ed. WB Saunders, Philadelphia, 1988
17. Ippoliti G, Rovati B, Graffigna A et al: Prophylactic use of rabbit ATG vs horse ALG in heart-transplanted patients under Sandimmun (CyA) therapy: clinical and immunological effects. Clin Transplant 3:1–5, 1989
18. Kohler G, Milstein C: Continuous culture of fused cells secreting antibodies of predefined specificities. Nature 256:495–7, 1975
19. Chatenoud L, Baudrihaye MF, Kreis H et al: Human in vivo antigenic modulation induced by the anti T-cell OKT3 monoclonal antibody. Eur J Immunol 12:979–82, 1982
20. Janssen O, Wesselborg S, Kabelitz D: Immunosuppression by OKT3-induction of programmed cell death (apoptosis) as a possible mechanism of action. Transplantation 53:233–5, 1992
21. Schroeder TJ, First MR, Mansour ME et al: Antimurine antibody formation following OKT3 therapy. Transplantation 49:48–51, 1990
22. MacDonald PS, Mundy J, Keogh AM et al: A prospective study of prophylactic OKT3 versus equine antilymphocyte globulins after heart transplantation—increased morbidity with OKT3. Transplantation 55:110–6, 1993
23. O'Connell JB, Renlund DG, Gay WA et al: Effi-

cacy of OKT3 retreatment for refractory cardiac allograft rejection. Transplantation 47: 608–11, 1989

24. Kirkman RL, Araujo JL, Busch GJ et al: Treatment of acute renal allograft rejection with monoclonal anti-T12 antibody. Transplantation 36:620–6, 1983

25. Hillebrand G, Rothaug E, Hammer G et al: Experience with a new monoclonal antibody in clinical kidney transplantation. Transplant Proc 21:1776–7, 1989

26. Waid TH, Lucas BA, Thompson JS et al: Treatment of acute cellular allograft rejection with T10 Bg. 1A–31A anti T-cell monoclonal antibody. Transplant Proc 21:1778–84, 1989

27. Soulillou JP, Cantarovitch D, Le Mauff B et al: Randomized controlled trial of a monoclonal antibody against the interleukin-2-receptor (33B3.1) as compared with rabbit antithymocyte globulin for prophylaxis against rejection of renal allografts. N Engl J Med 322:1175–82, 1990

28. Friend PJ, Hale G, Waldmann H et al: Campath-1M-Prophylactic use after kidney transplantation. Transplantation 48:248–53, 1989

29. Oei J, Cicciarelli J, Terasaki PI et al: Treatment of kidney graft rejection with CHAL1 and CBL1 monoclonal antibodies. Transplant Proc 6:2740–3, 1989

30. Tax WJM, Van de Heijden HMW, Willems HW et al: Immunosuppression with monoclonal anti-T3 antibody (WT 32) in renal transplantation. Transplant Proc 19:1905–7, 1987

31. Waldman H: Monoclonal antibodies for organ transplantation: prospects for the future. Am J Kidney Dis 11:154–8, 1988

32. Billingham ME, Cary NRB, Hammond ME et al: A working formulation for the standardization of nomenclature in the diagnosis of heart and lund rejection: heart rejection study group. J Heart Transplant 9:587–93, 1990

33. Youssem SA, Berry GJ, Brunt EM et al: A working formulation for the standardization of nomenclature in the diagnosis of heart and lung rejection: lung rejection study group. J Heart Transplant 9:593–601, 1990

5

Blood Flow During Cardiopulmonary Bypass: Alterations and Effects on Organ Function

John R. Cooper, Jr.

PURPOSE OF CARDIOPULMONARY BYPASS

The purpose of cardiopulmonary bypass (CPB) is to give the surgeon a motionless, relatively bloodless field in which to operate. In most cases, accomplishing this goal requires cardiac arrest and unventilated lungs. Support of the circulation during this period by an artificial device, the "heart-lung" machine, or pump oxygenator, subjects the patient to physiologic, and at times, pathophysiologic changes that may be unfamiliar. Many of these processes are understood now, although some do remain unclear after 40 years of use of the device. This chapter will serve as an introduction to this area. More exhaustive discussions may be found in recent texts.[1]

The physiology of blood flow during CPB is central to understanding the changes that occur during bypass. Understanding blood flow demands knowledge of four factors: the mechanics of bypass; the physiology of hemodilution, including basic physics of blood flow and rheology; how these all interact with specific pathophysiologic conditions; and what is "normal" or "acceptable" perfusion during CPB. This understanding will often make the etiology and therapy of postoperative complications clearer. The discussion will center on relatively short-term bypass (less than 3 hours). Long-term bypass, the use of univentricular or biventricular support devices, and extracorporeal membrane oxygenation are covered in Chapter 17.

MECHANICS

Extracorporeal Circuit

Support of the circulation first requires a mechanical pump; two types are currently employed. The positive displacement roller

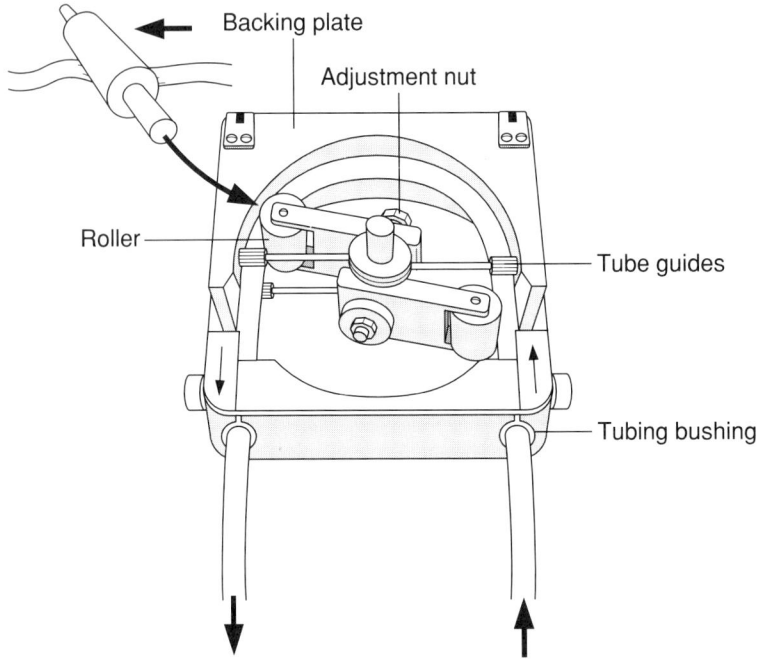

Fig. 5-1. Conventional roller pump. The rolling pin (upper left corner) shows the basic principle of the pump—positive displacement of blood as the roller compresses the tubing. The degree of roller occlusion is controlled by the adjustment nut. Lateral movement of tubing is prevented by the tube guides and the tube bushings prevent tube displacement or "creep" as the roller moves. (From Reed and Stafford,[62] with permission.)

pump, originally developed by Porter and Bradley in 1855,[2] is most commonly used. Blood is propelled by compression of tubing by rollers in a pump housing or "raceway" (Fig. 5-1). A constant speed motor drives the rollers, allowing stable perfusion despite varying resistance. The occlusion of the rollers against the housing wall is adjustable, and total occlusion of the tubing is avoided to decrease blood trauma.

The kinetic or centrifugal pump uses a series of rotating cones to move blood by centrifugal force (Fig. 5-2). This device is less traumatic to formed elements of blood and has achieved popularity in longer-term perfusion for this reason. It is, to some extent, compliance dependent, causing a decrease in perfusion when peripheral resistance increases.

The second component of the CPB circuits is the oxygenator. There are three types: bub-

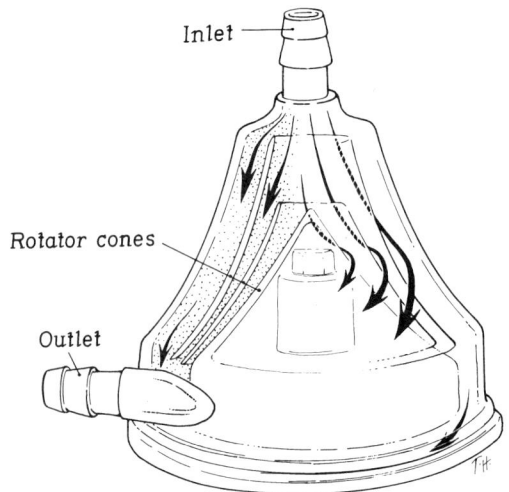

Fig. 5-2. Centrifugal force pump. Arrows demonstrate the blood flow path and the vaneless rotors. (From Reed and Stafford,[62] with permission.)

ble, membrane, and filming. The last is no longer in clinical use and is not discussed here. A bubble oxygenator uses a direct blood-gas interface. Gas exchange occurs by diffusion into and out of bubbles created when oxygen-rich gas passes through a scintillated plate in the base of the device. These bubbles are mixed with venous blood coming from the patient, and oxygenation occurs as the two are mixed. The blood-bubble mixture flows through a plastic mesh coated with an antifoaming substance to remove bubbles. The defoamed, oxygenated blood is collected into an arterial reservoir and is pumped from there back into the patient. A limited amount of trauma to the formed blood elements occurs because of the direct blood-gas interface. However, there are few clinical consequences of this if perfusion times are not prolonged. These oxygenators remain in common use because they are efficient at oxygenation and CO_2 removal, simple to operate, and relatively inexpensive.

A membrane oxygenator imposes a semipermeable plastic membrane between the blood and oxygen carrying gas. Diffusion occurs across this membrane and there is usually good oxygenation, but CO_2 removal is less efficient. The lack of a direct interface decreases blood trauma and has made these oxygenators popular for longer cases, pediatric perfusion, and extracorporeal membrane oxygenation. Unfortunately, they are more complex to set up and run, and are more expensive.

A typical CPB circuit is illustrated in Figure 5-3. The other major components of the circuit are the suction and venting devices that return blood to the pump from the surgical field. This blood is collected into a cardiotomy reservoir, defoamed, filtered, and returned to the venous side of the oxygenator. It should be noted that most of the trauma to blood occurs during this process (not in the oxygenator or pump) and that there is often a direct correlation between the amount of suctioning and the amount of hemolysis found.

Most of the tubing in the CPB circuit is polyvinyl chloride. Other plastics may be used in the oxygenator. Exposure of blood to this large foreign surface would produce massive thrombosis if the patient was not heparinized. This exposure does result in activation of the immune system, as discussed later.

Primes

Eliminating air and particulate matter from the pump oxygenator requires priming with fluid to provide a continuous fluid path from the venous to arterial side. Modern CPB techniques use crystalloid prime for this purpose, with the actual fluid and volume varying between institutions. Common fluids include Normosol, saline, dextrose in Ringer's lactate, and Ringer's lactate without glucose. These primes will obviously produce significant hemodilution.

Use of glucose in the prime is controversial because of recent work associating elevated glucose levels and worsened neurologic outcome in patients (not undergoing CPB) who have cerebral damage.[3] While it may seem logical to apply this finding to CPB, this has not been our experience. Glucose, by its osmotic effects, is known to reduce the volume of crystalloid markedly that must be added to the extracorporeal circuit, in order to maintain a constant flow rate. This decreases the constant loss of crystalloid solutions out of the vascular space into the interstitum and thus reduces the total amount of fluid required on CPB and with it, postoperative weight gain.[4] However, others avoid glucose completely.

Conduct of Cardiopulmonary Bypass

The pump oxygenator is operated by a specially trained perfusionist who controls blood flow by adjusting pump motor speed and oxygenation and CO_2 removal by changing gas flow into the oxygenator. The temperature of the perfusate, and often the administration of

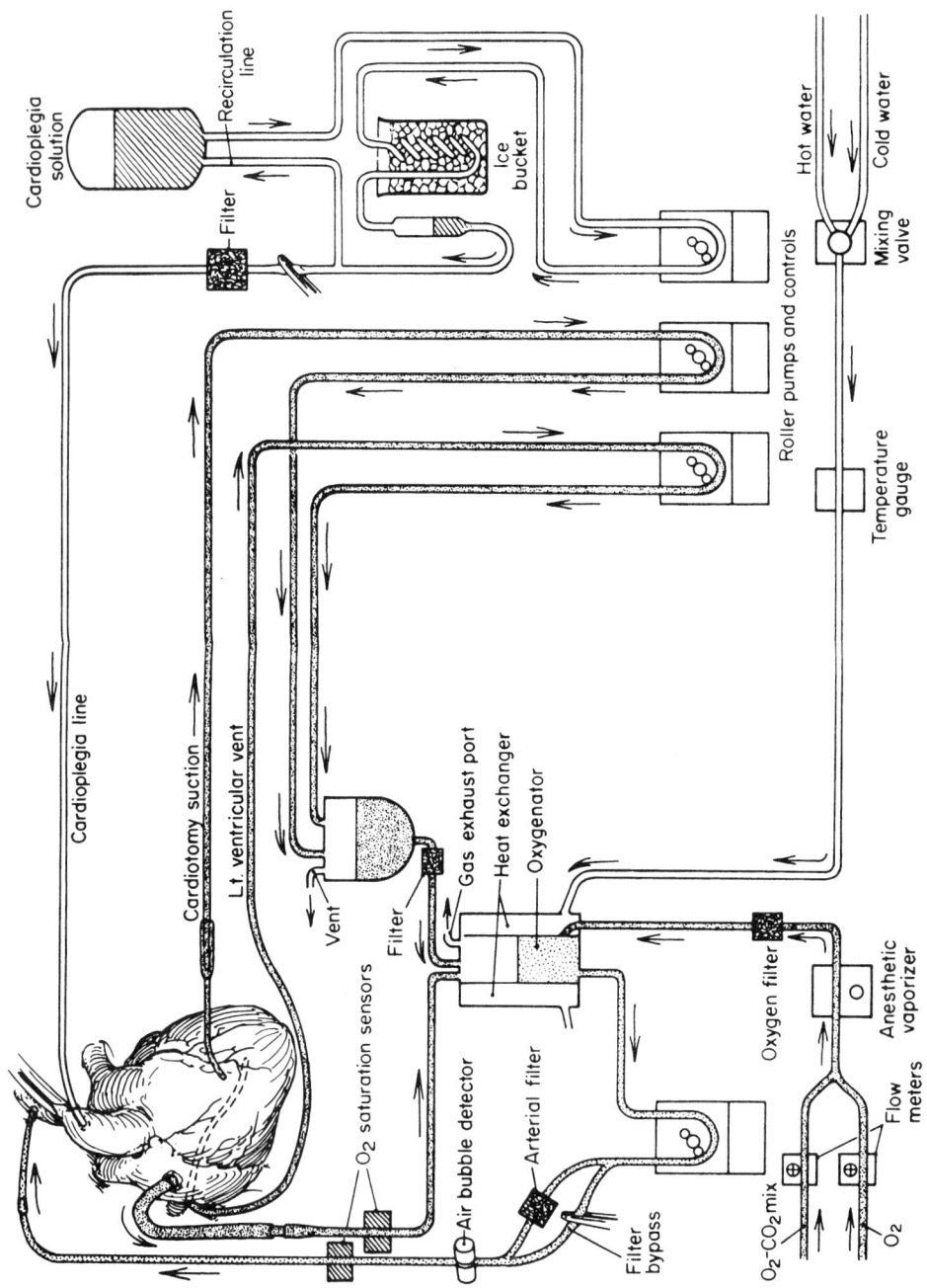

Fig. 5-3. Circuit diagram for a perfusion circuit using a bubble oxygenator, single venous cannulation, and cardioplegia administration. There are many variations in CPB circuits among institutions. (From Reed and Stafford,[62] with permission.)

cardioplegia, are also controlled by the perfusionist. Monitoring of perfusion pressure, urine output, and blood gases is part of the perfusionist's responsibilities as well (along with the anesthesiologist). The perfusionist will try to maintain flow and pressure within a range of "normal." This range has large institutional variations, but flows of 50 to 60 ml $\cdot$ kg^{-1} $\cdot$ min^{-1} or 2 L $\cdot$ m^{-2} $\cdot$ min^{-1} are common at normothermia. Target pressures are less well defined, although pressures of 30 to 100 mmHg are accepted at many institutions, at normothermia as well.

Venous blood returns to the oxygenator by gravity and must be constant for a constant flow to be generated. If venous return is interrupted and flow maintained, the reservoir of the oxygenator will be exhausted, and air may be pumped into the patient.

HEMODILUTION

Rheology of Blood

A complete discourse on rheology of human blood is beyond the scope of this chapter, but understanding elementary concepts is necessary. More complete reviews may be found elsewhere.[5]

A common model used to understand the forces governing blood flow involves a liquid contained between two parallel plates. If a force is applied to the top plate adequate to set it in motion and it moves with a certain velocity, the force required is proportional to the area of the plate. This force is known as the *shear stress*. The velocity at which the plate moves is proportional to the distance between the plates and is called *velocity gradient* or *shear rate*. The shear stress and velocity gradient are related by a constant known as the *fluid viscosity*. This may be expressed in the formula

Shear stress = viscosity $\times$ velocity gradient

Viscosity is constant for many fluids, such as water, at all shear rates; these are known as newtonian fluids. Blood, however, is a non-

newtonian fluid as its viscosity increases at lower shear rates. This results because the cellular components of blood tend to aggregate at low flow rates and inhibit flow by forming cellular clumps (rouleaux). Fibrinogen proteins form intracellular bridges between red cells causing rouleaux, and these bridges dissipate at higher flow rates.[6]

Lastly, when blood flow is zero, the force required to set it in motion is called the *yield stress*. This force influences viscous resistance to flow at low shear rates and is proportional to levels of fibrinogen and hematocrit. In contrast, the yield stress for newtonian fluids is essentially zero.

The cells influence flow not only by their interaction, but by their effect on the surrounding fluid as well, which behaves as it were part of the cell. The shape of red cells may be altered too, and as flow increases, they become ellipsoid and align their major axis in the direction of flow. This tends to decrease resistance to flow; thus, blood at higher flow rates behaves in a more newtonian manner.

Principles of Blood Flow

Cardiac output and thus organ blood flow are directly proportional to perfusion pressure and inversely proportional to the total peripheral resistance:

$$\text{Cardiac output} = \frac{\text{perfusion pressure}}{\text{total peripheral resistance}}$$

Total peripheral resistance is composed of the product of two additional components: vascular resistance and viscosity:

$$\frac{\text{Cardiac}}{\text{output}} = \frac{\text{perfusion pressure}}{\text{vascular resistance} \times \text{viscosity}}$$

The aorta and its major branches contribute little to vascular resistance; most of the resistance to flow resides in the arterioles, capillaries, and venules. As vessel diameter decreases and the kinetic energy of the blood falls, the shear rate decreases. Since viscosity is inversely related to the shear rate, it rises

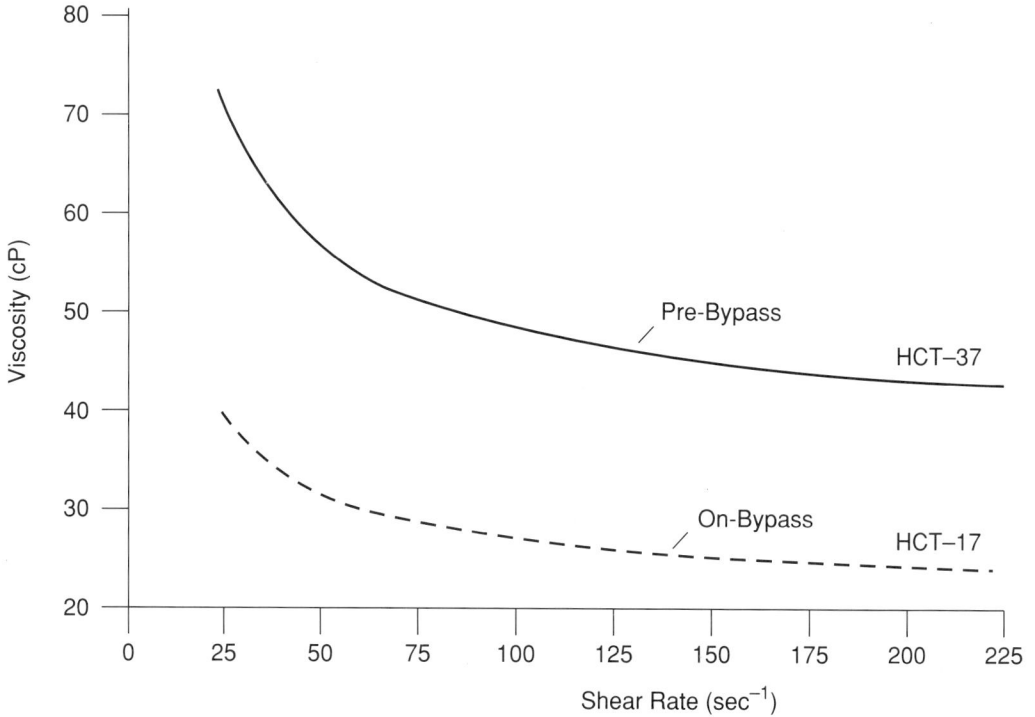

Fig. 5-4. Change in viscosity with hemodilution accompanying CPB. Viscosity is measured in centi-poise (cP). (Modified from Gordon et al.,[7] with permission.)

as velocity falls; therefore, peripheral resistance rises progressively as vessel diameter decreases. These effects are felt most severely in the post-capillary venules.

Another important principle is the direct, almost linear relationship between viscosity and hematocrit, so that a significant reduction in the hematocrit produces a profound reduction in viscosity, as shown in Figure 5-4 in a patient undergoing CPB.[7] This fall in hematocrit and viscosity produces a marked drop in peripheral resistance and an increase in tissue perfusion. In a dog model, a decrease in hematocrit from 42 percent to 25 percent produced a 50 percent increase in flow at the same perfusion pressure.[8] If hematocrit is lowered to less than 10 percent, blood behaves as a newtonian liquid.[9]

Hypothermia increases viscosity as temperature falls. This relationship is not as direct as with hematocrit and viscosity, but a 10°C fall in temperature produces a 20 to 25 percent increase in viscosity; therefore, tissue perfusion falls. Vasoconstriction, which normally accompanies hypothermia, also decreases blood flow to tissues. The decreased tissue perfusion resulting from these factors can be offset by the reduction in oxygen consumption of the hypothermic tissue, which is greater than the increase in viscosity. A 10°C fall in temperature causes a greater than 50 percent decrease in total body oxygen consumption.

Reduction of hematocrit below normal will by definition reduce oxygen-carrying capacity, but this reduction is only 10 percent when the hematocrit decreases from about 30 percent (maximum O_2 transport) to 20 percent.[10] In addition, during surgery other factors operative as compensatory mechanisms are present that either reduce oxygen demand or increase delivery. These include general

anesthesia, muscle relaxation, and normovo-
lemia, plus the improved microcirculatory
perfusion from decreased viscosity and hypothermia.

These principles have direct clinical application during CPB. The flow rates used
during conventional bypass are somewhat
lower than "normal" (50 ml $\cdot$ kg^{-1} $\cdot$ min^{-1}
or 2.0 L $\cdot$ m^{-2} $\cdot$ min^{-1}). In addition, hypothermia is used very commonly to permit reduc-
tion in flows to produce a dry operative field
and to promote myocardial and cerebral protection during reduced flows. The aggregate
effects of lowered flow rates and hypothermia
would tend to increase viscosity and conversely decrease tissue perfusion. Hemodilution counteracts these effects by reducing
blood viscosity.

The most noticeable clinical effect of the
marked fall in viscosity with hemodilution is
a significant fall in perfusion pressure at initiation of CPB. This fall is directly proportional
to the change in viscosity[7] (Fig. 5-5). Another
important and expected effect was described
by Guyton in animals—a significant passive
increase in venous return.[11] This is almost
certainly due to the increased flow in small
vessels, especially the post-capillary venules
where, as noted, viscosity is highest.

The general effects of hemodilution during
cardiopulmonary bypass reflect the interaction of these principles. When animals
undergo normovolemic hemodilution to a
hematocrit of 19 percent, there is an increase
in oxygen tension in liver, kidneys, pancreas,
small intestine, and skeletal muscle.[12] Cere-

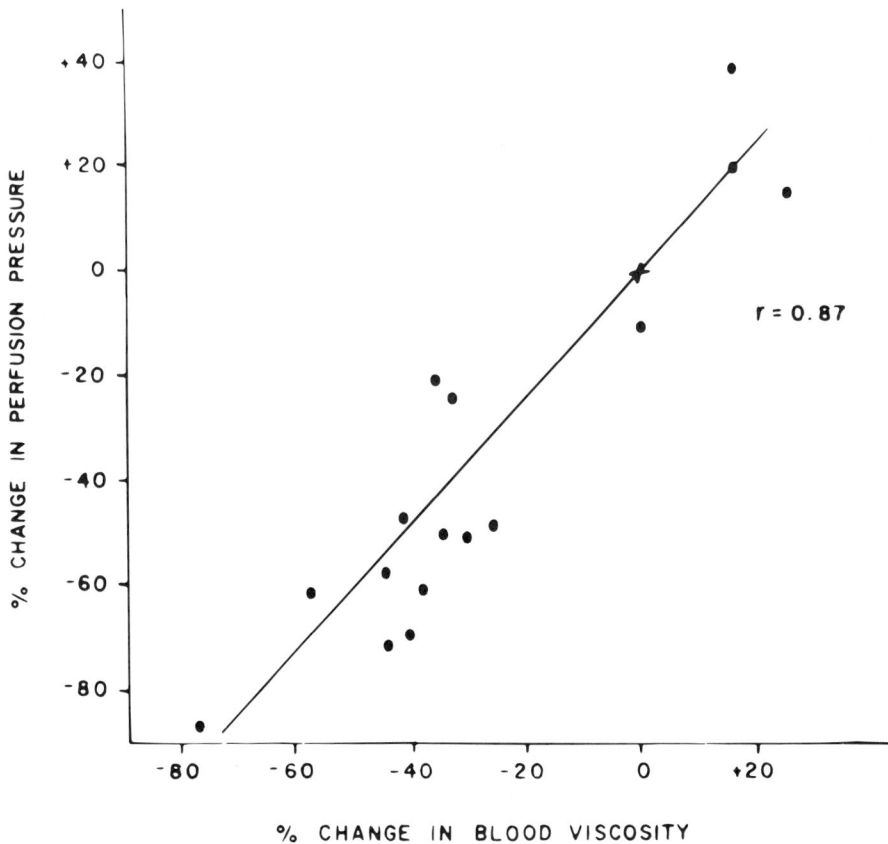

Fig. 5-5. Changes in perfusion pressure with changes in viscosity in a group of patients on CPB with
a constant flow rate. (Modified from Gordon et al.,[7] with permission.)

bral blood flow (CBF) also may increase 50 to 300 percent during hemodilution.[13] However, other factors significantly affect CBF, including autoregulation, carbon dioxide tension, and very high or very low perfusion pressure (see Ch. 12).

Hemodilution during CPB has salutory effects, but what are acceptable limits? There is a theoretical fall in microcirculatory flow with hematocrits over 30 percent and most institutions do try and achieve hematocrits below this level, although there is still considerable variation between institutions as to specific limits. Acceptable hematocrit ranges are also influenced by hypothermia. It is generally desirable to have hematocrits of less than 30 percent if temperature will be lowered to less than 30°C. If temperatures are to be less than 25°C, hematocrits of less than 25 percent are desirable. Hematocrits below 20 percent are clinically well tolerated with those in the 15 to 18 percent range quite common. Experimentally, abnormal distribution of organ blood flow has been found with hematocrits of less than 20 percent.[14] Clinically, this does not seem relevant, however, perhaps because of physiologic compensatory mechanisms, general anesthesia, and hypothermia. CPB hematocrits of less than 15 percent, while not common, as used in some circulatory arrest protocols and as occur in some Jehovah's Witness patients, are seemingly well tolerated.[15]

Acceptable hematocrits for separation from CPB is another subject demonstrating much institutional variation. There is evidence of a maldistribution of coronary blood flow with hematocrits of less than 15 percent.[16] Most would deem it wise to separate from bypass with hematocrits over this level, especially if coronary circulation is compromised or if there is evidence of myocardial ischemia or dysfunction. There is little hard evidence, however, and separation from CPB with hematocrits around 20 percent is common.

The possibility of dilutional coagulopathy also raised concerns with the initial use of hemodilution. In general, these concerns have proved unfounded, even in extreme cases. In fact, in polycythemic patients, a decrease in postoperative bleeding has been noted with adequate hemodilution.[17]

HISTORICAL LESSONS

The first successful open heart operation using CPB was performed by John Gibbon in 1953.[18] He attempted to duplicate normal human circulation in terms of flow rate (80 ml $\cdot$ kg^{-1} $\cdot$ min^{-1}) and perfusate (whole blood). After Gibbon retired from cardiac surgery, his methods were continued by Kirklin at the Mayo Clinic.[19] From these physicians' efforts the "high-flow" school of CPB was derived; that is, they accepted the concept that high flows mean better perfusion.

Another approach was taken by Lillehei et al.,[20] who used significantly lower flow rates (30 to 35 ml $\cdot$ kg^{-1} $\cdot$ min^{-1}) than did Gibbon and Kirklin. They based their approach on their knowledge of adequate flow rates in controlled cross-circulation experiments,[21] plus the observation that dogs with both superior and inferior cavas that were surgically occluded could survive for up to 1 hour.[22] This was possible because the azygos vein drains into a dog's right atrium directly and provided enough venous return (10 percent of normal) to allow adequate short-term perfusion. This lower flow technique proved popular because it mitigated the harmful effects of higher flows (trauma to formed elements and excessive suctioning). Both "high-flow" and "low-flow" schools achieved acceptance, and hypothermia was added to both by most surgeons to provide "organ protection." Both remain in use today.

The next major step in CPB came in the early 1960s with the introduction of asanguinous primes.[23] This produced immediate benefits. There was an immediate reduction in the amount of blood needed for CPB. Previously, with whole blood primes, 2 to 6 units of blood were needed to prime the CPB circuit alone. It became possible to perform

CPB without blood in some cases, markedly lessening the strain on blood banks, permitting surgery in Jehovah's Witnesses, and allowing CPB as an emergency procedure. Most importantly, there was a dramatic decrease in perioperative complications. This was noted by Cooley et al.,[24] reporting on the first large series (100 patients) using 5 percent dextrose in water as a priming fluid. These investigators noted an increase in venous return as would be expected from Guyton's work, and a fall in "neurologic, pulmonary and renal complications."

Until that time, complications had been attributed to low perfusion pressures and low flow rates (neurologic), low perfusion pressures, flow rates and low urine output (renal),[25] and the "pump" itself, plus parenchymal hypoxemia (pulmonary).[26] Especially illustrative is an often quoted paper by Stockard et al.,[27] who related neurologic complications to the time perfusion pressure was less than 50 mmHg.

Since that time, with hemodilution, no reliable study has been able to associate neurologic complications with any certain perfusion pressures, and several have shown no relationship between the two.[28-30] It is now apparent that the vast majority of these complications are due to embolic phenomena: atheromata from the cannulation site or ascending aorta, debris from diseased valves, thrombi from the left atrium or ventricle, or air retained in opened cardiac chambers or from the pump.[30]

Similar decreases in pulmonary and renal complications also occurred. Of note, the association between urinary output on CPB and postoperative renal function disappeared.[31] The most reliable predictor now of poor postoperative renal function is poor preoperative renal function (see Ch. 9). It also became clear that low cardiac output syndrome in the immediate post-CPB period was often associated not only with the above complications but also with untoward effects on other organ systems.[32]

The reason behind this large drop in the rate of complications associated with CPB was hemodilution itself, with its attendant fall in blood viscosity. It is apparent from the above formulas that as viscosity falls, flow (cardiac output) rises, even though perfusion pressure falls as well. Thus, it may be said that, under conditions of hemodilution, the relationship of adequate pressure equaling adequate perfusion is "uncoupled" and that adequate organ-preserving perfusion may be obtained at significantly lower pressures, and conversely, pressure no longer serves as an indicator of adequate flow.

BLOOD-GAS MANAGEMENT

Hypothermia affects blood flow to organs, as discussed above, with its effects on vasoconstriction and viscosity. It also affects blood-gas management. As temperature falls, CO_2 becomes more soluble in blood and the $PaCO_2$ falls to maintain the CO_2 stores constant. If a sample of hypothermic blood is taken for blood-gas measurement and analyzed at 37°C, as is standardly done, the PCO_2 and pH values will emerge as "normal." This does not reflect the actual state at the lowered temperature, however. If the blood-gas values are corrected to the specific temperature, the PCO_2 will be lowered and the pH elevated. It was thought in the first decades of CPB management that this reflected an abnormal state, so CO_2 was added to the gas inflow of oxygenators in order to elevate CO_2 stores and adjust the corrected pH value to "normal." This management of blood gases on CPB is known as the pH-stat technique.

This view was challenged in the early 1980s by physiologists who observed that over a wide range of temperatures poikilothermic animals maintained their intracellular acid-base balance, so there was a constant ratio of OH^- ions to H^+ ions.[33] This produces a constant relative alkalinity that parallels the pH changes of water. The buffering capacity of the imidazole group of histadine is responsible for this compensation. As temperature decreases, the pKa of the imidazole groups changes but the fraction of unprotonated histidine remains constant. CO_2 stores remain constant, with the result that pH changes with temperature. These unprotonated imidazole groups are known as "alpha" and this technique is known as alpha-stat. Many institutions adopted it. Practically, this is done by managing blood gases based on the uncorrected (37°C) laboratory values, rather than on those corrected back to the patient's temperature.

Clinically this has effects on CBF. With pH-stat strategy and the accompanying elevated CO_2 stores, cerebral vasodilation occurs and increased CBF results. This may obviously be considered desirable, but it has been suggested that the elevation of CO_2 may lead to loss of autoregulation, flow-metabolism uncoupling, and overperfusion of the brain. There is also speculation that significantly increased cerebral perfusion may lead to a higher incidence of embolic events. Conversely, alpha-stat management results in lower, but clinically adequate, CBF, preservation of autoregulation, and a decreased chance for emboli.

There are several experimental studies supporting the use of alpha-stat management; however, a clinical study comparing alpha- with pH-stat have shown no difference in neurologic outcome in adults.[34] Interestingly, recent laboratory[35] and retrospective clinical studies suggested that alpha-stat management may be detrimental in patients with cyanotic congenital heart disease who undergo deep hypothermia and circulatory arrest,[36] although this has not been our experience. (Cooper JR, Roughneen P, Ott DA: unpublished data).

PULSATILE PERFUSION

It was not possible to produce pulsatile perfusion in the early days of CPB. As technology has advanced, it has become possible to add pulsatile flow to conventional bypass. Clinical results have been very inconclusive, however. While significant physiologic effects such as lower peripheral vascular resistance and improved urine output have been reported, outcome studies examining cardiac, cerebral, and renal complications have been unable to demonstrate significant differences between pulsatile and nonpulsatile bypass.[37]

IMMUNE RESPONSE TO CARDIOPULMONARY BYPASS

In the mid-1980s, investigators noticed that CPB induced significant decline in lymphocyte count and function on the second postoperative day, which returned to normal by the seventh postoperative day. The various immunologic mechanisms responsible for this depressed immunoreactivity are better understood today. However, their clinical significance remains to be defined. This altered immunologic status could contribute to the commonly reported rise in temperature post-CPB that occurs in the absence of any recognized bacteriologic cause.[38] Altered immune function can enhance patients' susceptibility to postoperative infections, which are more frequent following cardiac surgery with CPB than with cardiac or major surgical procedures without CPB. Although most immunocompetent patients do not develop post-CPB viral infections (demonstrating their ability to defend themselves), occult defective immunoregulation may be exacerbated by the effects of open heart surgery. Severely ill (immunologically compromised) patients requiring CPB may be at higher risk of infectious complications during the postoperative period.

Early postoperative lymphopenia and inversion of the CD4+ to CD8+ ratio (see Ch. 11) were first explained by complement activation during CPB. The complement activation occurs because of blood exposure to the large foreign surface of the CPB circuit.[39] Both classical and alternate pathways may be activated with generation of both C3a and C5a anaphylotoxins. This activation in turn can cause chemotaxis of leukocytes, smooth muscle constriction, and arachidonic acid metabolic release. Leukocyte sequestration may occur in the pulmonary capillaries.[40] This entire process has been termed an inflammatory response to CPB and has been implicated in untoward effects of bypass on the entire body.[41]

Down-regulation of the immune response within the first few postoperative days can be restored by combined immunomodulatory regimens. In a study of 60 patients during the week after CPB, decreases in CD4+ T-cells and activated effector IL2R+ T-cells indicated impaired activation and regulation of the cell-mediated immunity.[42] Decreased interleukin (IL1 and IL2) synthesis, low γ-interferon serum concentrations, and in vivo delayed-type hypersensitivity response were also documented. In these patients, the use of indomethacin (which blocks prostaglandin E_2 [PGE_2] production), and thymopentin (the synthetic thymus hormone that enhances T-lymphocyte proliferation and maturation), effectively restored postoperative immune function. The observed monocytosis could be a key event in altering host defense, since restoration of altered immune function was obtained by blocking PGE_2 production. Monocytes synthesize PGE_2, which suppresses monocytic antigen presentation capacity, major HLA class II expression, and IL1 synthesis. In addition, PGE_2 blocks several T-cell functions by increasing CD8+ suppressor T-cell activity, which results in impaired T-cell function.

In addition, the confounding effects of intra- and postoperative hemorrhage, mediastinal exploration, and normal and abnormal cardiac output all may have significant immunologic effects in terms of suppression of immune function and further exposure to infective vectors. Conversely, removal of activated white blood cells and debris because of good cardiac output improves the immunologic state.[43]

Transfusion-Related Lung Injury

Transfusion may contribute to immunologic changes with further sustency effects. Although rare, the occurrence of noncardio-genic pulmonary edema (NCPE) caused by leukocyte antibodies after CPB is dramatic and often fatal. Several cases of transfusion-related acute lung injury have been reported.[44] Etiologic factors implicated in the development include white blood cell reaction, endotoxins, protamine reactions, and the use of a pump oxygenator. The lung is thought to be more susceptible than other organs. Specifically, neutrophil activation with pulmonary sequestration, generation of free radicals, and resultant increases in vascular permeability has been held responsible for "post-capillary leak." This is thought to produce interstitial edema and to cause or contribute to post-bypass respiratory failure.[45]

ORGAN BLOOD FLOW

Brain

CBF has probably been studied more extensively than any other organ flow during CPB because of fear and an incomplete understanding of neurologic complications. CBF and cerebral metabolism ($CMRO_2$) during CPB are influenced by each other and by temperature, $PaCO_2$, the anesthetic, hemodilution, and perhaps the age of the patient. The brain autoregulates flow based on its metabolism (flow-metabolism coupling) and also autoregulates flow in relation to perfusion pressure. Because of its high oxygen consumption relative to other tissues and its lack of energy stores, adequate oxygen delivery is critical. In general, CBF is reduced by general anesthesia, increased by hemodilution, and decreased by hypothermia. $CMRO_2$ is reduced by general anesthesia, not affected by hemodilution, and reduced by hypothermia. The net result is that oxygen delivery during standard CPB is more than adequate, although CBF is not "normal."[46,47]

One of the general fears concerning CBF is that pressure-flow autoregulation could be adversely affected under certain conditions. The debate over the appropriateness of pH-stat versus alpha-stat management of blood gases centers here, as discussed above. Autoregulation appears to also be impaired by deep hypothermia and circulatory arrest and perhaps by chronic hypertension. There is some evidence that diabetes impairs flow-metabolism autoregulation.[48] The clinical significance of any of autoregulatory disturbances, in terms of neurologic outcome, is unknown.

There is no question that the vast majority of neurologic complications attendant to CPB are due to embolic events that occur before, during, or after bypass.[30] The etiology may be particulate (atheromatous debris, calcium deposits from valves, thrombus from cardiac chambers) or air (from opened chambers or the oxygenation process). There is also the possibility that the jet of blood from the aortic cannula is directed at an atheromatous deposit on the aortic intima resulting in a "sand blasting" effect and particulate dislodgement. Preventive action against these CPB complications has included assessment of cannulation sites, including using echocardiography,[49] careful removal of air from cardiac chambers at procedure end, and the use of cerebral protection by a barbiturate.[50]

Special mention should be made of the patient with carotid stenosis undergoing CPB. Because of a reported increase in neurologic complications with symptomatic cardiac disease, many have assumed that all patients with carotid stenosis were at increased risk of cerebral compromise during CPB and reasoned that perfusion pressures needed to be maintained at a higher level during bypass in these patients. Studies of patients with significant cardiovascular disease found CBF to be normal, with no adverse outcome.[51]

Heart

It is necessary during almost all cardiac operations to cross-clamp the aorta and arrest coronary flow. This will lead to rapid depletion of energy stores and eventual myocardial necrosis; to conserve energy, many maneuvers have been used. Originally, systemic hy-

pothermia with intermittent cross-clamping or individual coronary perfusion was employed. Induced cardiac arrest with a cardioplegic solution was used by Melrose et al.[52] in the early days of cardiac surgery, but because of poor initial results, it was abandoned. The technique continued to be researched; it was eventually reintroduced clinically in the 1970s and has been used successfully since.

Most solutions are high in potassium and are administered at temperatures of 4° to 8°C into the aortic root after cross-clamping. In patients with aortic insufficiency, administration into each coronary artery may be necessary. Exact composition of the solution varied widely from hospital to hospital, as do techniques in administration. These include use of blood cardioplegia, retrograde administration via the coronary sinus, and warm cardioplegia.

Variation in techniques does not appear to have tremendous clinical significance in routine cases, as oxygen conservation comes from asystole and hypothermia. Removal of the aortic cross-clamp and renewed coronary perfusion wash out the cardioplegia solution, and often myocardial function is restored by this maneuver alone. This is especially true in coronary bypass operations in which proximal grafts can be done with a partial occluding clamp that isolates a section of aorta while flow resumes through the native coronary circulation.

Lung

Pulmonary injury following CPB has been known since the earliest use of the technique. The scope of this problem, however, is broad and multifactorial, with the etiology of some syndromes obscure even after 40 years of clinical use. Some explanations involve blood flow through the lungs while others invoke the more general effects of bypass. The reported incidence of respiratory failure after CPB varies, but this may be because the specific etiology may be difficult to determine, especially when separating cardiac from non-cardiac causes. Generally, though, the most common cause of respiratory failure is cardiac failure. Other etiologies are discussed below.

PARENCHYMAL HYPOXIA

The diversion of blood flow away from the lungs during total CPB leaves them supplied by the bronchial circulation. It was thought that lack of adequate perfusion during CPB would produce hypoxic damage to lung tissues. Strong evidence for this is lacking, although generally improved perfusion with hemodilution did produce a fall in pulmonary complications coincident to its use.

MECHANICAL DAMAGE

When the heart is arrested during CPB and all venous return is diverted to the oxygenator, blood still returns to the left side of the heart via the bronchial circulation. In operations such as coronary bypass, in which the cardiac chambers are not opened, this blood can accumulate and distend the left atrium and ventricle and can also elevate the pulmonary artery pressure. If left unvented this volume overload can damage not only the heart, but lung parenchyma as well. Use of an appropriate left atrial or aortic root vent is therefore common.

VOLUME OVERLOAD

Hemodilution with CPB produces a net loss of crystalloid perfusate to the body as a result of a fall in colloid osmotic pressure. Some of this loss may be to the pulmonary parenchyma, although because the lungs are isolated to a degree, this is uncommon. It is quite common, however, to see pulmonary volume overload post-bypass from cardiac causes and from mobilization of interstitial fluid from other sites. This may not occur until a few days postoperatively when a patient has been transferred out of intensive care. Colloid solutions, glucose, and prophylactic diuretics have been used in attempting to deal with this problem.

ATELECTASIS

Atelectasis represents the most common pulmonary problem after CPB. It may be contributed to by postoperative factors such as smoking, obesity, cardiac failure, and intraoperative factors, including volume overload, cardiac failure, and inadequate ventilation. Parenchymal collapse due to pleurotomy or compression by pleural fluid or blood are common as well. Left lung collapse is especially common during coronary bypass because of the left pleurotomy, which is often necessary to harvest the internal mammary artery.[53]

NONCARDIOGENIC PULMONARY EDEMA

Noncardiogenic pulmonary edema, an uncommon complex also known as adult respiratory distress syndrome, is ascribed to various etiologies, including the immunologic mechanisms noted above. Unfortunately, specific causes are often hard to identify in individual patients, and temporal relationship to a specific event or drug administration is often unreliable.

One cause, transfusion-related acute lung injury, is well described,[54] although it is rare and is often not recognized for what it is. This occurs when antileukocyte antibodies are transfused into a patient via red cell, plasma, or platelet components. Conversely, leukocytes may be transfused via the same components into patients who already have antileukocyte antibodies in their plasma. Whatever the case, the antibodies and leukocytes combine and the leukocytes are activated, aggregate, and are filtered by the lung. They release intracellular mediators, causing an anaphylactic like syndrome with hypotension, low filling pressures, but profound pulmonary capillary leak and proteinaceous pulmonary edema.

While this specific entity is perhaps the most dramatic type of transfusion-related lung injury, there is also evidence that decreasing exposure of patients to blood transfusions in general has been beneficial. Hemodilution techniques produced a fall in pulmonary complications, as did filtering of blood transfused during or post-bypass.[55] This presumably decreases the incidence of microemboli, including red cell debris and activated white blood cells.

Liver, Pancreatic, and Intestinal Perfusion

The intra-abdominal viscera, with the exception of the kidneys, have received relatively little attention as far as actual effects of CPB on them. This is partly because they are difficult to study directly, especially in intact humans, and also because postoperative complications due to hepatic failure or pancreatitis are relatively rare, at least as an isolated entity. Also, early studies concerning these organs involved CPB without hemodilution and are presently not applicable.

In general, experimental work shows that CPB with hemodilution increases liver, pancreatic, and intestinal blood flow, although this is not a universal finding. Function of the organs appears to remain intact, although suppressed in some instances; this suppression may be due to hypothermia in many cases. Liver failure or pancreatitis is usually associated with long perfusion times or low cardiac output following CPB. Endocrine function of the pancreas seems to be suppressed, with insulin secretion falling markedly during normal CPB and then recovering promptly once bypass is discontinued.[56] This has been attributed both to hypothermia and to a lack of pulsatile flow.

Kidney

In contrast to the liver and pancreas, the kidneys have received much attention since the early days of CPB because of the relatively high incidence of renal failure following cardiac operations. In the early days of cardiac surgery with blood primes, renal function post-bypass was correlated with function on bypass, as evidenced by the rate and amount of urine output.[25]

With hemodilution, there is increased flow to the kidneys as with other organs, and the association between urine output on CPB and postoperative function disappeared. In a recent study, Slogoff et al.[32] found that in the absence of evidence of low cardiac output (e.g., intra-aortic balloon pump [IABP], vasopressor usage), the only factor that correlated with poor postoperative renal function was poor preoperative function.

DRUG REACTIONS

Reactions to drugs are common throughout the scope of medical practice, but at least two types are more common with cardiac surgery.

Heparin-Induced Thrombocytopenia

Heparin-induced thrombocytopenia is a syndrome that results from the development of a heparin-dependent, antiplatelet antibody in a small number of patients exposed to heparin previously, usually after several days of therapy. There seems to be a higher incidence with bovine heparin than with porcine-derived heparin.[57] The antibody causes platelet aggregation and may progress to venous or arterial thromboembolism, disseminated intravascular coagulation (DIC), limb loss, or death. It should be suspected as a cause of continued bleeding in the post-CPB patient. Therapy consists of removal of continued exposure to heparin—usually the invasive pressure line flushing system.

Patients who carry the diagnosis, presenting for reoperation involving CPB, are at risk of re-exposure. The situation is compounded by the disappearance of the antibody in some patients. While extraordinary methods, such as anticoagulation with coumadin or other drugs, have been proposed,[58] short-term heparinization for CPB with no continuing exposure has been successful,[59] including several cases in my experience.

Protamine Reactions

Adverse effects of protamine administered to reverse heparin after CPB have been known since the earliest days of cardiac surgery. Three types are generally known: mild vasodilation related to histamine release, an immunologically mediated anaphylactic or anaphylactoid reaction in those patients with a prior exposure to protamine, and a syndrome of catastrophic pulmonary vasoconstriction associated with the heparin-protamine complex that also appears to be immunologically mediated.[60] The first type is common, the second rare, and the third very rare. The last two types often result in significant postoperative problems as a result of the resuscitative methods needed, including vasopressors and IABPs. These latter reactions are associated with noncardiogenic pulmonary edema, although this relationship is tenuous.

Another type of "reaction" associated with protamine is termed the "innocent bystander syndrome." This occurs in coronary bypass patients in whom it is impossible to perform a technically adequate graft and in whom the graft remains patent secondary to heparinization. Administration of protamine results in coagulation, myocardial ischemia, and cardiovascular collapse. Good documentation of this is lacking, although a similar mechanism has been proposed for patients receiving aprotinin.[61]

ASSESSING ADEQUACY OF PERFUSION

Adequate perfusion during CPB is the ultimate goal of every cardiovascular surgical team. Monitoring for adequate perfusion is not as easy as in the intact patient, as the usual signs of inadequate perfusion, especially the pressure-flow relationship, are uncoupled with modern hemodilution techniques.

Standard flow rates of $50 \text{ ml} \cdot \text{kg}^{-1} \cdot \text{min}^{-1}$ or $2 \text{ L} \cdot \text{m}^{-2} \cdot \text{min}^{-1}$ are a tested reference (as modified by the patient's age, weight, and hypothermia), but monitoring of perfusion-sensitive organs is the most reliable method. The brain and the kidneys are the organs most sensitive to inadequate flow. They are also the most easy to monitor: the electroencephalograph (EEG) can monitor global cerebral function, and urine output shows adequate perfusion of the kidneys, although the absence of urine output does not necessarily mean poor perfusion. Global monitoring includes arterial blood gases to examine oxygenator function, mixed venous gases can indicate adequate perfusion, although they do not ensure adequate regional perfusion.

REFERENCES

1. Gravlee G, Davis RF, Utley JR (eds): Cardiopulmonary Bypass: Principles and Practice, Williams & Wilkins, Baltimore, 1993
2. Cooley DA: Development of the roller pump for use in the cardiopulmonary bypass circuit. Tex Heart Inst J 13:114, 1987
3. Palsinelli WA, Levy DE, Sigsbee B et al: Increased damage after ischemic stroke in patients with hyperglycemia with or without established diabetic mellitus. Am J Med 74:540, 1983
4. Metz S, Keats AS: Benefits of a glucose-containing priming solution for cardiopulmonary bypass. Anesth Analg 72:428, 1991
5. Gordon RJ, Ravin MB, Daicoff GR: Blood rheology. p. 27. In Cardiovascular Physiology for Anesthesiologists. Charles C Thomas, Gordon R et al (eds): Springfield, IL, 1979
6. Merrill EW: Rheology of blood. Physiol Rev 49:863, 1969
7. Gordon RJ, Ravin MB, Rawitscher RE et al: Changes in arterial pressure, viscosity and resistance during cardiopulmonary bypass. J Thorac Cardiovasc Surg 69:552, 1975
8. Messmer K: Hemodilution. Surg Clin North Am 55:659, 1975
9. Laver MB, Buckley MJ: Extreme hemodilution in the surgical patient. p. 215. In Messmer K, Schmid-Schoenbein H (eds): Hemodilution. Theoretical Basis and Clinical Application. S Karger, Basel, 1972
10. LeVein HH, Ip M, Ahmed N et al: Lowering

blood viscosity to overcome vascular resistance. Surg Gynecol Obstet 150:139, 1980

11. Guyton AC, Richardson TQ: Effect of hematocrit on venous return. Circ Res 9:157, 1961

12. Race D, Dedichen H, Schenk WG: Regional blood flow during dextran-induced normovolemic hemodilution in the dog. J Thorac Cardiovasc Surg 53:578, 1967

13. Lundar T, Froysaker T, Lindegaard K et al: Some observations on cerebral perfusion during cardiopulmonary bypass. Ann Thorac Surg 39:381, 1985

14. Brazier J, Cooper N, Maloney JV et al: The adequacy of myocardial oxygen delivery in acute normovolemic anemia. Surgery 75:508, 1974

15. Cooper JR: Perioperative considerations in Jehovah's Witnesses. Int Anesthesiol Clin 28:210, 1990

16. Hagl S, Heimisch W, Meisner H et al: The effect of hemodilution on regional myocardial function in the presence of coronary stenosis. Basic Res Cardiol 72:344, 1977

17. Milam JD, Austin SF, Nihill MR et al: Use of sufficient hemodilution to prevent coagulopathies following surgical correction of cyanotic heart disease. J Thorac Cardiovasc Surg 89:623, 1985

18. Gibbon JH: Application of a mechanical heart and lung apparatus to cardiac surgery. Minn Med 37:171, 1954

19. Kirklin JW, Donald DE, Harshbarger HG et al: Studies in extracorporeal circulation. I. Application of Gibbon type pump oxygenator to human intracardiac surgery: 40 cases. Am Surg 144:2, 1956

20. DeWall RA, Lillehei RC, Sellers RD: Hemodilution perfusions for open heart surgery. N Engl J Med 266:1078, 1962

21. Lillehei CW, Cohen M, Warden HE et al: The results of direct vision closure of ventricular septal defects in eight patients by means of controlled cross circulation. Surg Gynecol Obstet 101:447, 1955

22. Cohen M, Lillehei CW: A quantitative study of the "azygos factor" during vena caval occlusion in the dog. Surg Gynecol Obstet 98:225, 1954

23. Green AE, Carey JM, Zuhdi N: Hemodilution principle of hypothermic perfusion. A concept of obviating blood priming. J Thorac Cardiovasc Surg 43:640, 1962

24. Cooley DA, Beall AC, Grondin P: Open heart operations with disposable oxygenators, 5 percent dextrose prime, and normothermia. Surgery 52:713, 1962

25. Bhat JG, Gluck MC, Lowenstein J et al: Renal failure after open heart surgery. Ann Intern Med 84:677, 1976

26. Tilney NL, Hester WJ: Physiologic and histologic changes in the lung of patients dying after prolonged cardiopulmonary bypass: an inquiry into the nature of post perfusion lung. Ann Surg 166:759, 1967

27. Stockard JJ, Bickford RG, Schauble JF: Pressure dependent cerebral ischemia during cardiopulmonary bypass. Neurology 23:521, 1972

28. Kolkka R, Hilberman M: Neurologic dysfunction following cardiac operation with low flow, low pressure cardiopulmonary bypass. J Thorac Cardiovasc Surg 79:432, 1980

29. Aren C, Blomstrand C, Wikkelso C: Hypotension induced by prostacyclin treatment during cardiopulmonary bypass does not increase the risk of cerebral complications. J Thorac Cardiovasc Surg 88:748, 1984

30. Slogoff S, Girgis KZ, Keats AS: Etiologic factors in neuropsychiatric complications associated with cardiopulmonary bypass. Anesth Analg 61:903, 1982

31. Abel RM, Buckley MJ, Austen WG et al: Acute postoperative renal failure in cardiac surgical patients. Surg Res 20:341, 1976

32. Slogoff S, Reul G, Keats AS et al: Role of perfusion pressure and flow in major organ dysfunction after cardiopulmonary bypass. Ann Thorac Surg 50:911, 1990

33. White FN: A comparative physiological approach to hypothermia. J Thorac Cardiovasc Surg 82:821, 1981

34. Bashein G, Townes BD, Nessley ML et al: A randomized study of carbon dioxide management during hypothermic cardiopulmonary bypass. Anesthesiology 72:7, 1990

35. Aoki M, Nomura F, Stromski ME et al: Effects of pH on brain energetics after hypothermic circulatory arrest. Ann Thorac Surg 55:1093, 1993

36. Jonas RA, Bellinger DC, Rappaport LA et al: Relation of pH strategy and developmental outcome after hypothermic circulatory arrest. J Thorac Cardiovasc Surg 106:362, 1993

37. Hickey PR, Buckley MJ, Philbin DM: Pulsatile and nonpulsatile cardiopulmonary bypass: re-

view of a counterproductive controversy. Ann Thorac Surg 36:720, 1983

38. Miholic J, Hiertz H, Hudec M et al: Fever, leukocytosis and infection after open heart surgery. A log-linear regression analysis of 115 cases. J Thorac Cardiovasc Surg 32:45, 1984

39. Chenoweth DE, Cooper SW, Hugle TE et al: Compliment activation during cardiopulmonary bypass. N Engl J Med 304:497, 1981

40. Westaby S: Compliment and the damaging effects of cardiopulmonary bypass. Thorax 38: 321, 1983

41. Kirklin JK: The post perfusion syndrome: inflammation and the damaging effects of cardiopulmonary bypass. In Tinker JH (ed): Cardiopulmonary Bypass: Current Concepts and Controversies. WB Saunders, Philadelphia, 1989

42. Markowitz A, Faist E, Lang S et al: Successful restoration of cell mediated immune response after cardiopulmonary bypass by immunomodulation. J Thorac Cardiovasc Surg 105:15, 1993

43. Kirklin JK, George JF, Holman W: The inflammatory response to cardiopulmonary bypass. p. 223 In Gravlee G, Davis RF, Utley JR (eds): Cardiopulmonary Bypass: Principles and Practice, Williams & Wilkins, Baltimore, 1993

44. Clifford A, Thomas S, Spenser F: Fulminating noncardiogenic pulmonary edema. J Thorac Cardiovasc Surg 80:868, 1980

45. Matthay MA, Wiener-Kronish JP: Respiratory management after cardiac surgery. Chest 95: 424, 1989

46. Schell RM, Kern FH, Greeley WJ et al: Cerebral blood flow and metabolism during cardiopulmonary bypass. Anesth Analg 76:849, 1993

47. Brusino FG, Reves JG, Smith LR et al: The effect of age on cerebral blood flow during hypothermic cardiopulmonary bypass. J Thorac Cardiovasc Surg 97:541, 1989

48. Croughwell N, Lyth M, Quill T et al: Diabetic patients have abnormal autoregulation during cardiopulmonary bypass. Circulation, suppl IV. 82:407, 1990

49. Wareng TH, Davila-Roman VG, Barzilai B et al: Management of the severely atheroscle-

rotic ascending aorta during cardiac operations. J Thorac Cardiovasc Surg 103:453, 1992

50. Nussmeier NA, Arlund C, Slogoff S: Neuropsychiatric complications after cardiopulmonary bypass, cerebral protection by a barbiturate. Anesthesiology 64:165, 1986

51. Johnsson P, Algotsson L, Ryding E et al: Cardiopulmonary perfusion and cerebral blood flow in bilateral carotid artery disease. Ann Thorac Surg 51:579, 1991

52. Melrose DG, Dreyer B, Bentall HH et al: Elective cardiac arrest. Lancet 2:21, 1955

53. Burgess GE, Cooper JR, Marino RJ et al: Pulmonary effects of pleurotomy during and after coronary artery bypass with internal mammary artery versus saphenous vein grafts. J Thorac Cardiovasc Surg 76:230, 1978

54. Hammerschmidt DE, Jacob HS: Adverse pulmonary reactions to transfusion. Adv Med 27: 511, 1982

55. Solis RT, Gibbs MB: Filtration of the microaggregates in stored blood. Transfusion 12:245, 1972

56. Kuntschen F, Galletti PM, Hahn C: Glucose insulin interactions during cardiopulmonary bypass. Hypothermia versus normothermia. J Thorac Cardiovasc Surg 91:451, 1986

57. Bell WR, Royall RM: Heparin induced thrombocytopenia: comparison of three heparin preparations. N Engl J Med 303:902, 1980

58. Kappa JR, Fisher CA, Todd B et al: Intraoperative management of patients with heparin-induced thrombocytopenia. Ann Thorac Surg 49:714, 1990

59. Olinger GN, Hussey CV, Olive JA et al: Cardiopulmonary bypass for patients with previously documented heparin induced platelet aggregation. J Thorac Cardiovasc Surg 87:673, 1984

60. Morel DR, Zapol WM, Thomas SR et al: C5a and thromboxane generation associated with pulmonary vaso and bronchoconstriction during protamine reversal of heparin. Anesthesiology 66:597, 1987

61. Cosgrove DM, Heric B, Lytle BW et al: Aprotinin therapy for reoperative myocardial revascularization: a placebo-controlled study. Ann Thorac Surg 54:1031, 1992

62. Reed CC, Stafford T: Cardiopulmonary Perfusion. 2nd Ed. Texas Medical Press, Houston, 1985

6

Ventilatory Management

Gregory Kerr
Stephen J. Thomas

Controlled mechanical ventilation for cardiac surgery patients became widespread in the 1960s when it was recognized that it promoted a smoother, more stable recovery.[1] Although advances have been made in ventilatory management, no one method has been determined to be "the best." Debate now centers on "late" versus "early" extubation, on ideal methods to treat poor oxygenation, and on the smoothest way to "wean" or separate a patient from mechanical ventilation. Factors particular to cardiac surgery that affect postoperative ventilatory management include the following:

Type of anesthesia delivered
Systemic hypothermia of varying degrees
Alterations in hemostasis
Blood and fluid volume shifts
Hemodynamic instability

In the past, patients undergoing surgery requiring cardiopulmonary bypass (CPB) typically received large doses of opiates and hypnotics as their main anesthetic. This was initially developed to facilitate prolonged mechanical ventilation. Conversely, some institutions continue to favor inhalation-based anesthesia, which allows for relatively early awakening and therefore relatively early extubation. Currently, the tide is turning toward techniques that foster earlier awakening and extubation. The rationale for this appears to be partly physiologic but predominantly economic.

These patients often undergo bypass with systemic hypothermia. Consequently, there is a very real concern of "afterdrop" in body temperature following separation from CPB. The traditional methods of keeping patients warm during surgery may not be as effective in these patients. Hypothermic patients are likely to be weaker in the postoperative period, making early extubation more difficult.[2]

Other problems include the large volume of fluid administered intraoperatively, postoperative bleeding and associated coagulopathies, as well as the hemodynamic instability and cardiac depression often present. All these issues must be taken into consideration during ventilatory management.

Postoperative ventilatory management attempts to preserve or improve pulmonary gas exchange and oxygenation. Adequate ventilation must be maintained and respiratory acidosis and its associated problems avoided. In the cardiac patient, in whom oxygen consumption is of the utmost concern, unnecessary increases in the work of breathing (WOB) and the associated oxygen costs must be avoided. These objectives must be met while preserving the function of other organ systems, yet preventing or avoiding pulmonary complications.

EFFECT OF CARDIOPULMONARY BYPASS ON PULMONARY FUNCTION

Cardiopulmonary bypass has itself been implicated in numerous changes that occur during the postoperative period. The changes can be such that the alveolar-arterial gradient may not return to normal for at least 7 days.[3] Studies have shown that a pulmonary inflammatory response has been associated with leukocytosis, fever, and the release of chemical mediators following CPB.[4] Alterations in renal and neurologic function have also been demonstrated. The mechanism for this phenomenon is unclear, but it appears to be related to complement activation, platelet aggregation and the effects of fibrinolysis resulting from exposure of blood to nonendothelial surfaces.[5–7] Biopsy and autopsy specimens have exhibited significant morphologic changes, revealing diffuse congestion with intra-alveolar and interstitial edema, as well as hemorrhagic atelectasis.[8]

Following CPB, lung compliance decreases,[9–11] resulting in an increase in peak airway pressures. An increase in both airway resistance and the work of breathing following CPB has also been demonstrated.[3,4] Clearly, one of the goals in managing these patients is to determine the etiology of the change in lung compliance and then to improve it, as well as the airway resistance.

It is well known that many cardiac patients develop atelectasis in the immediate postoperative period due either to manipulation of the lungs during surgery or to the presence of pleural effusions. Cardiac patients who have undergone coronary revascularization using the internal mammary arteries are particularly susceptible to these pulmonary problems.[12] When a patient develops an acute effusion during the immediate postoperative period, it is most likely secondary to bleeding, which may or may not be self-limited. This results in variable decreases in lung volume. General anesthesia alone can reduce functional residual capacity (FRC) as much as 20 percent.[4] This reduction may be due to the cephalad shifting of the diaphragm, which appears to be due to loss of tonic activity of the muscle.[13] The decrease in FRC as well as the ventilation-perfusion mismatch created by the atelectasis can result in a hypoxic state.

The decreased production of surfactant has been suggested as another possible cause for atelectasis in this group of patients. One theory suggests that an inadequate blood supply to the alveolar epithelium causes a reduction in the amount of surfactant released from type 2 alveolar epithelial cells.[4] Exposure of surfactant to plasma from normal adults has also been shown to inhibit its action.[14] Decreased surfactant production and function may also be related to hypothermia experienced during CPB.[15]

It had been speculated that phrenic nerve injury could in part explain the development of atelectasis. However, a prospective study by Markand et al.[16] failed to demonstrate a significant number of patients with phrenic nerve dysfunction.

Hachenberg et al.,[17] using a multiple inert gas technique, attempted to isolate and quantify the individual effects of intrapulmonary shunting, ventilation-perfusion mismatch, and low mixed venous oxygen tension on arterial oxygenation during cardiac surgery. These investigators found that gas exchange impairment was primarily due to intrapulmonary shunting, which was exacerbated by extracorporeal circulation. They also concluded that decreased cardiac output possibly contributed to perioperative hypoxemia.[17] Interestingly, one study suggested that the depression in cardiac output accompanying therapeutic interventions may be a significant factor leading to the decreases in intrapulmonary shunting seen during the treatment of adult respiratory disease syndrome (ARDS).[18]

Generally, overt respiratory failure during the postoperative period is not common, although there may be a slight deterioration in pulmonary function. Many reasons exist for both to occur, postoperative care must therefore take into consideration preventive care:

Atelectasis
Pulmonary edema
COPD exacerbation
Respiratory depressants
Neurologic injury
Cardiac dysfunction
Diaphragmatic dysfunction
Pain
Effusions
Pneumothorax
Mucous plugging

THE IMMEDIATE POSTOPERATIVE PERIOD: TRANSPORT TO AND ARRIVAL IN THE INTENSIVE CARE UNIT

Postoperative ventilatory management commences during transport to the intensive care unit (ICU). A problem often encountered upon arrival into the ICU is a widening of the alveolar-arterial oxygen gradient relative to that in the operating room. Adequate FiO_2, tidal volume, and positive end-expiratory pressure (PEEP) if necessary (e.g., if needed in the operating room) are therefore required during transport.

Upon arrival into the ICU, all routine monitors, including the pulse oximeter, should be sequentially connected. Meanwhile, the patient is attached to the mechanical ventilator. Typical ventilator settings are an FiO_2 of 70 to 100 percent, a tidal volume of 12 to 15,

$ml^{-1} \cdot kg^{-1}$, an intermittent mandatory ventilation (IMV) rate of 10, PEEP of 5, and pressure support of 5. After the endotracheal tube is attached to the ventilator, the patient's chest should be auscultated to ensure that both lungs are being well ventilated. Auscultation of the chest after arrival to the ICU is important, as it is not uncommon for mucous plugging, atelectasis, or endobrochial intubation to occur during transport. Chest radiographs are usually obtained in the immediate postoperative period to help detect these problems as well as the development of effusions and pneumothoraces.

Bergman[19] suggested that tidal volumes two to three times greater than the patient's predicted tidal volume can be safely administered without experiencing clinically important increases in the mean inspiratory airway pressure. The advantages of large tidal volumes include compensation for the increased deadspace ventilation that accompanies positive-pressure ventilation (PPV) and reduction in the amount of atelectasis seen with smaller tidal volumes.[20] Larger tidal volumes also allow lower respiratory rates. It is possible that these large tidal volumes can produce alveolar overdistension, which in turn can cause endothelial, epithelial, and basement membrane injuries. The result is an increase in microvascular permeability and lung rupture.[21]

Reduced respiratory rates have two advantages: the ensuing longer exhalation time often improves ventilation in patients with increased airway resistance, and reduction in the mean intrathoracic pressure has been associated with improved hemodynamics. An increase in alveolar pressure can develop when there is inadequate time for exhalation. This increase in pressure is often referred to as "auto-PEEP," the trapping (or "stacking") of gas in the alveoli, most frequently seen in patients with chronic obstructive pulmonary disease (COPD). Patients developing a significant amount of auto-PEEP may have difficulty initiating a ventilatory cycle because in order to do so the patient would have to create a negative pressure equal to the level of auto-PEEP. In relaxed patients, the amount of auto-PEEP is indicated on the ventilator's manometer when the expiratory port of the circuit is occluded at end exhalation.[22]

Hypoxemia is a concern that often presents early, and even during transport, as a result of treatment of hypertension in the postoperative period. Antihypertensive agents such as sodium nitroprusside, nitroglycerin, and the inhalation anesthetics inhibit hypoxic pulmonary vasoconstriction (HPV). Interfering with HPV can increase the alveolar-arterial gradient by creating ventilation-perfusion mismatch.[23,24] Studies have demonstrated that small residual levels of inhalation anesthetics affect venous admixture, resulting in postoperative hypoxemia.[25] This problem is more prevalent in patients with a history of chronic pulmonary disease.[24]

Although patients are rewarmed on CPB, it is not uncommon for the postoperative patient to arrive in the ICU with core temperatures in the range of 34° to 35°C,[26,27] followed by a period of warming in the range of 38° to 40°C (Fig. 6-1). Sladen[26] observed the response to ventilation of 73 patients with these changes in temperature. He noted that rewarming after hypothermic cardiopulmonary bypass is a consistent feature in the ICU. Also of note in this study was the fact that an acute respiratory acidosis occurred in 42 percent of patients during rewarming. This study emphasizes the importance of close carbon dioxide monitoring during this period following surgery.

VENTILATORY MODALITIES

A gamut of ventilatory patterns is available, each attempting to decrease the amount of work needed for breathing, to decrease the

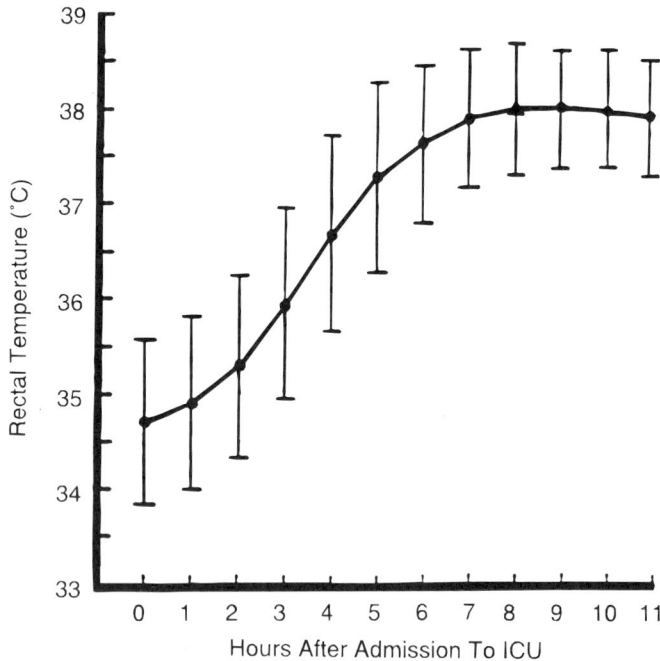

Fig. 6-1. Rectal temperature after admission to the ICU. Patients are admitted to the ICU cold (mean 34.7°C) and rewarmed to a mean of 38.3°C. Rewarming is completed by 8 hours after admission, but the most rapid rate of rewarming occurs 2 to 4 hours after admission. After 8 hours, temperature tends to settle back toward normal. Each point represents the mean rectal temperature $\pm$ SD. (From Sladen,[26] with permission.)

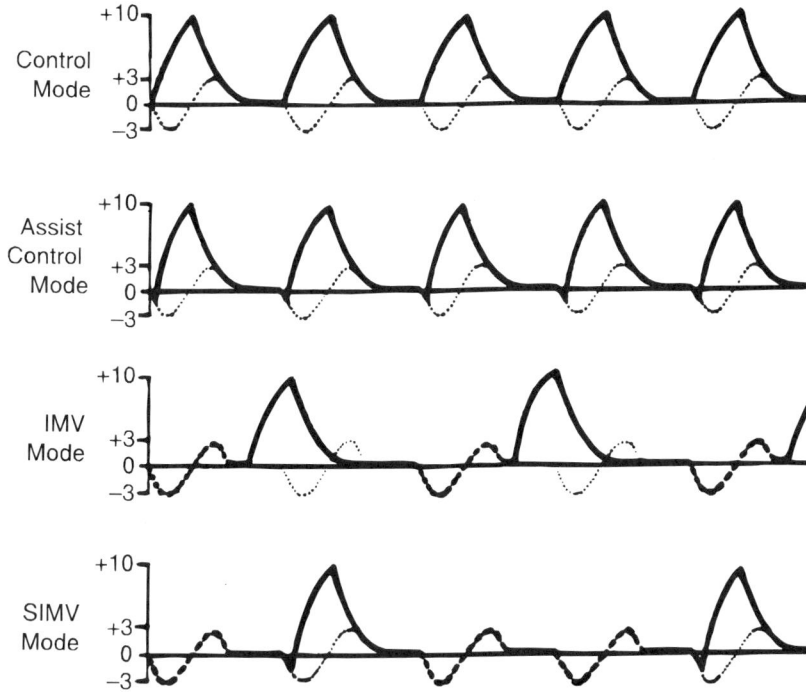

Fig. 6-2. Airway pressure tracings of the four standard volume preset modes. Thick solid lines represent ventilator breaths; thick dotted lines represent spontaneous breaths. Thin dotted lines indicate what the spontaneous pattern would have been without the ventilator breaths. (From Shapiro et al.,[117] with permission.)

amount of respiratory muscle atrophy, or to ease separation from mechanical ventilatory support (Fig. 6-2).

Control Mode Ventilation

Control mode ventilation (CMV) is rarely used today. In this mode, the ventilator delivers either a preset volume regardless of pressure generated (to an upper limit) or a variable volume according to a preselected pressure limit at a fixed rate. Historically, the resistance in the ventilator circuitry was great, requiring the patient to generate significant negative inspiratory pressure in order to breathe spontaneously. It was therefore necessary to paralyze the patient to avoid the increased WOB. Although a relatively simple mode of ventilation, CMV does not allow the patient to exercise the muscles of respiration,

making weaning from the ventilator more difficult.

Assist Control Ventilation

Assist control ventilation (A/C) has become popular in many critical care units. This mode allows the patient to breathe spontaneously and initiate a mechanical breath, enabling the patient to control minute ventilation above a preset minimum value. Each breath creates a negative inspiratory pressure, which activates the ventilator to deliver a set volume or pressure. When the patient's spontaneous respiratory rate drops below the preset backup rate, the machine automatically begins a respiratory cycle. The ventilator will continue to deliver controlled ventilation until the patient's own rate surpasses the preset minimum rate. In this way, the A/C mode allows the patient to use the muscles of respiration, while providing mechanical support when necessary.

Intermittent Mandatory Ventilation

IMV is a modality that competes with A/C in popularity. During the early 1950s, the development of the Engstrom ventilator made it possible for the patient to breathe spontaneously above the rate at which a ventilator was set.[28] During the 1960s, Emerson developed a volume limited ventilator that allowed the patient to breathe between the mechanical breaths of the ventilator. Following these developments, in 1973, Downs et al.[29] described IMV in which the patient receives a preset volume or volume determined by preset pressure limits at a preset rate. The innovation was that, while on IMV, a patient is able to breathe spontaneously, but generation of negative inspiratory pressure does not initiate a mechanical breath. Like A/C, IMV is a commonly used method for weaning patients from the ventilator. IMV improves intrapulmonary gas distribution, helps prevent muscle atrophy, and decreases the amount of sedation needed.[30] The effects of IMV on cardiac function are controversial. Some investigators suggest that spontaneous respiration during IMV lessens the deleterious effects of mechanical ventilation[31]; others report no difference.[32] Although its initial popularity was a result of its usefulness in the weaning process, today it is used for full ventilatory support as well. Interestingly, in a study by Tomlinson et al.[51] comparing weaning from T-piece trials versus IMV, no appreciable difference was found in the duration of weaning from the ventilator. Also, the data supporting the use of IMV over A/C are negligible.

Although the term IMV is frequently interchanged with SIMV (synchronized IMV), the two must be differentiated. IMV is essentially a CMV mode that allows the patient to take spontaneous breaths. Between mechanical breaths, the ventilator circuit is open allowing for the continuous flow of fresh gas. Mechanical breaths are delivered at a regular interval independent of the patient's own spontaneous respiratory pattern.

In 1976, Sahn and Lakshminarayan[33] were concerned that a mandatory mechanical breath simultaneous with a spontaneous inspiration might cause "stacking" of breaths or overdistension of the lungs. Therefore, SIMV was developed to avoid this problem; it is essentially A/C that allows for spontaneous respirations. Again, mechanical breaths are set for a specific time interval. Between the mechanical breaths, the patient is allowed to breathe spontaneously. Prior to the mechanical breath, the ventilator is designated to wait a predetermined "trigger period." Any spontaneous breath that occurs during this period will initiate the full predetermined breath. The ventilator will automatically give a full unassisted breath if no spontaneous breath is sensed during this period. A study by Heenan et al.[34] did not show any improvements in hemodynamics or reduced incidence of barotrauma in a comparison of IMV, with SIMV.[34]

Positive End-Expiratory Pressure

PEEP is a setting used to maintain alveolar patency and FRC, as well as redistribute extravascular lung water. PEEP has consistently been shown to have a favorable effect on the relationship between closing volume and FRC in various patient populations. However, assertions that PEEP decreases extravascular lung water have not been supported.[35,36] Nevertheless, it has been shown to redistribute water so as to improve oxygen diffusion across the alveolar-capillary membrane. It should be noted that in some reports "lung water" actually increased with PEEP.[37] Since there have been suggestions that noncardiogenic pulmonary edema may develop during procedures that require cardiopulmonary bypass as a result of white blood cell and platelet aggregation,[38] PEEP would appear to be appropriate when impairment of oxygenation is likely due to excess extravascular water.

Hypoxemia may develop whenever perfusion exceeds ventilation, so that blood leaving the alveolus has a lower oxygen content than blood leaving a well-matched alveolar capillary unit. When a low ventilation-to-perfusion ratio is present, hypoxemia is responsive to increasing the delivered oxygen concentration, since this increases alveolar PO_2. When hypoxemia is the result of true shunt (ventilation-to-perfusion ratio equal to zero), as with alveolar collapse, the administration of PEEP and PPV recruits these alveoli, increasing compliance and FRC. Downs and Mitchell[39] showed that PEEP was more effective than mechanical ventilation in maintaining near-normal functional expiratory lung volume and that PEEP may be indicated in the absence of significant pulmonary shunting or hypoxemia for patients with decreased expiratory lung volume.

PEEP has a complex effect on cardiovascular function. It is usually associated with a decrease in cardiac output, which appears to be the result of many interacting factors. In 1948, Cournand et al.[40] described the negative effect of positive pressure on venous return to the right side of the heart. Subsequent studies have supported the fact that the ability of PEEP to decrease venous return is probably the most important factor associated with decrease in cardiac output.[41] Increased levels of PEEP (as well as increased tidal volume) can be deleterious to right-sided cardiac output, as it increases pulmonary vascular resistance. This in turn can cause some degree of right-sided heart failure. The ensuing increase in right ventricular afterload also appears to cause a leftward shift of the intraventricular septum. This could cause the left ventricle to become less compliant, thereby limiting preload and decreasing cardiac output.[17]

Since high levels of PEEP (i.e., greater than 10 mmHg) may interfere with cardiac output, it is important to administer PEEP in such a way that it does not interfere with oxygen delivery. It is common practice to place most patients on 5 cmH_2O PEEP upon their arrival into the ICU and to increase PEEP incrementally if higher levels are desired. Hudson[42] recommends that PEEP be adjusted as follows: PEEP is the only variable being changed, stepwise increments of 3 to 5 cmH_2O are to be used, the time interval between changes should be minimized (e.g., 20 minutes), and the response to each change should be appropriately evaluated (i.e., cardiac output, mixed venous oxygen levels, PaO_2). The clinician should always be aware that if higher PEEP results in a deterioration in cardiac output, the use of inotropic support or increase in fluid volume should be considered to allow for continued administration of PEEP.

It has been suggested that PEEP be used to decrease bleeding in the postoperative cardiac patient, as it may act as a "venous pressure dressing."[43] More recent studies reveal data that do not support a decreased incidence of bleeding and subsequent transfusions in patients when PEEP is used.[44,45] It appears that PEEP is acceptable for postoperative bleeding as long as there is no hemodynamic compromise.

At the New York Hospital-Cornell Medical Center, patients are placed on 5 cmH_2O of continuous positive airway pressure (CPAP) prior to extubation. During CPAP, the patient's airway pressure remains above atmospheric pressure during inspiration and expiration with spontaneous breathing. Pressure support ventilation (PSV) may be used concomitantly to facilitate the weaning process. CPAP may also be administered by mask to extubated patients in circumstances in which the patient's clinical state might be improved with positive airway pressure. Since CPAP is in fact PEEP applied during spontaneous ventilation, its physiologic effects are similar to that of PEEP.

Pressure Support Ventilation

PSV has also become popular recently. The ventilator-dependent patient expends respiratory effort to breathe through the breathing circuit and its various attachments.[46,47] With the popularity of ventilation patterns that allow the patient to breathe spontaneously, the use of PSV as an adjuvant modality enables the patient to expend less energy to breathe, preventing respiratory fatigue. This is accomplished by delivering a certain preset pressure to the patient upon each spontaneous inspiration (Fig. 6-3). The ventilator is triggered upon inspiration to deliver this positive pressure continuously until the gas flow drops. By reducing fatigue, PSV should make weaning more comfortable.

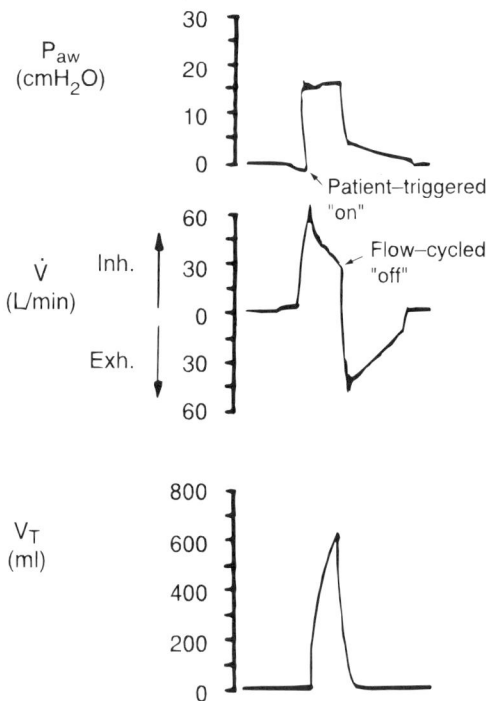

Fig. 6-3. Airway pressure (P_{aw}), flow rate ($\dot{V}$), and V_T tracings of pressure support ventilation (e.g., 15 cm H_2O). The ventilator is patient-triggered "on," and as long as inspiratory effort is maintained, airway pressure stays constant with a variable flow rate of gas from the ventilator. The ventilator cycles "off" when the patient's inspiratory flow rate demand decreases to a predetermined percentage of the peak inspiratory flow rate (i.e., the ventilator is flow-cycled "off"). (From Perel and Stock,[118] with permission.)

With a sufficiently high pressure support value, a patient should experience an increase in spontaneous tidal volumes, as well as a decrease in respiratory rate. MacIntyre[47] showed that PSV improved the patient's comfort of breathing compared with SIMV alone. He indicates that PSV be used on patients receiving full ventilatory support in order to improve gas exchange and recondition ventilatory muscles.

T-Piece

The T-piece has been used during the weaning process for some time. The basic design consists of an adapter in the shape of a T, which is attached to the endotracheal tube. One "limb" of the adapter is attached to an oxygen source that delivers a constant flow of oxygen. Upon inspiration, this fresh gas is delivered to the patient as well as some of the gas in the opposite (unattached) "limb." Upon expiration, the fresh gas as well as the gases being exhaled by the patient are allowed to escape through the unattached "limb." The T-piece allows the patient to breathe spontaneously through the endotracheal tube without PPS. Shapiro et al.[48] and Bolder et al.[49] and others have demonstrated the increased WOB associated with the presence of an endotracheal tube. They also noted the importance of the size and physical nature of the tube as factors that affect the work of breathing. A study by Brochard et al.[50] demonstrated that with an endotracheal tube in place, WOB is 27 percent greater than after extubation. It was further demonstrated that PSV effectively compensated for the increased WOB associated with the presence of an endotracheal tube. The aforementioned data imply that patients increase their WOB when they are placed on a T-piece, as opposed to a ventilator. However, Tomlinson et al.[51] studied weaning using T-piece trials versus IMV and found no appreciable difference in the timing of the process. It therefore appears that the use of a T-piece is acceptable in selected patients who would not be adversely affected by the increased WOB associated with the T-piece and in patients who would be extubated shortly or maintained on a T-piece for a relatively short period.

LESS CONVENTIONAL MODES OF VENTILATORY SUPPORT

Inverse Ratio Ventilation

Inverse ratio ventilation (IRV) implies that the inspiratory time is greater than the expiratory time during mechanical ventilation. IRV increases the mean airway pressure without increasing the peak inspiratory pressure as seen with other modes of ventilation. This characteristic of IRV allows it to improve oxygenation with minimal effects on cardiovascular function.[62] It is more commonly administered in a pressure-controlled mode, since it is difficult to administer with volume control. By prolonging the inspiratory phase and the time available for oxygen diffusion, oxygenation is improved, while theoretically the incidence of barotrauma is reduced. The longer inspiratory time may also allow for the recruitment of alveoli, while the shortened expiratory time would prevent the alveoli from collapsing. Several earlier case reports showed an improvement in oxygenation when IRV was applied,[53,54] as have more recent studies.[55] IRV is used in many ICUs when oxygenation poses a problem; however, there are insufficient data to prove the superiority of IRV over other ventilatory modes.

Although IRV seems to be a useful tool in certain clinical settings, it must be used cautiously. As the mean airway pressure increases, so does the possibility of air trapping in the alveoli. As stated earlier, the development of "auto-PEEP" can have deleterious effects on hemodynamics as well as ventilation.

High-Frequency Ventilation

High-frequency ventilation (HFV) is a mode of ventilation in which gases are delivered at frequencies of at least four times the normal rate. In 1915, Henderson et al.[56] suggested that patients could be ventilated by using small tidal volumes that still permit the transport of gas to the alveoli. Although the precise mechanism of gas transport is unclear, the combination of convective and diffusive mechanisms appears to play a key role. The mixing of gases due to the mechanical action of the heart against the lung may also be a factor.[57] HFV is typically used in patients who are hypoxic from diffuse lung injury or persistent bronchopleural fistulae when one of the crucial goals is avoiding high peak airway pressures.

Carbon dioxide removal may be problematic in the patient receiving HFV. At low frequencies (i.e., below 200 breaths/minute), $PaCO_2$ is inversely related to frequency and tidal volume. At higher frequencies, carbon dioxide removal is directly related to tidal volume, but not to frequency. Rates greater than 900 breaths/minute may cause air trapping and a subsequent decrease in gas flow. Because of the possibility of overdistending the lungs, HFV is contraindicated in patients with COPD or status asthmaticus. Increasing rates may also compromise hemodynamics.[58]

Airway Pressure-Release Ventilation

Airway pressure-release ventilation (APRV), introduced in 1987,[59] is a modality that has been likened to "variable CPAP." Carbon dioxide elimination occurs by both spontaneous ventilation and intermittent release of CPAP (an upper level of CPAP is selected to provide a mean airway pressure). To eliminate carbon dioxide and other gases, this airway pressure is intermittently released to a lower or zero CPAP level, as outlined earlier (Fig. 6-4 and Table 6-1). Therefore, ventilation is a function of how well the patient breathes spontaneously, as well as the frequency, duration, and pressure difference

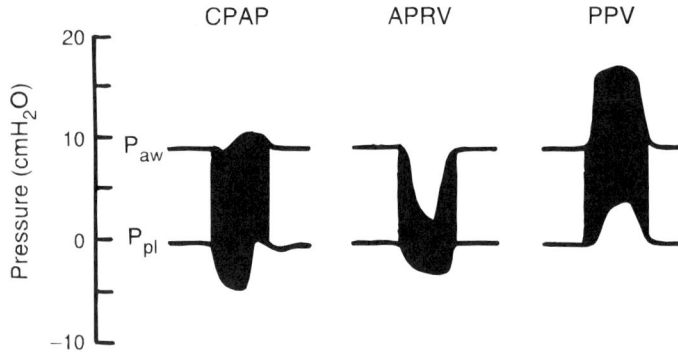

Fig. 6-4. Changes in peak airway pressure (P_{aw}) and intrapleural pressure (P_{pl}) during spontaneous breathing with CPAP, during APRV, and during conventional positive pressure ventilation (PPV). (From Rasanen et al.,[119] with permission.)

of each pressure release.[28] It was developed to decrease the incidence of barotrauma and hemodynamic compromise during mechanical ventilation. Patients with parenchymal lung injury would be most likely to benefit from this ventilatory technique since there is a marked decrease in airway pressure. Garner et al.[60] performed a study of patients who underwent CPB. These investigators showed that APRV, compared with CMV, resulted in similar oxygenation and ventilation with significantly lower peak airway pressures.

COMPLICATIONS OF VENTILATORY MANAGEMENT AND POSITIVE-PRESSURE VENTILATION

The use of PPV is associated with many complications. Studies by Kumar et al.[61] Steier et al.,[62] Petersen et al.,[63] and Gammon et al. suggest that there is a 4 to 20 percent incidence of barotrauma (pneumothorax, pneumomediastinum, or subcutaneous emphysema) with PPV. Conversely, a retrospec-

Table 6-1.   Data From Apneic Humans Receiving APRV and Conventional Ventilation After Cardiac Operations (X ± SD)

Variable	APRV	Conventional Ventilation
Peak P_{aw} (cmH$_2$O)	11 ± 1	32 ± 4[a]
pHa	7.38 ± .04	7.39 ± 0.04
PaCO$_2$ (mmHg)	38 ± 4	36 ± 3
PaO$_2$/FiO$_2$	281 ± 45	263 ± 0.40
(mmHg)	79 ± 16	79 ± 16
HR (beats · min^{-1})	5.2 ± 1.2	5.3 ± 0.9
CO (L · min^{-1})	67 ± 4	63 ± 10
SvO$_2$ (%)		

Abbreviations: P_{aw}, airway pressure; CO, cardiac output; SvO$_2$, mixed-venous oxyhemoglobin saturation; APRV, airway pressure-release ventilation.
 [a] $P < 0.01$ compared to APRV.
(From Perel and Stock,[118] with permission.)

tive study by Cullen and Caidera[64] reviewing the hospital course of 200 critically ill patients, revealed only one patient (0.5 percent incidence) who developed barotrauma. This patient was maintained on high peak airway pressures; other patients who had high peak airway pressures (greater than 40 cmH_2O) did not develop barotrauma. It was concluded that barotrauma secondary to mechanical ventilation with or without PEEP was a rare event.[64] Among later studies, Carlton et al.[65] showed that lung overexpansion increases pulmonary microvascular protein permeability and microvascular disruption in lambs. However, other investigators have refuted this finding.[66] Although it is unclear what the exact incidence of barotrauma is in patients who are being ventilated with positive pressure, it is clear that barotrauma is a complication that does exist and must be recognized.

Particular attention is required in patients with right heart failure, as increases in PEEP or large tidal volumes may increase PVR potentiating right ventricular failure dysfunction. When managing a postoperative patient whose hemodynamics are affected by PEEP, it must be remembered that inotropes, pressors, or fluid should be used as needed to maintain adequate hemodynamics.

The relationship between PPV and renal function is highly complex. Urine volume and sodium excretion appear to decrease as a consequence of changes in cardiovascular function (Fig. 6-5 demonstrates the effects of CMV on renal function). Indirect effects appear as a result of decreased venous return, resulting in a decreased cardiac output due to increased intrapleural pressure seen during mechanical ventilation. Another possible cause for a decrease in cardiac output is alterations in left ventricular distensibility due to PPV. Andrivet et al.[67] demonstrated that PPV with PEEP decreased plasma atrial natriuretic factor (ANF) caused by a reduction in atrial transmural pressure. This decrease in ANF is associated with a drop in urine output and urine sodium excretion. Direct effects are seen on renal perfusion through barore-

ceptors and the antidiuretic hormone (ADH), renin, and sympathetic systems[68] (see Ch. 10). Of note is the fact that although ADH levels are elevated during PPV, there may not be a direct correlation with the decrease in urine volume or free water clearance.[69] Nevertheless, it is important to understand the various factors that may be involved in order to best evaluate a patient's intravascular volume status.

The stress of surgery along with the many clotting derangements that exist in the postoperative period make the cardiac surgical patient a prime candidate for postoperative gastrointestinal bleeding. It has been demonstrated that as many as 40 percent of patients on mechanical ventilation for more than 3 days will develop gastrointestinal bleeding if not treated prohylactically.[70] There appears to be a drop in arterial pressure as well as an increase in venous pressure associated with PPV. The result could be low blood perfusion to the gastrointestinal mucosa, resulting in ischemia and subsequent ulcerations. This reasoning may also explain why ileus is frequently seen in patients who are dependent on mechanical ventilators.

The treating physician must be mindful of the oxygen toxicity associated with delivery of high oxygen concentration (FIO_2) levels.[71] Toxicity appears to be a function of both the dose of oxygen delivered and of the duration of delivery. Toxic oxygen metabolites are produced intracellularly throughout the body. Although most oxygen is reduced to water in the mitochondria,[72] some is metabolized to the superoxide anion (O_2^-), hydrogen peroxide, and reactive hydroxyl radicals.[73] Tissue damage results when the amount of metabolites produced exceeds the amount consumed. It appears that the metabolites are highly reactive and destroy intracellular components by oxidation and reduction reactions.[74] Injury most commonly involves the lungs, eyes, and central nervous system.[75] The most frequent manifestations of oxygen toxicity include pulmonary infiltrates, gas-exchange abnormalities, decreased tra-

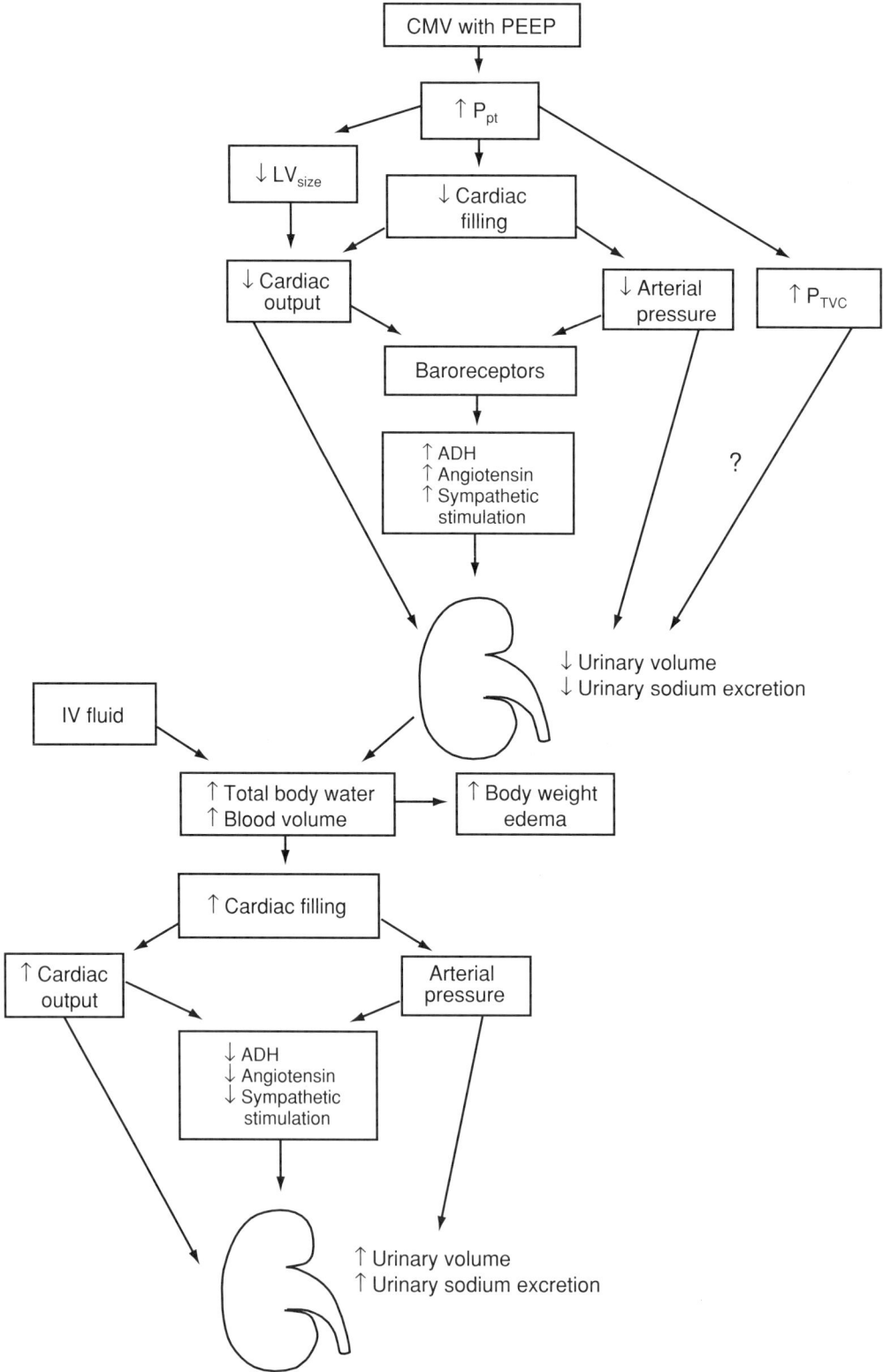

cheal mucous velocity, rales, tracheobronchitis, dyspnea, and pulmonary edema. It is unclear how much oxygen exposure results in pulmonary damage because of the difficulty distinguishing oxygen toxicity from the underlying disease for which the oxygen is being administered.[86] Generally, it is best to decrease the FIO_2 to 60 percent or below at the earliest possibility.

Oxygen concentration can be very important during the weaning process, especially in patients with COPD. The respiratory drive in these patients is exquisitely sensitive to peripheral chemoreceptors. The possibility exists for respiratory depression if the concentration of oxygen administered is excessively high.[76] It is therefore critical to be aware of carbon dioxide retention during the weaning process in patients who are not as dependent on it for their respiratory drive.

Pulmonary infection is associated primarily with mechanical ventilation and not with PPV. However, this problem may be a result not only of the effects of mechanical ventilation, but of the underlying disease state.[77]

RESPIRATORY DILEMMAS DURING THE POSTOPERATIVE PERIOD

Pulmonary edema is a common problem that must be managed during the postoperative period. The most common cause appears to be high pressure in the pulmonary microcirculation from elevated pressures in the left heart[78] due to valvular dysfunction, left ventricular dysfunction, or high intravascular fluid volume. Poor ventricular function may be secondary to incomplete surgical repair and/or ischemia or from a "stunned" myocardium that may last for a brief period after the operation[79] (see Ch. 7). Patients frequently require inotropic support until cardiac function returns to satisfactory levels. At the New York Hospital-Cornell Medical Center, most patients will receive a diuretic less than 24 hours after surgery, to help prevent the development of pulmonary edema. If the patient has developed pulmonary edema, extubation should be avoided until the edema has been adequately treated. The ventilator will assume the WOB while decreasing the preload to the heart. The clinician should consider echocardiography as part of the evaluation for pulmonary edema.

COPD is the most common cause of preoperative pulmonary dysfunction in cardiac surgical patients.[4] It is not uncommon for a patient to suffer from COPD-related symptoms such as bronchospasm during the postoperative period. It is therefore important to recognize these problems and be able to treat them as they arise. Many of these patients receive β_2-agonists administered by inhalation, not only for acute exacerbations, but also as part of their routine postoperative pulmonary care regimen. They have a rapid onset of action with minimal cardiovascular effects and are effective bronchodilators.[80] They have also been shown to help in mucociliary transport, helping to clear patients' secretions.[51] As a result, they have become the mainstay of treatment for patients with COPD during the postoperative period.

When patients do not respond readily to β_2-agonists, theophylline is often considered. Benefits of theophylline administration include relaxation of bronchial muscles,[81] decrease of pulmonary artery pressure,[82] improvement of right ventricular stroke

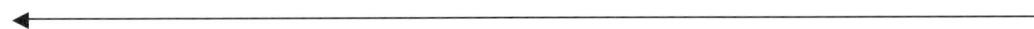

Fig. 6-5. Cardiovascular and hormonal changes affecting renal function during CMV with PEEP. The upper portion of the diagram indicates mechanisms by which CMV with PEEP leads to decreased urinary output and sodium excretion. The question mark indicates that there are data suggesting that increased P_{TVC} does not have direct renal effects. The lower portion proposes a mechanism whereby retention of water with sodium increases blood volume to restore renal function during prolonged mechanical ventilation. (From Berry,[120] with permission.)

volume, and improvement of respiratory muscle function.[83] Theophylline toxicity includes agitation, tachycardia with associated dysrhythmias, and gastrointestinal side effects. The use of theophylline in cardiac patients has been questioned because of these multiple side effects. Studies suggest there is no beneficial effect from the use of theophylline in patients having acute exacerbations of COPD when added to standard therapy.[84] Albert et al.[85] suggested that corticosteroids improve time of recovery from an acute exacerbation of COPD. Frequently, surgeons are concerned about postoperative healing in patients who are receiving steroids, but previous studies of its effects on wound healing have demonstrated that glucorticoids on the third day after surgery do not inhibit wound healing.[86]

WEANING

Although some authors discourage use of the term *weaning,* it is the most commonly used term describing the resumption of spontaneous ventilation and withdrawal of ventilatory support and therefore will be used in this section. Decisions concerning weaning should be carefully discussed by the medical and nursing staff in the ICU. Protocols should be devised and agreed upon to ensure a smooth and efficient process. The staff must also be aware of any problem that would contraindicate extubation. Such problems include the following:

Hypoxia
Hemodynamic instability
Bleeding
Hypothermia
Neurologic deficit
Poor weaning parameters (see Table 6-3)

The precise timing of extubation following cardiac surgery is very controversial. Many studies suggest that endotracheal extubation the same day of cardiothoracic surgery may enhance recovery, while reducing deleter-

ious respiratory and cardiovascular events. In a prospective study by Quasha et al.,[87] 38 patients were randomly assigned to one of two groups. One group was extubated within 2 ± 2 hours, the other within 18 ± 3 hours. The results suggested that cardiopulmonary morbidity in patients who underwent early extubation was less than for patients who underwent prolonged CMV. Although sedative and narcotic requirements were lower, the ICU stay was not shortened by early extubation.[87]

Butler et al.[88] observed 13 patients who underwent elective coronary artery bypass grafting (CABG) and then, after meeting certain extubation criteria, were weaned and extubated within 1 hour of the end of surgery. All patients tolerated the procedure without difficulty. Butler and colleagues indicated factors that might contribute to successful early extubation. These included short cardiopulmonary bypass times, reversal of muscle relaxation at the end of surgery, short-acting anesthetic drugs, and avoidance of postoperative hypothermia with its associated peripheral vasoconstriction and increased systemic vascular resistance. Although patients did experience respiratory acidosis, attentive care by the recovery staff prevented any adverse sequelae.[88]

Early extubation in selected patients may aid in reducing the costs of postoperative care by decreasing the use of sedatives and mechanical ventilation. Although Prakash et al.[89] and Klineberg et al.[90] recorded fewer ICU days, Quasha et al.[87] did not note a difference in time spent in the ICU. However, costs were significantly decreased in cases of early extubation. Early extubation may also help decrease the incidence of atelectasis, anatomic trauma, and other cardiopulmonary morbidity.

Studies have been done to determine which anesthetic method would be most effective for early extubation. In seeking to avoid the respiratory depression associated with narcotics, Lichtenthal et al.[91] administered inhalation agents as the primary anesthetic. It should be noted, however, that the inhalation technique may be associated with hemodynamic instability. Some studies have recommended the use of an adjuvant with the inhalation agent, such as epidural analgesia or more narcotics, in an effort to attain greater stability. The idea that the stress response and release of catecholamines may be suppressed with the use of narcotics raises the question of whether the patient should continue to receive high-dose narcotics during the postoperative period. It is unclear whether narcotics perform this task. It must be remembered the patient has yet to be awakened and extubated. Ramsay et al. demonstrated that use of narcotic reversal was not prudent, making it necessary to lower narcotic levels in a timely manner.

The use of propofol for cardiothoracic anesthesia as well as postoperative sedation may aid in early extubation. Roekaerts et al.[92] studied 30 ventilated patients in an open randomized study comparing propofol infusion versus midazolam. They concluded that, in the propofol-treated group, sedation was easier to control, and recovery from sedation and weaning from ventilation was faster. An observed drop in blood pressure in the propofol-treated group was deemed clinically acceptable.[92]

The argument set forth by those opposing early extubation is that the postoperative period is the most stressful time following cardiac surgery, requiring that the patient's stress response be controlled in order to avoid myocardial ischemia. While anesthesia suppresses the stress hormones (epinephrine, norepinephrine, adrenocorticotropic hormone [ACTH], and cortisol) during the procedure, levels of these hormones increase postoperatively.

Siliciano et al.[93] suggest that the cardiovascular effects of postoperative mechanical ventilation are overexaggerated in normovolemic patients. Ben-Haim et al. suggest that PPV with PEEP may improve the energy balance of the ischemic heart. They studied six dogs in which increasing levels of PEEP decreased aortic pressure, left ventricular (LV) pressure, aortic flow coronary blood flow (CBF), and myocardial oxygen consumption (MVO_2). However, the ratio of CBF to predicted MVO_2 increased with increasing PEEP. Siliciano and colleagues[93] also emphasizes that "personally relevant" mental stress has been shown to induce silent ischemia and ventricular dysfunction in patients with coronary artery disease.

Although clinical assessment is a very important tool to be used during the weaning process, weaning parameters provide objective data in deciding when to extubate. The New York Hospital-Cornell Medical Center employs the following criteria for extubation in the cardiothoracic ICU (Table 6-2). Institutions typically develop criteria based on their own experiences.

Most institutions obtain weaning parameters prior to extubation. This requires some degree of compliance from the patient and in some circumstances may be difficult to obtain. Our criteria for pulmonary function tests are included in Table 6-3.

Pulmonary function tests prior to extubation do not ensure that a patient will tolerate breathing without assistance. They do, however, provide objective data that help in decision-making. The negative inspiratory force measurement has traditionally been considered a good marker in determining neuromuscular function[94,96] and the patient's ability to cough. An important aspect of recovery following extubation is the ability to clear secretions and to maintain the patency of the alveoli. Coughing, which requires adequate muscular strength, is helpful under both cir-

Table 6-2. Extubation Criteria at New York Hospital-Cornell Medical Center

Parameters	Value
PO_2	$2 \times FiO_2$
PCO_2	<50 varies with history of lung disease
pH	7.35–7.45

Table 6-3. Routine Ventilatory Weaning Parameters

Parameter	Value
Negative inspiratory force	> -25 cmH$_2$O
Tidal volume	5–7 ml^{-1}·kg^{-1} body weight
Vital capacity	15 ml^{-1}·kg^{-1} body weight
Respiratory rate	<25·min^{-1}
Rapid shallow breathing index (RR/V$_T$(L)	<100

cumstances. Adequate coughing minimizes the need for devices such as inspiratory spirometers. In other studies, the validity of the negative inspiratory force came into question.[96] Tahvanainen's study revealed a high false-negative result (predicted failure but actual success), as well as a relatively high false-positive result (predicted success but actual failure).

The patient's vital capacity is another parameter helping determine whether the patient is ready to be extubated. Bendixen et al.[97] suggested that a vital capacity of 10 ml^{-1}·kg^{-1} should be sufficient in determining a patient's ability to sustain spontaneous breathing. Again, Tahvanainen et al.[96] showed a significant false-positive result in 18 percent of patients and a false-negative result in 50 percent of patients.

Thoracic compliance is a term that defines the elasticity of the chest wall and the lungs (Fig. 6-6). In order to ventilate effectively, the patient must overcome the elastic forces that determine thoracic compliance. Typically, static thoracic compliance (Cs) is calculated as

$$Cs = \frac{\text{volume delivered}}{(\text{static pressure} - \text{PEEP})}$$

Clinicians will assess compliance in order to determine the progress of therapy as well as predict weaning outcome. Normal static com-

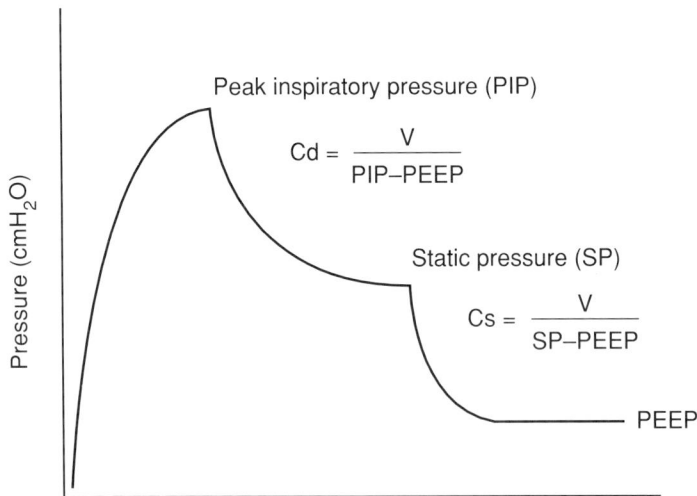

Fig. 6-6. Airway pressure trace with equations for dynamic (Co) and static (Cs) compliance. V is the tidal volume; SP is the static or plateau pressure. Normal dynamic compliance is not firmly established; however, it averages about 60 ml · cm H$_2$O in anesthetized patients receiving muscle relaxants. Normal static compliance for mechanically ventilated patients is approximately 50 to 100 ml · cmH$_2$O^{-1}. (Adapted from Karagianes,[121] with permission.)

pliance of mechanically ventilated patients is assumed to be within the range of 50 to 100 $ml \cdot cmH_2O^{-1}$. Pathologic states in the cardiac patient that will decrease compliance below this range include pneumothorax, pneumonia, effusion, atelectasis, pulmonary congestion, and pulmonary edema. In general, weaning outcome will most likely be unsuccessful if the endotracheal tube is removed with a compliance of $25 ml \cdot cmH_2O^{-1}$ or less. Dynamic compliance (Cd) is calculated as

$$Cd = \frac{volume\ delivered}{(peak\ inspiratory\ pressure\ -\ PEEP)}$$

It is not a true measure of thoracic compliance as the peak airway pressure includes the resistive component of applied pressure. A decrease in dynamic compliance is seen in patients with parenchymal disease as well as patients with airway disturbances. In fact, a decrease in dynamic compliance greater than static compliance suggests increased airway resistance.

The patient's overall clinical picture remains vitally important in assessing the feasibility of extubation. Is the patient using accessory muscles to breathe? What is the respiratory rate? Does the patient appear fatigued? Good objective pulmonary function tests and laboratory tests may not be sufficient indication for extubation.

Paradoxic motion of the abdomen has been studied as a clinical sign. Cohen et al.[98] studied 12 patients who were having difficulty weaning from the ventilator. Seven patients exhibited changes on the electromyographic (EMG) consistent with muscle fatigue. Six of these seven patients also showed signs of paradoxic motion of the abdomen. In four of the six patients, this was accompanied by a cyclical alteration in the contribution of the rib cage and abdomen to the tidal volume ("respiratory alternans"), while six patients developed an increase in respiratory rate. These signs were reportedly not present in patients who did not develop EMG changes.[98] Roussos and Macklem[99] in-

dicated that these changes in respiratory pattern provide a somewhat reliable diagnosis of inspiratory muscle fatigue. Some research indicated that abdominal paradoxic movement is a poor predictor of weaning outcome but that an index combining asynchronous and paradoxic motion of the rib cage and abdomen is a helpful predictor.[100]

Although respiratory rate has been underrated as an indicator of respiratory dysfunction, it has been shown to be a sensitive and specific marker for acute respiratory dysfunction.[101] Gravelyn and Weg[101] suggest that "as a measurement respiratory rate is simple, inexpensive and noninvasive, the utility of accurate routine respiratory measurements as a screening procedure is apparent."

Determining the respiratory rate and tidal volume provides an idea of the patient's lung compliance. Typically, the cardiac patient's postoperative compliance is worse than the preoperative due to increased intravascular fluid volume and atelectasis. The ratio of respiratory frequency to tidal volume during 1 minute of spontaneous breathing can be useful in predicting the patient's readiness for extubation. A value of less than 100 breaths $\cdot min^{-1} \cdot L^{-1}$ suggests that weaning will likely be successful.

Aspiration remains a concern, even when the awake and aware patient has a strong cough. Burgess et al.[102] studied 64 patients who underwent elective coronary bypass procedures. In the postoperative period, patients were instructed to swallow a radiopaque propliodine oil suspension immediately after extubation, after 4 hours and then after 8 hours. Chest radiographs were obtained 30 minutes after extubation. The radiographs revealed that all groups demonstrated some degree of aspiration, the severity decreasing as the elapsed time from extubation increased. This problem may be related to either sensory or motor impairment.[102] The managing physician must therefore be aware that even when criteria for extubation "are met," the risk of aspiration is still higher than normal.

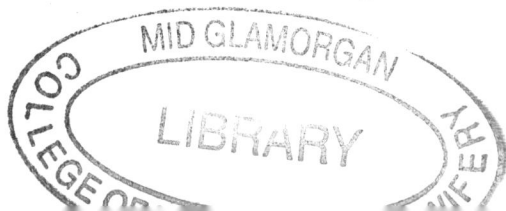

There are many ways to wean the patient from the ventilator. It is unclear what method will most efficiently wean the patient from the ventilator. The goals, however, are the same for all the methods. The various methods of partial support ventilation (assist control, IMV, and PSV) gradually allow the patient to assume the WOB. Weaning should allow the patient to use the respiratory muscles, to prevent atrophy from disuse. These methods involve decreasing the IMV rate to a point where the patient is breathing without the help of mechanical breaths (i.e., on CPAP or T-piece), decreasing assist control in the same manner, or placing the patient on CPAP and high levels of PSV and decreasing the PSV over time. The medical staff must avoid overexerting the patient and increasing the WOB should not become detrimental to the patient's recovery process.

Esteban et al.[103] prospectively studied 546 patients who received mechanical ventilation for a mean ($\pm$SD) of 7.5 $\pm$ 6.1 days and who were deemed ready for discontinuation from mechanical ventilation. The patients were assigned to undergo one of four weaning techniques: IMV, PSV, intermittent trials of spontaneous breathing (two to three times per day), or a once-daily trial of spontaneous breathing. The study demonstrated that once-daily trials of spontaneous breathing (as well as multiple daily trials) led to extubation about three times more quickly than IMV and about twice as quickly as PSV.[103] The results of this study cast doubt on the notion that the method of weaning does not affect the duration of weaning.

Many signs indicate that the patient is exerting too much effort to breathe. Although a respiratory rate below 20 to 25 breaths · min^{-1} would be ideal, a higher respiratory rate is acceptable in chronic patients, as long as they appear comfortable. However, an increase in heart rate and blood pressure, an increase in the use of accessory muscles, or the presence of diaphoresis are early signs indicating that longer ventilatory support may be required.

EXTUBATION

When preparing for extubation, the appropriate equipment must be made readily available for the eventuality of emergent reintubation, including an appropriate size endotracheal tube with stylet, a suction catheter attached to suction, an Ambu-bag, a laryngoscope, and muscle relaxant. Most importantly, the immediate presence of personnel skilled in endotracheal intubation is required.

At extubation, the patient is placed on 100 percent oxygen and instructed as to what will be taking place. Immediately after the patient is asked to take a deep breath, the endotracheal tube is removed while the patient coughs. A face mask delivering 50 to 100 percent oxygen is then placed. If necessary, inhaled bronchodilators are delivered at this time.

It is crucial for the nursing and medical staff to encourage coughing and deep breathing during the post-extubation period. The appropriate use of analgesics is emphasized to prevent the atelectasis that occurs when a patient splints the chest wall due to pain. Pain medications should not be avoided simply because the patient has already been extubated. (If there is concern about the patient's level of consciousness, a nonsteroidal anti-inflammatory drug such as ketorolac should be considered.) The nursing staff may also help by administering chest percussion and drainage.

DIFFICULT WEANING

Although most postoperative cardiac patients do relatively well with regard to ventilation, there are those who have difficulty being separated from the ventilator. Common problems that may interfere with the weaning process include a history of chronic or acute lung disease, intracranial pathology, inadequate cardiac function, inappropriate ventilator settings, malnutrition, or infection. Some of these problems can and should be avoided.

As malnutrition is a relatively common problem in cases involving mechanical ventilation, patients should receive either enteral or parenteral feedings at the earliest possibility[104,105] (see Ch. 8). It has been suggested that malnutrition interferes with regeneration of respiratory epithelium[106] with marked reductions of secretory immunoglobulin A (IgA) in respiratory fluids, as well as low serum levels of Ig complement.[107] The most notable effect of malnutrition is evident in muscular strength and respiratory drive. Previous studies have demonstrated the deleterious effects of malnutrition on respiratory muscular strength, as judged by maximum inspiratory and expiratory pressures.[108] Respiratory function measured as vital capacity and minute ventilation has been shown to decline in subjects that have been semistarved.[109] Interestingly, although nutritional support has been employed to help respiratory function, it tends to increase carbon dioxide production as well as the load on the respiratory system, which could interfere with the weaning process. When parenteral nutrition is being administered, it is crucial that excessive glucose be avoided as it increases carbon dioxide production.[106]

The incidence of cerebrovascular (CV) events in the cardiothoracic patient is approximately 1 to 5 percent[110] (see Ch. 12). Clearly, altered neurologic function may interfere with extubation. Patients who have suffered from intracerebral neurovascular events have varying degrees of impairment and must therefore be managed accordingly. Some patients who have suffered from CV events can protect their airways and do well when extubated. Others, however, will require prolonged ventilatory support as a result of the deleterious CV events.

Many patients require the aid of a ventilator for protracted periods. In general, however, one may wish to try to extubate a patient who seems to be heading toward a long course on the ventilator. The physician must be prepared for the fact that some patients who undergo cardiac surgery will require a tracheostomy; a quick decision to have the patient undergo placement of a tracheostomy may facilitate the recovery process.

RESPIRATORY DIFFICULTIES AFTER EXTUBATION

Following extubation, the postoperative cardiac patient will often develop difficulty breathing. This is commonly due to excess fluid sequestered in the lungs (pulmonary edema) secondary to high pressures in the pulmonary microcirculation. Aggressive administration of a diuretic may be all that is required. However, the treating physician must be aware that aggressive administration of diuretics such as furosemide or bumetanide may lead to hypokalemia, hypomagnesemia, and metabolic alkalosis. Although easily treated, these problems may be overlooked. The treating physician should consider the presence of an unsuccessful surgical repair or another untoward event resulting in ischemia to the myocardium. An echocardiogram at this point may be helpful in further evaluating the patient. It may be determined that the patient will require further inotropic support, afterload reduction, or even more surgical intervention.

Noncardiogenic pulmonary edema must be considered when cardiac function appears unimpaired and pulmonary artery "filling" pressures are low. Acute lung injury after CPB or ARDS may be present, requiring prolonged support with mechanical ventilation during the postoperative period. It appears that the acute lung injury may be related to the duration of CPB, protamine reaction or blood transfusion.[111,112] The management of these patients is similar to that of other patients with ARDS. Ventilatory support includes the administration of PEEP to maintain adequate oxygenation and to assist in avoiding the delivery of high oxygen concentrations (greater than 60 percent). Every effort must be made to avoid high airway pressures, using modalities previously discussed.

Diaphragmatic insufficiency occurs in a

small percentage of patients undergoing open heart surgery.[87] It is difficult to quantify the number of patients who develop diaphragmatic paresis or paralysis. It appears, however, that respiratory failure secondary to unilateral phrenic nerve injury is relatively rare.[113,114] Respiratory failure associated with bilateral diaphragmatic insufficiency after CPB is even less common and is probably related to significant hypothermia present during CPB.[115] The diagnosis of diaphragmatic insufficiency must be considered in patients who are difficult to wean from the ventilator or in patients who have persistent respiratory difficulties. The affected hemidiaphragm is typically "elevated" on the chest radiograph. This elevation is often associated with atelectasis in the same region. The diagnosis is difficult to make and may at times be a diagnosis of exclusion. The diagnosis can be made by using fluoroscopy or by obtaining upright posterior-anterior and lateral chest radiographs. Loh et al.[116] note that, for a number of reasons, in bilateral diaphragmatic paralysis or paresis, fluoroscopic examination is of little use. The measurement of transdiaphragmatic pressure is the only available test to make a definitive diagnosis of this problem. Therapy for these patients is typically supportive, with recovery of diaphragmatic function often taking many months. Prolonged mechanical ventilatory support is often necessary.

CONCLUSION

Ventilatory management of the postoperative cardiac patient presents many issues not seen in other patient groups. Much of what we know about ventilatory management in the critical care setting may be applied to the cardiac patient with "variations on the theme." It appears that many of the changes now being seen in postoperative care are being driven by the forces of economics and the incentive to bring down the cost of health care. Our efforts in this direction may be impeded as the average age of the cardiac

patient continues to rise. Nevertheless, research and technology continues to guide us into new areas of ventilatory management that will improve management of the postoperative patient.

REFERENCES

1. Lefemine AA, Harken DE: Postoperative care following open heart operations: routine use of controlled ventilation. J Thorac Cardiac Surg 52:207–16, 1966
2. Buzello W, Pollmacher T, Schluerman D, Urbanyi B: The influence of hypothermic cardiopulmonary bypass on neuromuscular transmission in the absence of muscle relaxants. Anesthesiology 64:279, 1986
3. Turnbull K, Miyagishima R, Gerein A: Pulmonary complications and cardiopulmonary bypass. A clinical study in adults. Can Anaesth Soc J 21:181–4, 1974
4. Matthay MA, Wiener-Kronish JP: Respiratory Management after cardiac surgery, Chest 95:424–34, 1989
5. Edmunds LH, Alexander JA: Effect of cardiopulmonary bypass on the lungs. In Fishman AP (ed): Pulmonary Disease and Disorders. McGraw-Hill, New York, 1980
6. Chenowith PE, Cooper SW, Hughli TE et al: Complement activation during cardiopulmonary bypass: evidence for generation of C3a and C5a anaphylotoxins. N Engl J Med 304: 497–503, 1981
7. Salama A, Hugo F, Heinrich D et al: Deposition of terminal C5b-9 complement complexes on erythrocytes and leukocytes during cardiopulmonary bypass. N Engl J Med 318:408–14, 1981
8. Asada S, Yamaguchi M: Fine structural changes in the lung following cardiopulmonary bypass. Its relationship to early postoperative course. Chest 59:478–83, 1971
9. Garzon AA, Seltzer B, Karlson KE: Respiratory mechanics following open-heart surgery for acquired valvular disease. Circulation, suppl. 33–34:57–64, 1964
10. Ghia J, Andersen N: Pulmonary function and cardiopulmonary bypass. JAMA 212:593–7, 1970
11. Ellis E, Brown A, Osborn JJ et al: Effect of altered ventilation patterns on compliance

during cardiopulmonary bypass. Anesth Analg 48:947–52, 1969

12. Kolef MH, Peller T, Knodel A, Cragun WH: Delayed pleuropulmonary complications following coronary artery revascularization with the internal mammary artery. Chest 94: 68–71, 1988

13. Froese AB, Sryan AC: Effects of anesthesia and paralysis on diaphragmatic mechanics in man. Anesthesiology 41:242–55, 1974

14. Phang P, Keough K: Inhibition of pulmonary surfactant by plasma from normal adults and from patients having cardiopulmonary bypass. Thorac Cardiovasc Surg 91:248–51, 1986

15. Nagao K, Ardila R, Sugiyama M, Hildebrandt J: Temperature and hydration: factors affecting increased recoil of excised rabbit lung. Respir Physiol 29:11–24, 1977

16. Markand ON, Moorthy SS, Mahomed Y et al: Postoperative phrenic nerve palsy in patients with open-heart surgery. Ann Thorac Surg 38:68–73, 1985

17. Hachenberg T, Tenling A, Nystrom S et al: Ventilation-perfusion inequality in patients undergoing cardiac surgery, Anesthesiology 80:509–19, 1994

18. Dantzker DR, Lynch JP, Weg JG: Depression of cardiac output is a mechanism of shunt reduction in the therapy of acute respiratory failure. Chest 77:636–42, 1980

19. Bergman NA: Effects of varying waveform on gas exchange. Anesthesiology 88:390, 1967

20. Shapiro BA, Vender JS: Postoperative respiratory management. p. 1149. In Kaplan JA (ed): Cardiac Anesthesia. WB Saunders, Philadelphia, 1993

21. Dreyfuss D, Soler P, Basset G, Saumon G: High inflation pressure pulmonary edema: respective effects of high airway pressure, high tidal volume and positive end expiratory pressure. Am Rev Respir Dis 137:1159–64, 1988

22. Pepe PE, Marini JJ: Occult positive end expiratory pressure in mechanically ventilated patients with airflow obstruction: the auto-PEEP effect. Am Rev Respir Dis 126:166–70, 1982

23. Marshall C, Lindgren L, Marshall BE: Effects of halothane and isoflurane in rat lungs in vitro. Anesthesiology 60:304, 1984

24. Benumof JL: One-lung ventilation and hypoxic pulmonary vasoconstriction: implica-

tions of anesthetic management. Anesth Analg 64:821, 1985

25. Marshall BE, Cohen PJ, Klingenmaier CH et al: Pulmonary venous admixture before, during and after halothane: oxygen anesthesia in man. J Appl Physiol 27:653, 1967

26. Sladen RN: Temperature and ventilation after hypothermic cardiopulmonary bypass. Anesth Analg 64:816–20, 1985

27. Noback CR, Tinker JH: Hypothermia after cardiopulmonary bypass in man. Anesthesiology 53:277–80, 1980

28. Bjork VO, Engstrom CG: The treatment of ventilatory insufficiency after pulmonary resection with tracheostomy and prolonged artificial ventilation. J Thorac Surg 30:356, 1955

29. Downs JB, Klein EF, Desautels D et al: IMV: a new approach to weaning patients from mechanical ventilators. Chest 64:331–5, 1973

30. Hershey MD: Ventilatory support of patients with respiratory failure. Int Anesthiol Clin 31: 149–68, 1993

31. Downs JB, Douglas ME, Sanfelippo PM et al: Ventilatory pattern intrapleural pressure and cardiac output. Anesth Analg 56:88–96, 1979

32. Zarins CK, Bayne CG, Rice CL et al: Does spontaneous ventilation with IMV protect from PEEP induced cardiac output depression? J Surg Res 22:299–304, 1977

33. Sahn SA, Lakshminarayan S, Petty TL: Weaning from mechanical ventilation. JAMA 235: 2208–12, 1976

34. Heenan TJ, Downs JB, Douglas ME et al: Intermittent mandatory ventilation: is synchronization important? Chest 77:598, 1980

35. Albert RK: Least PEEP: Primum non nocere. Chest 87:2–4, 1985

36. Rizk NW, Murray JF: PEEP and pulmonary edema. Am J Med 72:381–3, 1982

37. Caldini P, Leith JD, Brennan MI: Effect of continuous positive-pressure ventilation (CPPV) on edema formation in the dog lung. J Appl Physiol 39:672, 1975

38. Dantzker DR, Cowenhaven WN, Willoughby NJ et al: Gas exchange alterations associated with weaning from mechanical ventilation following coronary artery bypass grafting. Chest 82:674–7, 1982

39. Downs JB, Mitchell LA: Pulmonary effects of ventilatory pattern following cardiopulmonary bypass. Crit Care Med 4:295–300, 1976

40. Cournand A, Montly HL, Werko I: Physiologic studies of the effects of intermittent positive pressure breathing on cardiac output in man. Am J Physiol 152:162, 1948

41. Dorinsky PM, Whitcomb ME: The effect of PEEP on cardiac output. Chest 2:210–6, 1983

42. Hudson LD: Ventilatory managements of patients with adult respiratory distress syndrome. Semin Respir Med 2:128–39, 1981

43. Illabaca PA, Oschner JL, Mills NL: Positive end-expiratory pressure in the management of the patient with a postoperative bleeding heart. Ann Thorac Surg 30:281, 1980

44. Zurick AM, Urzua J, Ghattas M et al: Failure of positive end-expiratory pressure to decrease postoperative bleeding after cardiac surgery. Ann Thorac Surg 34:608, 1982

45. Hoffman WS, Tomasello DN, Mac Vaugh H: Control of postcardiotomy bleeding with PEEP. Ann Thorac Surg 34:71, 1983

46. Brochard L, Harf A, Lonino H, Lenair F: Inspiratory pressure support prevents diaphragmatic fatigue during weaning from mechanical ventilation. Am Rev Resp Dis 139:513–21, 1989

47. MacIntyre NR: Respiratory function during pressure support ventilation. Chest 89:677–83, 1986

48. Shapiro M, Wilson RK, Casar G et al: Work of breathing through different sized endotracheal tubes. Crit Care Med 14:1028–31, 1986

49. Bolder PM, Healy TEJ, Bolder AR et al: The extra work of breathing through adult endotracheal tubes. Anesth Analg 65:853–9, 1986

50. Brochard L, Rua F, Lorino H et al: Inspiratory pressure support compensates for the additional work of breathing caused by the endotracheal tube. Anesthesiology 75:739–45, 1991

51. Tomlinson JR, Miller KS, Lorah DG et al: A prospective comparison of IMV and T-piece weaning from mechanical ventilation. Chest 96:348–52, 1989

52. Ravizza AG, Caruga D, Cerchiari EL et al: Inversed ratio and conventional ventilation: comparison of the respiratory effects. Anesthesiology 59:523, 1983

53. Ravizza AF, Carugo D, Cuchian EL et al: Inverse ratio and conventional ventilations: comparison of the respiratory effects, abstracted. Anesthesiology 59:A523, 1983

54. Gurevitch MJ, VanDyke J, Young ES, Jackson K: Impaired oxygenation and lower peak airway pressure in severe adult respiratory distress syndrome. Chest 89:211–3, 1986

55. Tharatt RS, Allen RP, Albertson TE: Pressure controlled inverse ratio ventilation in severe adult respiratory failure. Chest 94:755–62, 1988

56. Henderson Y, Chillingsworth F, Whitney J: The respiratory dead space. Am J Physiol 38:1–19, 1915

57. Slutsky AS: Gas mixing by cardiogenic oscillations: a theoretical quantitative analysis. J Appl Physiol 51:1287–93, 1981

58. Jonson B, Lachmann B: Setting and monitoring of high-frequency jet ventilation in severe respiratory distress syndrome. Crit Care Med 17:1020–4, 1989

59. Stock MC, Downs JB, Frolicher DA: Airway pressure release ventilation. Crit Care Med 15:462, 1987

60. Garner W, Downs JB, Stock MC, Rasanen J: Airway pressure release ventilation (APRV): a human trial. Chest 94:779–81, 1988

61. Kumar A, Pontopiddan H, Falke KJ et al: Pulmonary barotrauma during mechanical ventilation. Crit Care Med 1:181–6, 1973

62. Steier M, Ching N, Roberts EB, Nealon TF: Pneumothorax complicating continuous ventilatory support. J Thorac Cardiovasc Surg 67:17–22, 1974

63. Petersen GW, Baier H: Incidence of pulmonary barotrauma in a medical ICU. Crit Care Med 11:67–9, 1983

64. Cullen DJ, Caidera DL: The incidence of ventilator induced pulmonary barotrauma in critically ill patients. Anesthesiology 50:185–90, 1979

65. Carlton DP, Cummings JJ, Scheerer RG et al: Lung overexpansion increases pulmonary microvascular protein permeability in young lambs. J Appl Physiol 69:577–83, 1990

66. Dreyfuss D, Soler P, Basset G, Saumon G: High inflation pressure pulmonary edema: respective effects of high airway pressure, high tidal volume and positive end-expiratory pressure. Am Rev Resp Dis 137:1159–64, 1988

67. Andrivet P, Adnot S, Brun-Buisson C et al: Involvement of ANF in the acute antidiuresis during PEEP ventilation. J Appl Physiol 65:1967–74, 1988

68. Berry AJ: Respiratory support and renal function. Anesthesiology 55:655–67, 1981
69. Khambatta HJ, Baratz RA: IPPB, plasma ADH, and urine flow in conscious man. J Appl Physiol 33:362–4, 1972
70. Geiger K, Goorgieff M, Lutz H: Side effects of positive pressure ventilation on hepatic function and splanchnic circulation. Int J Clin Monit Comput 12:103–6, 1986
71. Nahum A, Sznajder JI: Role of free radicals in critical illness. p. 672. In Hall JB, Schmidt GA, Wood LD (eds): Principles of Critical Care. McGraw-Hill, New York, 1992
72. Fridovich I: The biology of oxygen radicals. Science 210:875, 1978
73. Suzuki Y, Ford G: Mathematical model supporting the superoxide theory of oxygen toxicity. Free Radio Biol Med 16:63, 1994
74. Freeman B, Rosen G, Barber M: Superoxide perturbation of the organization of vascular endothelial cell membranes. J Biol Chem 261:5690, 1986
75. Jenkinson SG: Oxygen toxicity. J Intensive Care Med 3:137–52, 1988
76. Tenney SM: Ventilatory response to carbon dioxide in pulmonary emphysema. J Appl Physiol 6:477, 1954
77. Tobin MJ, Grenvik A: Nosocomial lung infection and its diagnosis. Crit Care Med 12:191–9, 1984
78. Matthay MA, Wiener-Kronish JP: Respiratory management after cardiac surgery. Chest 95:424–34, 1989
79. Kaplan JA: Treatment of perioperative left heart failure. p. 1058. In Kaplan JA (ed): Cardiac Anesthesia. 3rd Ed. WB Saunders, Philadelphia 1993
80. Weinberger M, Hendeles L, Ahrens R: Pharmacologic management of reversible obstructive airway diseases. Med Clin North Am 65:579–613, 1980
81. Paterson JW, Woolcock AJ, Shenfield GM: Bronchodilator drugs, Am Rev Respir Dis 120:1149–88, 1979
82. Matthay RA: Effects of theophylline in cardiovascular performance in chronic obstructive pulmonary disease. Chest 88:112S–7S, 1985
83. Aubier M, Roussos S: Effect of theophylline on respiratory muscle function. Chest 88:91S–7S, 1985
84. Rice KL, Leatherman JW, Duane PG et al:

Aminophylline for acute exacerbations of chronic obstructive pulmonary disease. Ann Intern Med 107:305–9, 1987
85. Albert RK, Martin TR, Lewis SW: Controlled clinical trial of methylprednisolone in patients with chronic bronchitis and acute respiratory insufficiency. Ann Intern Med 107:305–9, 1980
86. Sandberg N: Time relationship between administration of cortisone and wound healing in rats. Acta Chir Scand 127:446–55, 1964
87. Quasha AL, Loeber N, Feeley TW et al: Postoperative respiratory care: a controlled trial of early and late extubation following coronary-artery bypass grafting. Anesthesiology 52:135–41, 1980
88. Butler J, Cong GI, Pillai R et al: Early extubation after coronary artery bypass surgery: effects on oxygen flux and haemodynamic variables. J Cardiovasc Surg 33:276–80, 1992
89. Prakash O, Johnson B, Meij S et al: Criteria for early extubation after intracardiac surgery in adults. Anesth Analg 56:703–8, 1977
90. Klineberg PL, Geer RT, Hirsch RA et al: Early extubation after coronary artery bypass graft surgery. Crit Care Med 5:272–4, 1977
91. Lichtenthal PR, Wade LD, Niemyski PR, Shapiro BA: Respiratory management after cardiac surgery with inhalation anesthesia. Crit Care Med 11:603–5, 1983
92. Roekaerts PMHJ, Huygen FJPM, de Lange S: Infusion of propofol versus midazolam for sedation in the intensive care unit following coronary artery surgery. J Cardiothorac Vasc Anesth 7:142–7, 1993
93. Siliciano D, Hollenberg M, Goehner P, Mangano D: Use of continuous vs intermittent narcotic after CABG surgery: effects on myocardial ischemia, abstracted. Anesth Analg 70:S371, 1990
94. Black LF, Hyatt RE: Maximal respiratory pressures: normal values and relationship to age and sex. Am Rev Respir Dis 99:696–702, 1969
95. Black LF, Hyatt RE: Maximal respiratory pressures in generalized neuromuscular disease. Am Rev Respir Dis 103:641–50, 1971
96. Tahvanainen J, Salmenpera M, Nikki P: Extubation criteria after weaning from intermittent mandatory ventilation and continuous positive airway pressure. Crit Care Med 11:702–7, 1983

97. Bendixen HH, Egbert LD, Hedley-White J et al: Respiratory Care. CV Mosby, St. Louis, 1965, p. 149

98. Cohen CA, Zagelbaum G, Gross D et al: Clinical manifestations of inspiratory muscle fatigue. Am J Med 73:308–16, 1982

99. Roussos C, Macklem PT: The respiratory muscles. N Engl J Med 307:786–97, 1982

100. Tobin MJ, Guenther SM, Perez W et al: Konno-Mead analysis of rib cage abdominal motion during successful and unsuccessful trials of weaning from mechanical ventilation. Am Rev Respir Dis 135:1320–8, 1987

101. Gravelyn TR, Weg JG: Respiratory rate as an indicator of acute respiratory dysfunction. JAMA 244:1123–5, 1980

102. Burgess GE, Cooper JR, Marino RJ et al: Laryngeal competence after tracheal extubation. Anesthesiology 51:73–7, 1979

103. Esteban A, Frutos F, Tobin MJ et al: A comparison of four methods of weaning patients from mechanical ventilation. N Engl J Med 332:345–50, 1995

104. Driver AG, Le Brun: Iatrogenic malnutrition in patients receiving ventilatory support. JAMA 244:2195–6, 1980

105. Bassili HR, Deitel M: Effect of nutritional support on weaning patients off mechanical ventilators. JPEN 5:161–3, 1981

106. Askanazi J, Weissman C, Rosenbaum SH et al: Nutrition and the respiratory system. Crit Care Med 10:163–72, 1982

107. Stiehm ER: Humoral immunity in malnutrition. Fed Proc 39:3093–7, 1980

108. Arora NS, Rochester DF: Respiratory muscle strength and maximal voluntary ventilation in undernourished patients. Am Rev Respir Dis 126:5–8, 1982

109. Keys A, Brozek J, Henschel A et al: Biology of Human Starvation. University of Minnesota, Minneapolis, 1950, pp. 601–6

110. Furlan AJ, Breuer AC: Central nervous system complications of open heart surgery. Stroke 15:912, 1984

111. Swerdlow BN, Mihm FG, Getzl EJ, Matthay MA: Leukotrienes in pulmonary edema fluid after cardiopulmonary bypass. Anesth Analg 65:306–8, 1986

112. Maggart M, Stewart S: The mechanisms and management of noncardiogenic pulmonary edema following cardiopulmonary bypass. Ann Thorac Surg 43:231–6, 1987

113. Markand ON, Moorthy SS, Mahomed Y et al: Postoperative phrenic nerve palsy in patients with open heart surgery. Ann Thorac Surg 39:68–73, 1985

114. Wilcox P, Baile E, Hards J et al: Phrenic nerve function and its relationship to atelectasis after coronary artery bypass surgery. Chest 93:693–8, 1988

115. Chandler KW, Rozas CJ, Kory RC, Goldman AL: Bilateral diaphragmatic paralysis complicating local cardiac hypothermia during open heart surgery. Am J Med 77:243–9, 1984

116. Loh L, Golman M, Newsom DJ: The assessment of diaphragm function. Medicine, (Baltimore) 56:165–9, 1977

117. Shapiro BA, Kacmarek RM, Cane RD et al: Clinical Application of Respiratory Care. 4th Ed. CV Mosby-Year Book, Chicago, 1991

118. Perel A, Stock MC: Handbook of Mechanical Ventilatory Support. Williams & Wilkins, Baltimore, 1992

119. Rasanen J, Downs JB, Stock MC: Cardiovascular effects of positive pressure ventilation and airway pressure release ventilation. Chest 93:911–5, 1988

120. Berry AJ: Respiratory support and renal function. Anesthesiology 55:655, 1981

121. Karagianes TG: Pulmonary considerations. In Vanstrum GS (ed): Anesthesia in Emergency Medicine Little, Brown, Boston, 1989

7

Hemodynamic Management

S. Beloucif
D. Payen

The clinician's goal in the postoperative management of the patient following cardiac surgery is to optimize hemodynamics according to the modified physiology created by the surgery. Simultaneously, one must avoid exacerbating complications secondary to the duration of surgery or the ischemic period during aortic cross-clamping.

This chapter is conceptually separated into two areas. The first is the uncomplicated patient. This type of patient is typified by an otherwise healthy individual undergoing primary cardiac surgery. There are no ventricular disorders, organ impairment, or ancilliary disorders. The second portion of the chapter details the management of the complicated patient. This patient is typified by the elderly patient with organ impairment presenting for second- or third-time surgery.

The first step upon arrival in the intensive care unit (ICU) is to review the patient's general physiologic status prior to surgery, current hemodynamic status, and quality of the surgical repair. Hemodynamic function prior to and following surgical repair in addition to the management of weaning from cardiopulmonary bypass are useful indicators of the postoperative prognosis.

As a general rule, the aim of hemodynamic intervention is to provide adequate peripheral tissue and organ oxygenation while maintaining global cardiac function. In most cases, the decision-making process is summarized with a few simple guidelines. However, in the complicated patient, knowledge of the pathophysiologic mechanisms involved in each condition is useful to help determine which specific therapeutic interventions are required. In principle, these guidelines include optimization of myocardial loading conditions, restoration of myocardial contractility without deleterious effects on cardiac rate or rhythm, and ideally a reduction in myocardial oxygen consumption.

THE UNCOMPLICATED PATIENT

In an uncomplicated course, weaning from cardiopulmonary bypass (CPB) and postoperative hemodynamic management requires only an adjustment of preload. The goal of therapy is to assist the myocardium in adapting to the modifications induced by the ischemic period (aortic cross-clamp period) and often the surgical procedure.

Following hypothermic CPB, the rewarming period is often accompanied by a decrease in systemic vascular resistance. Close monitoring and control of preload are mandatory for the reasons enumerated below. As the patient emerges from general anesthesia, serial analyses of the general hemodynamic status (systemic blood pressure, ventricular filling pressures such as central venous pressure [CVP] or pulmonary capillary wedge pressure [PCWP] and cardiac output [CO] or central [either CVP or pulmonary artery] venous oxygen saturation) will help minimize myocardial oxygen consumption while maximizing peripheral oxygen delivery. Close attention to the postoperative hemoglobin level will also avoid unnecessary hemodynamic "stress" by ensuring adequate oxygen delivery (both myocardial and peripheral). An excessive postoperative diuresis may result in hypovolemia in the post-CPB period (possibly due to perioperative use of diuretics or isovolemic hemodilution). The occurrence of hypokalemia is frequent in this setting, and potassium replacement is often required.

The pathophysiology of aortic stenosis (see Ch. 1) results in a dramatic reduction in left ventricular (LV) compliance. Ventricular output becomes heavily dependent on an adequate volume status with elevated LV filling pressures necessary to maintain LV volume. The presence and quality of atrial contraction are so important that a sequential atrioventricular temporary pacemaker may be required to maintain an effective cardiac output. Hypertension may be a problem postoperatively. This is secondary to the pre-existing chronic decrease in perfusion and may persist for days or weeks.

In contrast, the pathophysiology of chronic aortic regurgitation (see Ch. 2) may result in ventricular dysfunction, which surgery may not alleviate. Postoperatively, regurgitant flow is eliminated and LV end-diastolic volume is usually decreased. Maintenance of an adequate preload is necessary, however, in a dilated, highly compliant LV. Some patients are hypotensive after surgery as the chronic decrease in systemic vascular resistance (SVR) (an adaptive mechanism aimed to facilitate forward flow) may persist after the surgery. They may require α-adrenergic support to reverse this derangement in SVR, as well as inotropic drugs to address the impairment of cardiac function. Utilization of the intra-aortic balloon pump in the postoperative period is useful, in contrast to the preoperative period, in which it is contraindicated because of an increase in regurgitant flow.

After the surgical repair of mitral stenosis, most patients usually have an uncomplicated course, as LV function is generally preserved. However, the preoperative progression of this disorder is usually prolonged, and the chronic pressure overload present in the left atrium often results in chronic pulmonary hypertension. Pulmonary hypertension will increase right ventricular (RV) afterload and may result in RV failure either preoperatively or acutely during the postoperative period.

The pre-existing pathophysiologic changes of chronic mitral regurgitation (see Ch. 2) may require the maintenance of relatively high left atrial pressures to fill a distended left atrium adequately. Following mitral valve replacement, the disappearance of the "low-pressure pop-off" into the left atrium may impose an increased load to the LV, since the entire stroke volume (SV) is now ejected into the higher-pressure arterial system. Afterload reducing drugs and/or inotropic drugs can be beneficial in these patients.

THE COMPLICATED PATIENT

A complicated patient implies the existence of circulatory dysfunction sufficiently severe to induce peripheral organ dysfunction. Although multiple causes may complicate the postoperative course, one can schematically separate these into cardiac and noncardiac groups. The cardiac factors include (1) primary myocardial failure of ischemic or nonischemic origin, and (2) cardiac failure resulting from poorly matched loading conditions. The subsequent clinical consequences are then classified into "backward" or "forward" failures, which reflect either congestive or hypoperfusion syndromes, respectively. The noncardiac factors include pre-existing renal, hepatic, or pulmonary dysfunction (see detailed discussion in Chs. 10 and 7, respectively).

Cardiac Factors

MYOCARDIAL FAILURE

It is imperative in the complicated patient to recognize the existence of myocardial dysfunction as a participant in circulatory impairment as early as possible. Even if therapeutic management will not entail infusing inotropic drugs prior to optimizing loading conditions, knowledge of possible myocardial dysfunction is essential. Following cardiac surgery, myocardial ischemia may be secondary to an increased myocardial oxygen demand (or stress-induced myocardial ischemia), without resultant increase in myocardial oxygen delivery. One frequent cause of this oxygen deficit is postoperative hypertension, which should be treated by arterial vasodilators after control of aggravating factors such as pain or shivering. This type of myocardial ischemia (demand related) is not a major therapeutic concern, since correction of the causative agent is definitive therapy.

More frequently, however, decreased oxygen supply without a resultant increase in myocardial oxygen demand is the cause of ischemic episodes (supply related). These episodes may be secondary to coexisting coronary artery disease, perizonal ischemia following infarction, coronary emboli following surgery, sympathetic activation, or defects in myocardial protection. If LV dysfunction secondary to myocardial ischemia is suspected, two particular conditions—the "stunned"

and the "hibernating" myocardium—must be distinguished. "Stunned myocardium" refers to a transient myocardial contractile dysfunction following an ischemia-reperfusion episode (e.g., emergency coronary artery bypass graft [CABG] surgery following a complicated percutaneous transluminal coronary angioplasty). In this case, inotropic drugs can be used without deleterious effect upon myocardial energetics.[1-3] In contrast, the "hibernating myocardium" is an adaptive and protective mechanism. Myocardial contractile function is reduced because of a chronic decrease in myocardial blood flow (i.e., chronic ischemia).[4] Treatment relies on both increasing coronary blood flow and reducing myocardial oxygen demand. In this situation, inotropic drugs improve the contractile status of the heart, but at the expense of an oxygen deficit secondary to limitations in coronary blood flow.

Early diagnosis and treatment of myocardial ischemia is mandatory, especially during the first 72 hours after coronary revascularization. The appearance of ischemia during this period is associated with an increased incidence of perioperative myocardial infarction, although no data exist to suggest that treatment reduces the incidence of infarction. The diagnosis of myocardial ischemia can be difficult because of a number of "silent" or nonpainful episodes, with hypotension or ST segment alterations as the only premonitory sign. Buffington[5] proposed the maintenance of a rate-pressure ratio (heart rate divided by mean arterial pressure) less than one as an appropriate goal. Although not validated in clinical studies, keeping the value of heart rate in beats per minute lower than mean arterial pressure in mmHg is a readily available clinical indicator of subendocardial perfusion and may be more predictive than the rate-pressure product.

However, at the extremes of heart rate (i.e., less than 40 or greater than 128 beats · min^{-1}) it is neither useful or desirable. The rate-pressure ratio would lead the clinician to focus on maintaining an adequate coronary perfusion pressure primarily by controlling heart rate, an important determinant of both myocardial oxygen consumption and supply. However, in those patients with limited contractile function, stroke volume may be fixed, thus making cardiac output heart rate dependent.

Since coronary artery disease concerns both macro- and microvessels, coronary resistance might remain high (particularily in the presence of an elevation in sympathetic tone) even after the proximal stenoses have been bypassed. In this situation, sufficient coronary perfusion pressure has to be maintained. Arterial hypotension secondary to peripheral vasodilation and/or hypovolemia may precipitate or aggravate myocardial ischemia. Vasoconstrictors are required to increase coronary perfusion pressure, even though they increase LV afterload and myo-

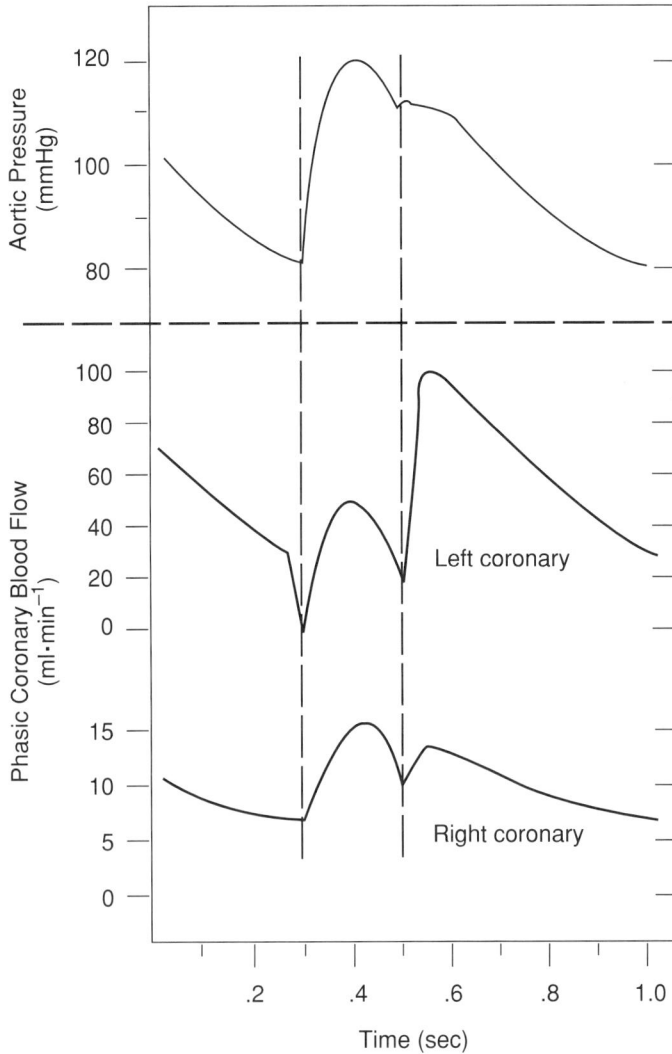

Fig. 7-1. Comparison of left and right coronary blood flow patterns. (From Berne and Levy,[34] with permission.)

cardial oxygen consumption. By contrast, in the absence of hypotension, arterial vasodilators such as calcium channel entry blockers are widely used to prevent vasospasm (especially for internal mammary artery grafts), although evidence for efficacy in this use is lacking.

Myocardial ischemia is also a frequent occurrence in patients suffering from aortic stenosis. The hypertrophic LV is easily transformed into an ischemic myocardium, and myocardial preservation can be compromised during CPB. Postoperatively, aggressive pharmacologic therapy is needed to preserve adequate coronary perfusion.

RV failure is more frequent in the hypertrophied RV associated with pulmonary hypertension and is potentiated by inadequate RV protection during aortic cross-clamping. The normal anatomic location of the RV is anterior to the LV; thus, the infrared component of the surgical lighting warms it to a greater degree. RV failure does occur, however, in the absence of pre-existing RV hypertrophy.

Two physiologic concepts are important guides to therapy. First, the thin-walled RV is a pump better adapted to volume loads than to pressure loads. Thus, a reduction in preload is poorly tolerated, but a reduction in afterload is usually beneficial. RV myocardial failure is characterized by the existence of congestive signs affecting the liver and the kidney. Inotropes are also useful to further reduce the "backward" pump failure. Second, RV coronary perfusion, in the absence of chronic hypertrophy, is present during both the systole and the diastole (Fig. 7-1). Thus, systolic coronary flow is impaired if a reduction in aortic pressure is associated with systolic pulmonary hypertension. Therapy should be directed toward improving coronary perfusion pressure by increasing aortic systolic pressure and lowering systolic pulmonary artery pressure. The recent demonstration of the effectiveness of nitric oxide inhalation as a selective pulmonary vasodilator could achieve this improvement in RV myocardial oxygen balance.[6-8]

VENTRICULAR FAILURE DUE TO LOADING CONDITIONS

Influence of Preload
Similar to the uncomplicated course, routine adjustment of preload is necessary throughout the first 24 hours. Hypovolemia is commonly a result of bleeding, excessive diuresis, and vasodilation. Optimizing preload is an easy and efficient way to enhance global ventricular function in acute heart failure. Clinically, ventricular filling pressures are

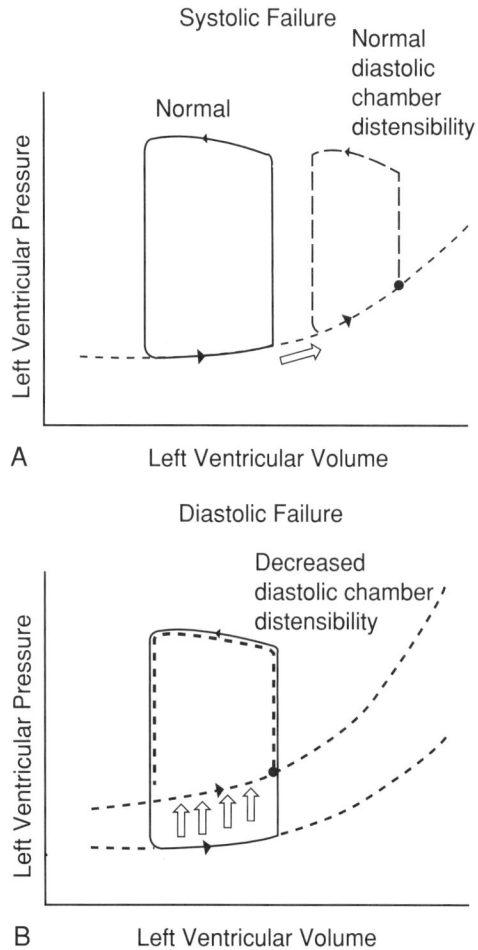

Fig. 7-2. (A & B) Diastolic left ventricular pressure-volume relationships and the influence of an increased preload or of a change in ventricular diastolic compliance on left ventricular end-diastolic pressure. (From Lorell,[35] with permission.)

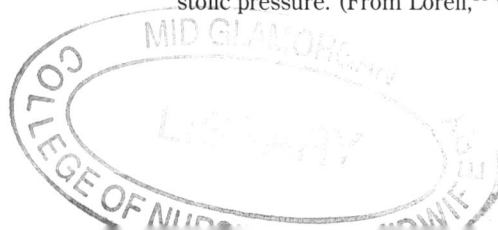

taken as an estimate of preload. The relationship between ventricular diastolic pressure and volume (i.e., ventricular diastolic function) is defined by the ventricular compliance curve. This relationship may be altered either "chronically" because of the evolution of the disease (e.g., increased diastolic stiffness in a patient suffering from aortic stenosis with a concentric hypertrophy), or "acutely" as seen during acute ventricular ischemia, which impairs LV relaxation and may elevate diastolic filling pressure without changing end-diastolic volume (LV diastolic dysfunction with reduced compliance) (Fig. 7-2).

In order to define an "adequate" level of preload for a given patient, one must be mindful of a patient's diastolic function curve if pressures are taken as an estimate of ventricular volume. For example, chronic aortic regurgitation is usually associated with an increase in compliance accompanied by eccentric hypertrophy (Fig. 7-3). In these patients, changes in LV volume are poorly correlated with changes in LV filling pressure. In contrast, during acute aortic insufficiency, as seen in acute aortic endocarditis, the destruction of the aortic valves induces a sud-

den and massive LV volume overload. Since insufficient time exists to allow for LV adaptation, severe congestive heart failure with pulmonary edema and hypotension is common. Similarly, during chronic mitral regurgitation, the LV is volume expanded with an increase in LV compliance (LV filling pressures are only slightly elevated despite an extremely high LV end-diastolic volume). As a consequence of the regurgitant flow, the left atrium enlarges to "absorb" this regurgitant energy. This "protects" the pulmonary vasculature against large increases in pressure; however, during acute mitral regurgitation (e.g., papillary muscle dysfunction following myocardial infarction), the left atrium cannot accommodate the sudden regurgitant flow. This requires the pulmonary venous and capillary beds to dissipate the excess energy. The result is often noted clinically as "giant v-waves" seen on the pulmonary artery capillary wedge pressure tracing. (For a more complete discussion of these changes see Ch. 2.)

Influence of Afterload

For any set of contractility and preload conditions, afterload is an important determinant

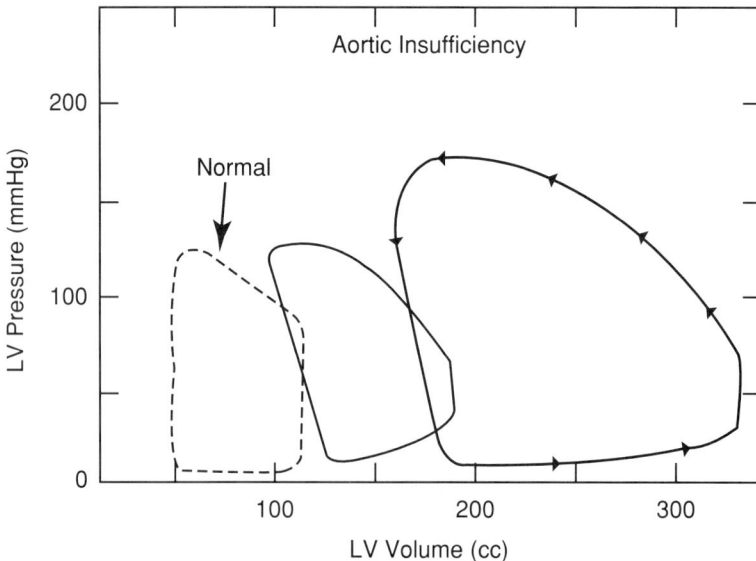

Fig. 7-3. Left ventricular pressure-volume relationships in normal (left loop), acute (center loop), and chronic (right loop) aortic regurgitation. (From Jackson et al.,[36] with permission.)

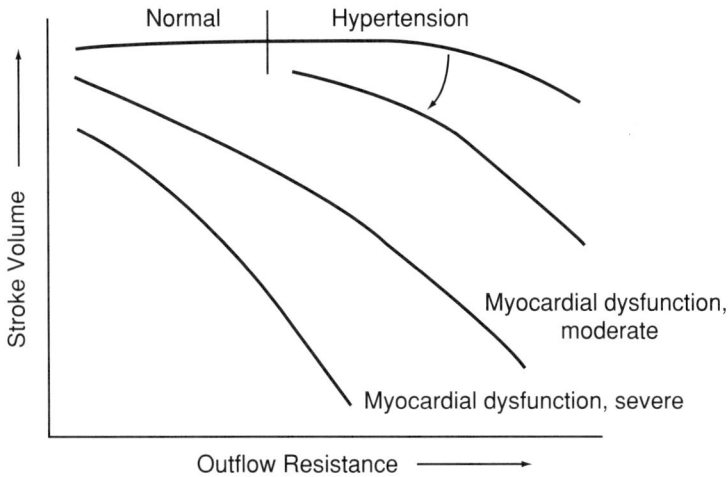

Fig. 7-4. Changes in left ventricular stroke volume with increased afterload. (From Cohn and Franciosa,[37] with permission.)

of CO. SV is inversely related to ventricular afterload (i.e., CO decreases as afterload increases) and the relationship is steeper in the presence of poor contractility (i.e., LV failure) (Fig. 7-4). Thus, if one administers an arterial vasodilator, the improvement in SV is a direct function of the baseline ventricular function.

Afterload is routinely envisioned as a single parameter, SVR. Strictly speaking, however, afterload is a combination of elastance, resistance, and inertance. While afterload is usually considered a parameter influencing LV function, it is also a mechanical characteristic of the arterial circulation. That is to say, for each SV, there is a corresponding increase in arterial pressure (Fig. 7-5). The slope of this vascular pressure-volume relationship represent the arterial elastance (E_a) of the system. The left ventricle and the arterial circulation are joined together during ejection, forming a "coupled" biologic system. This interaction is described as "ventriculo-arterial coupling" and is analyzed in a format proposed by Sunagawa et al.[9] The slope of the arterial elastance E_a (which joins the end-systolic pressure-volume point to the end-diastolic pressure-volume point is added to the classic ventricular pressure-volume loop (Fig. 7-5). "Flipping" the systemic arte-

rial pressure-volume relationship such that the stroke volume parameter decreases from left to right (Fig. 7-5C), allows one to superimpose on a single diagram the interaction of the ventricular and systemic arterial pressure-volume relationships. The end-systolic pressure-volume point represents the intersection between E_{es} (the ventricular systolic maximum elastance derived from the end-systolic pressure-volume relationship) and E_a. E_{es} is also known as E_{max}, the term used for the remainder of this discussion.

Using the relationships between preload (i.e., end-diastolic volume), afterload (i.e., E_a), and contractility (i.e., E_{max}) enables one to better understand the expected hemodynamic modifications following the administration of a venous or arterial vasodilator. The application of this method of graphic analysis is also useful in comprehending the vasodilator therapy in patients with heart failure.

When a venodilator is administered, a decrease in SV (from SV to SV' in Fig. 7-6) occurs simultaneously with a decrease in arterial pressure (P_{es}) (assuming a constant inotropic state). If a pure arterial vasodilator is used, a similar decrease in P_{es} is achieved through selective afterload reduction. As the

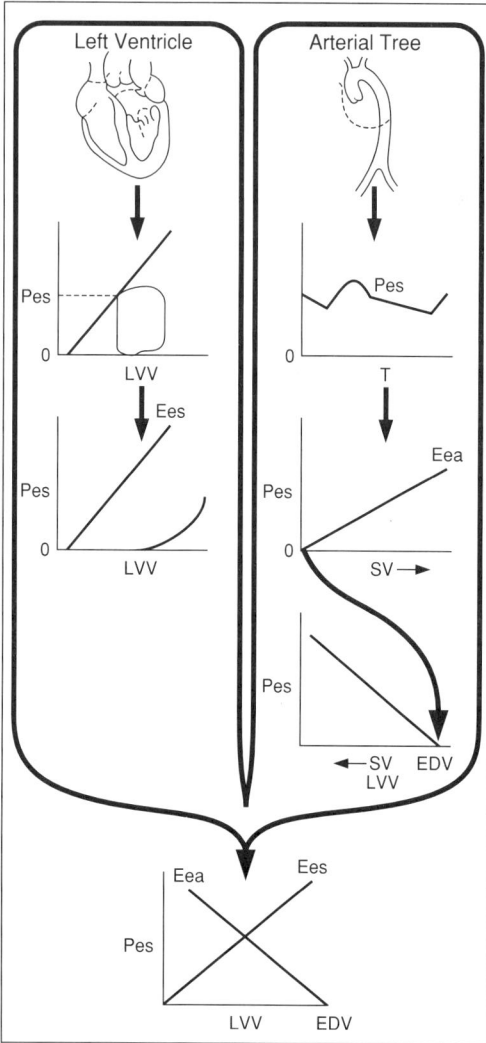

Fig. 7-5. Pressure-volume relationships for the left ventricle and the arterial tree. E_{es} reflects the slope of the end-systolic pressure-volume relationship (*left*), and E_{ea} the elastance of the arterial tree. Rearranging these relations allows representation on a single diagram (*bottom*) of the ventricular and arterial parameters, E_{es} and E_{ea}, intersecting at the end-systolic pressure end-systolic volume point. (From Sunagawa et al.,[9] with permission.)

slope of the arterial elastance relationship decreases from E_a to E_a' (Fig. 7-6B), if preload (i.e., same end-diastolic volume) is unaltered, SV will increase from SV to SV″ (Fig. 7-6B).

As an example of this "coupling" effect in clinical practice, vasodilating drugs result in combined reductions in preload and afterload. Thus, the resultant effect is an interaction between preload and afterload.[10] The failing ventricle is relatively preload independent but very afterload dependent. This interaction of pathophysiology and pharmacology results in different quantitative changes following vasodilator therapy in heart failure when compared to normal individuals.[11,12] When LV failure is present, E_{max} (the slope of the end-systolic pressure-volume relationship) is decreased. If one examines the E_{max} to E_a relationship in heart failure (low E_{max}), one notes that the decrease in SV induced by a venous vasodilator will be of lesser magnitude than that observed with a normal heart (Fig. 7-7). Conversely, the administration of an arterial vasodilator (moving from point E_a to E_a' in Fig. 7-8) in a patient with a similar decrease in E_{max} will induce a greater increase in SV than in a patient with a normal heart.[13]

If, despite correction of both preload and afterload, inadequate perfusion persists, impairment of myocardial contractility is usually the culprit. Impaired contractility may be due to pre-existing degradation of cardiac function, preoperative treatment with negative inotropic drugs, perioperative myocardial infarction, coronary emboli, or spasm. Since a pure inotropic drug (i.e., one devoid of vasoactive action) is not currently available, one must consider an inotrope's effect on afterload, when support is required. For instance, dobutamine, (an inotropic drug with vasodilating properties[14,15]) or the combination of dobutamine and a vasodilator, are two alternatives when hypoperfusion is associated with normo- or hypertension, respectively.

By contrast, inotropic drugs with vasoconstrictive properties such as dopamine or epi-

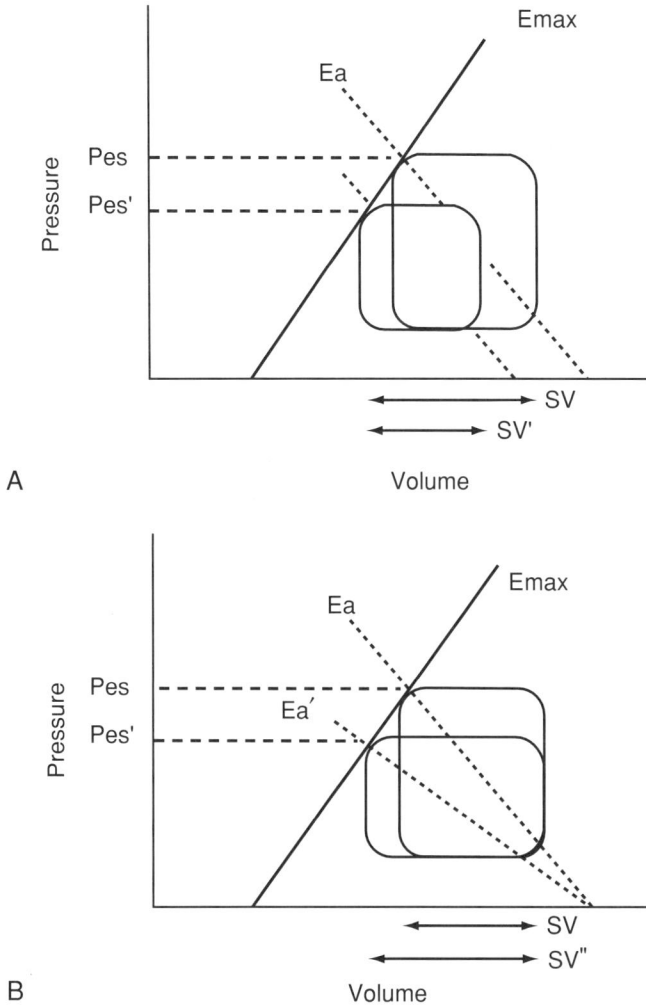

Fig. 7-6. Changes in stroke volume induced by **(A)** the administration of a pure venous vasodilator or **(B)** a pure arterial vasodilator. (From Payen and Beloucif,[38] with permission.)

nephrine can elevate afterload and coronary perfusion pressure, which may be useful in hypoperfused patients with "peripheral vascular failure" or low SVR. However, if the elevation in afterload is out of proportion to the positive inotropic effect, little or no increase in SV is expected.

Cardiac Tamponade
In cardiac tamponade, the transmural ventricular filling pressures are very small because of the significant compressive effect of blood or blood clots in the mediastinum. Compared

to the classic signs of tamponade seen in "medical" diseases (increased CVP equal to PCWP, decreased CO with pulsus paradoxus), following cardiac surgery, tamponade can present with the association of a low CO and hypotension in a patient who was formerly suffering from excessive postoperative bleeding. Fluid loading in this scenario will induce a marked increase in ventricular filling pressures without correcting hypotension.

While the equalization of RV and LV filling

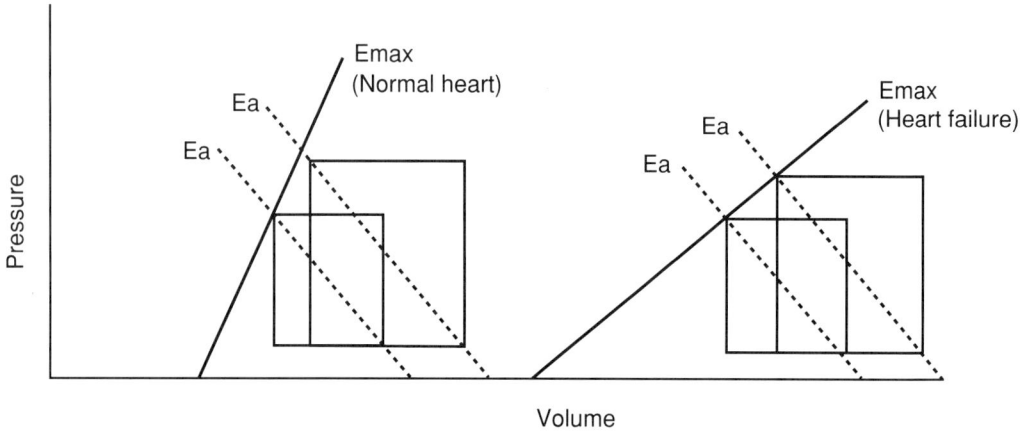

Fig. 7-7. Changes in stroke volume induced by the administration of a pure venous vasodilator in a patient with a normal heart or the presence of left ventricular failure.

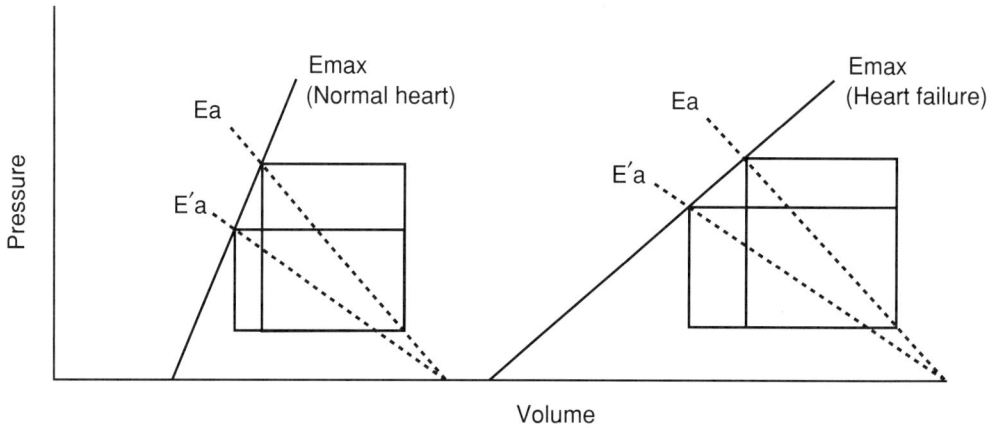

Fig. 7-8. Changes in stroke volume induced by the administration of a pure arterial vasodilator in a patient with a normal heart or in the presence of a left ventricular failure.

pressures may help differentiate this diagnosis from acute heart failure, echocardiography is especially helpful (see Ch. 14). In particular, cases of localized compression of the atrium (regional tamponade) are difficult to diagnose by any other means. Recently, the disappearance of a positive diastolic venous inflow in the superior vena cava or hepatic veins has proved a reliable echocardiographic sign of cardiac tamponade.[16–18] On the CVP trace, this sign will correlate with a diminished or absent diastolic y-descent (Fig. 7-9) contrasted with a maintained systolic x-descent.[19] Finally, in some patients diagnosis can prove very difficult, and a high index of suspicion is required for patients with an

Fig. 7-9. Modifications in venous flows in a pulmonary vein (Q_{PV}), the superior vena cava (Q_{SVC}), the inferior vena cava (Q_{IVC}), and in left ventricular (P_{LV}), right atrial (P_{RA}), and pericardial (P_{PE}) pressures (**A**) before and (**B**) after production of cardiac tamponade in a dog. (From Beloucif et al.,[19] with permission.)

Systole Diastole

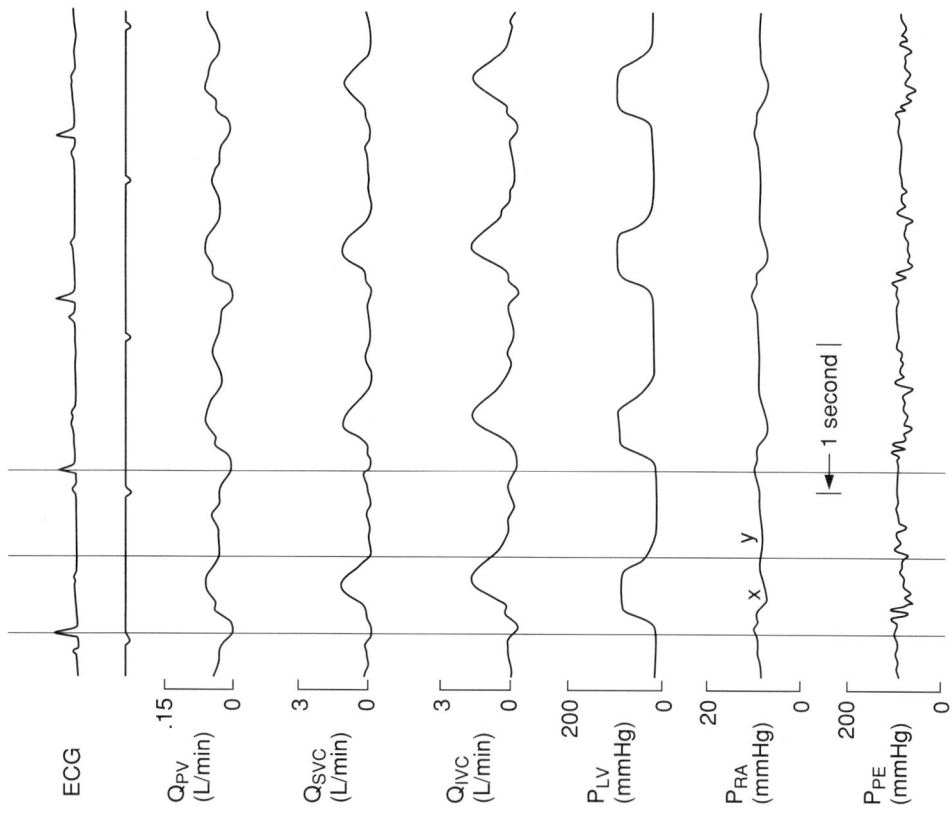

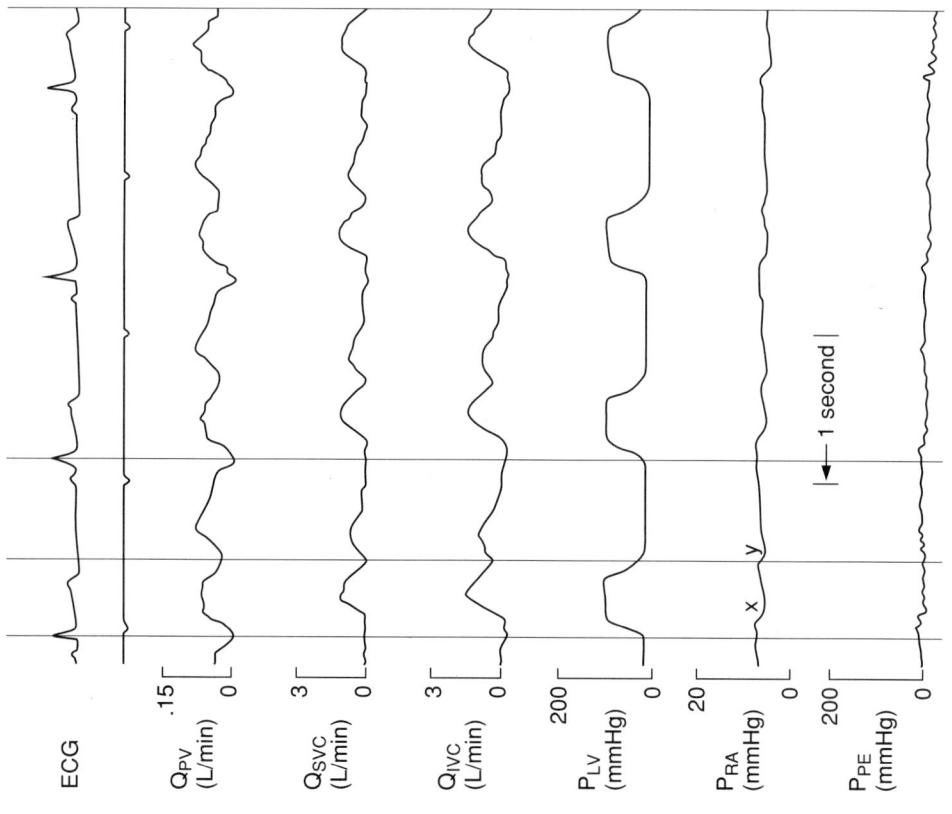

ECG

Q_{PV} (L/min)

Q_{SVC} (L/min)

Q_{IVC} (L/min)

P_{LV} (mmHg)

P_{RA} (mmHg)

P_{PE} (mmHg)

A

B

ECG

Q_{PV} (L/min)

Q_{SVC} (L/min)

Q_{IVC} (L/min)

P_{LV} (mmHg)

P_{RA} (mmHg)

P_{PE} (mmHg)

133

increase in CVP associated with "unexplained" progressive oliguria.

Treatment is surgical, with reopening of the chest and evacuation of the blood and blood clots present in the mediastinum. Emergent therapy includes maintenance of elevated venous pressure by either fluid loading or MAST (Military Anti-Shock Trousers) suit combined with small doses of vasopressors. Ketamine or etomidate are the anesthetic agents of choice, as both maintain systemic venous compliance, thus preventing a precipitous fall in blood pressure.

The Body

Once the diagnosis of myocardial insufficiency is entertained and the etiology of this dysfunction elucidated, attention is next drawn to the organ-specific consequences of heart failure. The clinical symptoms can be separated into (1) "backward failure," with signs of congestion of blood upstream from the LV (acute pulmonary edema) or the RV (jugular venous distension and congestive hepatomegaly); and (2) "forward failure," the reduced ability of the myocardium to deliver blood downstream from the LV, leading to acute circulatory failure, systemic hypoperfusion, oliguria, and altered mentation. Finally, some patients present with both syndromes, indicating a grave prognosis.

PATHOPHYSIOLOGIC CONSEQUENCES OF BACKWARD FAILURE (CONGESTION)

When RV dysfunction predominates, signs of backward failure will mainly include renal or hepatic dysfunction. For the kidney, increased vena caval pressure will aggravate any pre-existing reduction in renal perfusion pressure and may rarely initiate such a reduction in the otherwise uncomplicated patient. Although elevated ventricular filling pressures trigger an increase in the secretion of atrial natriuretic factor (ANF) and vasodilatory prostaglandins, the relentless progression to renal failure frequently occurs in this setting. Besides usual symptomatic treatment (forced diuresis or continuous hemofiltration), improvement in systemic hemodynamics (i.e., relief of the signs of venous congestion and increasing CO) is mandatory.

In the case of acute hepatic dysfunction following cardiac surgery, the latter considerations (i.e., increasing CO) are of paramount importance, as there are no similar strategies for improving hepatic excretory function. Often in this setting, hepatic venous congestion is superimposed on decreased arterial inflow. Marked elevation in hepatic transaminases are noted, indicative of centrilobular hepatic necrosis.[20] Subsequently, increased coagulation times and lactate production result as hepatocellular function further deteriorates. Although continuous hemofiltration controls the deleterious increases in venous pressures, primary therapy is aimed at improving organ perfusion and cardiac function.

The introduction of inhaled nitric oxide following mitral valve replacement can ameliorate the increased pulmonary vascular resistance and possibly decrease RV afterload.[6-8] As previously discussed, decreasing RV afterload improves RV function, resulting in improved CO for a lower CVP. In a patient with overwhelming RV dysfunction and distension with secondary hepatic dysfunction, inhaled nitric oxide reportedly increased both mixed venous and hepatic venous oxygen saturations, resulting in normalization of hepatic function (Fig. 7-10).

LV failure elevates left atrial and pulmonary artery occlusion pressure and may lead to pulmonary edema and pleural effusion. This would be potentiated by any alterations in permeability of the alveolo-interstitial membrane. CPB results in activation of the complement and cytokine cascade systems (see Ch. 5), which alter alveolar permeability. Following cardiac surgery, acute respiratory failure (an "ARDS-like lung") is often associated with cardiogenic pulmonary edema. This condition may require the initiation of therapeutic maneuvers (titration of optimal positive end-expiratory pressure [PEEP])

11 AM   3 PM

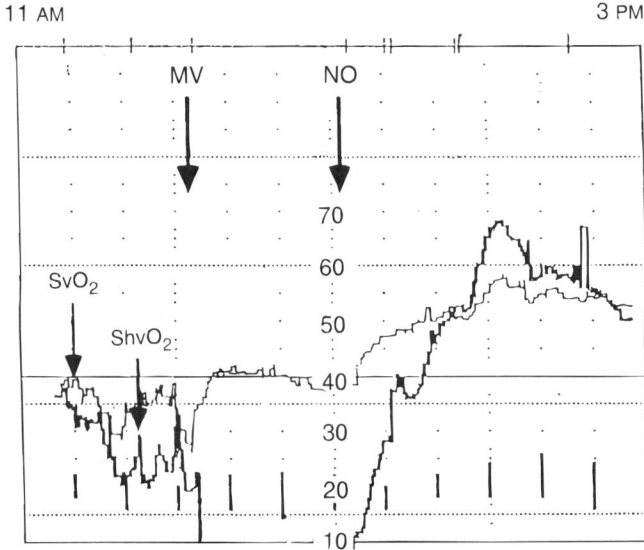

Fig. 7-10. Effect of nitric oxide (NO) administration on the evolution of mixed venous ($S\bar{v}O_2$) and hepatic venous oxygen saturations ($ShvO_2$) in a patient with severe right ventricular failure. "MV" denotes initiation of mechanical ventilation. (From Gatecel et al.,[40] with permission.)

(see Ch. 6), which aggravate the existing myocardial dysfunction. Thus, pulmonary congestion secondary to LV failure may exacerbate pulmonary hypertension in patients with borderline RV function. This not only worsens pulmonary gas exchange but also causes an additional workload for the RV.

PATHOPHYSIOLOGIC CONSEQUENCES OF FORWARD FAILURE (ISCHEMIA)

Compensatory mechanisms for acute LV decompensation typically result in hyperstimulation of the sympathetic system. This usually results in the elevation of SVR to maintain arterial blood pressure. However, as previously discussed, LV function further deteriorates only as a consequence of the increase in workload.[12,21]

Forward failure with shock induces both splanchnic ischemia (reduced portal blood flow) and decreased hepatic arterial inflow. If this decrease in hepatic blood flow is amplified (by hepatic venous congestion), marked decreases in hepatic perfusion pressure are the result. The kidney is also sensitive to similar alterations in perfusion pressure. The cli-

nician is faced with the necessity of improving both systemic arterial pressure and forward flow in a patient with low-CO syndrome.

If overall organ perfusion is not improved by the optimization of loading conditions, the administration of an inotrope might restore blood pressure by improving forward flow. However, in cases of refractory LV dysfunction, systemic hypotension may persist despite inotropic therapy, because of inability to perfuse the coronary vascular bed. In these cases, the utilization of vasopressors is necessary in order to treat this refractory hypotension. The aim is to interrupt the vicious circle of severe cardiac dysfunction and hypotension, aggravating the decrement in cardiac performance via secondary coronary and systemic ischemia.

Dopamine and norepinephrine are effective as vasopressors, and epinephrine in higher dosages is useful when additional inotropic effect is desired. These drugs must be progressively titrated. Rather than relying on a predetermined blood pressure level as the goal (e.g., systolic blood pressure of 100 mmHg), one might choose to consider the lowest blood pressure, restoring urine output or decreasing blood lactate levels as a more appropriate endpoint.

TREATMENT

Besides purely cardiac parameters (i.e., intrinsic contractile state), CO is also determined by peripheral factors. As previously discussed, the failing heart is relatively preload independent but is very sensitive to alterations in afterload. In the postoperative management of the cardiac surgical patient, one must consider both inotropes and vasopressors.

A Simplified Algorithm for Hemodynamic Management After Cardiac Surgery

The hemodynamic management of patients after cardiac surgery relies on simultaneous measurements of preload (pulmonary artery occlusion pressure-PA catheter, central venous pressure-CVP catheter, or end-diastolic volume echocardiography) and myocardial performance (cardiac output-PA catheter, central venous PO_2-CVP catheter, or ejection fraction echocardiography). This leads to four different situations according to a "low" or "normal" myocardial performance and a "low" or "high" preload. The remainder of this section refers to data generated from a PA catheter, but similar tables can be constructed using the other parameters (Fig. 7-11). Compared to the normal pulmonary artery occlusion pressure (PAOP)-normal CO situation, a decreased CO associated with a low PAOP would reflect a hypovolemic status, whereas an elevated PAOP, even if it is not always a reliable indicator of preload, would indicate the possibility for pulmonary congestion.

In addition to this classical format, clinical decisions based on CO and mean systemic arterial pressure (MAP) values could be used. Hemodynamic patterns are more readily assessed, rather than requiring the calculation of SVR:

$$SVR = [MAP - CVP]/CO$$

This recommendation is based on the following observations. First, compared to MAP, the value of CVP is small and can be neglected. Second, calculation of the true resistance of the arterial system would require measurement of the critical arterial closing pressure. Critical arterial closing pressure cannot be measured in clinical practice but can be as high as 30 or 35 mmHg (much higher than the typical CVP). Additionally, rather than considering a value of CO as "normal," "low," or "high," one should consider a given CO as adequate or not, as it relates to peripheral oxygen requirements. Such a distinction is usually easily obtained after cardiac surgery from $S\bar{v}O_2$ values. Since a normal (greater than 75 percent) $S\bar{v}O_2$ usually reflects a normal peripheral extraction of oxygen by the organism, it is assumed to reflect an adequate CO compared to the peripheral tissue needs.

Figure 7-12 describes such a format considering the possible values of MAP and CO, in which six theoretical hemodynamic situations can be considered.

1. *Systemic hypertension with a low CO:* In this case, arterial vasodilators are usually considered in order to decrease the LV afterload, thus lowering arterial pressure while simultaneously correcting the decreased CO. This situation is the most frequent hemodynamic profile following cardiac surgery. However, before initiating therapy with an arterial vasodilator, one should eliminate hypovolemia as a possible etiology, as postoperative hypertension is a frequent presentation of hypovolemia. Fluid loading in such patients will result in normalization of blood pressure with marked increases in CO. If the diagnosis of hypovolemia is not considered, the administration of an arterial vasodilator will be poorly tolerated; resulting in sig-

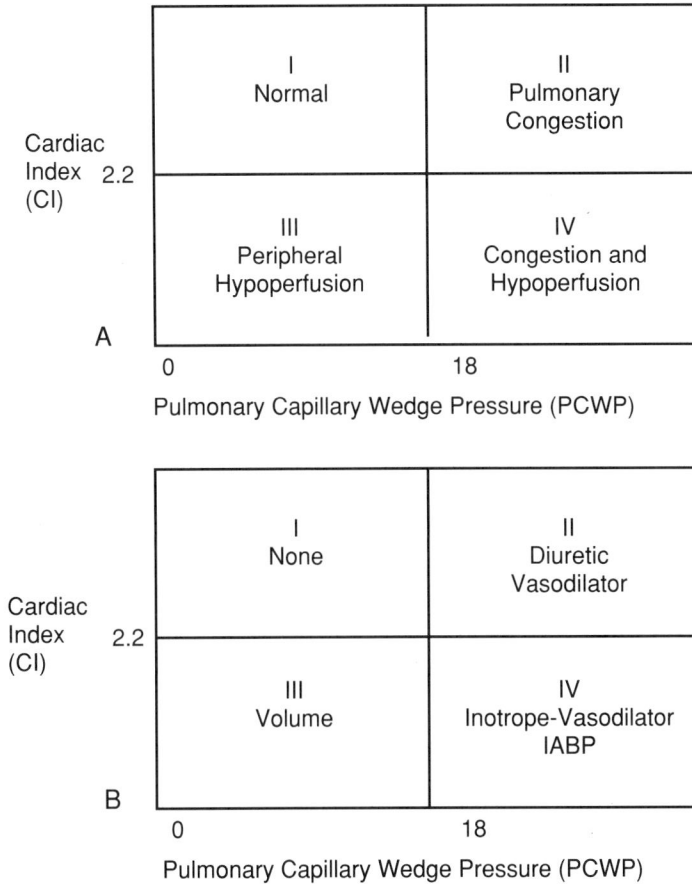

Fig. 7-11. (A & B) Hemodynamic management derived from simultaneous PAOP and CO measurements. (From Kaplan and Guffin,[39] with permission.)

nificant decreases in arterial pressure without simultaneous improvement in stroke volume. If the patient is hypertensive and normovolemic, however, arterial vasodilators are very effective, with regard to both peripheral (CO will increase) and myocardial (since myocardial oxygen consumption will decrease) oxygen utilization.

2. *Systemic hypertension with a high or normal CO:* Before prescribing a vasodilator, an etiology must be sought, such as postoperative pain or shivering. Primary treatment of the etiologic agent rather than the hypertension per se must always be considered first. Symptomatically lowering arterial pressure at a time when the patient

has a high oxygen consumption would serve little or no purpose and could result in deleterious changes in myocardial oxygen utilization. As this scenario is typically associated with a hyperadrenergic state, central α_2-agonists (clonidine, dexmedetomidine, ivascerol), and peripheral β-adrenergic blockers are often helpful in ablating sympathetic tone.

3. *Hypotension associated with a low CO:* The initial management of a patient with this condition requires optimizing the PAOP. A low PAOP (or low CVP/end-diastolic volume) ideally reflects a small ventricular filling volume (hypovolemic state), and this patient must receive fluid loading. If

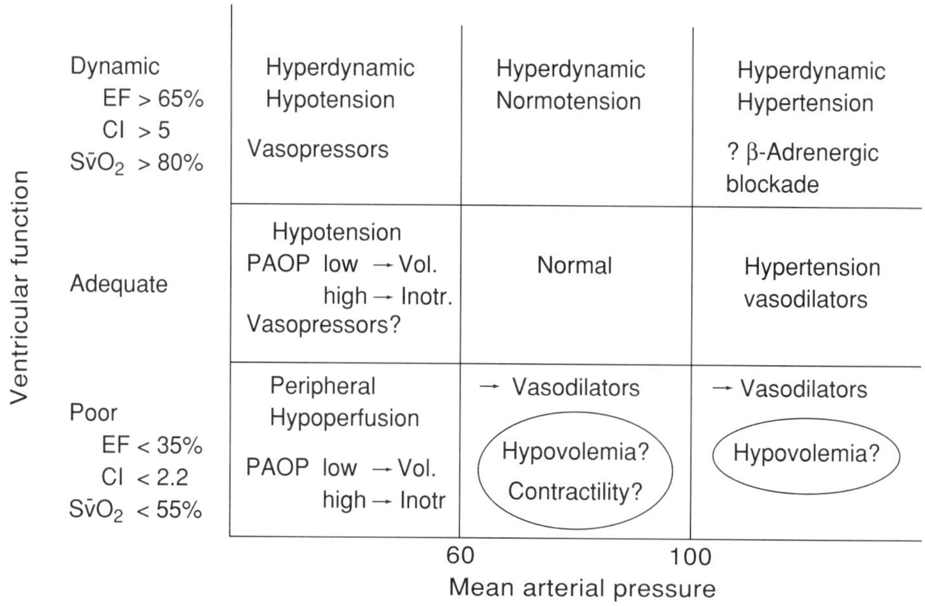

Fig. 7-12. Simplified algorithm for hemodynamic management after cardiac surgery.

PAOP is markedly increased (i.e., higher than 18 mmHg), a cardiogenic component is the problem and inotropic administration is usually indicated. It is, however, important to ensure that there is no component of diastolic dysfunction. The most direct route is by transesophageal echocardiography (TEE) (see Ch. 14). If the end-diastolic ventricular chamber size is large and the contractile function poor, the requirement for inotropic support is ensured. When a persistent low CO syndrome is present despite "maximal" medical pharmacologic support, placement of an intra-aortic balloon pump should be considered[22] (see Ch. 17).

4. *Low CO at a normal systemic blood pressure:* Measurement of ventricular filling will aid in the delineation of hypovolemia or impaired contractility. The existence of normotension allows one to reduce afterload selectively with lesser (but not absent) concerns regarding associated hypovolemia. If the low output syndrome is associated with normal or elevated ven-

tricular filling, the selection of inotropic drugs with arterial vasodilating properties such as dobutamine, amrinone, or enoximone is important.

5. *Hyperdynamic hypotension (systemic hypotension at a high CO):* Significant concern for coronary perfusion pressure must exist in this subgroup. This hemodynamic profile (resembling the hyperdynamic state of septic shock) might respond simply to vasopressors. The goal is to both increase systemic blood pressure to adequate levels and improve peripheral perfusion. One must be careful to avoid increasing the workload to the heart. This profile seems to occur more frequently when warm cardioplegia is used. Estimation of ventricular function is mandatory when vasopressors are considered, as the addition of a pure α-agonist such as phenylephrine is poorly tolerated if baseline cardiac function is impaired. In borderline cases, epinephrine or norepinephrine, which combine α and β effects, is more appropriate. The inotropic effect induced by stimula-

tion of cardiac β-receptors will mitigate the potentially deleterious effect of increased afterload on cardiac function. In cases of refractory hypotension, placement of an intra-aortic balloon pump should be discussed in order to augment diastolic coronary blood flow and reduce myocardial oxygen consumption.

6. *Hyperdynamic normotension:* There is little to be gained from hemodynamic manipulation of this patient. The principal goal is to monitor the hemodynamic situation frequently. If the patient returns to a normal state (adequate ventricular function and normotension), no other therapy is indicated. If, however, the patient develops hyperdynamic hypertension as the effects of anesthetic drugs become less marked, vasodilators, analgesic agents, or sympatholytic agents are the front-line defense. Finally, if the patient's condition changes to a hyperdynamic hypotensive state, vasoconstrictive agents are required.

Specific Therapeutic Agents

VOLUME LOADING

In patients with acute heart failure, early detection and treatment of associated hypovolemia are mandatory before starting more aggressive therapy with inotropic or vasodilating drugs. Volume replacement is especially important in cases of acute rather than chronic heart failure because the acutely failing heart is relatively preload sensitive (unlike the chronic scenario). This condition is common when symptoms of acute heart failure develop in a patient with previously normal ventricular function or following inappropriate diuretic or vasodilation therapy.

If myocardial function was previously impaired, hypovolemia presents without signs of congestion in the pulmonary vascular bed, low pulmonary artery occlusion pressures, or CVP (classically less than 15 mmHg) and a normal or slightly small ventricular cavity on echocardiography. The diagnosis is confirmed with rapid infusions of 300 to 500 ml of fluid while observing changes in PAOP or

CVP and CO. If pulmonary artery occlusion or central venous pressure rise without a corresponding increase in cardiac output, then additional strategies are warranted to increase CO.

DRUGS WITH PREDOMINANTLY CARDIAC EFFECTS

Dobutamine is a synthetic catecholamine with predominantly β_1-adrenergic agonist properties and slight α_1-adrenergic effects. The normal α_1-vasoconstrictor effects are partially offset by peripheral β_2 actions; thus, the effect of intravenous dobutamine is generally an inotropic effect, with little or no peripheral effect. Dobutamine can affect both heart rate and rhythm but is generally without a deleterious elevation in arterial blood pressure. This results in a beneficial effect of dobutamine on the balance between myocardial oxygen consumption and myocardial oxygen supply (coronary blood flow). The use of inotropic agents that are oxygen utilization "neutral" is especially important following coronary bypass graft surgery.[23]

DRUGS WITH CARDIAC AND VASCULAR EFFECTS

Dopamine is a natural catecholamine, a precursor of epinephrine and norepinephrine. Dopamine, like dobutamine, possesses potent β_1-adrenergic effects that induce an increase in contractility; however, dopamine also stimulates peripheral α_1-adrenergic receptors (directly and indirectly by stimulation of the release of endogenous norepinephrine) that may lead to vasoconstrictive side effects. The venoconstrictive effects may reduce systemic venous compliance and increase ventricular filling pressures when the vasoconstrictive properties of dopamine override the beneficial inotropic effects. As discussed earlier, this situation may result in myocardial oxygen imbalance.

The primary clinical advantage of dopamine is the stimulation of dopaminergic-specific receptors in the renal and mesenteric vascular beds at low doses (2 to 3 $\mu g \cdot kg^{-1}$

$\cdot$ min^{-1}). Mesenteric and renal blood flows are increased, with salutory effects on glomerular filtration rate and sodium excretion. The dose-response curves for the α-, β-, and dopamine receptors are not identical from patient to patient. One must carefully define the effect before titrating the dose. It is possible for α-constrictive effects to overlap with "dopaminergic" effects or for the "dopaminergic" effect not to occur.

Norepinephrine is one of the endogenous catecholamines that serve as chemical mediators of the sympathetic nervous system. Norepinephrine has a predominantly vasoconstrictive effect. It stimulates β_1-cardiac receptors increasing cardiac force and rate but is devoid of β_2 peripheral vasodilating activity. When this absence of β_2 effect is combined with a strong affinity for the α_1-receptor, vasoconstriction is the inevitable result. Accordingly, the indication is to raise very low blood pressure values (as in the systemic inflammatory response syndrome/septic shock) that can compromise coronary perfusion. The doses of norepinephrine used should be carefully titrated to maintain coronary perfusion pressure without a resultant decrease in cardiac output. The intense peripheral vasoconstriction induced by norepinephrine may adversely affect organ perfusion while increasing cardiac work, thus perpetuating myocardial ischemia.

Epinephrine is the other endogenous catecholamine. It stimulates cardiac β_1-receptors, with effects on β_2- and α_1-peripheral adrenergic receptors. At low doses (1 to 2 μg $\cdot$ min^{-1} or 15 to 30 ng $\cdot$ kg^{-1} $\cdot$ min^{-1} in a 70-kg individual), epinephrine acts mainly on β_1- and β_2-receptors, with an increased CO secondary to enhanced contractility and systemic vasodilatation. From 2 to 10 μg $\cdot$ min^{-1} (30 to 150 ng $\cdot$ kg^{-1} $\cdot$ min^{-1}), stimulation of the peripheral α_1-receptors increases with concomitant vasoconstriction despite stimulation of the β_1-cardiac receptors. At higher doses (10 to 20 μg μg $\cdot$ min^{-1} or 150 to 300 ng $\cdot$ kg^{-1} $\cdot$ min^{-1}), the cardiac β_1 effects are overwhelmed and an intense vasoconstrictive reaction may occur.

Epinephrine is more frequently effective for weaning from cardiopulmonary bypass than dopamine or dobutamine.[24] Epinephrine is also useful following cardiac surgery when a state similar to that observed with septic shock is accompanied by a decreased inotropic state. Finally, in patients with RV failure due to pulmonary hypertension, the vasoconstrictive properties of epinephrine are intensified when infused through a left atrial catheter. This is especially advantageous when combined with an intravenous pulmonary vasodilator such as isoproterenol or the prostaglandin (PGE$_1$) administered via a right atrial catheter.

Isoproterenol is a synthetic catecholamine with β_1 and β_2 activity. Isoproterenol has inotropic properties, but with a vasodilating action that decreases arterial pressure and is associated with a marked chronotropic effect. It may precipitate a myocardial oxygen imbalance as coronary perfusion pressure is reduced, whereas the tachycardia and the increased inotropic stimulation increase myocardial oxygen consumption. Its primary indications are to reverse the effects of therapy with β-blockers or to treat complete atrioventricular (AV) heart block pharmacologically. Finally, isoproterenol may be useful as a treatment for acute RV failure secondary to acute pulmonary hypertension.[25] The decrease in PVR with isoproterenol therapy is generally more pronounced than the decrease in SVR.

DRUGS WITH PREDOMINANTLY VASCULAR EFFECTS

Nitroprusside is a potent nitrosovasodilator, leading to both arterial and venous vasodilation.[10,11] It is a short-acting drug that is titrated to enhance cardiac function by decreasing afterload and is especially helpful in patients with LV failure. Nitroprusside is a potentially toxic drug when infused for long durations (greater than 24 to 48 hours), because of cyanide toxicity. The primary use of nitroprusside is to "test the hypothesis" that a reduction in afterload is advantageous. Once the hypothesis is examined, therapy should either be continued with a long-acting agent (hydralazine, Ca^{++}-channel blocker, angiotensin-converting enzyme [ACE] inhibitor) or discontinued as unhelpful.

Nitroglycerin is a systemic vasodilator acting predominantly on the capacitive venous compartment. This increase in venous capacitance results in peripheral venous blood pooling and a decrease in ventricular filling pressures. This reduction in ventricular filling pressure is useful in congestive heart failure, reducing myocardial oxygen consumption while maintaining stable CO and blood pressure. Overzealous administration can result in hypotension with a baroreflex-mediated increase in heart rate.[26,27] Nitroglycerin may be administered as prophylactic therapy following coronary revascularization. Although the incidence of perioperative hypertension is reduced, an increased incidence of hypotensive episodes is observed. Furthermore, prophylactic administration did not prevent the occurrence of myocardial ischemia or decrease the incidence of postoperative myocardial infarction.[28]

DRUGS WITH VASCULAR AND CARDIAC EFFECTS

A new class of agents, the phosphodiesterase inhibitors (i.e., amrinone, milrinone, or enoximone), combine inotropic and vasodilating properties. These drugs act on the phosphodiesterase enzymes that usually metabolize cAMP. Intracellular cAMP levels are increased in cardiac muscle and peripheral vascular smooth muscle, thus explaining their inotropic and vasodilating properties. Compared to dobutamine, a similar increase in cardiac index is achieved, but at a lower PAOP and without the deleterious increase in heart rate.[29] Compared to nitroprusside, for a similar decrease in PAOP and SVR, cardiac index and MAP are higher after intravenous enoximone administration.[30] These drugs also improve ventricular relaxation,

which may explain how a decrease in pulmonary artery occlusion pressure is accompanied by an increase in cardiac output. As ventricular relaxation improves, ventricular compliance improves, resulting in a higher end-diastolic volume for any ventricular pressure.[31]

The therapeutic application of the phosphodiesterase inhibitors could be limited after cardiac surgery because of their duration of action compared to catecholamines (long versus short). Although there is a theoretical concern regarding the release of hypoxic pulmonary vasoconstriction, in practice, aggravation of hypoxemia is not a common problem. This latter effect may be minimized by the resulting increase in CO after treatment. As CO increases, mixed venous saturation would also increase, possibly counteracting any increase in venous admixture.[32] Finally, synergistic effects are described in association with epinephrine, especially in severe heart failure patients during weaning from cardiopulmonary bypass.[33]

CONCLUSION

Care of the complicated patient requires recognition of the independent effects of afterload, preload and contractile state alterations, as well as their mutual interdependence. Additionally, the management goals must incorporate previous pathophysiologic organ dysfunction when one is choosing a therapeutic strategy. Cardiac hypertrophy or dilation may already be present as part of the chronic adaptation to pressure or volume overload that accompanied the cardiac disease that necessitated surgery (see Ch. 1). Postoperatively, if acute heart failure develops, additional compensatory mechanisms are mainly the consequence of sympathetic stimulation. This increase in catecholamine release will change myocardial metabolism dramatically. This pathophysiologic adaptation may induce dysrhythmias, cause peripheral vasoconstriction, and increase LV afterload and myocardial oxygen consumption.

All these factors have a deleterious effect on ventricular performance. The etiology of complications following cardiac surgery are multifactorial. Treatment is directed toward improving heart function while simultaneously adjusting the peripheral circulation. Detrimental alterations in cardiac function may be ascendant after cardiac surgery and may precipitate peripheral hypoperfusion. Conversely, dramatic reductions in arterial tone may lead to ventricular failure by decreasing coronary perfusion. These two elements must be examined when contemplating therapeutic options and consequences.

REFERENCES

1. Bolli R: Mechanism of myocardial "stunning." Circulation 82:723–38, 1990
2. Bolli R, Zhu WX: Beta-Adrenergic stimulation reverses postischemic myocardial dysfunction without producing subsequent functional deterioration. Am J Cardiol 56:964–8, 1985
3. Braunwald E, Kloner RA: The stunned myocardium: prolonged postichemic ventricular dysfunction. Circulation 66:1146–9, 1982
4. Rahimtoola SH: The hibernating myocardium. Am Heart J 117:211–21, 1989
5. Buffington CW: Hemodynamic determinants of ischemic myocardial dysfunction in the presence of coronary stenosis in dogs. Anesthesiology 63:651–62, 1985
6. Girard C, Lehot JJ, Pannotier JC et al: Inhaled nitric oxide after mitral valve replacement in patients with chronic pulmonary artery hypertension. Anesthesiology 77:880–3, 1992
7. Rich GF, Lowson SM, Johns RA et al: Inhaled nitric oxide selectively decreases pulmonary vascular resistance without impairing oxygenation during one-lung ventilation in patients undergoing cardiac surgery. Anesthesiology 80:57–62, 1994
8. Rich GF, Murphy GD Jr, Ross CM, Johns RA: Inhaled nitric oxide. Selective pulmonary vasodilation in cardiac surgical patients. Anesthesiology 78:1028–35, 1993
9. Sunagawa K, Maughan W, Burkhoff D, Sagawa K: Left ventricular interaction with arterial load studied in isolated canine ventricle. Am J Physiol 245:H773–80, 1983
10. Packer M, LeJemtel T: Physiologic and pharmacologic determinants of vasodilator response: a conceptual framework for rationale drug therapy for chronic heart failure. Prog Cardiovasc Dis 244:275–92, 1982
11. Miller R, Fennell W, Young J et al: Differential systemic arterial and venous actions and consequent cardiac effects of vasodilator drugs. Prog Cardiovasc Dis 245:353–74, 1982
12. Ross J: Afterload mismatch and preload reserve. Prog Cardiovasc Dis 184:255–70, 1976
13. Pouleur H, Covell J, Ross J: Effect of nitroprusside on venous return and central blood volume in the absence and presence of acute heart failure. Circulation 61:328–37, 1980
14. Tuttle RR, Mills J: Dobutamine: development of a new catecholamine to selectively increase cardiac contractility. Circ Res 36:185–96, 1975
15. Vatner SF, McRitchie RJ, Braunwald E: Effects of dobutamine on left ventricular performance, coronary dynamics and distribution of cardiac output in conscious dogs. J Clin Invest 53:1265–73, 1974
16. Appleton C, Hatle L, Popp R: Cardiac tamponade and pericardial effusion: respiratory variation in transvalvular flow velocities studied by Doppler echocardiography. J Am Coll Cardiol 11:1020–30, 1988
17. Burstow, D, Oh J, Bailey K et al: Cardiac tamponade: characteristic Doppler observations. Mayo Clin Proc 64:312–24, 1989
18. Byrd B III, Linden R: Superior vena cava Doppler flow velocity patterns in pericardial disease. Am J Cardiol 65:1464–70, 1990
19. Beloucif S, Takata M, Robotham JL: Influence of pericardial constraint on atrioventricular interactions. Am J Physiol 263:H125–34, 1990
20. Birgens HS, Hendricksen J, Poulsen H: The shock liver: clinical and biological findings in patients with centrilobular liver necrosis following cardiogenic shock. Acta Med Scand 204:417–23, 1978
21. Mason DT: Afterload reduction and cardiac performance. Am J Med 65:106–25, 1978
22. Macciolo G, Lucas W, Norfleet E: The intraaortic balloon pump: a review. J Cardiothorac Anesth 2:365–73, 1988
23. Beloucif S, Laborde F, Beloucif L et al: Determinants of systolic and diastolic flow in coronary bypass grafts with inotropic stimulation. Anesthesiology 73:1127–35, 1990

24. Steen P, Tinker J, Pluth J: Efficiency of dopamine, dobutamine and epinephrine during emergence from cardiopulmonary bypass in man. Circulation 57:378–84, 1978

25. Daoud F, Reeves J, Kelly D: Isoproterenol as a potential pulmonary vasodilator in primary pulmonary hypertension. Am J Cardiol 42: 817–22, 1978

26. Vatner S, Higgins C, Braunwald E: Sympathetic and parasympathetic components of reflex tachycardia induced by hypotension in conscious dogs with and without heart failure. Cardiovasc Res 8:155–61, 1974

27. Vatner S, Pagani M, Rutherford J et al: Effects of nitroglycerine on cardiac function and regional blood flow distribution in conscious dogs. Am J Physiol 2343:H244–52, 1978

28. Gallagher J, Moore R, Jose A et al: Prophylactic nitroglycerin infusion during coronary artery bypass surgery. Anesthesiology 64: 785–9, 1986

29. Installe E, Gonzalez M, Jacquemart J et al: Comparative effects on hemodynamics of enoximone (MDL-17,043), dobutamine and nitroprusside in severe congestive heart failure. Am J Cardiol 60:46C–52C, 1987

30. Amin D, Shah P, Hulse S, Shellock F: Comparative acute hemodynamic effects of intravenous sodium nitroprusside and MDL-17,043, a new inotropic drug with vasodilator effects, in refractory congestive heart failure. Am Heart J 109:1006–12, 1985

31. Kereiakes D, Viquerat C, Lanzer P et al: Mechanisms of improved left ventricular function following intravenous MDL-17,043 in patients with severe chronic heart failure. Am Heart J 108:1278–84, 1984

32. Vincent J, Carlier E, Berre J et al: Administration of enoximone in cardiogenic shock. Am J Cardiol 62:419–23, 1988

33. Boldt J, Kling D, Moosdorf R, Hempelmann G: Enoximone treatment of impaired myocardial function during cardiac surgery: combined effects with epinephrine. J Cardiothorac Anesth 4:462–8, 1990

34. Berne RM, Levy MD: Cardiovascular Physiology. CV Mosby, St. Louis, 1972

35. Lorell BH: Left ventricular diastolic pressure-volume relations: understanding and managing congestive heart failure. Heart Failure 4: 206, 1988

36. Jackson JM, Thomas SJ, Lowenstein E: Anesthetic management of patients with valvular heart disease. Semin Anesth 1:232–52, 1982

37. Cohn J, Franciosa J: Vasodilatory therapy of cardiac failure. N Engl J Med 297:27–31, 254–8, 1977

38. Payen D, Beloucif S: Acute left ventricular failure. p. 230. In Pinsky MR, Dharnaut JF (eds): Pathological Foundations of Critical Care. Williams and Wilkins, Baltimore, 1993

39. Kaplan JA, Guffin AV: Treatment of perioperative left ventricular failure p. 1058. In Kaplan JA (ed): Cardiac Anesthesia. 3rd Ed. Grune & Stratton, Orlando, FL, 1993

40. Gatecel C, Mebazaa A, Kong R et al: Inhaled nitric oxide improves hepatic tissue oxygenation in right ventricular failure: value of hepatic venous oxygen saturation monitoring. Anesthesiology 82:588–90, 1995

8

Nutritional Support

Darryl T. Hiyama

Historically, the coexistence of malnutrition and chronic cardiac disease has been recognized for many years. Indeed, Hippocrates himself may have been one of the first individuals to record his observations: "the flesh is consumed and becomes water . . . the abdomen fills with water; the feet and legs swell; the shoulders, clavicles, chest, and thighs melt away."[1] Fortunately, this classic severe form of so-called cardiac cachexia is uncommon in medicine today. Instead, the prevalent types of malnutrition seen in a modern cardiac surgery practice are the less severe forms of protein-calorie malnutrition common among elderly or hospitalized patients and among those with chronic illnesses.

A number of recent studies would suggest that the presence of malnutrition substantially increases the risk of postoperative morbidity and mortality following both cardiac and noncardiac surgical procedures. With the ready availability of nutritional support, in the form of either enteral or parenteral formulations, the assumption that the risk of postoperative complications can be modified by treating malnutrition is understandable and even logical. However, the validity of this assumption remains to be proven in randomized and prospective evaluation. In an era of

cost-containment, shortened hospital stays, third-party payor reviews, and capitation contracts, the benefit of nutritional support will have to be proved and the indications for its use judiciously determined. In the absence of definitive information, the decision regarding the use of nutritional support becomes the responsibility of the physicians involved in the perioperative care of the cardiac surgery patient.

It is hoped that the information provided in this chapter will provide some guidance in this decision. This chapter reviews the current understanding of the relationship between malnutrition and cardiac surgery, the effects of malnutrition on cardiac structure and function, and the circumstances in which nutritional support may be of benefit for patients undergoing cardiac operations.

CARDIAC DISEASE AND MALNUTRITION

The actual incidence of malnutrition among cardiac surgery patients appears to be related to the characteristics of this subpopulation of patients and to the type of cardiac disease. The elderly, generally accepted as those patients over 65 years of age, have a well-recognized risk of malnutrition and rep-

145

resent a significant proportion of cardiac surgery candidates. A national survey conducted in Great Britain documented an incidence of malnutrition of 6 and 5 percent in men and women, respectively, between the ages of 70 and 80 years. In men and women over the age of 80 years, the incidence was 12 and 8 percent, respectively.[2] Although there are few data regarding the incidence of malnutrition among the free-living elderly in the United States, the incidence among elderly nursing home residents may be as high as 52 to 85 percent.[3,4] Even among elderly patients considered previously healthy but hospitalized for an acute surgical problem (e.g., appendicitis), the incidence of malnutrition may be as high as 22 percent.[5] Therefore, the risk of malnutrition is substantial in the patient over 65 years of age and probably increases with advancing age.

A number of separate studies report that 30 to 50 percent of adult general medicine and surgery patients exhibit enough biochemical or anthropometric abnormalities to suggest the presence of protein-calorie malnutrition.[6–10] Importantly, among these patients, malnutrition was not suspected by clinical assessment or biochemical abnormality. Only because of directed nutritional screening was malnutrition considered. Among patients with cardiac disease, Heymsfield et al.[11] dubbed this latter form of malnutrition "nosocomial cardiac cachexia," which can arise in previously well-nourished patients due to inadequate nutritional intake during the pre- or postoperative period. At risk are patients experiencing a complex or atypical postoperative course or those hospitalized prior to operation.

Atherosclerotic coronary artery disease, unless complicated by ischemic cardiomyopathy or valvular disease, does not appear to be associated with significant malnutrition. In a prospective study of 100 adult patients undergoing cardiac operations, Abel et al.[12] reported few abnormal anthropometric, biochemical, or cell-mediated measurements. The average age of the patients was 55 years,

the majority were slightly overweight, and 90 percent had arteriosclerotic heart disease. It was concluded that arteriosclerotic heart disease was not associated with malnutrition.

In contrast, severe, chronic congestive heart failure (CHF) is the condition most likely to be complicated by malnutrition. Heymsfield and colleagues[13] noted a prevalence of significant malnutrition in 37 percent of ambulatory cardiac patients, New York Heart Association (NYHA) class III or greater. Carr et al.[14] similarly found clinical evidence of malnutrition in 50 percent of patients with severe chronic CHF due to ischemic or dilated cardiomyopathy.[14] Blackburn and co-workers,[15] in screening 350 hospitalized patients, reported an incidence of protein-calorie malnutrition in 53 percent of patients with a primary cardiac diagnosis. Thus, among cardiac surgery patients, the presence of advanced age, hospitalization, and severe chronic CHF should be considered risk factors for malnutrition.

Cardiac Cachexia

Originally associated with long-standing rheumatic valvular disease, cardiac cachexia, in varying degrees of severity, may be associated with valvular disease, congenital malformations, or cardiomyopathy. Central to this syndrome is the development of malnutrition secondary to metabolic changes related to chronic cardiac decompensation. Although a number of causes of cardiac-related malnutrition have been proposed, only a few have been well studied or elucidated.[16] Decreased intake of protein and calories is clearly a major factor. Appetite may be affected by medications, sodium- and fat-restricted diets, as well as fatigue and malaise. Recently, elevated serum levels of tumor necrosis factor (TNF) have been reported in patients with chronic congestive heart failure.[17,18] Levine et al.[17] noted elevated levels of TNF in a significantly higher number of patients with heart failure compared to healthy control subjects. These investigators further noted that patients with elevated TNF levels had lower body weight, more advanced heart failure, anemia, and hyponatremia than cardiac patients without increased TNF levels. However, TNF is only a partial explanation for both the anorexia and hypermetabolism characteristic of this condition.

Early satiety may result from extrinsic gastric compression due to hepatomegaly or ascites or delayed gastric emptying. Malabsorption may also play a role. Moderate incidences of steatorrhea have been reported in small groups of patients with CHF.[19,20] Splanchnic, hepatic, and pancreatic hypoxia may impair the synthesis of pancreatic exocrine enzymes and bile salts. In addition, intestinal hypoxia may depress active transport mechanisms for glucose and amino acids.

It is important to note the hypermetabolic condition of these patients, in addition to the difference between cardiac cachexia and uncomplicated total or semistarvation. In simple starvation, the primary metabolic response to diminished nutrient intake is *hypometabolism,* mediated by a reduction in cortisol and catecholamine secretion and decreased production of triiodothyronine, renin, angiotensin, and aldosterone.[21] The physiologic changes are marked by bradycardia, lowered systolic and diastolic blood pressure, and reduced plasma volume and anemia.[22–24] In addition, there is effective conversion of primary fuel substrate to keto acids for the myocardium. The cumulative effect of these changes is an overall reduction in oxygen consumption and myocardial work. In cardiac cachexia, malnutrition occurs in a setting of increased metabolic demands,[16] arising from augmented respiratory and cardiac work requirements,[25,26] activation of the sympathetic nervous system,[27,28] and possibly cytokine activity.[17]

The clinical result of these conditions is a loss of skeletal muscle mass, a reduction in subcutaneous and visceral fat stores, and a decrease in visceral protein production. Peripheral edema and ascites develop, both from the heart failure and from hypoproteine-mia.[16] However, as noted earlier, clinical and biochemical parameters may not be sufficient to identify malnourished patients. Body weight measurements are confounded by edema, unless adequate diuretic therapy has been achieved. Visceral protein level, particularly albumin, may be relatively preserved, despite other evidence of malnourishment.[29] Although the application of advanced techniques for measuring lean body mass such as total body potassium or magnetic spectroscopy would be useful, their cost and logistical difficulties make them impractical at this time. At present, the use of anthropometric measurements of somatic protein stores such as the mid-arm muscle circumference and fat stores such as the triceps skinfold test provide as useful addition to screening process.[14,15,29,30] Immunologic testing at present offers little clinical utility due to both a low prognostic value as well as extremely slow response following nutritional repletion.[31,32]

EFFECTS OF MALNUTRITION UPON CARDIAC STRUCTURE AND FUNCTION

Structure

Early in the twentieth century, it was erroneously, but widely, believed that the heart is "spared" the muscle-wasting effects of starvation. Foster,[33] in 1895, interpreted a report by Voit,[34] published in 1866, regarding a single starved cat whose heart weight was only 2.6 percent smaller than that of a single nonstarved animal. Unfortunately, this "overinterpretation" was perpetuated by a number of investigators and in a number of prominent textbooks of physiology. Subsequent studies have proved that the heart can undergo significant atrophy in both starved animals and humans.[35–39] Kuykendall et al.[39] indicated that the heart undergoes glycogenolysis and proteolysis similar to other metabolically active tissues during starvation, and these changes may account for some of the reduction in heart size in early starvation. Chauhan and coworkers,[35] using a model of isolated protein deficiency in rhesus monkeys, noted fiber degeneration progressing from minimal atrophy to frank necrosis, fibrosis, and scarring. The extent of the myocardial damage correlated with the duration of protein deficiency. Similar findings have also been reported in children with fatal kwashiorkor, suggesting that similar changes occur in humans.[38]

Although vulnerable to atrophy, the heart may be relatively "spared" compared to skeletal muscle and fat stores. Keys and colleagues[24] studied healthy men for a 6-month period of controlled starvation. During the first 3 months, the reduction in heart size paralleled the decrease in body weight; however, by the sixth month, the heart size had decreased by 17 percent compared to a reduction in body weight of 24 percent. Heymsfield et al.[29] reported similar results, using radiographic and echocardiography techniques to determine cardiac volume and mass in cachectic and normal patients. This study noted an absolute reduction in heart volume and a left ventricular (LV) mass in cachectic patients; however, when indexed to body weight, both total heart volume and LV mass were found to be increased in comparison to the control group. This finding suggests a relatively greater loss of skeletal muscle mass than cardiac mass during starvation.

Electrophysiologic Changes

Electrocardiographic (ECG) changes in malnutrition are not unique. In malnourished rhesus monkeys, T-wave flattening and inversion was a common finding.[40] In humans, decreased voltage may be seen if atrophy has occurred. Instances of fatal ventricular dysrhythmias have been reported following starvation. Low ECG voltage and prolonged QT intervals were found in young, otherwise healthy patients following therapeutic starvation. These changes appear to resolve following nutritional repletion.

Myocardial Function

Of greater relevance to the perioperative care of cardiac surgery patients is the effect of malnutrition upon cardiac function. Early reports, based on observations of normal clinical cardiac status in children with untreated kwashiorkor, suggested that cardiac function is not affected by protein-calorie malnutrition.[38,41] However, a number of studies involving various techniques of cardiac output measurement indicate that cardiac output is decreased under conditions of prolonged starvation[24,42] and cachexia associated with chronic illness.[29] Because cardiac atrophy was noted in each of these studies, it might be assumed that the decreased cardiac output is due to decreased myocardial contractility. However, this assumption may be erroneous, and the effect of malnutrition on cardiac function may be modified by a number of conditions.

Under conditions of simple starvation, Keyes et al.[24] noted a reduction in pulse rate and stroke volume, and therefore cardiac output, although none of the subjects developed clinical evidence of heart failure. These findings are consistent with the hypometabolism and reduced plasma volume associated with uncomplicated starvation. Heymsfield and coworkers[29] reported dissimilar findings in a group of cachetic hospitalized patients with malignancy, cirrhosis, and inflammatory bowel disease. Compared to a control group of healthy, height-matched volunteers, end-diastolic volume (EDV) and stroke volume (SV) were significantly decreased, 37 and 32 percent, respectively. Cardiac output was reduced by 17 percent, but this difference was not statistically significant. Of interest, ejection fraction (EF), mean rate of LV circumferential fiber shortening, left posterior wall thickening, and left posterior wall excursion were not significantly different between the study and control groups. This latter finding suggests that systolic ejection phase indices were not altered despite evidence of decreased heart volume and LV mass in this study. In fact, the minimal reduction in cardiac output and decreased EDV would indicate that LV systolic function would be normal, or even increased. It was concluded that the increased cardiac work may be due to disease processes (e.g., anemia, liver disease, cancer) or as a compensatory mechanism for a decreased EDV due to reduced blood volume.

Animal studies that allow the direct measurement of myocardial contractility performance indicate that protein malnutrition does result in a decrease in myocardial contractility. Kyger et al.[43] reported significant decreases in overall myocardial contractility in protein-depleted rats. Similarly, Abel et al.[36] noted decreased cardiac compliance and lower peak developed pressures during systole in malnourished dogs.

In the setting of CHF, malnutrition is secondary to the effects of decreased cardiac output. Hypertrophy of the myocardium is a compensatory mechanism in many instances of cardiac failure. However, the increased metabolic rate found in severe CHF, combined with inadequate caloric and protein intake to support net protein synthesis, probably leads to worsening myocardial atrophy. Therefore, in this situation, malnutrition not only affects myocardial performance but also precludes a useful compensatory mechanism.

IMPLICATIONS OF MALNUTRITION IN CARDIAC SURGERY

In addition to the effects of protein and calorie deprivation on the heart itself, malnutrition is recognized to have an impact on several clinical aspects of cardiac surgery. As is true of surgical patients in general, moderate to severe malnutrition has been associated with increased morbidity and mortality among cardiac surgery patients. Abel and coworkers[44] noted a higher incidence of pneumonia, mediastinitis, acute renal failure, and a higher number of days of mechanical ventilation in malnourished cardiac surgical patients compared to a well-nourished control group. It is significant that, in this study, the mortality in the malnourished group was 16 percent compared to no mortality in the control group. In a retrospective study, Rich and coworkers[45] reported that a serum albumin level of less than $3.5 \text{ g} \cdot \text{dl}^{-1}$ alone in elderly cardiac surgery patients was associated with an increased frequency of postoperative confusion, congestive heart failure, renal dysfunction, gastrointestinal complications, and prolonged lengths of hospital stay. Mortality also tended to be higher in the low albumin group.

In theory, the provision of nutritional support to support metabolic activity and to restore lean body mass may have some influence on the prevention or elimination of the complications noted above. From a clinical standpoint, nutritional support has two potential roles: (1) nutritional repletion prior to cardiac operation to improve clinical outcome, and (2) metabolic support during the postoperative course.

It has been shown that, in humans, nutritional repletion can reverse some of the effects of malnutrition on the heart itself. Keyes et al.[24] noted that heart dimensions and hemodynamic parameters were restored to normal using an oral ad libitum diet, although complete restoration required up to 20 weeks of therapy. Heymsfield et al.[29] reported a 15 percent increase in LV mass after 2 weeks of parenteral nutrition and a 31 percent increase after 3 to 5 weeks of nutritional support. In this latter study, cardiac output and EDV were restored with 2 weeks of parenteral nutrition. Gibbons et al.[46] successfully treated three patients with cardiac cachexia with 3 weeks of preoperative oral nutritional supplement. Receiving $40 \text{ kcal} \cdot \text{kg}^{-1} \cdot \text{day}^{-1}$, these patients achieved positive nitrogen balance and improved serum albumin levels before undergoing operation. One patient developed postoperative hemolysis; however, there were no other complications and no deaths in this small series. Gibbons and colleagues concluded that preoperative nutritional support could be successfully administered but would require 3 weeks of therapy based on the whole body net protein synthesis rate.

Recently, Otaki[47] reported a lower postoperative mortality rate in patients with cardiac cachexia who received preoperative nutritional support. In a retrospective evaluation, he noted that use of a 6- to 7-week course of hypocaloric parenteral nutrition in addition to an oral diet significantly increased serum albumin, total protein, and potassium levels and decreased serum creatinine, demonstrating that net protein synthesis was achieved. Following operation, operative mortality in the group receiving nutritional support was 17 percent, significantly lower than the 57 percent mortality in the group that did not receive nutritional support. A further potential benefit of preoperative nutritional support has been identified by a number of studies.[48–50] Lolley and coworkers[48] reported that elevation of myocardial glycogen levels using both fat and glucose loading prior to cardiac bypass resulted in a lowered incidence of vasopressor dependence, myocardial infarction, and serious ventricular dysrhythmias.

This evidence suggests that preoperative nutritional support may be of some benefit in severely malnourished patients, although further evaluation is needed. This is analogous to the experience in noncardiac surgical patients, in whom a reduction in postoperative morbidity has been demonstrated in patients with moderate to severe malnutrition using perioperative parenteral nutrition. The single greatest limitation is the time required to achieve net protein synthesis, on the order of several weeks. While this may seem impractical in cardiac surgery, the decrease in perioperative complication rates will more than compensate for the delay in nonemergent surgery.

The alternative role of nutritional support in the postoperative period is one of metabolic support. If preoperative support was used, this should be continued into the postoperative period until adequate oral intake is achieved. In well-nourished patients who have uneventful postoperative courses, no support is indicated if mechanical ventilation is discontinued within 48 hours and if there is no active sepsis or renal or hepatic organ failure. The period of hypermetabolism after operation and cardiopulmonary bypass appears to resolve within the first week after operation unless complications occur. In the event that this period is extended, nutritional support is indicated to preserve lean body mass.

Both the enteral[51] and parenteral routes[46,47,52] have been demonstrated to be safe and effective means of delivering nutritional support. Although glucose administration does increase energy expenditure, this increased need for oxygen delivery has not proved clinically significant. The use of fat as a caloric source may have significant benefit in terms of increasing myocardial glycogen and allowing significant caloric delivery with minimal fluid administration. Negative cardiopulmonary effects associated with lipid administration can be avoided by not exceeding $3 \text{ mg} \cdot \text{kg}^{-1} \cdot \text{min}^{-1}$.[53] Estimated doses of 30 $\text{kcal} \cdot \text{kg}^{-1}$ body weight per day should be adjusted by the level of stress, though not exceeding 30 to 40 percent of the calculated resting energy expenditure. Ideally, indirect calorimetry should be used to avoid the deleterious effects of overfeeding.

SUMMARY

There is good preliminary information to support the use of nutritional support in the moderate to severely malnourished cardiac surgical patient, to reverse the effects of malnutrition prior to operation. This may improve patient outcome, although this hypothesis remains to be proved with further investigation.

REFERENCES

1. Katz AM, Katz PB: Diseases of the heart in works of Hippocrates. Br Heart J 24:257, 1962
2. Department of Health and Social Security: A

nutrition survey of the elderly. Rep Health Soc Subj (Lond) 16:1, 1979

3. Pinchcofsky-Devin GD, Kaminski MV: Incidence of protein-calorie malnutrition in nursing home population. J Am Coll Nutr 6:109, 1987

4. Shaver HS, Loper JA, Lutes RA: Nutritional status of nursing home patients. J Parenter Enteral Nutr 4:367, 1980

5. Arnbjornsson E: Nutritional assessment and postoperative complications in elderly patients undergoing emergency appendectomy. Curr Surg 20:457, 1985

6. Bistrian BR, Blackbum GL, Hallowell E, Heddle R: Protein status of general surgical patients. JAMA 230:858, 1974

7. Bistrian BR, Blackburn GL, Vitale J et al: Prevalence of malnutrition in general medical patients. JAMA 235:1567, 1976

8. Hill GL, Blackett RL, Pickford I et al: Malnutrition in surgical patients: an unrecognised problem. Lancet 1:689, 1977

9. Weinsier RL, Hunker EM, Krumdieck CL, Butterworth CE Jr: Hospital malnutrition: a prospective evaluation of general medical patients during the course of hospitalization. Am J Clin Nutr 32:418, 1979

10. Willard MD, Gilsdorf RB, Price RA: Protein-calorie malnutrition in a community hospital. JAMA 243:1720, 1980

11. Heymsfield SB, Smith J, Redd S, Whitworth HB: Nutritional support in cardiac failure. Surg Clin North Am 61?5,

12. Abel RM, Fisch D, Horowitz J et al: Should nutritional status be assessed routinely prior to cardiac operation? J Thorac Cardiovasc Surg 85:752, 1983

13. Heymsfield S, Bleier J, Wenger N: Detection of protein-calorie undernutrition in advanced heart disease, abstracted. Circulation, suppl III. 55/56:102, 1977

14. Carr JG, Sevenson LW, Wolden JA, Heber D: Prevalence and hemodynamic correlation of malnutrition in severe congestive heart failure secondary to ischemic or idiopathic dilated cardiomyopathy. Am J Cardiol 63:709, 1989

15. Blackburn GL, Gibbons GW, Bothe A et al: Nutritional support in cardiac cachexia. J Thorac Cardiovasc Surg 73:489, 1977

16. Pittman JG, Cohen P: The pathogenesis of cardiac cachexia. N Engl J Med 271:403, 1964

17. Levine B, Kalman J, Mayer L et al: Elevated circulating levels of tumor necrosis factor in severe chronic heart failure. N Engl J Med 323:236, 1990

18. McMurray J, Abdullah I, Dargie JH, Shapiro D: Increased concentrations of tumour necrosis factor in "cachectic" patients with severe chronic heart failure. Br Heart J 66:356, 1991

19. Davidson JD, Goodman DS, Walsmann TA, Gordon RS Jr: Protein-losing gastroenteropathy in congestive heart-failure. Lancet 2:899, 1961

20. Jones RV: Fat-malabsorption in congestive cardiac failure. BMJ 1276, 1961

21. Landsberg L, Young JB: Fasting, feeding and the regulation of the sympathetic nervous system. N Engl J Med 298:1295, 1978

22. Sowers JR, Myby M, Stern N et al: Blood pressure and hormone changes associated with weight reduction in the obese. Hypertension 4:686, 1982

23. Einhom D, Young JB, Landsberg L: Hypotensive effect of fasting: possible involvement of the sympathetic nervous system and endogenous opiates. Science 217:727, 1982

24. Keys A, Henschel A, Taylor HL: The size and function of the human heart at rest in semistarvation and in subsequent rehabilitation. Am J Physiol 150:153, 1947

25. McParland C, Krishnan B, Wang Y, Gallagher CG: Inspiratory muscle weakness and dyspnea in chronic heart failure. Am Rev Respir Dis 146:467, 1992

26. Rochester DF, Esau SA: Malnutrition and tbe respiratory system. Chest 85:411, 1984

27. Levine TB, Francis GS, Goldsmith SR et al: Activity of the sympathetic nervous system and renin-angiotensin system assessed by plasma hormone levels and their relation to hemodynamic abnormalities in congestive heart failure. Am J Cardiol 49:1659, 1982

28. Chidsey CA, Braunwald E, Morrow AG: Catecholamine excretion and cardiac stores of norepinephrine in congestive heart failure. Am J Med 39:442, 1965

29. Heymsfield SB, Bethel RA, Ansley JD et al: Cardiac abnormalities in cachectic patients before and during nutritional repletion. Am Heart J 95:584, 1978

30. Murray MJ, Marsh HM, Wochos DN et al: Nutritional assessment of intensive-care unit patients. Mayo Clin Proc 63:1106, 1988

31. Negro F, Cerra FB: Nutritional monitoring in

the ICU: rational and practical application. Crit Care Clin 4:559, 1988

32. Ulicny KS, Hiratzka LF, Williams RB et al: Sternotomy infection: poor prediction by acute phase response and delayed hypersensitivity. Ann Thorac Surg 50:949, 1990

33. Foster M: A Textbook of Physiology. Macmillan, New York, 1895

34. Voit C: Uber die verschiedenheiten der Erweisszersetzing beinHungem. Z Biol 2:309, 1866

35. Chauhan S, Nayak NC, Ramalingaswami V: The heart and skeletal muscle in experimental protein malnutrition in rhesus monkeys. J Pathol 90:301, 1965

36. Abel RM, Grimes JB, Alonso D et al: Adverse hemodynamic and ultrastructural changes in dog hearts subjected to protein calorie malnutrition. Am Heart J 97:733, 1979

37. Smythe PM, Swanepoel A, Campbell JAH: The heart in kwashiorkor. BMJ 1:67, 1962

38. Wharton BA, Balmer SE, Somers K, Templeton AC: The myocardium in kwashiorkor. Q J Med 149:107, 1969

39. Kuykendall RC, Rowlands BJ, Taegtmeyer H, Walker WE: Biochemical consequences of protein depletion in the rabbit heart. J Surg Res 43:62, 1987

40. Garnett ES, Barnard DL, Ford J et al: Gross fragmentation of cardiac myofibrils after therapeutic starvation for obesity. Lancet 1:914, 1969

41. Edozien JC, Rahim-Khan MA: Anaemia in protein malnutrition. Clin Surg 34:315, 1968

42. Alleyne GAO: Cardiac function in severely malnourished Jamaican children. Clin Sci 30: 553, 1966

43. Kyger ER, Block WJ, Roach G, Dudrick SJ: Adverse effects of protein malnutrition on myocardial function. Surgery 97:147, 1978

44. Abel RM, Fischer JE, Buckley MJ et al: Malnutrition in cardiac surgical patients. Arch Surg 111:45, 1976

45. Rich MW, Keller AJ, Schectman KB et al: Increased complications and prolonged hospital stay in elderly cardiac surgical patients with low serum albumin. Am J Cardiol 63:714, 1989

46. Gibbons GW, Blackburn GL, Harken DE et al: Pre- and postoperative hyperalimentation in the treatment of cardiac cachexia. J Surg Res 20:439, 1976

47. Otaki M: Surgical treatment of patients with cardiac cachexia: an analysis of factors affecting operative mortality. Chest 105:1347, 1994

48. Lolley DM, Myers WO, Ray JF et al: Clinical experience with preoperative myocardial nutrition management. J Cardiovasc Surg 26:236, 1985

49. Oldfield GS, Commerford PJ, Opie LH: Effects of preoperative glucose-potassium on myocardial glycogen levels and on complications of mitral valve replacement. J Thorac Cardiovasc Surg 91:874, 1984

50. Girard C, Quentin P, Bouview H et al: Glucose and insulin supply before cardiopulmonary bypass in cardiac surgery: a double-blind study. Ann Thorac Surg 54:259, 1992

51. Heymsfield SB, Casper K: Congestive heart failure: clinical management by use of continuous nasoenteric feeding. Am J Clin Nutr 50: 539, 1989

52. Paccagnella A, Calo MA, Caenaro G et al: Cardiac cachexia: preoperative and postoperative nutrition management. J PEN J Parenter Enteral Nutr 18:409, 1994

53. Fiaccodori E, Tortorella G, Gonzi G et al: Hemodynamic, respiratory, and metabolic effects of medium-chain triglyceride-enriched lipid emulsions following valvular heart surgery. Chest 106:1660, 1994

9

Renal Function After Cardiopulmonary Bypass

Tiong H. Liem

Renal dysfunction is not unusual after cardiac surgery and cardiopulmonary bypass (CPB). This chapter focuses on the pathogenesis and diagnosis of postoperative renal dysfunction and acute renal failure (ARF) and presents strategies to prevent their development.

INCIDENCE AND RISK

The frequency of a transient decline in renal function is approximately 30 percent,[1-3] while ARF requiring hemodialysis is observed in 3 percent of all patients following CPB. The mortality rate of those patients requiring hemodialysis is very high, ranging from 24 percent to 70 percent.[4,5] ARF occurs more commonly following pediatric than adults cardiac surgery.[4,6-8]

Of 1,988 patients undergoing cardiac surgery, Frost et al.[9] found that 2.5 percent of adult and 8.3 percent of pediatric patients developed ARF requiring dialysis. The mortal-

---

* To convert $\mu mol * L^{-1}$ to $mg \cdot dl^{-1}$, divide by 88.4.

ity rate of these patients was as high as 63 percent. In this same study, perioperative low cardiac output and preoperative renal insufficiency (serum creatinine greater than 110 $\mu mol \cdot L^{-1}*$) were the most important risk factors for developing postoperative ARF.

The incidence of postoperative ARF is higher after valvular surgery (2.7 percent) than after coronary artery bypass graft (CABG) surgery (1.1 percent), although the mortality rate is similar (61 percent and 51 percent, respectively).[10] ARF occurs most frequently in patients with active endocarditis (8.1 percent versus 2.5 percent), peripheral vascular disease (5.7 percent versus 2.3 percent), and a history of prior cardiac surgical procedures (3.8 percent versus 2.5 percent).

Zanardo et al.[11] described, in a prospective study of 775 patients without pre-existing renal dysfunction (mostly adults, mean age 57.5 ± 11 years), an 11.4 percent incidence of renal dysfunction (serum creatinine level of 1.5 to 2.5 $mg \cdot dl^{-1}$), and a 3.7 percent incidence of ARF (serum creatinine level higher than 2.5 $mg \cdot dl^{-1}$) following cardiac surgery using CPB. Within this same patient

153

group, the mortality rate was 0.8 percent in "normal" patients, 9.5 percent in patients with renal dysfunction, and 44.4 percent once ARF developed. The following were risk factors for developing postoperative renal impairment: use of the intra-aortic balloon pump, need for deep hypothermic circulatory arrest, low cardiac output syndrome, advanced age, need for emergency operation, and low urinary output during CPB.

However, hemodynamic instability is not the sole prognosticator of ARF. Ghattas et al.[12] reviewed 2,468 patient charts following cardiac surgery and found a surprisingly high incidence of ARF after CPB in the absence of low cardiac output or hemodynamic instability. Only 20 (38 percent) of their 58 patients defined as having severe hemodynamic failure developed postoperative ARF. Furthermore, of the 29 patients (1.2 percent) who required dialysis in the first week after surgery, 9 patients (31 percent) had stable perioperative hemodynamics.

In summary, those patients undergoing repeat cardiac procedures or presenting with preoperative renal dysfunction, low cardiac output, endocarditis, or peripheral vascular disease are predisposed to postoperative renal dysfunction. Pediatric and valvular cardiac surgery also augment the risk of postoperative renal dysfunction. It is these cases in which additional measures for renal protection during and after surgery should provide added benefit. The remainder of this chapter discusses alternatives for providing effective protection.

PATHOGENESIS

Normal Physiology

As this chapter focuses on renal function following cardiac surgery, interactions between the cardiovascular and renal systems are outlined in brief.

The baroreceptors in the carotid sinus continuously signal the arterial pressure to the vasomotor center in the central nervous system (CNS) via the ninth nerve. When the blood pressure falls, the vasomotor center in the CNS increases efferent sympathetic tone with the following effects: (1) an increase in heart rate, (2) an increase in peripheral vascular resistance, and (3) activation of the β-adrenergic receptors in the kidney by locally released norepinephrine. This renal β-adrenergic activation increases renal renin secretion.

Renin is released from renal juxtaglomerular cells of the distal afferent arteriole of the kidney, where release is stimulated by increases in intracellular cAMP and inhibited by increases in cytosolic calcium. Renin, in turn, catalyzes the conversion of angiotensinogen to angiotensin I, a relatively inactive decapeptide prohormone. Angiotensin I is converted via angiotensin converting enzyme to angiotensin II, an octapeptide with potent vasoconstrictive properties. Angiotensin-converting enzyme (ACE) is a rather nonspecific metalloenzyme (containing zinc) widely distributed throughout the body, including the lungs, kidney, brain, and blood vessels.

Angiotensin II stimulates the adrenal cortex to synthesize and secrete aldosterone, which subsequently acts on the cortical collecting tubules of the kidney to promote reabsorption of sodium and water and increase excretion of potassium. The presence of angiotensin II, and its degradation product angiotensin III, normally inhibits further release of renin via a negative feedback loop. Angiotensin II formation therefore results in both vasoconstriction as well as expansion of blood volume, which usually produce an increase in systemic blood pressure.

In the kidney, the actions of angiotensin II lead to an increase in prostaglandin secretion, particularly PGE_2 (a potent vasodilator), which may counteract the renal vasoconstrictive properties of angiotensin II. When prostaglandin synthesis is blocked by indomethacin, renal blood flow (RBF) falls sharply, presumably due to the effect of unopposed angiotensin II renal vasoconstriction.[13] An additional loop in this network of regulation is the release of atrial natriuretic peptide from the cardiac atria. When the volume in the atria is too high, stretch receptors located in the atrial wall sense this expansion and release atrial natriuretic peptide, which opposes aldosterone.

In conclusion, a fall in blood pressure activates a cascade of events that result in renal and systemic vasoconstriction with subsequent retention of both salt and water.

Pathophysiology

The period of CPB during cardiac surgery represents a significant departure from normal physiology: mean arterial pressure and hematocrit decline concomitantly as a result of hemodilution by the pump priming, pulsatile pressure becomes nonpulsatile (when the nonpulsatile mode of CPB is used), blood and body temperatures decline, and platelets and leukocytes are activated as the patient's blood makes contact with CPB tubes and the oxygenator. Plasma concentrations of epinephrine and norepinephrine increase significantly immediately after starting CPB.[14–17] The levels of plasma renin activity (PRA)[18–23] and plasma endothelin (a vasoconstricting substance released by the endothelium that is a potent renal vasoconstrictor)[24–28] increase significantly following onset of CPB.[29]

Given the magnitude of these physiologic and hormonal changes during CPB, a 3 percent incidence of renal failure appears rather low. However, the high mortality of these patients is sufficient evidence that preventive efforts are likely to be effacacious. Many preventive measures are available for the prevention of ARF following cardiac surgery. Unfortunately, many different definitions were used in these studies for the determination of postoperative renal dysfunction and ARF. Comparison of the results is therefore difficult, and conclusions are drawn with some circumspection.

DIAGNOSIS

Common Indicators of Renal Dysfunction

Urine output, serum creatinine level, peak serum creatinine level, endogenous creatinine clearance, water and sodium reabsorp-tion, urine concentration of microalbumin, urine N-acetyl β-D-glucosaminidase (NAG) level,[30] free water clearance, fractional excretion of sodium, renal functional reserve, urine β_2-microglobulin (β_2-M) level, and renal failure index (RFI) are the most reported tests for postoperative renal dysfunction.

URINE MICROALBUMIN

The kidneys play an important role in preventing protein and albumin loss. In the adult, approximately 70 kg of plasma albumin passes through the kidneys each day. Only approximately 8 g (0.011 percent) reaches the tubules, which reabsorb most of the albumin, leaving only 8 mg to appear in the urine. At this level of activity, the tubular protein absorption mechanism is near saturation; thus, small increases in glomerular permeability result in large increases in albuminuria.

NAG AND β_2-MICROGLOBULIN

NAG and (β_2-M) level in the urine is a sensitive test for renal tubular damage.[31] From a variety of enzymes excreted into the urine by the kidney, NAG has emerged as the most widely measured because of its stability, relative high molecular mass (MW 130,000), which precludes glomerular filtration, and the presence in the tubular lysosomes. Thus, an increase in urinary NAG is a sensitive indicator for renal tubular damage.

An increase of urine concentration of microalbumin with normal urinary NAG and β_2-M concentrations indicates an increase in glomerular permeability. The lack of rise of NAG and β_2-M indicates little or no renal tubular involvement.

Renal Blood Flow and Glomerular Filtration Rate

The measurement of RBF and the glomerular filtration rate (GFR) using the clearance of inulin and hippurate or radionuclides is desirable but is too labor and time intensive. The use of serum and urinary concentrations

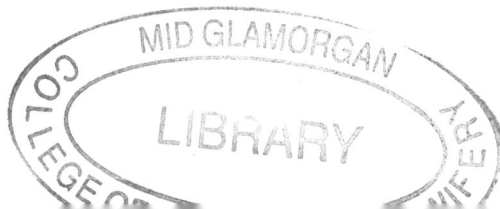

of creatinine, with calculations of endogenous creatinine clearance, as estimates of GFR is unsuitable for clinical research purposes. This unsuitablity is related to the numerous errors that can be made and is therefore poorly reproducible.[32] In patients with renal insufficiency, estimation of GFR using this method usually overestimates the measured GFR when compared to inulin or hippurate clearance. This discrepancy occurs as a consequence of proximal tubular creatinine secretion increasing progressively as GFR declines.[33-36] Additional errors inherent in the use of serum creatinine or creatinine clearance as determinants of GFR include interindividual variability in muscle mass, dietary protein intake, and the hyperbolic relationship between rates of change in serum creatinine concentration and GFR.[32,33,37]

A new and easy method for the determination of GFR is available using urographic contrast agents. Urographic contrast media is similar to inulin in that it is cleared predominantly by the kidneys (less than 2 percent of excretion extrarenal—predominantly biliary—in patients with normal function). It is freely filtered by the glomerulus, neither reabsorbed nor secreted to any significant degree by renal tubules, and not protein bound.[38-41] Elimination of urographic contrast media conforms to a first-order kinetic model that permits determination of GFR by x-ray fluorescence measurement of the rate of decline of plasma iodine content. The plasma samples are derived from sequentially obtained peripheral venous blood specimens ("slope-intercept" technique) or a single blood specimen ("single sample" technique) drawn at precisely determined time(s) following administration. No urine collection is necessary, and the length of time required to process each plasma specimen is less than 10 minutes. In one study,[42] in which healthy patients and patients with renal insufficiency were included, x-ray fluorescence results were in good correlation with inulin (r = 0.86) and radionuclide clearances (r = 0.89).

However, further evaluation of this method is necessary.

In summary, comparing the results of different studies is difficult. The incidence of renal dysfunction is dependent on the definition used in the study. A "standard" description of postoperative renal dysfunction is therefore desirable.

PREVENTION

Many factors influence RBF and GFR during CPB. High plasma concentrations of renin, catecholamines, and endothelin will certainly influence RBF and GFR during CPB. Many strategies to prevent ARF after CPB are available. Later in this section we will discuss the use of (1) low "renal" dose dopamine, (2) mannitol, (3) calcium channel blockers, (4) ACE inhibitors, and (5) blockade of the sympathetic outflow for preventing postoperative ARF following CPB and heart surgery. All these physiologic endocrine responses have been caused by an "unphysiologic" state—CPB. Modifications that attempt to return the CPB pattern to as physiologic a state as possible are (1) pulsatile versus nonpulsatile flow of the CPB, and (2) high versus low flow rate and high versus low perfusion pressure during CPB. Each of these alternatives is examined below.

Modification of Cardiopulmonary Bypass

PULSATILE VERSUS NONPULSATILE FLOW

Nonpulsatile perfusion during CPB may induce increases in vasomotor tone (because of reasons described earlier) with a subsequent decrease in organ perfusion, resulting in renal dysfunction.[43] During pulseless perfusion, some investigators report that plasma renin activity (PRA) increases, while it remains unchanged during pulsatile perfusion.[18-21] Other workers cannot confirm these findings.[22,23] Although they did not measure PRA, Canivet et al.[21] were unable to document any difference in urine β_2-M levels (see preceding section) comparing pulsatile to nonpulsatile groups. These results concur with those of Manche et al.,[44] who found similar increases in urine β_2-M levels in patients undergoing CPB with pulsatile and nonpulsatile perfusion. However, this study included only 11 patients and, since the incidence of ARF is low, this study cannot distinguish between a clinical renal outcome and pulsatile or nonpulsatile perfusion. In a clinical study of 100 patients with normal preoperative renal function, Badner et al.[45] concluded that the mode of perfusion, pulsatile or nonpulsatile, did not influence perioperative renal function.

In summary, although the PRA level seems to increase less during pulsatile perfusion, no study is able to show improved renal outcome as a result.

PERFUSION PRESSURE AND FLOW RATE

Controversies continue over whether low perfusion pressures with high flow rates during CPB alter intraoperative and especially postoperative renal outcome. In adults, the CPB circuit is generally primed with crystalloids or colloids, which result in some degree of hemodilution. The hematocrit will usually decline to 20 to 25 vol percent. In patients with normal body temperature (37°C), higher flow rates are needed to maintain oxygen transport. At lower body temperatures, however, total body oxygen consumption declines. Now lower flow rates deliver sufficient oxygenated blood to prevent anaerobic metabolism in vital organs. Indeed, lower flow rates may provide luxury perfusion because muscular activity is responsible for about 20 percent of the total body oxygen consumption, and these patients are chemically paralyzed.

The mixed venous oxygen saturation (monitored during CPB), is ideally a reflection of the total body oxygen consumption. It is not capable of distinguishing venous oxygen consumption of the different vital organs.

Mixed venous oxygen saturations cannot provide estimates of sufficient flow rates for oxygen transport to individual vital organs.

In a dog model, Lazenby et al.[46] demonstrated that blood flow during hypothermic CPB is shunted to skeletal muscle. As pump flows increase, an increasing percentage of this flow is shunted to skeletal muscle. Thus, if an increase in flow is the only mode used to compensate for low systemic perfusion pressure, it is very unlikely to prevent postoperative renal dysfunction. Valentine et al.[47] could not find any differences in renal outcome in 122 patients between fixed flow rates (2.4 L · min^{-1}) or tailored flow rates (1.3 L · min^{-1} · m^{-2}) during hypothermia, while the venous oxygen saturation was kept at 75 to 80 percent at any time.

The advantages cited by those using low-flow rates include a decrease in trauma to blood constituents, a decrease in emboli formation, minimization of bronchial collateral flow (i.e., return to the left ventricle), decrease in tissue edema, and a decrease in CPB tubing and connector failures.

Urzua et al.[48] investigated 21 patients with normal renal function. These patients were divided into two groups. The first group consisted of 14 patients who received no treatment for perfusion pressure during CPB (average 57.7 ± 8.2 mmHg); a second group consisted of (7 patients) where low perfusion pressure was treated with phenylephrine to maintain perfusion pressure above 70 mmHg (average 71.1 ± 3.1 mmHg). Flow rate was maintained at 2.2 L · min^{-1} · m^{-2} in both groups throughout CPB. No significant differences were found in hematocrit during CPB between groups. They found a significantly higher creatinine clearance in the higher perfusion pressure group intraoperatively, but not postoperatively, and no patient in either group developed postoperative ARF. However, patients with lower perfusion pressure during CPB presented with higher osmolal clearances postoperatively.

Postoperative renal function is as important as intraoperative renal function, as renal failure most frequently develops several hours or days postoperatively. A study of 504 adult patients[49] estimated the correlation between low perfusion pressures and low flow rates during hypothermic CPB and the development of postoperative ARF. Fifteen of the 504 patients (3 percent) developed ARF postoperatively. The TM^{-50} (mmHg of MAP less than 50 mmHg multiplied by the minutes that the MAP remains less than 50 mmHg) in patients who developed ARF postoperatively was not significantly different than those patients without renal dysfunction. There was also no difference found in the LF^{-40} (the difference between a perfusion flow of 40 ml · kg^{-1} · min^{-1} and a lesser flow, multiplied by the minutes of flow less than 40 ml · kg^{-1} · min^{-1}) between the two groups. However, in those patients who developed ARF postoperatively, a significantly lower MAP was noted during the pre-bypass, weaning, post-CPB, and ICU periods. The presence of preoperative renal dysfunction, neurologic disease, peripheral vascular disease, and diabetes were the most important risk factors for developing ARF after CPB.

However, in a retrospective study of 428 open heart operations, Yeboah et al.[1] showed that when the perfusion pressure was maintained above 80 mmHg, the incidence of renal failure was significantly reduced. Unfortunately, the variable definition of postoperative renal failure may be responsible for much of the discrepancies observed in these two studies.

In summary, there are still many unanswered questions with regard to flow and pressure, but it seems that renal function of patients at high risk of postoperative ARF (preoperative renal disease, diabetes, and peripheral vascular disease) would be better preserved if normal perfusion pressure and flow are used during CPB.

Theoretically, augmentation of perfusion pressure with α-adrenergic agonist is not desirable physiologically. This is because α-agonists cause vasoconstriction of the renal arteries. No study has been able to document a detrimental effect of α-adrenergic agonists on postoperative renal function.

Pharmacologic Prevention

RENAL DOSE DOPAMINE

A renal dose (2 to 5 μg · kg^{-1} · min^{-1}) of dopamine is traditionally used to protect the kidneys during heart surgery. Dopamine, an endogenous catecholamine, is known to cause an increase in RBF, GFR, urine flow, and sodium excretion.[50–53] This increase in GFR and sodium excretion is interpreted as an increase in RBF secondary to afferent and efferent arteriolar vasodilation, mediated by the action of dopamine on specific vascular receptors.[54,55] Additionally, a renal dose of dopamine has the added benefit of increasing the cardiac index, which may offer an advantage in preventing renal failure, especially during the pre- and post-CPB periods.

However, natriuresis after low-dose dopamine was demonstrated in the absence of changes in RBF and GFR, suggesting a specific tubular effect.[51,55,56] Recently, specific dopamine (DA1)-receptors in the proximal tubule were identified.[57,58] In healthy volunteers, Olsen et al.[59] investigated the effects of low-dose dopamine on renal hemodynamics and renal tubular reabsorption of sodium and water. Sodium clearance increased by 128 percent, while RBF and GFR increased only by 43 percent and 9 percent, respectively. They concluded that natriuresis during low-dose dopamine infusion is caused by an increase in outflow of sodium from the proximal tubules that is not fully compensated for in the distal tubules.

Despite the theoretical advantages attributed to low-dose dopamine, very few studies are available that investigate this therapy for preventing renal failure after cardiac surgery using CPB. Costa et al.[60] investigated the value of low doses of dopamine during cardiac surgery using CPB in patients with preoperative renal dysfunction. Unfortunately, only 21 patients were included in this study (12 control patients and 8 low-dose dopamine patients), there was no anesthetic protocol, and many different medications were used (lasix, phentolamine, phenylephrine, digoxin, and vasodilators) during and after CPB. Despite these reservations, they found significantly higher ratios of sodium output/intake and free water output/intake in the low-dose dopamine group during CPB. Their conclusion was that low-dose dopamine infusion increases water and sodium excretion during CPB. The mechanism was presumed to be the renal vasodilator effect of low-dose dopamine; however, since dopamine augments natriuresis, this conclusion is unsupported by their data. Furthermore, there is no evidence from this study that increased water and sodium excretion improve renal outcome.

In a double-blind randomized study, Myles et al.[61] investigated the renal outcome of 52 patients undergoing CABG surgery. All patients were normal with respect to renal function preoperatively. They failed to document any differences in urine output, creatinine clearance, and free water clearance between patients receiving dopamine 200 $\mu g \cdot min^{-1}$ or placebo, despite a statistically significant improvement in hemodynamics in the dopamine group.

In summary, low-dose dopamine improves general hemodynamics, but a renal protective effect during cardiac surgery is still questionable.

MANNITOL

Mannitol is an osmotic diuretic widely used during CPB.[62] The purpose is to modify the nature of postischemic injury favorably[63] by lowering renal vascular resistance and preserving tubular integrity. However, the effectiveness of this drug in preventing renal insufficiency in patients undergoing cardiac surgery and CPB remains controversial. In an animal model of norepinephrine-induced reversible ARF, Burke et al.[64] documented that prophylactic administration of mannitol was protective. These workers suggest that by increasing proximal tubular pressure,

mannitol keeps the glomerular capillary pressure stable and thereby prevents tubular obstruction. Trimble et al.[65] confirmed that mannitol reduces mechanical hemolysis in an vitro study but were unable to confirm this in a controlled clinical study.

Free radicals, including the superoxide anion, hydrogen peroxide, and hydroxyl radical, may be generated during CPB and reperfusion.[66] Mannitol can reduce the plasma hydrogen peroxide free radical in patients undergoing CABG surgery.[67] Although the link between renal dysfunction and free radical activity during CPB is unknown, experimental studies have demonstrated the ability of free radical scavengers, such as mannitol, to reduce ischemia-induced protein leakage across vessel walls in rabbit kidney.[68] Mannitol is also known to offer protection against free radical-induced injury in the mouse renal brush border membrane.[69]

In a clinical study, Ip-Yam et al.[70] failed to show any effect of prophylactic mannitol on postoperative renal function (creatinine clearance, fractional sodium excretion, microalbuminuria, urinary NAG, and urine output).

In summary, while mannitol is capable of protecting against renal free radical injury, the link between free radical damage and renal dysfunction is unknown. Additionally, there is no clinical evidence to document the efficacy of mannitol as a renal protective agent.

CALCIUM CHANNEL BLOCKERS

Calcium Channel Blockers and Renal Hemodynamics

The action of calcium channel blockers on renal hemodynamics is very complex. Calcium channel blockers, in the presence of vasoconstrictive agents such as norepinephrine or endothelin markedly augment the GFR while producing only modest improvements in RBF. The predominant influence of calcium channel blockers on GFR suggests that they antagonize the afferent arteriolar effects

of sympathetic agonists such as norepinephrine.

In the hydronephrotic isolated perfused
kidney, the afferent and the efferent arterioles are visualizable using videomicros-
copy.[71] This technique permits direct visualization of these arterioles following
pharmacologic intervention. Using this
method, calcium channel blocker administration does preferentially dilate the afferent ar-

teriole during angiotensin II administration.
The vasodilating effect of calcium channel
blockers on the efferent arterioles is significantly less than the vasodilating effect on the
afferent arterioles.[72]

In order to obtain a better understanding
of the interaction between the renal vascular
effects of angiotensin II and calcium channel
blockers, RBF and GFR responses to angiotensin II infusions into the dog renal artery

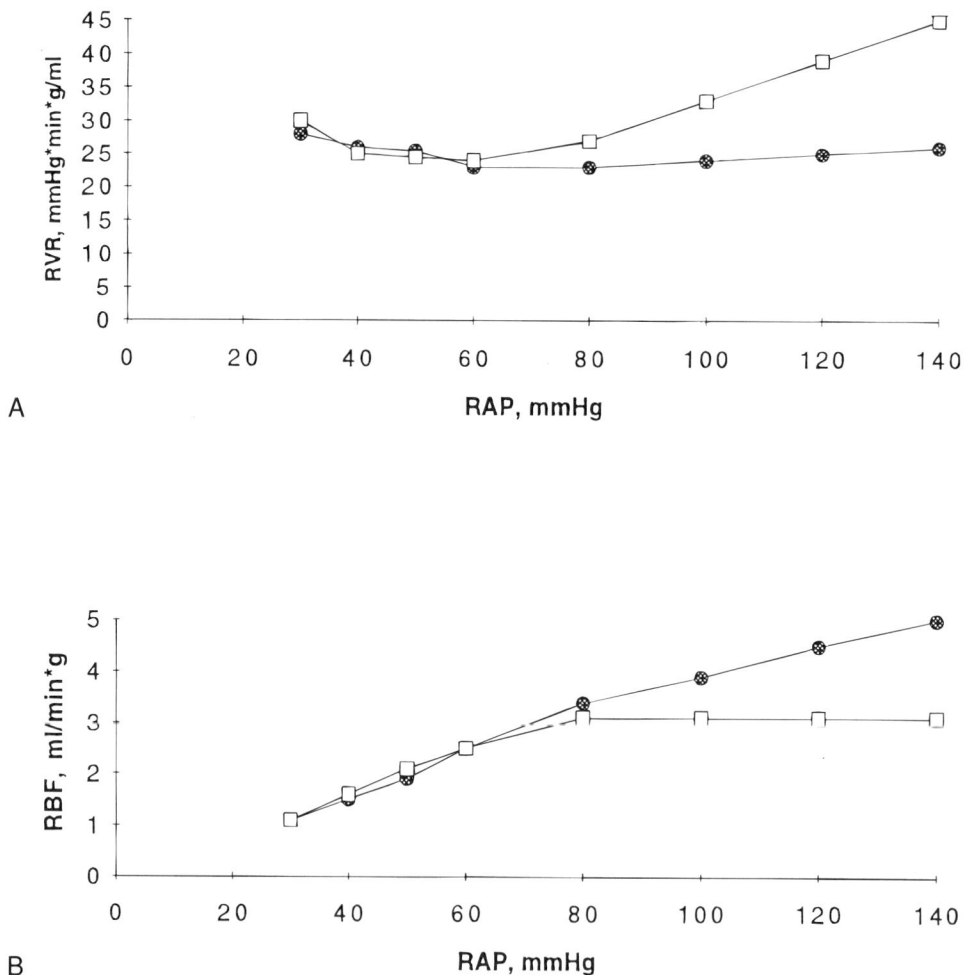

Fig. 9-1. Effects of verapamil on renal autoregulatory behavior in the anesthetized dog. **(A)** Relationship between renal arterial pressure (RAP) and renal vascular resistance (RVR) before and during
infusion of verapamil (5 to 7 $\mu g \cdot min^{-1} \cdot kg^{-1}$) into the renal artery. **(B)** Relationship between RAP
and renal blood flow (RBF) before and during verapamil infusion. *Key:* ⊕, verapamil; □, control.
(From Carmines et al.,[73] with permission.)

were evaluated either before or during infusion of a calcium channel blocker[73] (Fig. 9-1). In addition, the dogs were pretreated with an ACE inhibitor in order to reduce the contribution of endogenous angiotensin II levels to the responses observed. Before infusion of the calcium channel blocker, angiotensin II infusion was accompanied by a 19 percent reduction in GFR.

During infusion of a calcium channel blocker, the effects of angiotensin II on GFR were completely eliminated, indicating that most if not all of the effects of angiotensin II were reversed by calcium channel blockers. The effects of angiotensin II on RBF were not reversed by calcium channel blockers, which substantiates evidence that calcium channel blockers antagonize the vasoconstrictive effects of angiotensin II on the afferent arterioles, but not the efferent arterioles. This also implies that angiotensin II exerts vasoconstrictor actions on afferent and efferent arterioles through different mechanisms. These results suggest a complex interaction between angiotensin II and calcium channel blockers in the control of glomerular hemodynamics.

Calcium channel blockers interfere with appropriate autoregulatory resistance adjustments in the renal vasculature.[74-76] Under normal autoregulatory conditions, RBF will remain stable, and renal vascular resistance will increase as renal arterial pressure increases. Calcium channel blockers influence renal autoregulatory behavior by attenuating the increase in renal vascular resistance. Therefore, RBF will increase at increasing renal arterial pressures. This is the probable explanation for the ability of calcium channel blockers to increase the RBP within the autoregulatory range of systemic arterial pressure. At arterial pressures below the autoregulatory range, however, there is little or no difference between RBF under control conditions and during calcium channel blockade.

Furthermore, calcium channel blockers are known to influence the tubuloglomerular feedback mechanism.[73] Under normal conditions, increasing delivery of solute to the macula densa segment (an increased GFR) activates the tubuloglomerular feedback mechanism. As a result, vasoconstrictor signals from the macula densa increase the afferent arteriolar resistance to reduce glomerular pressure and GFR. Calcium channel blockers hinder the responsiveness of the afferent arterioles to signals from the macula densa cells.

Natriuretic Effects of Calcium Channel Blockers
Evidence indicates that calcium channel blockers are natriuretic. Numerous investigations have evaluated the direct effect of calcium channel blockers on sodium homeostasis in experimental animals.[77,78] An increase in urinary sodium excretion was a prominent feature in all these studies. The increase in sodium excretion, however, is not explained solely by increased GFR, because GFR increased in only 50 percent of cases. Interestingly, the increases in sodium excretion occurred despite decreases in blood pressure, which would ordinarily favor increased sodium reabsorption because of the reduction in RBF.

These observations indicate that the natriuretic effects of calcium channel blockers cannot be attributed solely to their hemodynamic effects. In a study using anesthetized normotensive rats,[79] amlodipine (a calcium channel blocker) lowered blood pressure by an average of 10 percent. This fall in blood pressure did not affect RBF or GFR. Thus, sodium load to the tubules was unchanged; however, the excretion of fluid and sodium increased about twofold. The fractional sodium excretion increased from 2.4 to 5.3 percent of the filtered load. These and other confirmatory observations[80,81] strongly support the conclusion that calcium channel antagonists act directly on the tubular system to augment natriuresis.

Calcium Channel Blockers and Cardiopulmonary Bypass
The CPB period is very unphysiologic: pulseless circulation, hypothermia, hemodilution, no circulation through the lungs, and

contact of circulating blood with foreign surfaces (e.g., oxygenator). All these factors combine to provoke the varied reactions within the human endocrine system. High plasma levels of norepinephrine, endothelin, renin, and angiotensin are repeatedly described during CPB.

Myers and Moran[82] suggested that the hypothermic, nonpulsatile cardiopulmonary bypass state is associated with a mild degree of renal ischemia, affecting both glomerular and tubular function. Although isolated insult may predispose the renal system to the development of ARF, ARF supervenes only if other types of ischemic injuries (low output syndrome, nephrotoxins) are superimposed. Only 3 percent of patients undergoing heart surgery with CPB develop ARF postoperatively; thus, there are few patients for clinical studies to impute the effects of calcium channel blockers on postoperative renal outcome.

In a study by Hashimoto et al.[83] the efficacy of the calcium channel blocker nicardipine was evaluated for amelerioration of renal damage following CPB. In patients treated with nicardipine during surgery ($5 \mu g \cdot kg^{-1} \cdot min^{-1}$), the plasma endothelin concentration during and after CPB was lower and there was a significant reduction in N-acetyl-β-D-glucosaminidase and γ-glutamyltranspeptidase (markers of renal tubular damage) concentrations in the urine compared with control group.

Endothelin, a recently characterized 21-amino acid peptide, is synthesized by vascular endothelial cells.[25,84] It is a potent renal vasoconstrictor,[24-28] and elevated circulating levels of endothelin may play a pathophysiologic role in conditions such as hypertension and postischemic renal hypoperfusion.[85] Loutzenhiser et al.[86] described the effects of endothelin on the renal microvasculature in isolated perfused hydronephrotic and normal kidneys. In both kidney types, endothelin was found to be a potent vasoconstrictor of the afferent arteriole, with lesser effects on the efferent arteriole. More importantly, endothelin reduced GFR in both groups. These findings indicate that endothelin is a potent renal vasoconstrictor that decreases GFR predominantly by vasoconstriction of the afferent arteriole. In contrast, both the vasoconstriction of the afferent arteriole and the reduction in GFR were completely reversed by nifedipine. The authors conclude that endothelin elicits renal vasoconstriction via a mechanism involving dihydropyridine-sensitive calcium channels and that such calcium channels play a prominent role in the activation of the afferent arteriole.

Amenta et al.[87] investigated the interaction between endothelin and nicardipine in the human renal artery using a radioligand and autoradiographic study. They found the highest density of nicardipine binding sites in the tunica media of the renal artery. A lower density was also noticeable in the tunica adventitia. Endothelin, reduced nicardipine binding as a function of concentration, a 10-nM endothelin concentration reduced nicardipine binding by about 85 percent. These findings indicate an interaction (probably at the receptor level) between nicardipine binding and endothelin. This interaction may account for the attenuation by nicardipine of endothelin vasoconstriction.

The effects of a continuous diltiazem infusion on renal function during cardiac surgery were described by Zanardo et al.[88] Thirty-five patients scheduled for CABG surgery, all with normal renal function preoperatively (serum creatinine less than 0.133 mmol $\cdot L^{-1}$), were randomly assigned to three groups: control group (C), diltiazam $1 \mu g \cdot kg^{-1} \cdot min^{-1}$ group (D1), and diltiazam $2 \mu g \cdot kg^{-1} \cdot min^{-1}$ group (D2). Diltiazam was infused throughout surgery and continued for 36 hours postoperatively. The GFR of the C and the D1 groups showed a significant fall during CPB compared to the pre-bypass period but returned to baseline values postoperatively. No change in GFR was observed in the D2 patients. Furthermore, after CPB, urinary output was significantly greater in the D2 patients compared to either of the other groups. This was more impressive in light of a lower mean arterial pressure in the D2 group. This suggests that a continuous infusion of diltiazem improves GFR and urine output during and after CPB, but it does not affect postoperative renal outcome (renal failure).

Similar to studies regarding ACE inhibitors (see next section), study size and composition are a continuing problem. Patients included in these studies of calcium channel blockers are not high-risk patients for postoperative ARF. Further studies, which not only increase patient enrollment but also specifically include patients at high risk of developing ARF postoperatively, are necessary to clarify adequately the calcium channel blocker's role in ARF prophylaxis during CPB. Although calcium channel blockers are effective in preventing renal insufficiency from a variety of insults (i.e., radiocontrast agents, aminoglycosides, chemotherapeutic agents, and cyclosporine), the value of calcium channel blockers in preventing ARF following cardiac surgery and CPB remains uncertain.

ANGIOTENSIN-CONVERTING ENZYME INHIBITORS

ACE inhibitors are frequently prescribed by cardiologists for patients with systemic hypertension or congestive heart failure. While the use of ACE inhibitors in cardiac anesthesia is increasing, it is not common practice to use ACE inhibitors for treating hypertension or preventing renal ischemia. In contradistinction, the literature describes severe hypotension and bradycardia during induction of anesthesia in patients receiving ACE inhibitor therapy.[89–92] (A more in-depth description of the renin-angiotensin system [RAS] is presented under the section, Pathogenesis.)

In the well-hydrated, sodium-replete patient, anesthesia is not a significant stimulus to the circulating RAS. However, the estimation of a relative fluid deficit during surgery closely correlates with the previously described rise in plasma-renin activity, indicating RAS activation.[93] Surgery (or nociception) is also a potent activation stimulus in the RAS. Plasma-renin activity increases threefold from baseline values, irrespective of blood loss[94] due solely to sympathetic stimulation during surgery.

Stimulation of β_1-adrenoceptors in the juxtaglomerular apparatus by either endogenous catecholamines or exogenous β-receptor agonists stimulates the release of renin, leading to angiotensin II production (see the section, Pathogenesis). In contrast to endothelin, angiotensin II has a preferential constrictor effect on efferent arterioles.[95] Therefore, angiotensin II helps stabilize GFR during periods of hypotension or water and sodium deficits. Simultaneously, angiotensin II-mediated efferent arteriolar constriction causes changes in peritubular capillary hemodynamics that lead to increased sodium reabsorption.

The excretion of most metabolic waste products, such as urea and creatinine, is directly proportional to GFR. Thus, RAS activation allows unaltered excretion of these products during periods of hypotension. The direct actions of angiotensin II on tubular transport in addition to direct effects caused by aldosterone secretion augment sodium retention without impairing the excretion of metabolic waste products.[96]

Carmines et al.[73] investigated the effects of angiotensin II on renal vascular hemodynamics. In a dog model in which an ACE inhibitor was used to inhibit endogenous angiotensin II release, exogenous angiotensin II was then infused followed by an examination of renal vascular function. Carmines and colleagues concluded that an infusion of angiotensin II causes decreases in RBF (21 percent) and in GFR (19 percent). This result is consistent with work done by Navar and Rosivall,[97] which indicates that angiotensin II reduces RBF and GFR by constricting both afferent and efferent renal arterioles.

The influence of ACE inhibitors per se on renal hemodynamics is very hard to describe. The effects are often determined in patients with pre-existing increases in angiotensin II plasma concentration. For example, in patients with renal artery stenosis, GFR is dependent on high concentrations of angiotensin II to constrict the efferent glomerular arterioles and therefore to generate adequate filtration pressure. If production of angiotensin II is prevented by ACE inhibition, GFR can fall dramatically, leading to a rapid detorioration in renal function.[98,99]

Conversely, there are specific circumstances in which ACE inhibition is beneficial to patients who are at high risk of renal damage. Proteinuria in patients with renal diseases of diverse etiology (i.e., glomerulonephritis, systemic lupus erythematosus and nephrotic syndrome) is significantly reduced by ACE inhibitor therapy.[100,101] ACE inhibitors are also effective at reducing the microalbuminuria associated with diabetes mellitus.[102]

Following CPB, plasma angiotensin II is increased significantly for several hours.[103] In patients without pre-existing cardiac or renal disease, pretreatment with ACE inhibitors, 2 days prior to heart surgery, results in improvements in RBF, GFR, and urinary sodium excretion when compared with placebo.[104] However, there was no difference in renal outcome of the patients postoperatively. This is primarily related to small sample size (18 patients) and the exclusion of patients with prior renal dysfunction. Additionally, the mechanism of action of ACE inhibitors is impossible to ascertain because all patients in this study were pretreated with calcium channel blockers. Without pretreatment with calcium channel blockers, the known elevation in plasma levels of endothelin during CPB (a vasoconstrictor of the afferent arterioles) combined with ACE inhibitor therapy should decrease RBF and GFR.

The influence of calcium channel blockers on whole kidney and arteriolar responsiveness to angiotensin II is well described. The renal vasoconstrictive action of angiotensin II is either abolished[105] or markedly attenuated by prior calcium channel blockade.[106] Other studies demonstrate that treatment with an ACE inhibitor during calcium channel blockade causes additional renal vasodilation, which can be reversed by exogenous administration of angiotensin II.[107]

In summary, since calcium channel blockers reduce[106] or abolish[105] the renal vascular effects of angiotensin II, in addition to counteracting the renal effects of endothelin, it seems probable that ACE inhibitors offer little value in renal protection during CPB.

Sympathetic Neural Blockade by Epidural Anesthesia

Efferent sympathetic nerve fibers innervating the kidneys emerge from the cord between T10 and L2.[108] Electrostimulation of the peripheral stump of renal nerves in dogs increases plasma-renin activity.[109] A circulatory challenge such as arterial hypotension evokes renin release both in humans and in animals with intact sympathetic systems, but it is unknown whether this is mediated by a decrease in arterial pressure per se or by reflex activation of sympathetic renal efferent nerves. During extensive thoracic and lumbar epidural anesthesia, sympathetic outflow is attenuated by preganglionic neural blockade.

In nonpremedicated awake patients without cardiovascular diseases, Hopf et al.[110,111] investigated the influence of thoracic epidural blockade on the renin and vasopressin plasma concentrations in response to induced arterial hypotension by sodium nitroprusside. Sensory blockade, 50 minutes after the institution of thoracic epidural anesthesia, extended from T1 to T11 (pinprick method). However, since regional temperatures on both hand and foot increased significantly (using infrared thermography) at constant ambient and rectal temperatures, it must be assumed that the sympathetic blockade was more extensive.

In patients with intact sympathetic innervation, a decrease in mean arterial pressure from 90 to 67 mmHg resulted in an increase in plasma renin and no change in plasma vasopressin concentrations. Conversely, during sympathetic blockade by epidural anesthesia, plasma renin concentrations remained unchanged, but plasma vasopressin concentrations increased significantly. The authors suggest that renal sympathetic nerve fibers play an important role in mediating renin release during hypotension, while release of vasopressin is probably a secondary compensatory mechanism.

This assumption was confirmed by Carp et al.[112] When epidural anesthesia was administered to patients treated with one of the following agents: placebo, ACE inhibitors, or an arginine vasopressin (AVP) type-V_1 antagonist, there was no significant change in blood pressure. However, combined treatment with ACE inhibitors and AVP type-V_1 antagonist resulted in a significant decrease in blood pressure following the institution of epidural anesthesia.

During CPB, plasma angiotensin II, plasma epinephrine, and norepinephrine concentrations all increase significantly.[103] These factors may exert a negative effect on renal function. Using high thoracic epidural anesthesia during CABG surgery prevents the increase in plasma epinephrine and norepinephrine concentrations. However, the interaction of plasma angiotensin II levels (renal outcome) during CPB (and the influence of high thoracic epidural analgesia) is unknown.

ANESTHETIC MANAGEMENT OF CARDIAC SURGICAL PATIENTS WITH TERMINAL RENAL FAILURE

Patients on maintenance hemodialysis for end-stage renal failure are at risk of accelerated atherosclerosis resulting from hypertension, increased cardiac output, hypertriglyceridemia, and elevated parathyroid hormone levels.[113] With the "progress" in medical management, increasing numbers of patients with chronic renal disease are becoming candidates for cardiac surgery.

These patients are highly sensitive to changes in fluid balance, and levels of serum potassium represent a high-risk group for cardiac surgery.[114,115] Schmid et al.[116] have described the management and outcome of cardiac surgery in 31 patients requiring chronic hemodialysis. All patients but one survived the surgery (3.3 percent mortality); this perioperative death was not associated with renal failure, however. Schmid et al. recommend performing preoperative hemodialysis on the day before surgery. To avoid admixture of cardioplegic solution (with its high potassium concentration) with blood returning to the pump, they recommend double cannulation to avoid returning the coronary sinus effluent to the pump.

A hemofiltration set is connected to the extracorporeal circuit for ultrafiltration, which facilitates intraoperative management of fluids and electrolytes. It is possible to remove as much as 1,500 to 2,000 ml of fluid using this method, and serum potassium levels rarely exceed 6.0 mmol $\cdot$ L^{-1}.[117] If, despite ultrafiltration, the potassium plasma level exceeds 6.0 mmol $\cdot$ L^{-1}, insulin-glucose infusion can be administered for temporary relief.

Unlike patients with normal renal function, catecholamines are preferred to the administration of large volumes of fluid to prevent pulmonary edema. The routine intravenous administration of potassium enriched mixtures is eschewed. Despite all the above measures, hyperkalemia or pulmonary edema often respond solely to hemodialysis; however, hemodialysis in the immediate postoperative period increases both the risk of postoperative hemodynamic instability and postoperative bleeding.

In these patients, continuous arteriovenous hemodialysis (CAVHD) is a better strategy than conventional hemodialysis. Although peritoneal dialysis is an alternative for patients with hemodynamic instability, it is not recommended for patients with compromised pulmonary status (an increasingly common problem in today's aging patient population).

CAVHD was described by Geronemus and Schneider[118] in 1984. This technique offers patients the chief advantage of reducing cardiovascular complications because of the decreased rate of reduction in the intravascular volume.

With conventional hemodialysis, the dialysis membrane is a potent activator of the intrinsic coagulation pathway and complement cascade. This cascade leads to leukocyte sequestration and activation in the lung. Hypoxemia and an elevation in pulmonary artery pressure often result.[119] The hypoxemia or pulmonary pressure elevation may further aggravate previously compromised cardiac function. Complement activation does not occur to the same extent with the more biocompatible membranes used in a CAVHD dialyzer. Another advantage of CAVHD is the ability to provide adequate parenteral nutrition to the patient without fluid overloading.

The urgency of the surgery in patients with terminal renal insufficiency has been found[120,121] to be an important variable associated with increased perioperative mortality (36 percent). Preoperative hemodialysis (PHD) is often associated with dysrhythmias or hypotension. If these complications occur in a patient with unstable angina, the result is dramatic and many times fatal. Therefore, PHD is contraindicated in patients undergoing emergency CABG.

Ilson et al.[121] have evaluated the postoperative outcome of patients treated with intraoperative hemodialysis (IHD) compared with the outcome of patients treated with PHD. Postoperatively, patients treated with IHD have lower mean serum potassium, creatinine, and blood urea nitrogen concentrations. The mean serum bicarbonate concentration was unchanged compared with the mean preoperative value, while the mean serum bicarbonate in patients treated with PHD was significantly decreased. In addition, IHD patients were hemodialyzed 2 days after surgery, while the PHD patients needed hemodialysis on the first postoperative day.

These findings are consistent with those of Soffer et al.[122] Zawada et al.,[123] and Hakim et al.,[124] in which postoperative hemodialysis could easily be delayed in IHD patients until the third postoperative day. Figure 9-2 shows the intraoperative hemodialysis setup as described by Ilson et al.[121] However, no evidence exists to show that IHD improves postoperative outcome or reduces the mortality of patients with end-stage renal disease requiring emergency cardiac surgery.

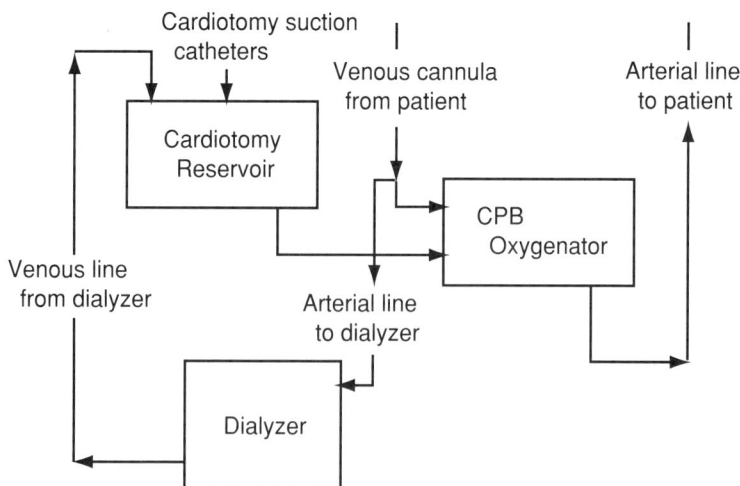

Fig. 9-2. Intraoperative hemodialysis setup.

POSTOPERATIVE MANAGEMENT OF CARDIAC SURGICAL PATIENTS WITH TERMINAL RENAL FAILURE

Patients with terminal renal failure who have undergone cardiac surgery require special postoperative management, with particular attention to the following issues: peritoneal dialysis, CAVHD versus hemodialysis, coagulation disorders (platelet dysfunction), infection, and aspirin after surgery.

The use of peritoneal dialysis has several advantages over hemodialysis or CAVHD. It needs minimal equipment and does not require the presence of a specialized technician. Most importantly, the hemodynamic instability and the risk of bleeding with heparin is avoided. Several contraindications exist for peritoneal dialysis: impaired pulmonary function (low PaO_2), peritoneal adhesions or a history of previous laparotomies, and an open connection between the thorax and the abdomen. Ko et al.[120] initiate peritoneal dialysis immediately upon arrival to the ICU to relieve the fluid load and to maintain a normal serum potassium level. Antibiotics are routinely added to the peritoneal dialysate. Peritoneal dialysis is continued for the first 7 postoperative days and is then switched to hemodialysis for those who are dependent preoperatively. When peritoneal dialysis is contraindicated, hemodialysis or CAVHD can be performed.

Patients with end-stage renal failure are known to have platelet dysfunction with subsequent defect in coagulation. Their platelets demonstrate both adhesion and aggregating deficiencies, and in addition, serum levels of factor III are low.[125] To achieve hemostasis following CPB, platelets and fresh frozen plasma are required more frequently than in patients without chronic renal dysfunction. The use of deamino-8-d-arginine vasopressin (DDAVP) has been shown to improve bleeding time (a measure of platelet function) in uremic patients.[126]

Renal failure patients are susceptible to infection, which is attributed to leukocyte dysfunction. Leukocytes are deficient in both absolute numbers[125] as well as function (decreased chemotactic response). Decreased intrinsic clearance rates and the type of dialysis are important determinants of antibiotic choice and dosing.

The peri- and postoperative use of aspirin prolong aortocoronary graft patency.[127] The risk/benefit ratio of perioperative aspirin use in this patient population is unclear.[125] However, the pathogenesis of intimal hyperplasia and atherogenesis involves the endothelium and other cell types in addition to platelets. Therefore, the judicious application of postoperative aspirin in renal insufficiency patients may be helpful, but not immediately postoperatively.

CONCLUSIONS AND RECOMMENDATIONS

Renal dysfunction occurs in a high percentage (30 percent) of patients undergoing cardiac surgery with the use of CPB. Although the incidence of acute renal failure requiring hemodialysis is low (3 percent), the mortality rate is very high (50 percent). Preventive measures are especially indicated for patients at high risk of ARF postoperatively; that is, those patients with preoperative renal dysfunction, peripheral vascular disease (diabetes), endocarditis, valvular disorders, prior operative performances, and congenital lesions.

Although controversies abound, efforts to ameliorate low perfusion pressure and low flow during CPB seem prudent. Whether the intra-CPB administration of an α-agonist (to treat periods of hypotension) has any influence on the renal outcome is unknown.

From the medications mentioned above, calcium channel blockers are probably the best means for preventing postoperative renal failure. If calcium channel blockers are used, their intravenous administration must begin after the induction of anesthesia and continue throughout and following surgery for at least 24 hours. Although no study documents a beneficial effect of a "renal dose" of dopamine on the postoperative renal outcome, its use during surgery is unlikely to harm the patient.

The value of thoracic epidural anesthesia for preventing postoperative renal dysfunction is unknown. Prevention of high catecholamine and renin plasma concentrations during CPB might prove beneficial for renal outcome. However, one cannot give specific recommendations concerning prevention of renal failure after cardiac surgery because no clinical studies are able to show beneficial effects of a particular drug or anesthetic technique on renal outcome.

In summary, we require many additional investigations to evaluate the effects of drugs and anesthestic techniques on the postoperative renal outcome in patients undergoing cardiac surgery.

REFERENCES

1. Yeboah ED, Petrie A, Pead JL: Acute renal failure and open heart surgery. BMJ 1:415–8, 1972
2. Bhat JG, Gluck MC, Lowenstein J et al: Renal failure after open heart surgery. Ann Intern Med 84:677–82, 1976
3. Abel R, Buckley J, Austen W et al: Etiology, incidence, and prognosis of renal failure following cardiac operations. Results of a prospective analysis of 500 consecutive patients. J Thorac Cardiovasc Surg 71:323–33, 1976
4. Hanson J, Loftness S, Clarke D et al: Peritoneal dialysis following open heart surgery in children. Pediatr Cardiol 10:125–8, 1989
5. Kron IL, Joob AW, Meter V: Acute renal failure in the cardio-vascular surgical patient. Ann Thorac Surg 39:590–8, 1985
6. Baxter P, Rigby ML, Jones OD et al: Acute renal failure following cardiopulmonary bypass in children: result of treatment. Int J Cardiol 7:235–43, 1985
7. Böök K, Öhqvist G, Björk VO et al: Peritoneal dialysis in infants and children after open heart surgery. Scand J Thorac Cardiovasc Surg 16:229–33, 1982
8. Rigden SPA, Barratt TM, Dillon MJ et al: Acute renal failure complicating cardiopulmonary bypass surgery. Arch Dis Child 57: 425–30, 1982
9. Frost L, Pedersen RS, Lund O et al: Prognosis and risk factors in acute, dialysis requiring renal failure after open-heart surgery. Scand J Thorac Cardiovasc Surg 25: 161–6, 1991
10. Hammermeister KE, Burchfiel C, Johnson R et al: Identification of patients at greatest risk for developing major complications at cardiac surgery. Circulation, suppl IV. 32: IV380–9, 1990
11. Zanardo G, Michielon P, Paccagnella A et al: Acute renal failure in the patient undergoing cardiac operation. Prevalence, mortality rate, and main risk factors. J Thorac Cardiovasc Surg 107:1489–95, 1994
12. Ghattas MA, Sethna DH, Rezkana H et al: Patterns of acute renal failure (ARF) requiring dialysis after open heart surgery. Anesth Analg 65:S57, 1986
13. Terragno NA, Terragno DA, McGiff JC: Contribution of prostaglandines to renal circulation in conscious, anesthetized, and laparotomized dogs. Circ Res 40:590–5, 1977
14. Lacoumenta S, Yeo TH, Paterson JL et al: Hormonal and metabolic responses to cardiac surgery with sufentanil-oxygen anesthesia. Acta Anaesthesiol Scand 31:258–63, 1987
15. Howie MB, McSweeney TD, Lingram RP et al: Comparison of sufentanil-O_2 and fentanyl-O_2 for cardiac anesthesia. Anesth Analg 64: 877–87, 1985
16. Sebel PS, Bovil JG: Cardiovascular effects of sufentanil anesthesia. Anesth Analg 61: 115–9, 1982
17. Liem TH, Booij LHDJ, Hasenbos MAWM et al: Coronary artery bypass grafting using two different anesthetic techniques. Part III. Adrenergic responses. J Cardiothorac Vasc Anesth 6:156–61, 1992
18. Landymore RW, Murphy DA, Kinley CE et al: Does pulsatile flow influence the incidence of postoperative hypertension? Ann Thorac Surg 28:261–8, 1979
19. Goodman TA, Gerard DF, Bernstein EF et al: The effects of pulseless perfusion on the distribution of renal cortical blood flow and on renin release. Surgery 80:31–9, 1976
20. Taylor KM, Bain WH, Russell M: Peripheral vascular resistance and angiotensin II levels

during pulsatile and non-pulsatile cardiopulmonary bypass. Thorax 34:594–8, 1979

21. Canivet JL, Larbuisson R, Damas P et al: Plasma renin activity and urine β_2-microglobin during and after cardiopulmonary bypass: pulsatile vs non-pulsatile. Eur Heart J 11:1079–82, 1990

22. Philbin DM, Levine FH, Kono K et al: Attenuation of the stress response to cardiopulmonary bypass by the addition of pulsatile flow. Circulation 64:808–12, 1981

23. Salerno TA, Henderson M, Keith FM et al: Hypertension after coronary operation: can it be prevented by pulsatile perfusion? J Thorac Cardiovasc Surg 81:396–9, 1981

24. Loutzenhiser R, Epstein M, Hayashi et al: Direct visualization of effects of endothelin on renal microvasculature. Am J Physiol 258: F61–8, 1990

25. Whittle BJR, Moncada S: The endothelium explosion. A pathophysiological reality or biological curiosity? Circulation 81:2022–5, 1990

26. Goetz KL, Wang BC, Madwed JB et al: Cardiovascular, renal, and endocrine responses to intravenous endothelin in concious dogs. Am J Physiol 255:R1064–8, 1988

27. Lopez-Farre A, Montanes I, Millas I et al: Effect of endothelin on renal function in rats. Eur J Pharmacol 163:187–9, 1989

28. Badr KF, Murray JJ, Breyer MD et al: Mesangial cell, glomerular and renal vasculature responses to endothelin in the rat kidney. Elucidation of signal transduction pathways. J Clin Invest 83:336–42, 1989

29. Knothe C, Boldt J, Zickmann B et al: Endothelin plasma levels in old and young patients during open heart surgery: correlations to cardiopulmonary and endocrinology parameters. J Cardiovasc Phar 20:664–70, 1992

30. Price RT: Urinary enzymes, nephrotoxicity and renal disease. Toxicology 23:99–134, 1982

31. Price RG: Measurement of N-acetyl-β-glucosaminidase and its isoenzymes in urine. Methods and clinical applications. Eur J Clin Chem Clin Biochem 30:693–705, 1992

32. Bauer JH, Brooks CS, Burch RN: Clinical appraisal of creatinine clearance as measurement of glomerular filtration rate. Am J Kidney Dis 2:337–46, 1982

33. Bastl C, Katz MA, Shear L: Uremia with low

serum creatinine—an entity produced by marked creatinine secretion. Am J Med Sci 273:289–92, 1977

34. Shemesh O, Golbetz H, Kriss JP et al: Limitations of creatinine as a filtration marker in glomerulopathic patients. Kidney Int 28: 830–8, 1985

35. Carrie BJ, Golbetz HV, Michaela AS et al: Creatinine: an inadequate filtration marker in glomerular disease. Am J Med 69:177–82, 1980

36. Tomlanovich S, Golbetz H, Perlorth M et al: Limitations of creatinine in quantifying the severity of cyclosporin-induced chronic nephropathy. Am J Kidney Dis 8:322–37, 1986

37. Mitch WE: The influence of diet on progression of renal function. Annu Rev Med 35: 249–64, 1984

38. Cattell WR: Excretory pathways for contrast media. Invest Radiol 5:473–97, 1970

39. Dure-Smith P: The dose of contrast media on intravenous urography: a physiologic assessment. AJR 108:691–7, 1970

40. Saxton HM: Urography, review article. Br J Radiol 42:321–46, 1969

41. Denneberg T: Clinical studies on kidney function with radioactive sodium diatrizoate (Hypaque). Acta Med Scand, suppl. 442: 1–134, 1966

42. Lewis R, Kerr N, Van Buren C et al: Comparative evaluation of urographic contrast media, inulin, and ^{99m}Tc-DTPA clearance methods for determination of glomerular filtration rate in clinical transplantation. Transplantation 48:790–6, 1989

43. Mandelbaum I, Burns WH: Pulsatile and non pulsatile blood flow. Am Med Assoc 191: 121–4, 1965

44. Manche AR, Walesby RK, Goode AW et al: β_2-Microglobin excretion as an index of renal function on pulsatile and non pulsatile cardiopulmonary perfusion. Perfusion 2:195–203, 1987

45. Badner NH, Murkin JM, Lok P: Differences in pH management and pulsatile/nonpulsatile perfusion during cardiopulmonary bypass do not influence renal function. Anesth Analg 75:696–701, 1992

46. Lazenby WD, Ko W, Zelano JA et al: Effects of temperature and flow rate on regional blood flow and metabolism during cardiopul-

monary bypass. Ann Thorac Surg 53:957–64, 1992

47. Valentine S, Barrowcliffe M, Peacock J: A comparison of effects of fixed and tailored cardiopulmonary bypass flow rates on renal function. Anaesth Intensive Care 21:304–8, 1993

48. Urzua J, Troncoso S, Bugedo G et al: Renal function and cardiopulmonary bypass: effect of perfusion pressure. J Cardiothorac Vasc Anesth 6:299–303, 1992

49. Slogoff S, Reul GJ, Keats AS et al: Role of perfusion pressure and flow in major organ dysfunction after cardiopulmonary bypass. Ann Thorac Surg 50:911–8, 1990

50. Goldberg LI, McDonald RH, Zimmerman AM: Sodium diuresis produced by dopamine in patients with congestive heart faillure. N Engl J Med 269:1060–4, 1963

51. Mc Donald RH, Goldber LI, McNay JL et al: Effect of dopamine in man: augmentation of sodium excretion, glomerular filtration rate, and renal plasma flow. J Clin Invest 43:1116–25, 1964

52. Meyer MB, McNay JL, Goldberg LI: Effects of dopamine on renal function an hemodynamics in dog. J Pharmacol Exp Ther 156:186–92, 1967

53. Goldberg LI: Cardiovascular and renal actions of dopamine: potential clinical application. Pharmacol Rev 24:1–29, 1972

54. Chapmaan BJ, Horn NM, Munday KA et al: The actions of dopamine and of sulpiride on regional blood flows in the rat. J Physiol (Lond) 298:437–52, 1980

55. Davis BB, Walter MJ, Murdaugh KA et al: The mechanism of increase in sodium excretion following dopamine infusion. Proc Soc Exp Biol Med 129:210–3, 1968

56. Wasserman K, Huss R, Kullmann R et al: Dopamine induced diuresis in the cat without changes in renal hemodynamics. Arch Pharmacol 312:77–83, 1980

57. Felder RA, Blecher M, Calcagno PL et al: Dopamine receptors in the proximal tubules of the rabbit. Am J Physiol 247:F499–505, 1984

58. Felder RA, Jose PA: Dopamine 1-receptors in rat kidneys identified with ^{125}I-Sch 23982. Am J Physiol 255:F970–6, 1988

59. Olsen NV, Hansen JM, Ladefoged SD et al: Renal tubular reabsorption of sodium and water during infusion of low-dose dopamine in normal man. Clin Sci 78:503–7, 1990

60. Costa P, Ottino GM, Matani A et al: Low-dose dopamine during cardiopulmonary bypass in patients with renal dysfunction. J Cardiothorac Anesth 4:469–73, 1990

61. Myles PS, Buckland MR, Schenk NJ et al: Effect of "renal dose" dopamine on renal function following cardiac surgery. Anaesth Intensive Care 21:56–61, 1993

62. Dobernak RD, Reiser MP, Lillehie CW: Acute renal failure after open heart surgery utilizing extracorporeal circulation and total body perfusion. Analysis of 1000 patients. J Cardiovasc Surg 43:441–52, 1962

63. Meyers BD: Nature of postischaemic renal injury following aortic or cardiac surgery. p. 167. In Bihari D, Neild G (eds): Acute Renal Failure in the Intensive Therapy Unit. Springer-Verlag, Berlin, 1990

64. Burke TJ, Cronin RE, Duchin KL et al: Ischemia and tubule obstruction during acute renal failure in dogs: mannitol in protection. Am J Physiol 238:F305–14, 1980

65. Trimble AS, Hait MR, Osborn JJ et al: Mannitol and extracorporeal circulation. J Thorac Cardiovasc Surg 49:307–12, 1965

66. Utley JR: Pathophysioloy of cardiopulmonary bypass: current issues. J Cardiovasc Surg 5:177–89, 1990

67. Yang MW, Lin CY, Hung HL et al: Mannitol reduces plasma hydrogen peroxide free radical in patients undergoing coronary artery bypass graft surgery. Ma Tsui Hsueh Tsa Chi 30:65–70, 1992

68. Bratell S, Folmerz P, Hansson R et al: Effects of oxygen free radical scavengers, xanthine oxidase inhibition and calcium entry blockers on leakage of albumin after ischemia. An experimental study in rabbit kidneys. Acta Physiol Scand 134:35–41, 1988

69. Kaur A, Sethi AK, Ganguly NK et al: Concentration dependent function of superoxide dismutase in oxygen free radicals mediatedtissue injury in renal brush border membrane. Biochem Int 19:385–95, 1989

70. Ip-Yam PC, Murphy S, Baines M et al: Renal function and proteinuria after cardiopulmonary bypass: The effects of temperature and mannitol. Anesth Analg 78:842–7, 1994

71. Steinhausen M, Snoei H, Parekh N et al: Hydronephrosis: a new method to visualize vas

afferens, efferens and glomerular network. Kidney Int 23:794–806, 1983

72. Loutzenhiser RD, Epstein M: Renal hemodynamic effects of calcium antagonists. J Cardiovasc Pharmacol, suppl 6. 12:S48–52, 1988

73. Carmines PK, Mitchell KD, Navar LG: Effects of calcium antagonists on renal hemodynamics and glomerular function. Kidney Int, suppl. 36. 41:S43–8, 1992

74. Ono H, Kokubun H, Hashimoto K: Abolition by ccalcium antagonists of the autoregulation of renal blood flow. Naunyn Schmiedebergs Arch Pharmacol 285:201–7, 1974

75. Navar LG, Champion WJ, Thomas CE: Effects of calcium channel blockade on renal vascular resistance response to changes in perfusion pressure and angiotensin-converting enzyme inhibition in dogs. Circ Res 58: 874–81, 1986

76. Ogawa N: Effect of nicardipine on the relationship of renal blood flow and of renal vascular resistance to perfusion pressure in dog kidney. J Pharm Pharmacol 42:138–40, 1990

77. Luft FC, Aronoff GR, Sloan RS et al: Calcium channel blockade with nitrendipine: effects on sodium homeostasis, the renin angiotensin system, and the sympathetic nervous system in humans. Hypertension 7:438–42, 1985

78. Luft FC, Weiberger MH: Calcium antagonists and renal sodium homeostasis p. 203. In Epstein M, Loutzenhiser R (eds): Calcium Antagonists and the Kidney. Hanley & Belfus, Philadelphia, 1990

79. Johns EJ: A study of renal actions of amlodipine in the normotensive and spontaneously hypertensive rat. Br J Pharmacol 94:311–8, 1988

80. Romero JC, Raij L, Granger JP et al: Multiple effects of calcium entry blockers on renal function in hypertension. Hypertension 10: 140–51, 1987

81. Osswald H, Weinheimer G, Kapp JF: Renal action of calcium antagonists. J Neural Transm, suppl. 31:39–53, 1990

82. Myers BD, Moran SM: Hemodynamically mediated acute renal failure. N Engl J Med 314:97–105, 1986

83. Hashimoto K, Nomura K, Nakano M: Pharmacological intervention for renal protection during cardiopulmonary bypass. Heart Vessels 8:203–10, 1993

84. Yanagisawa M, Kurihara H, Kimura S et al: A novel potent vasoconstrictor peptide produced by vascular endothelial cells. Nature 332:411–5, 1988

85. Kon V, Yoshioka T, Fogo A et al: Glomerular actions of endothelin in vivo. J Clin Invest 83: 1762–7, 1989

86. Loutzenhiser R, Epstein M, Hayashi et al: Direct visualization of effects of endothelin on renal microvasculature. Am J Physiol 258: F61–8, 1990

87. Amenta F, Rossodivita I, Ferrante F: Interactions between endothelin and dihydropyridine-type calcium antagonist nicardipine in the human renal artery: a radioligand and autoradiographic study. J Autonomic Pharmacol 14:129–36, 1994

88. Zanardo G, Michielon P, Rosi P et al: Effects of continuous diltiazem infusion on renal function during cardiac surgery. J Cardiothorac Vasc Anesth 7:711–6, 1993

89. Kataja JH, Kaukinen S, Viinamäki OVK et al: Hemodynamic and hormonal changes in patients pretreated with captopril for surgery of abdominal aorta. J Cardiothorac Anesth 3: 425–32, 1989

90. McConachie I, Healy TEJ: ACE inhibitors and anaesthesia. Postgrad Med J 65:273–4, 1988

91. Selby DG, Richards JD, Marshman JM: ACE inhibitors. Anaesth Intensive Care 17:110–1, 1989

92. Russel RM, Jones RM: Postoperative hypotension associated with enalapril. Anesthesiology 6:394–9, 1989

93. Robertson D, Michelakis AM: Effect of anesthesia and surgery on plasma renin activity in man. J Clin Endocrinol Metab 334:831–6, 972

94. Miller EDJ: The renin angiotensin system in anesthesia. p. 19. In Brown BR (ed): Anesthesia and the Patient With Endocrine Disease. FA Davis, Philadelphia, 1980

95. Kellow NH: The renin-angiotensin system and angiotensin converting enzyme (ACE) inhibitors. Anesthesia 49:613–22, 1994

96. Hall JE: The renin-angiotensin system: renal actions and blood pressure regulation. Compr Ther 17:8–17, 1991

97. Navar LG, Rosivall L: Contribution of renin-angiotensin system to the control of intrarenal hemodynamics. Kidney Int 25:857–68, 1984

98. Davidson R, Wilcox CS: Diagnostic usefulness of renal scanning after angiotensin converting enzyme inhibitors. Hypertension 18: 299–303, 1991

99. McGrath BP, Matthews PG, Johnstone CI: Use of captopril in the diagnosis of renal hypertension. Aust NZ J Med 111:359–63, 1983

100. Heeg JE, De Jong PE, Van der Hem GK et al: Reduction of proteinuria by angiotensin converting enzyme inhibition. Kidney Int 32: 78–332, 1987

101. Lagrue G, Robeva R, Laurent J: Antiproteinuric effect of captopril in primary glomerular disease. Nephron 46:99–100, 1987

102. Taguma Y, Kitamato Y, Futaki G et al: Effect of captopril on heavy proteinuria in azotemic diabetes. N Engl J Med 313:1617–20, 1985

103. Taylor KM, Morton JJ, Brown JJ et al: Hypertension and renin angiotensin system following open heart surgery. J Thorac Cardiovasc Surg 74:840–5, 1977

104. Colson P, Ribstein J, Mimran A et al: Effect of angiotensin converting enzyme inhibition on blood pressure and renal function during open heart surgery. Anesthesiology 72:23–7, 1990

105. Loutzenhiser R, Epstein M: Effects of calcium channel antagonists on renal hemodynamics. Am J Physiol 232:F619–29, 1985

106. Ichikaw I, Miele JF, Brenner B: Reversal of renal cortical actions of angiotensin II by verapamil and magnese. Kidney Int 16:137–47, 1979

107. Navar L, Champion WJ, Thomas CE: Effects of calcium channel blockade on renal vascular resistance responses to changes in perfusion pressure and angiotensin converting enzyme inhibition in dogs. Circ Res 58:874–81, 1986

108. Bonica JJ: Autonomic innervation of the viscera in relation to nerve block. Anesthesiology 29:79–813, 1968

109. Osborne JL, Holdaas H, Thames MD et al: Renal adrenoceptor mediation of antinatriuretic and renin secretion responses to low frequency renal nerve stimulation in the dog. Circ Res 53:298–305, 1983

110. Hopf HB, Schlaghecke R, Peters J: Sympathetic neural blockade by thoracic epidural anesthesia suppresses renin release in response to arterial hypotension. Anesthesiology 80:992–9, 1994

111. Hopf HB, Arand D, Peters J: Sympathetic blockade by thoracic epidural anaesthesia suppresses renin release in response to hypotension, but activates the vasopressin system. Eur J Anaesth 9:63–9, 1992

112. Carp H, Vadhera R, Jayaram A et al: Endogenous vasopressin and renin angiotensin systems support blood pressure after epidural block in humans. Anesthesiology 80:1000–7, 1994

113. Lindneer A, Charra B, Sherrard DJ et al: Accelerated atherosclerosis in prolonged maintenance hemodialysis. N Engl J Med 290: 697–701, 1974

114. Deutch E, Bernstein RC, Addonizio P et al: Coronary artery bypass surgery in patients on chronic hemodialysis. Ann Intern Med 110:369–72, 1989

115. Laws KH, Merril WH, Hammon JW et al: Cardiac surgery in patients with chronic renal disease. Ann Thorac Surg 42:152–7, 1986

116. Schmid C, Ziemer G, Laas J et al: Open heart surgery in patients requiring chronic hemodialysis. Scand J Thorac Cardiovasc Surg 26: 97–100, 1992

117. Kramer P, Seegers A, DeVivie R et al: Therapeutic potential of hemofiltration. Clin Nephrol 11:145–9, 1979

118. Geronemus P, Schneider N: Continuous aarteriovenous hemodialysis: a new modality for treatment of acute renal failure. Trans Am Soc Artif Inter Organs 30:60–7, 1984

119. Jacob AI, Gavellas G, Zarco R et al: Leukopenia, hypoxia and complement function with different hemodialysis membranes. Kidney Int 17:571–6, 1980

120. Ko W, Kreiger KH, Isom OW: Cardiopulmonary bypass procedures in dialysis patients. Ann Thorac Surg 55:677–84, 1993

121. Ilson BE, Bland PS, Jorkasky DK et al: Intraoperative versus routine hemodialysis in end-stage renal disease patients undergoing open heart surgery. Nephron 61:170–5, 1992

122. Soffer O, MacDonell RC, Finlayson DC et al: Intraoperative hemodialysis during cardiopulmonary bypass in chronic renal failure. J Thorac Cardiovasc Surg 77:789–91, 1979

123. Zawada ET, Stinson JB, Done G: New perspectives on coronary artery disease in hemodialysis patients. South Med J 75:694–6, 1982

124. Hakim M, Wheeldon D, Bethune DW et al: Hemodialysis and hemofiltration on cardiopulmonary bypass. Thorax 40:101–6, 1985

125. Brenner BM, Lazarus JM: Chronic renal failure. p. 1150. In Wilson JD, Braunwald E, Isselbacher KJ et al (eds): Harrison's principles of internal medicine. McGraw-Hill, New York, 1991

126. Mannucci PM, Remuzzi G, Pusineri F et al: Deamino-8-D-arginine vasopressin shortens bleeding time in uremia. N Engl J Med 308: 8–12, 1983

127. Goldman S, Copeland J, Moritz T et al: Stastine aspirin therapy after operation. Effects on early grafts patency. Circulation 24:520–6, 1991

10

Coagulation Dysfunction After Cardiopulmonary Bypass

Bruce D. Spiess

BLEEDING AND TRANSFUSION BEHAVIOR

Hemorrhage after cardiopulmonary bypass (CPB) is a much feared complication. All patients have some chest tube drainage for at least the first 24 hours, but there is considerable variability in quantity and quality (i.e., hematocrit) of the drainage.[1-4] Such numbers are institution dependent because the protocols for bypass are different in each hospital. Each institution uses a different combination of CPB circuit, heparin and protamine protocol, oxygenator, filter and cannula system, and perfusion temperature. The length of CPB is also highly variable and is at least somewhat dependent on whether an institution has physicians in training. There is no doubt that the length of time on CPB is related to a number of postoperative complications.[5] Postoperative hemorrhage is an outcome variable common to most reports.

Abnormal or excessive postoperative bleeding is again somewhat hard to define, and each institution defines its own accept-

able limits. Unacceptable blood loss varies from anything greater than $100 \text{ ml} \cdot \text{h}^{-1}$ in any time period to patients requiring more than 10 units of blood. It is probably fair to say that approximately 20 percent of CPB cases will violate institutional "norms" with regard to chest tube output.

Three to 14 percent of all CPB patients are returned to the operating room for re-exploration of the mediastinum within the first 24 hours of surgery.[1] It is difficult to ascertain what percentage of these patients have true coagulopathic bleeding versus surgical hemorrhage. In a recent study of postoperative bleeding, thromboelastography (TEG) was used as the arbiter for surgical versus component therapy and resulted in a 50 percent reduction in the rate of reoperation.[6] It would seem reasonable to assume that at centers not using TEG, roughly 50 percent of bleeding cases may represent surgical and 50 percent coagulopathic events. The puzzle that remains is how to predict which patients are susceptible to excessive hemorrhage and how they can be most appropriately treated.

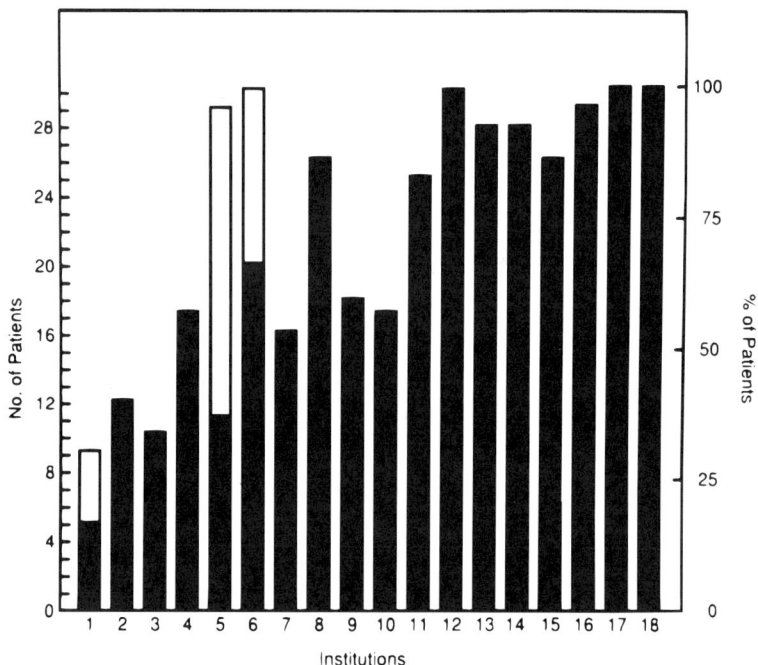

Fig. 10-1. Variability in red cell transfusion after CABG surgery at 18 major U.S. institutions. (From Goodnough et al.,[7] with permission.)

This chapter examines some of the causes of coagulopathy development, techniques to assess and treat these complications, as well as strategies for prophylaxis against excessive hemorrhage.

The immense variability in transfusion practice is the result of concern and anxiety regarding postoperative hemorrhage and an inability to do timely and accurate coagulopathic diagnosis.[7,8] Work from the late 1980s showed that the use of red blood cell products varied widely across some 18 major medical centers performing coronary artery bypass graft (CABG) surgery.[8] More variable was the use of fresh frozen plasma and platelet components. At some centers, less than 10 percent of patients received these components, whereas at other institutions more than 75 percent were transfused (Figs. 10-1 and 10-2). Recently almost 2,500 patients undergoing CABG at 24 institutions were analyzed for the occurrence of transfusion and hemorrhage events.[8] Although there have

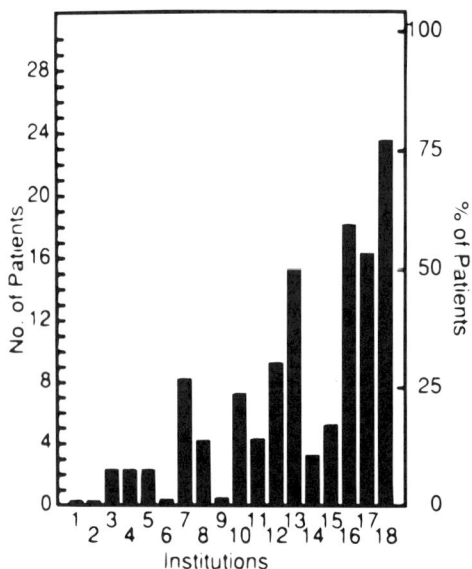

Fig. 10-2. Variability in platelet transfusion after CABG surgery at 18 major U.S. institutions. (From Goodnough et al.,[7] with permission.)

been some changes from the earlier data, the same variability is present, even though the lay public has exerted pressure on the medical community to reduce heterologous transfusions. Chest tube outputs in centers with the largest transfusion requirements versus those with the lowest was not different either in the earlier or the contemporary study.

CAUSES OF COAGULOPATHY

CPB creates changes that can lead to a complex sequence of events resulting in coagulopathic bleeding.[9-14] These changes include hemodilution of pro-coagulant proteins and platelets, drug effects of heparin and protamine, platelet activation, platelet inhibition, thrombin generation, fibrinolysis activation, and the effects of hypothermia. Many of these are discussed in detail in this section.

Hemodilution of proteins and platelets is an obligatory event with acellular priming of the CPB machine. Even if blood primes are used, and these may contain some plasma, the platelets will be diluted. The arithmetic computation of the effects of dilution predicts that a dilutional decrease of one-third occurs in the normal 70-kg adult. However, platelet stores, predominantly in the spleen and liver, can be released quickly in response to stress. Regardless, as soon as the CPB run is begun, platelet consumption begins. The dilution of proteins does occur, but the serine proteases (e.g., factors VII and IX) as nonconsumed enzymes are required in concentrations of only 25 to 30 percent of normal for adequate function.[15] This of course assumes all other factors are normal. The consumable coagulation proteins, fibrinogen, and factors V and VIII are again present in enough excess that the usual dilution with prime alone is rarely an independent cause of hemorrhage. Protein dysfunction as a sole cause of bleeding probably occurs in less than 5 percent of all patients undergoing CPB.[16] This explains why there is no difference in the chest tube output in institutions that use a great deal of fresh frozen plasma versus those that use very little.

Platelet changes during CPB are widely implicated as a common link to postoperative hemorrhagic dysfunction.[9-14] One can argue whether fibrinolysis or platelet abnormalities are the major problem, but activation of the fibrinolytic system does inhibit or, during hypothermia, activate platelets.

Following an injury, platelets are responsible for the initial closure of capillaries and vessels smaller than 30 to 50 μm. The competency of the platelet plug is of paramount importance in arresting the capillary ooze. The protein cascade, activated during normal coagulation, must interact with the phospholipid component of the activated platelet surface. Once the coagulation cascade is complete and the formation of fibrin final, the platelets bind with fibrinogen/fibrin strands at glycoprotein binding sites (GBIIb/IIIa).

Platelets undergo a series of changes following the initiation of CPB that may ultimately result in a later coagulopathic syndrome. The CPB circuit binds platelets and within 10 minutes of instituting extracorporeal circulation, up to 30 percent of platelets are bound. They probably bind due to an electromagnetic attraction between the plastic and platelet glycoproteins and phospholipids. As CPB time continues, more platelets interact with the artificial surface. Therefore, there is good evidence that the length of CPB is linearly related to the degree of platelet dysfunction. Once platelets bind to the artificial surface they are activated.

Although platelets can undergo graded activation during CPB, many become so activated that they disgorge the contents of their α- and dense granules.[17,18] These granules contain a number of vasoactive compounds and coagulation activators, including fibrinogen, thromboxane, serotonin, epinephrine, adenosine diphosphate (ADP), and thrombin, as well as others. What contribution the release of these compounds may have to a postoperative coagulation abnormality is unclear. Once these activated platelets undergo an active, adenosine triphosphate (ATP)-consuming phase change (associated with the contraction of active myosin), they can no longer participate in coagulation.

The surface of platelets is covered with binding sites for activators, inhibitors, and others (to other platelets, surfaces, glycoprotein Ib, von Willebrand binding site, fibrinogen/fibrin-glycoprotein IIb/IIIa). These latter glycoprotein binding sites may be damaged by the CPB system.[17–19] Recent work using platelet flow cytometry has shown that after CPB, the population of platelets with normal binding sites is greatly reduced and a substantial variability in reactivity ensues.[18] Other researchers using flow cytometry with different assay methods have concluded that the binding sites remain relatively intact but that there are substantial changes in the substrates available to those binding sites.[17]

Certainly this debate may go on for some time, but the practitioner can be certain that platelet surface interactions are abnormal even after short periods on CPB. However, the population of platelets within a given individual will show variation; some may be spared whereas others are greatly affected. Also, some patients demonstrate a more exaggerated response to CPB than others. Recent work in animal models with new agents that specifically bind and protect but do not activate these glycoprotein binding sites shows that coagulation function post-CPB is better preserved if they are used.[20]

Fibrinogen/fibrin has the ability to bind to six different platelet binding sites.[21] This is due to the repeat sequence of three key amino acids. It is possible for fibrin to bind to the same platelet or, conceivably, up to six different platelets. If the binding sites are partially destroyed during CPB, it would seem that overall clot integrity is degraded, as fewer interactions between fibrin and platelets take place.

FIBRINOLYSIS

The interaction between platelets and the fibrinolytic system has been mentioned. The reader should realize that, although the discussions are presented in a compartmentalized function, they are truly interactive. The fibrinolytic system is universally activated during CPB.[22,24] There is a rapid rise in tissue plasminogen activator (TPA) within minutes of commencing bypass.[24,25] Some definition of terms is required when discussing TPA.

TPA is released from the endothelium in response to a number of stimuli, including thrombin, complement, kallikrein, bradykinin, and activated factors XII and XI. TPA is inhibited in its action upon plasminogen (a plasma circulating zymogen manufactured by the liver) by another hepatically manufactured protein: plasminogen activator inhibitor-1 (PAI-1). TPA and PAI-1 bind and TPA becomes active in creating fibrinolysis only after it overwhelms circulating PAI-1.

Although TPA changes during CPB, it is very important to distinguish TPA antigen from TPA activity. TPA antigen rises throughout CPB and actually achieves its highest level immediately after the administration of protamine (usually at the conclusion of CPB).[25] However, TPA antigen is not what is important for the formation of the actual lytic state. PAI-1 decreases as TPA-PAI-1 complexes are formed following initiation of CPB and reaches very low levels during the first 30 minutes.[26] Following the decline in PAI-1 complexes and the surge in TPA, the highest TPA activity occurs in the first 10 minutes after the onset of CPB. Concomitantly, the greatest decline in platelet activity occurs and possibly the zenith in thrombin generation.[27]

Plasmin, the end product of the action of TPA on plasminogen, is a platelet inhibitor at normothermia.[12,28] However, below 30° to 32°C, plasmin actively changes and it becomes a platelet activator.[29] Unfortunately, the end result of platelet activation is that when rewarming occurs and the patient is separated from CPB, there will be fewer functional platelets available for normal coagulation. The biochemistry of the plasmin shift from platelet inhibitor to activator at these hypothermic temperatures is unclear.

One can speculate that plasmin acting on both fibrinogen and fibrin effects changes at the glycoprotein IIb/IIIa binding site. If fibrinogen or fibrin are bound to the platelet surface, they are rendered incapable of further reactivity by plasmin; however, that platelet binding site is now inactive. The decrease in circulating thrombin (which acts as activator) is also cited as a possible cause for the down-regulation of platelet activation.[17] It appears that plasmin itself does not destroy glycoprotein binding sites.

PAI-1 decreases within the first few minutes of commencing CPB.[25,26,30] However, it increases as CPB continues and surges to levels 50 to 100 times normal during the first 24 hours postoperatively.[26] Since PAI-1 rises during the late CPB period, even though TPA antigen may be rising the overall effect is that TPA activity is on the decline, even though it is still high in comparison to normal non-CPB levels.[26] TPA antigen and activity decline rapidly after the conclusion of CPB. This leaves PAI-1 as the dominant force in the fibrinolytic coagulation system.

PAI-1 is a very pro-thrombotic protein via its regulation of TPA activity.[31–34] By binding and inhibiting TPA it inhibits that enzyme to avoid "run-away" primary fibrinolysis. PAI-1 controls the early disaggregation of small platelet microaggregates. Platelets then adhere and form tighter bonds with the fibrin strands interlinking them. If TPA is allowed to proceed unchecked, these microaggregates are broken apart. PAI-1 therefore promotes platelet aggregation and early clot formation. It is found in elevated levels in a number of hypercoagulable or pro-thrombotic states, including unstable angina, acute myocardial infarction, deep venous thrombosis, pulmonary embolism, and pre-eclampsia/eclampsia.[33–36]

Postoperatively, in noncardiac surgery, PAI-1 surges as well, and in peripheral vascular surgery (a population of patients that are quite hypercoagulable) this PAI-1 surge is detrimental (an increase in graft thrombosis and myocardial infarction). Interestingly, this surge can be attenuated or prevented by the use of postoperative epidural pain therapy for 24 to 72 hours.[37]

Platelets are commonly located in close proximity to the highest concentrations of PAI-1. Those patients with the highest surge in PAI-1 had the longest myocardial ischemia times.[26] Some researchers have found that platelets adhere to vascular endothelium after aortic cross-clamp removal and depression of platelet adherence with dipyridamole and aspirin will decrease perioperative infarction.[38,39] Is the surge in PAI-1 after CPB a marker for, or the cause of, early coronary graft thrombosis, graft spasm, or myocardial infarction? That is a pertinent question that is not answerable at this writing.

The interaction of platelets, plasmin, TPA, and PAI-1 has been described. Most research represents data as means and standard deviations; however, what is important for the clinician in the operating room is how an individual patient will respond to the bypass stimulus. The changes in levels of fibrinolytic proteins are also highly variable. In one study of 38 patients there was a 100-fold variation in TPA activity and a 200-fold variation in PAI-1 levels.[26] Most importantly, the biochemical events causing release of these proteins do not appear to be linked. Indeed, the patients with the greatest increase in TPA are not associated with the greatest rise in PAI-1. Therefore, the stimulus for the production/release of these key proteins must be different. To date we do not know what modulates the level of release of either TPA or PAI-1.

HEPARIN AND PROTAMINE

Even if a CPB circuit with a completely biocompatible surface is created and tested, anticoagulation in some form is required as stasis of blood in any portion of the circuit during CPB would be disadvantageous. Heparin is the most widely used anticoagulant. It is a conglomerate of multiple mucopolysaccharides that have the potential to bind to the

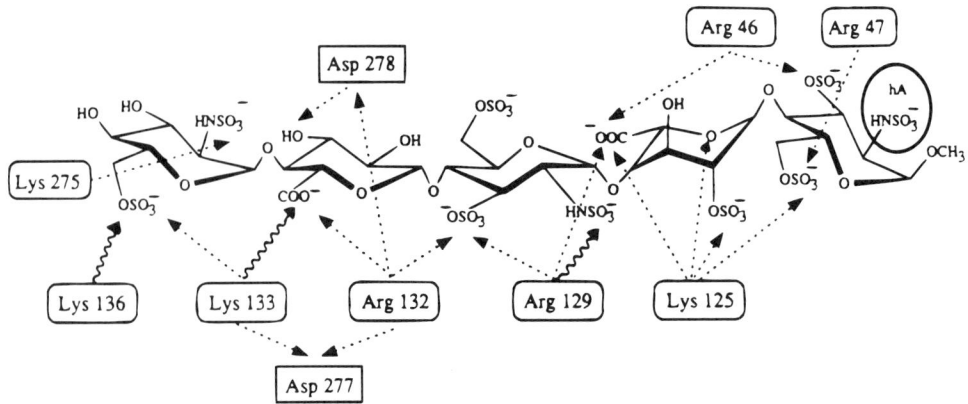

Fig. 10-3. Specific pentasaccharide sequence that binds heparin to antithrombin III. (From Grootenhuis and van Boeckel,[107] with permission.)

circulating anticoagulant protein, antithrombin III (ATIII).

The binding site of heparin is a well-known specific pentasaccharide sequence[40] (Fig. 10-3). It contains three glycosamine residues and two hexuronic acid units. With that sequence bound to ATIII, the protein/mucopolysaccharide complex acts as a key, unlocking a binding site on ATIII for thrombin. The capability of ATIII for inhibiting thrombin's action upon fibrinogen is enhanced 10,000-fold by binding with heparin.[41]

Thrombin is a key enzyme in overall coagulation and acts as an amplifier for many reactions, including platelet activation and fibrinolysis. It makes very good sense to decrease thrombin activity; however, even with very high levels of heparin administration, some thrombin activation does occur.[42] The reactions forming thrombin are never completely inhibited.[43]

Heparin has a number of actions other than as an anticoagulant, including actions on white blood cells and as an inhibitor of vascular muscularis growth.[44] The implications of these lesser investigated effects for individuals undergoing CPB are yet to be determined. Heparin protocols for anticoagulation during CPB are widely investigated and are summarized elsewhere.

At the conclusion of CPB, the high level of anticoagulation achieved with heparin must be quickly and effectively reversed. The expectation by many practitioners is that coagulation will immediately revert to a normal pre-CPB baseline. Of course, from the previous discussions regarding platelet and fibrinolytic changes during CPB, that is not possible, even for the shortest CPB run. Protamine sulfate, a polycationic histone protein, is administered to bind ionically to the anionic sites of heparin. These two compounds bind quickly and irreversibly, causing a precipitate (if done outside the bloodstream).

Removal of heparin-protamine complexes is carried out by the reticuloendothelial system. Protamine also causes wide-ranging disturbances, including hypotension due to histamine release, allergic reaction (IgG or IgE mediated), and rarely thromboxane-related cardiovascular and pulmonary collapse.[45] Once again, the management and causes of these protamine-mediated complications are widely publicized.

Are heparin or protamine ever the cause of postoperative coagulopathy? Heparin is reversed quite effectively by protamine; however, this means that heparin must be free in the plasma. Heparin is largely protein bound (in excess of 90 percent); thus, when protamine is administered, the protein-bound fraction will not ionically bind to protamine.[46]

Thankfully, the dissociation of heparin from its protein-bound fraction is quite slow and therefore, there is no sudden release, although heparin rebound is a possibility. Clinically, heparin rebound as the sole cause of excessive postoperative hemorrhage is rare.[47]

Unfortunately, the activated clotting time (ACT), which is the one test that clinicians associate with heparin administration, will not show the effects of this low-level release of heparin from the protein binding sites. The ACT uses either kaolin or cellite as a stimulator in such massive quantities that they will overcome very large doses of heparin (i.e., to increase the accuracy of the test during CPB). The ACT is not designed to be sensitive to the low-level or trace heparin effect, as the level of activation of the extrinsic cascade is too powerful.

The activated partial thromboplastin time (aPTT) is often used to follow moderate-dose heparin on the clinical ward, but after CPB it is usually elevated to 1.5 to 1.8 times normal.[48] The cause of that elevation is unclear, but some have suggested that the heparin-protamine complex interferes with the activator in the test. Perhaps the thrombin time would be the best test to assess trace amounts of heparin. Recent studies have shown, however, that when using routine amounts of heparin in patients with normal renal and hepatic function, heparin rebound is not a common cause of major postoperative bleeding.[49] The use of ACT titration (i.e., dose-response curves) of heparin followed by protamine dosing based on heparin activity will lead to lower dosages of protamine being administered than with empiric therapy. There appears to be no increase in bleeding from decreasing protamine dosages.[50]

Protamine was also studied as a cause of postoperative bleeding.[51–53] Protamine is known to be an in vitro anticoagulant. It possesses antithrombin properties and may competitively bind to the sites that ATIII would occupy.[53] Concentrations of 100 μM protamine decrease fibrin conversion from fibrin-ogen by up to 50 percent.[53] Protamine alone given to volunteers not undergoing CPB prolonged their Lee-White clotting time.[54] This is a nonstimulated whole blood test of the rate of clot formation. It would follow that a compound has a mild antithrombin effect if it shows mild prolongation of the time required for initiation of clot formation.

More impressive is the effect of the heparin-protamine complex on platelet number and perhaps function. In dogs, sheep, and humans after heparin administration, subsequent protamine administration will cause a rapid decrease in platelet count.[55–57] In sheep, which appear to be very sensitive to thromboxane-mediated events, the decrease can be as great as 90 percent within 3 to 5 minutes.[56,57] Indeed, sheep are used as a model for studying severe pulmonary vascular dysfunction after protamine administration.

In humans, an approximately 30 percent platelet drop occurs immediately after protamine administration.[55] This appears to be a transient effect, as the numbers begin to climb within 30 to 45 minutes and are normal by 2 hours. The biochemical reason for this effect is unknown; however, this author will conjecture a cause. If heparin interacts with the coagulation protein complex bound to the GpIIb/IIIa binding site (where fibrinogen, thrombin, and the macromolecular complex of factor Xa-calcium and factor VII are working), protamine is binding to and coating that site. It appears that the reticuloendothelial system actively removes platelets bound to heparin and protamine complexes. Other research would support the view that the platelets being removed from the circulation by this process are the platelets that had fairly normal active GpIIb/IIIa sites. Those are exactly the platelets that are required for normal coagulation function in the patient after CPB.

Does this supposition fit the clinical picture encountered daily in the operating rooms? Indeed it does. Shortly after protamine is administered, there is a rapid change in coagulation and the surgical field improves. Sometimes one can actually see gross clot formation; however, often within minutes, there is a recrudescence of oozing. Is the protamine-heparin complex interaction with platelet surface the cause of that effect? It seems quite possible. This effect may actually be largely responsible for the unique transfusion behavior encountered at the many institutions.

If a patient begins to ooze after the initial formation of clot, there is a natural tendency to try to fix the problem proactively. Hence, fresh frozen plasma and platelet concentrates are ordered from the blood bank. Some 45 minutes later (when these componenets arrive), the natural course of events is such that the platelet count is recovering from the effects of the heparin-protamine complex. If these components are administered, and the oozing improves, there is a reward established for the behavior pattern (ordering coagulation components).

Would time have simply been enough to handle the problem? It is impossible to ascertain clinically, as once a coagulopathy is established, the ongoing loss of precursors results in rapid deterioration. This author remains convinced that the effect of the heparin-protamine complex alone can cause significant and dangerous decreases in platelet number and probably function, although it should be noted that platelet number alone does not correlate well with postoperative bleeding.

These are sufficient reasons to view protamine as a potentially hazardous agent and to therefore limit its dosage. Although studies have shown that protamine is rapidly metabolized and that moderate increases in dosage are well tolerated, these studies have been done with the Lee-White clotting test. This test is relatively insensitive to the platelet effects previously discussed. Routine practice has been that heparin is administered to maintain an ACT above some arbitrarily determined number, such as 450 seconds, although there is no evidence to suggest this

is a "magical" level for CPB. Institutions then select their protamine dose based on either the heparin administered or the last ACT. If the protamine dose is based on total heparin administered and administered in a 1.3 to 1 ratio, it is likely to result in excesses of protamine (i.e., the generation of potential antithrombins). An in vitro ratio of 0.3–0.5 to 1 (protamine to heparin) is required to remove all traces of heparin activity.[54,58] Because of the side effects of protamine and its intrinsic capability to cause anticoagulation, a slow infusion with the dosage tailored to the patient's requirements appears best.

PROPHYLAXIS: DRUGS TO PREVENT BLEEDING

There is a temptation to try to find a single agent that, when administered prior to CPB, will prevent the problems of postoperative hemorrhage. As suggested above, however, the hemorrhagic complications and their etiologies are neither unifactorial nor easily solved. Therefore, it is far too simplistic and quite unrealistic to think that one drug will solve all the problems. However, a number of therapeutic options are available and are being employed to reduce these complications.

The first prophylactic maneuver to examine is the preoperative withdrawal of agents that may potentiate a coagulopathy after CPB. The literature brings extensive focus on aspirin and other prostanoid-affecting drugs (nonsteroidal anti-inflammatory drugs [NSAIDs]) that affect platelet function. Aspirin is a widely prescribed mild platelet inhibitor. Aspirin exerts its effects by poisoning the cyclo-oxgenase enzyme system during thrombopoiesis.[59] Platelets exposed to small amounts of aspirin during the megakarocyte production phase do not have the ability to produce thromboxane. This does not mean that they are nonfunctional. It only means that when stimulated (as they are by exogenous thromboxane, ADP, or thrombin), they are unable to participate in further platelet recruitment by releasing thromboxane.

A controversy exists as to the importance of the effect of aspirin on postoperative blood loss. A number of studies substantiate that aspirin ingestion preoperatively is associated with increased chest tube output and administration of coagulation components; unfortunately, most of these studies are not blinded.[60,61] Recent data from a very large database as well as other recent reports disagree and have shown little or no difference between those patients exposed to aspirin and those not so exposed.[62,63] Today, patients move rapidly from diagnosis to intervention with the mean time from catheterization to operation greatly reduced. As surgical delay to accommodate aspirin withdrawal is no longer an option, this entire controversy may be moot.

The list of other medications administered to patients undergoing CPB that cause platelet dysfunction includes calcium channel blockers, β-blockers, antibiotics, nitroprusside, nitroglycerin, and methylxanthines.[64] Inhibition of platelet function with cephalosporins appears to be very real, but is probably not related to thromboxane release.[65] The use of such agents at many institutions approaches 100 percent; however, concern for perioperative hemorrhage is never entertained. Although in theory, aspirin may be a platelet inhibitor, undue concern regarding the withdrawal of patients from aspirin is unlikely to result in clinical benefit.

D-8-Arginine vasopressin (DDAVP) is an analogue of vasopressin with fewer vasoreactive properties that has historically offered some promise in reducing perioperative blood loss.[66] In patients with demonstrated platelet dysfunction (e.g., renal failure) DDAVP increases platelet affinity.[67] In von Willebrand's disease and hemophilia A, DDAVP may be the treatment of choice.[68] It produces an increase in the release of von Willebrand's fraction of factor VIII from the endothelium. Therefore, in susceptible patients, bleeding times after its administration

are shortened. DDAVP is also effective in uremic and end-stage hepatic failure patients.[69]

Since the platelet dysfunction after CPB is pivotal to the cause of hemorrhage, it makes intuitive sense that administering an agent to improve platelet function may decrease postoperative hemorrhage. One widely publicized study performed largely in complex or reoperative cases showed a significant decrease in blood loss in patients treated with DDAVP.[66] Other investigators repeated these studies but used groups of patients at lower risk of bleeding and did not find the same significant reduction in hemorrhage.[70,71] However, one study with DDAVP administered in patients receiving aspirin did show a reduction in postoperative bleeding.[67] It was suggested that in those patients whose platelet dysfunction is unrelated to von Willebrand's factor, the endothelium is stimulated following CPB. Thus, adding an external stimulus with DDAVP does little to increase either the production or release. This suggests there is a subpopulation of people who can benefit from this drug.

A study was conducted to prospectively identify patients using TEG into groups with normal or abnormal platelet function.[72] Within these groups, patients were randomly allocated to receive either DDAVP or placebo in a double-blind fashion. In the group with normal platelet function, the effect of DDAVP was negligible and there was no difference in postoperative blood loss. However, in the group of patients with decreased platelet function, the administration of DDAVP after separation from CPB resulted in a significant decrease in postoperative blood loss (similar to those with normal platelet function). Conclusions drawn from this study are that there is a subpopulation that responds to DDAVP, that TEG is useful as a platelet function monitor, and that without prior identification of patients with platelet dysfunction, DDAVP offers no value. It makes little sense to administer DDAVP randomly to all patients undergoing CPB in the hope of finding this special population. Unfortunately, the study was not large enough to see if DDAVP administration could convert or prevent patients from becoming members of the subgroup with extensive hemorrhage.

The fibrinolytic system, as stated earlier, is both active and interactive with other causes of depressed platelet function during CPB. The rationale for seeking control of this activation seems intuitively obvious. Multiple pharmacologic agents are available to control the fibrinolytic process, including εamino-caproic acid (EACA), tranexamic acid (TA), and p-aminobenzoic acid (PABA). All these compounds are essentially analogues of the amino acid lysine. Lysine offers a very important binding site on a number of coagulation proteins. It is at lysine binding sites that plasmin binds to fibrinogen and fibrin, and it is also at lysine binding sites that plasminogen interacts with TPA. These lysine analogues competitively inhibit the binding of plasmin to fibrinogen and fibrin. To a lesser extent, they also decrease the conversion of plasminogen to plasmin. What they do to the production of TPA and its subsequent effects is less clear.

In the very early days of CPB, it was known that prophylactic administration of lysine analogues (EACA) decreased postoperative hemorrhage.[73] A number of largely retrospective or uncontrolled studies were published showing that bleeding was decreased. More recently, focus has been on the usage of TA, which is, milligram for milligram, at least 10 times as potent as EACA.[74] In multiple studies using routine CABG patients, there are good demonstrations that postoperative bleeding is reduced by approximately 33 percent.[74,75] Unfortunately, the manner in which these studies were conducted rarely translates into a significant reduction in blood transfusion.[74,75] If one studies patients at relatively low risk of large amounts of blood loss, it is not surprising that large differences in transfusion are not forthcoming. The effect of using lysine analogues in a high-risk group of patients remains unanswered. Nor do we know a great deal about the effects of these drugs on TPA, PAI-1, complement, and the other mediators of the inflammatory reaction to CPB.

Aprotinin is also a fibrinolytic inhibitor, but it is not a lysine analogue. It is a 58-amino acid bovine lung protein with multiple effects. It was originally intended as a drug to reduce pulmonary injury from CPB. The dosage of aprotinin was calculated to inhibit kallikrein production. During this early work on pulmonary injury, it was noted that postoperative bleeding was markedly reduced.[76] Therefore, clinical trials examining the relationship of aprotinin administration to postoperative hemorrhage were undertaken. Like the lysine analogue drugs, aprotinin was effective. In every trial to date, aprotinin has decreased bleeding in amounts ranging from 30 percent to 88 percent.[76–80] These reductions, unlike the lysine analogue work, do translate into similar reductions in blood or component usage.

The mechanism of action of aprotinin has been extensively investigated. TPA production is completely inhibited with the pre-CPB administration of 2,000,000 kallikrein inhibiting units (KIU), followed by an infusion of $1,000,000 \text{ KIU} \cdot \text{h}^{-1}$.[80] Serum urokinase activity, an agent similar to TPA, is also effectively inhibited. PAI-1 surges during CPB, as there is no TPA-PAI-1 complex formed resulting in the clearance of PAI-1.[80] It is unclear whether there is a higher than normal surge of PAI-1 after CPB if aprotinin is used than in normal subjects. There are no data regarding the extreme variability in fibrinolysis seen in the routine population.

Platelet function is better preserved in patients who receive aprotinin.[78] Perhaps glycoprotein binding sites are well preserved; certainly, electron micrographic studies have shown better preservation of the intracellular granules with aprotinin pretreatment. Aprotinin was originally targeted to suppress some of the inflammatory responses to CPB. There are data suggesting that both complement and white blood cell activation are decreased as well.

Why should not every patient receive such a drug? At certain centers outside the United States, that indeed happens. In Europe and Canada, aprotinin is not as expensive as it is in the United States. In our increasingly cost-conscious medical world, monetary considerations play a major role. EACA and TA are considerably less expensive. A comparison between the two agents was carried out in France albeit in a relatively small number of patients.[81] Unfortunately, most of the patients were undergoing routine CABG surgery and therefore not at high risk of perioperative bleeding or transfusion. As expected, there was no significant difference in bleeding between those given EACA and aprotinin.

Another recent but retrospective study of chest tube output and transfusion requirements in patients undergoing reoperative CABG, combined CABG and valve replacement, thoracic aortic aneurysm repair, or multiple valve replacements did show significant differences.[82] The groups analyzed were patients who had undergone these procedures in the 6 months prior to and after the approval of aprotinin by the FDA. The dose of aprotinin used was the one-half Hammersmith dose consisting of 1,000,000 KIU as a loading dose followed by an infusion of 500,000 KIU per hour. Also, 1,000,000 KIU is added to the CPB pump prime. The mean hemorrhage in EACA patients was approximately 1,600 ml for the first 24 hours, whereas that seen with aprotinin was 900 ml. Furthermore, the length of time in the operating room after completion of CPB was 34 minutes shorter in the aprotinin group than in the EACA group.

All medications have side effects and the agents mentioned above are no different. DDAVP can cause significant hypotension and vasodilation.[83] EACA and TA appear to have the fewest potential adverse events, although significant adverse events were never investigated. Furthermore, these drugs have not undergone the scrutiny of an FDA series of trials. Aprotinin has been very heavily scrutinized. It is a bovine protein (a recombinant DNA-produced product is in development) and therefore carries some risk of anaphylaxis. The size and type of this protein are similar to those of protamine, so one might expect roughly similar rates of reaction to administration. If aprotinin is administered to large populations of first-time CABG patients, many of whom will require reoperation, the risk of anaphylaxis will increase. Aprotinin can cause transient renal dysfunction with elevation of the creatinine and blood urea nitrogen. But most controversial has been a worry that aprotinin may increase the risk of myocardial ischemia (MI). Claims of no increase in the rate of MI with EACA and TA are based on absence of evidence not evidence of absence.

If coagulation is better preserved, and platelets in conjunction with low-flow characteristics are responsible for either early graft thrombosis, it is theoretically possible for aprotinin to increase the rate of MI. The first human trial of aprotinin in the United States bolstered this concern, as there was a trend toward more MIs in the group receiving aprotinin.[84] At autopsy, the number of grafts thrombosed in the aprotinin group was higher than in the control group; however, no denominator was given by which to adequately judge those data. The small number of autopsy patients also added to the inconclusiveness of the data.[84]

An animal study performed in swine was published with regard to the problem of hypercoagulation and aprotinin.[85] In this animal model, the femoral arteries were injured with a clamp to simulate endothelial damage. Animals were given either aprotinin or saline as a placebo, and vessels were inspected for patency and histology. The group that received aprotinin had more thromboses than those that received saline. Unfortunately, this work has little implication for CPB, as the animals neither underwent CPB nor received heparin. One would expect these results to occur in normal animals. If antifibrinolytic agents are administered in the presence of significant endothelial damage, platelet aggregation and thrombosis are enhanced. Further human work in this area does not support the increased risk of thrombosis following CPB.

At the Munich Heart Center (which has the world's largest experience with aprotinin), more than 1,784 patients received aprotinin with no increase in MI rate, length of stay in the intensive care unit (ICU), or hospital or mortality.[86] Many of these patients also underwent recatheterization after recovery from CABG surgery, which showed no increase in the rate of graft thrombosis.[87] In similar assessments of graft patency with either ultrafast magnetic resonance imaging (MRI) or contrast computed tomography (CT), the incidence of patent grafts is equal in groups that did and did not receive aprotinin.

A recently completed Food and Drug Administration (FDA) phase III study on 287 patients at six major academic centers also focused on the possibility of an increased risk of MI.[88] Three different dosages of aprotinin were administered and compared to placebo in a randomized and double-blind fashion. The medications administered were aprotinin at full Hammersmith, one-half Hammersmith, pump prime only (1,000,000 KIU only) dosages, or normal saline. Blood loss and transfusion requirements were significantly lower in the Hammersmith and one-half Hammersmith groups. MI was determined by a blinded, third-party cardiologist's reading of electrocardiography (ECG) and independently blinded laboratory CPK measurements. The rate of MI was 8 percent across all groups. Substantial evidence shows that aprotinin does not unduly increase the risk of MI. Nonetheless, there will certainly be forthcoming case reports in the literature stating that a patient died, secondary to a graft thrombosis and aprotinin administration.

BIOCOMPATIBLE SURFACES

The platelet and fibrinolytic abnormalities previously described are due to the blood's reactions to the artificial surfaces of the CPB circuit and oxygenator. Recently, covalently bonded heparin circuits have become available for both research and clinical use.[89,90] The endothelial surface of all blood vessels is coated with a complex mixture of proteins, eicosanoids, glycosaminoglycans, and heparin. Heparin coating of a bypass circuit cannot hope to mimic completely all the actions of a biologically interactive cell layer. However, there is some encouraging work in animals showing that prolonged CPB can be carried out without systemic administration of heparin. Using these systems, there appears to be less activation of complement than with routine CPB, and platelet number and presumably function are also better preserved.[90,91] In humans, this heparin-coated surface, when combined with full systemic heparinization, totally inhibits the production TPA during CPB (Spiess BD: unpublished data). Some early reports noted that postoperative blood loss is not decreased in those patients in whom a heparin-coated surface was used. However, this study did not coat the oxygenator with heparin.[92] Much more work is required before any conclusions can be drawn, but it would make sense that a reduction in TPA production is associated with a decrease in the incidence of coagulopathy.

MONITORING

The monitoring of coagulation following CPB is different from coagulation monitoring in operative situations. A number of laboratory tests are affected by the process of CPB; therefore, "normal ranges" are not established. In particular, the prothrombin time (PT) and aPTT are elevated after CPB by at least 1.5 to 1.8 times normal. It is not known how long that elevation persists and whether it occurs in all or only certain patients. Perhaps it is those patients with the greatest changes in TPA levels or heparin-protamine interaction that have the greatest artificial elevation in PT and aPTT.

The ACT is used to ensure reversal of heparin's anticoagulation with protamine. However, even a normal ACT level does not ensure that all heparin effect was reversed. The ACT overstimulates the intrinsic system such that trace amounts of heparin cannot be detected. The ACT after the patient is weaned from CPB should actually be lower than the baseline ACT if that baseline is drawn prior to sternotomy. The explanation for this phenomenon is probably related to the release of tissue thromboplastin during surgery that enhances coagulation; however, the ACT is very insensitive to these low levels of tissue thromboplastin.

The inability to return the ACT to baseline following an appropriate dose of protamine is often a problem. Commonly, extra protamine is administered; however, if the ACT either stays the same or becomes prolonged there are other problems. Further administration of protamine will exacerbate the problem, as excess protamine functions as an antithrombin agent. If either after or during CPB the ACT is greater than or equal to 999, either extreme levels of heparinization have been given or a more complex coagulopathy has occurred. Our experience has shown that the latter most often represents a platelet deficiency, either thrombocytopenia itself or a severe platelet dysfunction. Finally, following protamine administration of the ACT, complete normalization is of little use in predicting postoperative hemorrhage.

During the postoperative period, the coagulation profile, including the PT, aPTT, thromboplastin time (TT), fibrin-split products (FSPs), fibrinogen, and platelet count, may be of some value.[1,48,93–95] Although each of the individual coagulation profile tests or the entire profile together are quite inaccurate in predicting postoperative hemorrhage. With regard to sensitivity and specificity profiles, the platelet count has the best profile but it is still inaccurate.[93] FSPs are nearly universally elevated. Although one might expect patients with the highest rate of fibrinolysis and production of FSPs to be associated with the highest incidence of hemorrhage, this is not the case.[22–24] The level of FSPs is dependent on several factors, including the amount of TPA stimulation, available plasmin and antiplasmin, fibrinogen level, and the hepatic clearance of FSPs. There have been no studies demonstrating that there is a direct relationship between the concentration of FSP and chest tube output.

Since platelet function is an important contributor to abnormal bleeding, one would anticipate the bleeding time to be predictive of excessive hemorrhage. In recent reviews of the literature regarding the use of the bleeding time, the conclusions are uniform. The bleeding time has no predictive value in defining patients at risk of hemorrhage either following general or cardiovascular surgery.[96] Studies focusing only on patients who had undergone CPB are also unimpressive with regard to the predictive power of the bleeding time.[97]

The bleeding time is dependent on skin tissue turgor, blood flow, skin temperature, vascular vasoreactivity, and multiple other factors. Immediately after CPB, all these factors are abnormal. Following CPB, most patients are hypothermic, with resultant redistribution of their cutaneous blood flow. Many patients are receiving vasoactive drips and have significant extracellular edema. The test for bleeding time requires trained personnel and is very observer dependent. Although it is possible to demonstrate changes in the bleeding time in a controlled situation, this is insufficient justification for its use in assessing platelet function following CPB.

The foregoing factors make the diagnosis of platelet dysfunction a diagnosis of exclusion. The coagulation profile, if used systematically, will achieve this purpose. A recently developed and tested algorithm for diagnosis and treatment based on the coagulation profile noted a significant reduction in transfusion[48,98] (Fig. 10-4). This algorithm diagnoses platelet dysfunction by the systemic application of the various tests in the coagulation profile.

With the advent of bedside PT and aPTT testing, data acquisition is quite rapid. A test

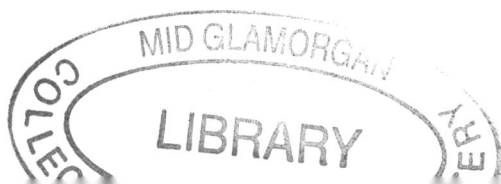

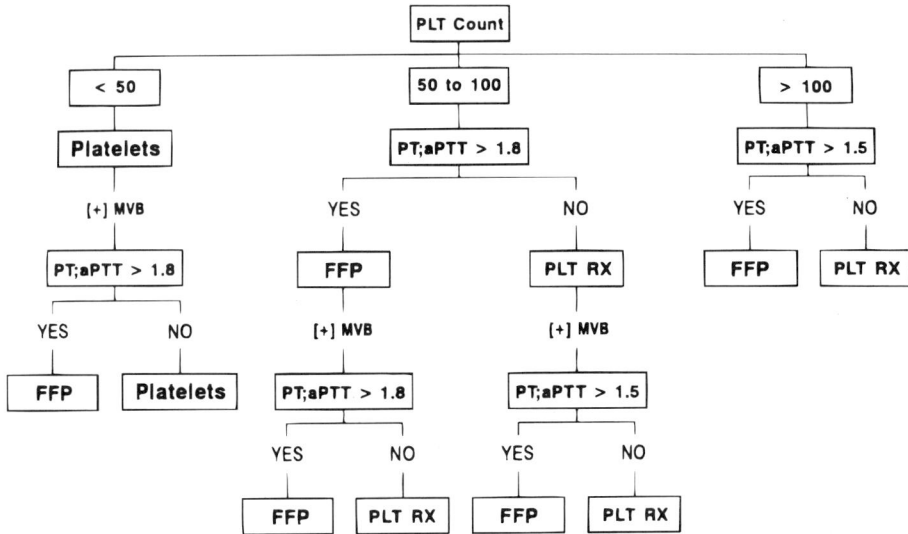

Fig. 10-4. Algorithm for treating coagulopathies using the coagulation profile. Note that platelet function abnormalities are proven by a process of elimination. (From Despotis et al.,[1] with permission.)

that offers the immediate availability of fibrinogen concentrations is undergoing testing at this time. Unfortunately, a rapid platelet assay remains beyond the ken of the operating room. While platelet counts greater than $50,000 \ ml^{-1}$ are sufficiently accurate on commercially available counter systems, below that number accurate counts are done by hand counting. This is a time-consuming practice and if $50,000 \ ml^{-1}$ is the clinical limit for platelet transfusion, attempts to determine platelet counts below this level provide excessive accuracy.

Whole blood clot testing of viscoelastic parameters has recently gained popularity for both hepatic transplantation and CPB.[93–95,99,100] Two types of tests are available: the TEG and the Sonoclot. The TEG is dealt with in some detail because there is more research available with that instrument. The Sonoclot is a viscometer that uses whole blood maintained at 37°C to assess clot integrity.[101] A vertically vibrating plastic probe is suspended in a small crucible of whole blood, and the impedance to vibration is traced on paper over time. Blood viscosity changes as clot formation proceeds, and a relationship

exists between viscosity function and platelet-fibrinogen interaction. Clinical work has shown that the Sonoclot is a better predictor of major hemorrhage than routine coagulation profile testing, although less so than the TEG. Unfortunately, the inflection points of the Sonoclot test are not well defined, and therefore quantitative research is very difficult.

The TEG is a measure of clot strength (not viscosity) over time.[102] Intuitively, it would seem that if major changes in clot strength occur, those patients with lower clot strength would be more susceptible to bleeding than those with normal clot strength. The TEG measures clot strength by adding whole blood to a warmed cuvette into which a suspended piston is placed. That piston rotates in a 4.5-degree arc with a 1-second pause at the end of each rotation. As a clot forms between the wall of the cuvette and the suspended piston, the elastic shear modulus (clot strength) is measured. A paper tracing of this interaction is produced at a constant speed ($2 \ mm \cdot min^{-1}$). The amplitude of the paper tracing at any time is the shear modulus, and the amount of pen deflection (in mm) can be related to the physical force of deformation by the following equation:

$$G = \frac{100 \times A}{100 - A}$$

where A is the amplitude and G is shear modulus in dynes $\cdot$ cm^{-2}. The maximum amplitude (MA) of the TEG is the point of maximum clot strength.

The TEG measurement, in whole blood, is dependent on the interaction of platelets, fibrinogen, and fibrin. It is also probably dependent on the amount of cross-linking of fibrin within the clot matrix as well. Recent work from patients not undergoing CPB has shown that a mathematical model of the MA can be constructed if the fibrinogen concentration and platelet count are known. Such a mathematical model has shown that both factors are important but that platelets are probably weighted twice as heavily in the effect as compared to fibrinogen.

TEG testing in CPB is the best predictor of abnormal postoperative chest tube output.[93–95] In work from the late 1980s using a binary decision system (TEG was either normal or abnormal, and bleeding was normal or abnormal), the TEG had a greater than 80 percent predictive accuracy for abnormal bleeding.[94,95] Routine coagulation profile testing, either in its entirety or by individual tests, was less than 50 percent accurate. The TEG had an approximately 20 percent false-positive test rate (i.e., the test determined that coagulation was normal, yet patients bled) and no false-negative results.

A recent study specifically examining the issue of sensitivity and specificity has shown that TEG has the best overall sensitivity and specificity rating for predicting abnormal hemorrhage. Sensitivity was 71.4 percent and specificity 89.3 percent.[93] Of interest, and in stark contrast to others, this study did show that the bleeding time had a reasonable sensitivity and specificity grouping.[93] Platelet count, although 100 percent sensitive, was only about 50 percent specific. The other routine coagulation profile tests were very poorly

represented in their combination of sensitivity and specificity.

Other researchers, when examining both adult and pediatric patients who had undergone CPB, have shown that the TEG is capable of predicting abnormal hemorrhage.[93–95,103] Only one study stands in contradiction.[100] That study attempted to create a linear correlation between individual TEG parameters and chest tube output. One would not expect a close correlation because the MA is a linear representation of a nonlinear function (shear elasticity). While there is a population of patients who have markedly abnormal TEG-MA values associated with postoperative hemmorhage, that relationship is not linear. There is, however, a cutoff for clot strength (or MA) below which bleeding becomes truly excessive. This study did not control coagulation therapy that occurred continuously from the time of TEG measurement until the assessment of 24-hour total chest tube output. Nonetheless, the platelet count and the TEG-MA offered the closest correlations with abnormal hemorrhage.[100] Wang and colleagues also noted that the TEG, when normal, always separated those patients with surgical bleeding from those without.

All reports agree that the TEG is very effective for separating surgical from coagulopathic bleeding. In the previous article examining sensitivity and specificity, the TEG was found to have a 92.3 percent negative predictive value.[93] That means that if the TEG was normal (i.e., a negative test) and the patient was bleeding, a surgical cause would be found (92.3 percent of cases).[100] The bleeding patient either in the operating room or the intensive care unit always presents the physicians with a tough decision. Is the bleeding coagulopathic or is it surgical? The TEG provides a single test that can be used with greater than 90 percent confidence to judge whether the bleeding requires reopening the chest or treating it with drugs and coagulation components.

Recent research with the TEG has shown that when performed during full heparinization the results obtained are similar to those following the administration of protamine.[104] Either heparinase or a small amount of protamine is added to the blood sample in vitro to allow TEG testing following removal of the aortic cross-clamp.[104,105]

Using this strategy, an algorithm (similar to the one devised based on the coagulation profile) was devised for the TEG (Fig. 10-5). This algorithm uses the platelet count, fibrinogen concentration, and the TEG. If the platelet count is below 50,000 ml, platelet concen-

trates are transfused after protamine administration. If the fibrinogen is below 100 mg · dl^{-1} cryoprecipitate is administered. If the platelet and fibrinogen levels are above target levels, TEG is used to examine the level of platelet dysfunction.

Prior work has shown that TEG-MA levels below 35 mm are associated with an increased propensity for hemorrhage, and therefore platelets are administered. Also, prior work with DDAVP and TEG has shown it to be effective below 45 mm MA. Thus,

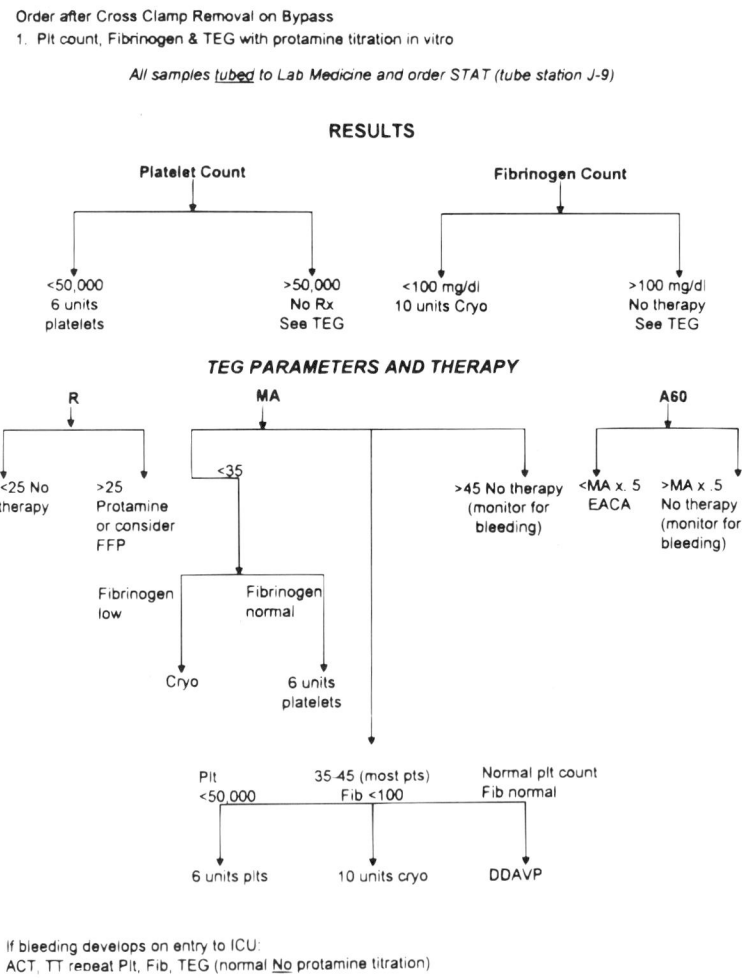

Order after Cross Clamp Removal on Bypass
1. Plt count, Fibrinogen & TEG with protamine titration in vitro

All samples tubed to Lab Medicine and order STAT (tube station J-9)

RESULTS

Platelet Count

<50,000
6 units
platelets

>50,000
No Rx
See TEG

Fibrinogen Count

<100 mg/dl
10 units Cryo

>100 mg/dl
No therapy
See TEG

TEG PARAMETERS AND THERAPY

R

<25 No
therapy

>25
Protamine
or consider
FFP

MA

<35

Fibrinogen
low

Fibrinogen
normal

Cryo

6 units
platelets

>45 No therapy
(monitor for
bleeding)

A60

<MA x .5
EACA

>MA x .5
No therapy
(monitor for
bleeding)

Plt
<50,000

35-45 (most pts)
Fib <100

Normal plt count
Fib normal

6 units plts

10 units cryo

DDAVP

If bleeding develops on entry to ICU:
ACT, TT repeat Plt, Fib, TEG (normal No protamine titration)

Fig. 10-5. Treatment algorithm for coagulopathies after cardiopulmonary bypass based on platelet count, fibrinogen concentration, and thromboelastography. Note that platelet dysfunction is identified by thromboelastography.

35 to 45 mm MA, DDAVP is administered.[72] Above 45 mm, there is no medical risk for hemorrhage and if the patient is bleeding then surgical causes are suspected and remedied.

Data acquired from patients undergoing reoperative CABG procedures who received aprotinin before and during CABG had better preservation of their TEG than did those patients receiving a placebo (saline). No test is consistently able to predict the risk of perioperative hemorrhage when performed in the preoperative period. Data acquired from patients undergoing valve replacement assessed by TEG showed that patients entering the operation with abnormal TEG values had a higher risk of bleeding than did those with normal values. A "hemorrhage index" of risk is not available, but future work may help further the discriminatory ability of the TEG.

PEDIATRICS

Hemorrhage after CPB in the pediatric age group is especially worrisome. The smaller chest cavity means that the total volume into which blood collects is considerably less than in adults. More importantly, the congenital abnormalities for which patients seek surgical therapy are such that the margin for error is very small. Those patients in whom the surgical repair requires the creation of an atrial baffle or those with hypokinetic and distended right ventricles will not tolerate extrinsic compression of these key structures. In this group of patients in particular, tamponade can be an early catastrophic event from which there is literally no recovery.

Dilutional coagulopathies are a much greater problem as the body surface area gets smaller. Red cell pump primes are often used, and in some cases whole blood may be available. There are good data to suggest that fresh, warm whole blood is very effective in this group for decreasing postoperative hemorrhage.[106] In a study of 161 infants and children, each subject received one of three types of therapy. Group I had transfusion requirements met after surgery with whole blood collected within 6 hours of infusion. Group II had whole blood collected for transfusion within 24 to 48 hours of infusion. Group III had packed red cells, fresh frozen plasma, and platelets given as individual components. Blood loss was followed for 24 hours, and a number of coagulation tests were performed, including bleeding time, platelet count, PT, aPTT fibrinogen, fibrin degradation products, von Willebrand factor level, and platelet aggregation response to ADP, epinephrine, ristocetin, and collagen. The blood loss of the groups was presented (in $ml \cdot kg^{-1}$) and was 50.9 (9.3) for group I, 44.8 (6.0) group II, and 74.2 (8.9) group III.

The data were further segregated into children under 2 years of age and those undergoing complex surgery. In some of these subgroupings the differences became quite profound. The coagulation tests revealed abnormal platelet responses in the group that received component therapy. The overall conclusion was that in children under 2 years of age expected to undergo complex cardiac repair, there is a significant benefit to the use of fresh whole blood. Not every center has the capability to deliver fresh whole blood 24 hours per day, but it is something that should be considered in advance.

Patients with right heart failure may have hepatic dysfunction and splenomegaly. Children with cyanotic heart disease are expected to exhibit enhanced fibrinolytic activity. It is unclear whether this is a low-grade, chronic, diffuse intravascular coagulation (DIC) or represents up-regulation of plasmin activators.

The effects of profound hypothermia and circulatory arrest on fibrinolytic activity are poorly described. Hypothermia depresses both serine protease functions as well as platelet function. Earlier work in animal models documented a decrease in platelet count with profound hypothermia. The suggestion was that platelets were sequestered in the spleen. All these defects should be reversible upon rewarming, yet patients subjected to profound hypothermia are more hypocoagulable than those undergoing the identical operation at normothermia. A secondary issue is that cyanotic children are more ill prior to the operation. Their pre-existing morbid state exacerbates the potential for coagulopathy following CPB.

APPROACH TO THE BLEEDING PATIENT

When confronted with the patient who is bleeding after CPB, it is important to evaluate the problem in a systematic manner. As is generally true in medicine, history is the most important consideration. A patient who is oozing immediately after being weaned from bypass presents a completely different problem than the patient who begins to bleed several hours after a previously normal recovery.

The quantity and quality of the blood being lost are important. A quiet postoperative period broken with a sudden increase in chest tube output suggests a surgical cause. If the blood is bright red in color, the possibility of an arterial source is very high. The presence of clotted blood in the chest tubes also supports the diagnosis of surgical bleeding.

Normally, blood from the chest tube has undergone fibrinolysis; thus, it should not clot. If blood clots in the chest tubes, it is either being shed faster than the rate of coagulation or the mediastinum is already filled with clot. Finally, if the blood is clotting, it should also stop all small vessel "ooze."

If the hemodynamic state suggests the presence of tamponade, a return to the operating room or immediate opening of the chest in the intensive care unit is lifesaving. Generally, patients with profound coagulopathy do not experience tamponade, as their coagulation function is insufficient to form clot in the mediastinum.

Transport from the ICU to the operating room is a serious event. Movement of critically ill patients with vasoactive drips, endotracheal tubes, and intra-aortic balloon pumps or other hardware is a logistical prob-

lem. Morbidity and mortality occur from alterations in the infusion rates of vasoactive compounds or inadvertant extubation. The risk of infection and probably the risk of peripheral neuropathy is increased every time the sternum is opened. Therefore, it makes great sense to use all the monitoring possible to avoid returning to the operating room. The TEG is very helpful in making that decision. In its absence, a platelet count, fibrinogen, and TT is a reasonable battery of tests. If this battery of tests is normal and one is still suspicious of a coagulopathy, platelet dysfunction should be suspected and treated. Prophylactic transfusion of components does not decrease chest tube output in any published series. Postoperative intervention with antifibrinolytics is far less effective than prophylactic usage, but it does little harm. DDAVP, if administered without appropriate indications, is not effective.

Unfortunately, the fear of worsened bleeding or persistent hemorrhage is so great that patients often receive multiple therapies. If the bleeding ceases, the clinician does not know what improved the condition. The technique of giving everything possible is more common than not, but it has never been investigated for negative impacts. Potential negative impacts include an increase in thrombosis rate and MI (hypercoagulability), an increase in acute infection rate (immunosuppressive effects of blood transfusion), and the potential for viral transmission by the use of allogeneic blood products (see Ch. 11).

One consideration that is rapidly causing widespread concern is cost. Blood products are very costly and if prophylactic transfusion therapy is not efficacious, it only increases the hospital bill. Perhaps prophylactic therapy will cease to be used when capitated payment schemes become the norm and the cost of transfusion is deducted directly from the physician's fee.

REFERENCES

1. Despotis GJ, Santoro SA, Spitznagel E et al: Prospective evaluation and clinical utility of on-site monitoring of coagulation in patients

undergoing cardiac operation. J Thorac Cardiovasc Surg 107:271, 1994

2. Jobes DR, Nicholson SC, Steven JM: Inhibition and restoration of hemostasis in the young cardiac surgical patient. Cardiol Young 3:370, 1993

3. Hardy JF, Perrault J, Tremblay N et al: The stratification of cardiac surgical procedures according to use of blood products: a retrospective analysis of 1480 cases. Can J Anaesth 38:511, 1991

4. Verska JJ, Lonser ER, Brewer LA III: Predisposing factors and management of hemorrhage following open heart surgery. J Cardiovasc Surg 13:361, 1972

5. Harker LA: Bleeding after cardiopulmonary bypass. N Engl J Med 314:1446, 1986

6. Spiess BD, Gillies BSA, Chandler W, Verrier E: Changes in transfusion therapy and reexploration rate after institution of a blood management program in cardiac surgical patients. J Cardiothorac Vasc Anesth 9:168, 1995

7. Goodnough LT, Johnston MF, Toy PT et al: The variability of transfusion practice in coronary artery bypass surgery. Transfusion Medicine Academic Award Group. JAMA 265:86, 1991

8. Stover EP, Siegel LC, Parks R et al: Variability in transfusion practice for coronary artery bypass surgery persists despite national consensus guidelines. McSPI Research Group. Anesthesiology 81:A1224, 1994

9. Bick RL: Hemostasis defects associated with cardiac surgery, prosthetic devices, and other extracorporeal circuits. Semin Thromb Hemost 11:249, 1985

10. Holloway DS, Summaria L, Sandesara J et al: Decreased platelet number and function and increased fibrinolysis contribute to postoperative bleeding in cardiopulmonary bypass patients. Thromb Haemost 59:62, 1988

11. Mammen EF, Koets MH, Washington BC et al: Hemostasis changes during cardiopulmonary bypass surgery. Semin Thromb Hemost 11:281, 1985

12. Khuri SF, Wolfe JA, Josa M et al: Hematologic changes during and after cardiopulmonary bypass and their relationship to bleeding time and nonsurgical blood loss. J Thorac Cardiovasc Surg 104:94, 1992

13. Páramo JA, Rifóu J, Llorens R et al: Intra- and

postoperative fibrinolysis in patients undergoing cardiopulmonary bypass surgery. Haemostasis 21:58, 1991

14. Harker LA, Malpass TW, Branson HE et al: Mechanisms of abnormal bleeding in patients undergoing cardiopulmonary bypass: acquired transient platelet dysfunction associated with selective α-granule release. Blood 56:824, 1980

15. Spiess BD: Perioperative coagulation concerns: function, monitoring and therapy. p. 4:1. In Barash PG, Cullen BF, Stoelting RK (eds): Clinical Anesthesia Updates. JB Lippincott, Philadelphia, 1993

16. Spiess BD, Tuman KJ, McCarthy R et al: Thromboelastographic diagnosis of coagulopathies in patients undergoing cardiopulmonary bypass. Anesth Analg 68:S273, 1989

17. Kestin AS, Valeri CR, Khuri SF et al: The platelet function defect of cardiopulmonary bypass. Blood 82:107, 1993

18. Rinder CS, Mathew JP, Rinder HM et al: Modulation of platelet surface adhesion receptors during cardiopulmonary bypass. Anesthesiology 75:563, 1991

19. Rinder CS, Bohnert J, Rinder HM et al: Platelet activation and aggregation during cardiopulmonary bypass. Anesthesiology 75:388, 1991

20. Uthoff K, Zehr KJ, Geerling R et al: Inhibition of platelet adhesion during cardiopulmonary bypass reduces postoperative bleeding. Circulation 90:II-269, 1994

21. Nichols AJ, Ruffolo RR Jr, Huffman WF et al: Development of GP IIb/IIIa antagonists as antithrombotic drugs. TIPS 13:413, 1992

22. Kucuk O, Kwaan HC, Frederickson J et al: Increased fibrinolytic activity in patients undergoing cardiopulmonary bypass operation. Am J Hematol 23:223, 1986

23. VanderSalm TJ, Ansell JE, Okike ON et al: The role of epsilon-aminocaproic acid in reducing bleeding after cardiac operation: A double-blind randomized study. J Thorac Cardiovasc Surg 95:538, 1988

24. Stibbe J, Kluft C, Brommer EJ: Enhanced fibrinolytic activity during cardiopulmonary bypass in open heart surgery in man is caused by extrinsic (tissue-type) plasminogen activator. Eur J Clin Invest 14:375, 1984

25. Tanaka K, Takao M, Yaka I et al: Alterations in coagulation and fibrinolysis associated

with cardiopulmonary bypass during open heart surgery. J Cardiothorac Anesth 3:181, 1989

26. Chandler WL, Fitch JCK, Wall MH et al: Individual variations in the fibrinolytic response during and after cardiopulmonary bypass. Thromb Haemost (submitted) 1995

27. Teufelsbauer H, Proidl S, Havel M et al: Early activation of hemostasis during cardiopulmonary bypass: evidence for thrombin mediated hyperfibrinolysis. Thromb Haemost 68:250, 1992

28. Gouin I, Lecompte T, Morel MC: In-vitro effect of plasmin on human platelet function in plasma. Inhibition of aggregation caused by fibrinogenolysis. Circulation 85:935, 1992

29. Kowalski E, Kopec M, Wegrzynowicz Z: Influence of fibrinogen degradation products (FDP) on platelet aggregation, adhesiveness, and viscous metamorphosis. Thromb Haemost 10:406, 1963

30. van Oeveren W, Jansen NJ, Bidstrup BP et al: Effects of aprotinin on hemostatic mechanisms during cardiopulmonary bypass. Ann Thorac Surg 44:640, 1987

31. Cortellaro M, Cofrancesco E, Boschetti C et al: Increased fibrin turnover and high PAI-1 activity as predictors of ischemic events in atherosclerotic patients. Arterioscler Thromb 13:1412, 1993

32. Margaglione M, DiMinno G, Grandone E et al: Abnormally high circulation levels of tissue plasminogen activator and plasminogen activator inhibitor-1 in patients with a history of ischemic stroke. Arterioscler Thromb 14: 1741, 1994

33. Hamsten A, Walldius G, Szamosi A et al: Plasminogen activator inhibitor in plasma: risk factor for recurrent myocardial infarction. Lancet 2:3, 1987

34. Risberg B: Fibrinolysis and trauma. p. 149. In Sawaya R (ed): Fibrinolysis and the Central Nervous System. Hanley and Belfus, Philadelphia, 1990

35. Kluft C, Verheijen JH, Jie AF et al: The postoperative fibrinolytic shutdown: A rapidly reverting acute phase pattern for the fast-acting inhibitor of tissue type plasminogen activator after trauma. Scand J Clin Lab Invest 45:605, 1985

36. Sautter RD, Myers WO, Ray JF III, Wenzel FJ: Relationship of the fibrinolytic system to postoperative thrombotic phenomena. Arch Surg 107:292, 1973

37. Rosenfeld BA, Beattie C, Christopherson R et al: The effects of different anesthetic regimens on fibrinolysis and the development of postoperative arterial thrombosis. Anesthesiology 79:435, 1993

38. Feinberg H, Rosenbaum DS, Levitsky S et al: Platelet deposition after surgically induced myocardial ischemia: an etiologic factor for reperfusion injury. J Thorac Cardiovasc Surg 84:815, 1982

39. Chesebro JH, Clements IP, Fuster V et al: A platelet-inhibitor-drug trial in coronary-artery bypass operations: benefit of perioperative dipyridamole and aspirin therapy on early postoperative vein-graft patency. N Engl J Med 307:73, 1982

40. Choay J, Lormeau JC, Petitou M et al: Structural studies on a biologically active hexasaccharide obtained from heparin. Ann NY Acad Sci 370:644, 1981

41. Hemker HC, Beguin S: Mode of action of heparin and related drugs. Semin Thromb Hemost, suppl. 17:29, 1991

42. Okajima Y, Kanayama S, Maeda Y et al: Studies on the neutralizing mechanisms of antithrombin activity of heparin by protamine. Thromb Res 24:21, 1981

43. Wagner WR, Johnson PC, Thompson KA, Marrone GC: Heparin-coated cardiopulmonary bypass circuits: hemostatic alterations and postoperative blood loss. Ann Thorac Surg 58:734, 1994

44. Frebelius S, Hedin U, Swedenborg J: Thrombogenicity of the injured vessel wall—role of antithrombin and heparin. Thromb Haemost 71:147, 1994

45. Horrow JC: Protamine: A necessary evil. p. 15. In Ellison N, Jobes DR (eds): Effective Hemostasis in Cardiac Surgery. WB Saunders, Philadelphia, 1988

46. Mahadoo J, Heibert L, Jaques LB: Vascular sequestration of heparin. Thromb Res 12:79, 1978

47. Ellison N, Beatty CP, Blake DR et al: Heparin rebound. Studies in patients and volunteers. J Thorac Cardiovasc Surg 67:723, 1974

48. Despotis GJ, Grishaber JE, Goodnough LT: The effect of an intraoperative treatment algorithm on physicians' transfusion practice in cardiac surgery. Transfusion 34:290, 1994

49. Gravlee GP, Rogers AT, Dudas LM et al: Heparin management protocol for cardiopulmonary bypass influences postoperative heparin rebound but not bleeding. Anesthesiology 76:393, 1992

50. Wright SJ, Murray WB, Hampton WA, Hargovan H: Calculating the protamine-heparin reversal ratio: A pilot study investigating a new method. J Cardiothorac Vasc Anesth 7:416, 1993

51. Kresowik TF, Wakefield TW, Fessler RD II, Stanley JC: Anticoagulant effects of protamine sulfate in a canine model. J Surg Res 45:8, 1988

52. Dutton DA, Hothersall AP, McLaren AD et al: Protamine titration after cardiopulmonary bypass. Anaesthesia 38:264, 1983

53. Cobel-Geard RJ, Hassouna HI: Interaction of protamine sulfate with thrombin. Am J Hematol 14:227, 1983

54. Ellison N, Ominsky AJ, Wollman H: Is protamine a clinically important anticoagulant? Anesthesiology 35:621, 1971

55. Heyns A, Lotter MG, Badenhorst PN et al: Kinetics and in-vivo redistribution of III Indium-labelled human platelets after intravenous protamine sulphate. Thromb Hemost 44:65, 1980

56. Morel DR, Zapol WM, Thomas SJ et al: C5a and thromboxane generation associated with pulmonary vaso- and broncho-constriction during protamine reversal of heparin. Anesthesiology 66:597, 1987

57. Morel DR, Costabella PM, Pittet J-F: Adverse cardiopulmonary effects and increased plasma thromboxane concentrations following the neutralization of heparin with protamine in awake sheep are infusion rate-dependent. Anesthesiology 73:415, 1990

58. Glass DD: Plasma heparin activity and antagonism during cardiopulmonary bypass with hypothermia. Anesth Analg 56:569, 1977

59. Roth GJ, Siok CJ: Acetylation of the NH_2-terminal serine prostaglandin synthetase by aspirin. J Biol Chem 253:3782, 1978

60. Ferraris VA, Ferraris SP, Lough FC, Berry WR: Preoperative aspirin ingestion increases operative blood loss after coronary artery bypass grafting. Ann Thorac Surg 45:71, 1988

61. Bashein G, Nessly ML, Rice AL et al: Preoperative aspirin therapy and reoperation for bleeding after coronary artery bypass surgery. Arch Intern Med 151:89, 1991

62. Karwande SV, Weksler BB, Gay WA, Subramanian VA: Effect of preoperative antiplatelet drugs on vascular prostacyclin systhesis. Ann Thorac Surg 43:318, 1987

63. Taggart DP, Siddiqui A, Wheatley DJ: Low-dose preoperative aspirin therapy, postoperative blood loss, and transfusion requirements. Ann Thorac Surg 50:424, 1990

64. Campbell FW, Addonizio VP: Platelet function alterations during cardiac surgery. p. 85. In Ellison N, Jobes DR (eds): Effective Hemostasis in Cardiac Surgery. WB Saunders, Philadelphia, 1988

65. Baeuerle JJ, Mongan PD, Hosking MP: An assessment of the duration of cephapirin-induced coagulation abnormalities as measured by thromboelastography. J Cardiothorac Vasc Anesth 7:422, 1993

66. Salzman EW, Weinstein MJ, Weintraub RM et al: Treatment with desmopressin acetate to reduce blood loss after cardiac surgery. N Engl J Med 314:1402, 1968

67. Dilthey G, Dietrich W, Spannagl M, Richter JA: Influence of desmopressin acetate on homologous blood requirements in cardiac surgical patients pretreated with aspirin. J Cardiothorac Vasc Anesth 7:425, 1993

68. Kobrinsky NL, Israels ED, Gerrard JM et al: Shortening of bleeding time by 1-desamino-8-D-arginine vasopressin in various bleeding disorders. Lancet 1:1145, 1984

69. Mannucci PM, Remuzzi G, Pusineri F et al: Desamino-8-D-arginine vasopressin shortens the bleeding time in uremia. N Engl J Med 308:8, 1983

70. Sarraccino S, Adler E, Gibbons PA et al: DDAVP does not decrease post bypass bleeding in acyanotic children. Anesthesiology 70:A1057, 1989

71. Hackmann T, Gascoyne RD, Naiman SC et al: A trial of desmopressin (1-desamino-8-d-arginine vasopressin) to reduce blood loss in uncomplicated surgery. N Engl J Med 321:1437, 1989

72. Mongan PD, Hosking MP: The role of desmopressin acetate in patients undergoing coronary artery bypass surgery. A controlled trial with the thromboelastographic risk stratification. Anesthesiology 77:38, 1992

73. Sterns LP, Lillehei CW: Effect of epsilon

aminocaproic acid to reduce bleeding during cardiac bypass in children with congenital heart disease. Anesthesiology 40:604, 1974

74. Horrow JC, Hlavacek J, Strong MD et al: Prophylactic tranexamic acid decreases bleeding after cardiac operations. J Thorac Cardiovasc Surg 99:70, 1990

75. Horrow JC, Van Riper DF, Strong MD et al: The dose-response relationship of tranexamic acid. Anesthesiology 82:383, 1995

76. Royston D, Bidstrup B, Taylor KM et al: Effect of aprotinin on need for blood transfusion after repeat open heart surgery. Lancet 2:1289, 1987

77. Dietrich W, Barankay A, Dilthey G et al: Reduction of homologous blood requirements in cardiac surgery by intraoperative aprotinin application—clinical experience in 152 cardiac surgical patients. J Thorac Cardiovasc Surg 37:92, 1989

78. van Oeveren W, Harder MP, Roozendaal KJ et al: Aprotinin protects platelets against the initial effect of cardiopulmonary bypass. J Thorac Cardiovasc Surg 99:788, 1990

79. Royston D: High dose aprotinin therapy: the first five years' experience. J Cardiothorac Vasc Anesth 6:76, 1992

80. Van Oeveren W, Jansen NJ, Bidstrup BP et al: Effects of aprotinin on hemostatic mechanisms during cardiopulmonary bypass. Ann Thorac Surg 44:640, 1987

81. Trinh-Duc P, Wintrebert P, Boulfroy D et al: Comparison des effects de l'acide E-aminocaproique et de l'aprotinine sur le saignement per et post-opératoire en chirurgie cardiaque. Ann Chir 46:677, 1992

82. VanNorman G, Lu J, Spiess BD et al: Aprotinin vs aminocaproic acid in moderate-to-high risk cardiac surgery: relative efficacy and costs, abstract. Anesth Analg 80(suppl. 1):19, 1995

83. Salmenperä M, Kuitunen A, Hynynen M, Heinonen J: Hemodynamic responses to desmopressin acetate after CABG: a double-blind trial. J Cardiothorac Vasc Anesth 5:146, 1991

84. Cosgrove DM, Heric B, Lytle BW et al: Aprotinin therapy for reoperative myocardial revascularization: a placebo-controlled study. Ann Thorac Surg 54:1031, 1992

85. Samama CM, Mazoyer E, Bruneval P et al: Aprotinin could promote arterial thrombosis in pigs: A prospective randomized, blind study. Thromb Haemost 71:663, 1994

86. Dietrich W, Barankay A, Hähnel C, Richter JA: High-dose aprotinin in cardiac surgery: three years' experience in 1,784 patients. J Cardiothorac Vasc Anesth 6:324, 1992

87. Bidstrup BP, Underwood SR, Sapsford RN: Effect of aprotinin (Trasylol) on aortocoronary bypass graft patency. J Thorac Cardiovasc Surg 105:147, 1993

88. Levy JH, Pifarre R, Schaff HV et al: A multicenter, double-blind, placebo-controlled trial of aprotinin for reducing blood loss and the requirement of donor blood transfusion in patients undergoing repeat coronary artery bypass grafting. Circulation 92:2236, 1995

89. Von Segesser LK, Weiss BM, Turina MI: Perfusion with heparin-coated equipment: potential for clinical use. Semin Thorac Cardiovasc Surg 2:373, 1990

90. Nilsson L, Storm KE, Thelin S et al: Heparin-coated equipment reduces complement activation during cardiopulmonary bypass in the pig. Artif Organs 14:46, 1990

91. Videm V, Svennevig JL, Fosse E et al: Reduced complement activation with heparin-coated oxygenator and tubings in coronary bypass operations. J Thorac Cardiovasc Surg 103:806 1992

92. Wagner WR, Johnson PC, Thompson KA, Marrone GC: Heparin-coated cardiopulmonary bypass circuits: hemostatic alterations and postoperative blood loss. Ann Thorac Surg 58:734, 1994

93. Essell JH, Martin TJ, Salinas J et al: Comparison of thromboelastography to bleeding time and standard coagulation tests in patients after cardiopulmonary bypass. J Cardiothorac Vasc Anesth 7:410, 1993

94. Spiess BD, Tuman KJ, McCarthy RJ et al: Thromboelastography as an indicator of post cardiopulmonary bypass coagulopathies. J Clin Monit 3:25, 1987

95. Tuman KJ, Spiess BD, McCarthy RJ et al: Comparison of viscoelastic measures of coagulation after cardiopulmonary bypass. Anesth Analg 69:69, 1989

96. Rodgers RP, Levin J: A critical reappraisal of the bleeding time. Semin Thromb Hemost 16:1, 1990

97. Gluszko PR, Maring JK, Edmunds LH Jr:

Bleeding time test. J Thorac Cardiovasc Surg 101:173, 1991

98. Goodnough LT, Johnston MF, Ramsey G et al: Guidelines for transfusion support in patients undergoing coronary artery bypass grafting. Ann Thorac Surg 50:675, 1990

99. Kang YG, Martin DJ, Marquez J et al: Intraoperative changes in blood coagulation and thromboelastographic monitoring in liver transplantation. Anesth Analg 64:888, 1985

100. Wang JS, Lin CY, Hung WT et al: Thromboelastogram fails to predict postoperative hemorrhage in cardiac patients. Ann Thorac Surg 53:435, 1992

101. Saleem A, Blifeld C, Saleh SA et al: Viscoelastographic measurement of clot formation: a new test of platelet function. Ann Clin Lab Sci 13:115, 1983

102. Hartert H: Blutgerinnungstudieu wit der thromboelastographic, eineru neuen untersuchingsverfahren. Klin Wochenschr 16:257, 1948

103. Martin P, Horkay F, Rajah SM et al: Monitoring of coagulation status using thromboelastography during paediatric open heart surgery. Int J Clin Monit Comput 8:183, 1991

104. Spiess BD, Wall M, Gillies BS et al: A comparison of thromboelastography with heparinase or protamine sulfate added in-vitro during heparinized cardiopulmonary bypass: and subsequent development of an algorithm for coagulation treatment. Anesth Anal (submitted) 1995

105. Tuman KJ, McCarthy RJ, Djuric M et al: Evaluation of coagulation during cardiopulmonary bypass with a heparinase-modified thromboelastographic assay. J Cardiothorac Vasc Anesth 8:144, 1994

106. Manno CS, Hedberg KW, Kim HC et al: Comparison of the hemostatic effects of fresh whole blood, stored whole blood, and components after open heart surgery in children. Blood 77:930, 1991

107. Grootenhuis PDJ, van Boeckel CAA: Constructing a molecular model of the interaction between antithrombin III and a potent heporin analogue. J Am Chem Soc 113:2743–7, 1991

11

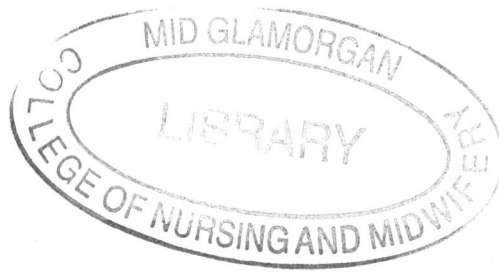

Infectious Disease

Dominique Farge
Catherine Amrein

Cardiac surgery is noncontaminated clean surgery and belongs to category I of the Altemeier classification (Table 11-1). However, patients in the early postoperative period are highly susceptible to infection, which will affect both early and late morbidity and mortality. Several risk factors contribute to infection: the patient's medical condition, the use of multiple invasive devices (indwelling catheters, chest tubes, and intubation), the immunologic consequences of cardiopulmonary bypass, and risk of infection from blood transfusions. In addition, in heart and heart-lung transplant recipients, for whom infection is the first cause of death in the early postoperative period, immunosupressive therapy enhances these risk factors.

Whatever the cardiac surgical procedure, all types of nosocomial infections can be observed during the early postoperative period. The most frequently observed are respiratory infections, septicemia, operative site infections, and urinary tract infections. Antibiotic prophylaxis reduces the risk of infection, but the specific guidelines for prevention vary according to a particular intensive care unit's (ICU) bacterial ecology and surgical team. Early diagnosis of nosocomial infections can

be difficult despite appropriate patient monitoring. Nevertheless, prompt effective therapy is mandatory to reduce subsequent morbidity, especially in transplant recipients.

A particular type of early postoperative infection is related to blood transfusions. Although their clinical manifestations are often delayed, their consequences may be severe. Bacterial infections are rare, while viral infections, despite careful screening of transfused blood products, are still a major threat. The best preventive measure is to rely on an autologous blood donation program and to avoid the transfusion of heterologous blood products.

NOSOCOMIAL INFECTIONS

Despite strict prevention and careful follow-up evaluation, nosocomial infections are still observed in 8 to 14 percent of patients after cardiac surgery with cardiopulmonary bypass (CPB).[1,2] They increase the hospital stay and cost of care and impair postoperative outcome and prognosis.

The bacterial inoculum responsible for nosocomial infections is either endogenous (skin, chest wall, or lower limbs) or exoge-

199

Table 11-1. Classification of Operative Wounds in Relation to Contamination and Increasing Risk of Infection

Clean
    Elective, primarily closed, and undrained
    Nontraumatic, uninfected
    No inflammation encountered
    No break in aseptic technique
    Respiratory, alimentary, genitourinary, or oropharyngeal tracts not entered

Clean-contaminated
    Alimentary, respiratory, or genitourinary tracts entered under controlled conditions and without unusual contamination
    Appendectomy
    Oropharynx entered
    Vagina entered
    Genitourinary tract entered in absence of culture-positive urine
    Biliary tract entered in absence of infected bile
    Minor break in technique
    Mechanical drainage

Contaminated
    Open, fresh traumatic wounds
    Gross spillage from gastrointestinal tract
    Entrance of genitourinary or biliary tracts in presence of infected urine or bile
    Major break in technique
    Incisions in which acute nonpurulent inflammation is present

Dirty and infected
    Traumatic wound with retained devitalized tissue, foreign bodies, fecal contamination, or delayed treatment, or from a dirty source
    Perforated viscus encountered
    Acute bacterial inflammation with pus encountered during operation

(From Altemeier et al.,[84] with permission.)

nous (contamination from the operating room). The two largest composite risk factors for nosocomial infections include patient demographics and surgical procedures.

An example of a patient demographic risk factor is tobacco consumption and/or chronic obstructive pulmonary disease (COPD). Either of these factors increases the risk of nosocomial pneumonia. In addition to CPB,[3] cachexia, malnutrition, and severe heart failure all contribute to decreased immune function. An example of the influence of surgical procedures is the use of bilateral internal mammary artery grafts. The risk of mediastinitis is increased in all patients and is considered a relative contraindication in diabetic patients. Infection is also enhanced by perioperative bleeding, since early reintervention may be necessary and coagulum is an excellent medium for bacterial growth. Prolonged use of invasive monitoring, as well as placement of intra-aortic balloon counterpulsation or other mechanical circulatory support devices significantly increase the risk of infection (see Ch. 17).

In the early postoperative period, daily investigation for possible infected sites is mandatory. Clinical examination includes inspection of surgical wounds, catheter insertion sites, drainage from chest tubes, as well as urinary analysis, body temperature, chest radiographs, and white blood cell (WBC) count. Suspicion of septicemia necessitates a minimum of four to six blood cultures with added bacteriologic examinations performed systematically or in accordance with the clinical context.

Diagnosis of infection can be difficult. There is a poor correlation between fever and infection during the early postoperative period[4]; sepsis can also manifest with hypothermia. Hyperpyrexia may be related to the administration of blood products or to drug-induced immunoallergic reactions. However, antibiotic-related fever is exceptional and can only be diagnosed after ruling out all other causes. Leukocytosis is common in the early postoperative period. Only sustained leukocytosis deserves attention, but severe sepsis can also induce leukopenia. Monitoring C-reactive protein levels is a good indicator of ongoing infection. Typically, these proteins remain elevated in the postoperative period or undergo further elevation if a clinical infection is present. Chest radiographic analysis is often difficult due to the lower quality when performed at bedside in the ICU. Moreover, both cardiogenic edema and post-bypass pulmonary lesions induce a diffuse interstitial pulmonary infiltrate that may be mistaken for infection.

The site of infection is difficult to determine when clinical symptoms are misleading, such as with lymphangitis or surgical wound erythema unrelated to fever. An infectious etiology is a high probability when weaning from ventilatory support or cardiotonic drugs becomes impossible. Altered liver function tests and cholestasis can be explained by low cardiac output, hemolysis, infection, or a combination of all three. Other investigations, such as an abdominal ultrasound, thoracic, and/or abdominal computed tomography (CT) scan and sinus radiographs or a cranial CT scan, offer great diagnostic value. A Doppler ultrasound examination allows detection of infected thrombophlebitis. In the absence of fever or chills, septic shock, while in the hypodynamic phase, is difficult to distinguish from cardiogenic shock.

Early treatment requires empiric antibiotic therapy at first, which is then subjugated to the cultured pathogens. Careful monitoring of serum antibiotic levels is necessary to adjust dosing in the presence of hepatic or renal dysfunction (especially true with aminoglycosides and vancomycin). The measurement of antibiotic levels in wound drainage or bronchial secretions is also helpful. Efficacy of treatment is assessed by negative blood cultures or bacteriologic specimens, defeverscence, and hemodynamic improvement. Sustained clinical symptoms or positive cultures despite antibiotic therapy is due to either antibiotic underdosage, resistance to therapy, or an unsuspected pathogen.

Prevention of nosocomial infections starts in the operating room with strict asepsis while placing indwelling arterial, venous, and urinary catheters. Asepsis must be maintained throughout the surgical procedure and thereafter in the ICU for dressing changes, endotracheal aspirations, and catheter manipulations. The number of invasive devices should be limited and should be removed as early as possible. Hand washing by medical and paramedical staff members is fundamental (and in our opinion is always

insufficiently practiced). This low-cost procedure is highly efficient in preventing nosocomial infections,[5] and sinks must be available at the bedside.[6] These simple hygenic rules must include stethoscopes and electrocardiographic (ECG) pads, as they are recognized vectors for nosocomial outbreaks with multiresistant bacteria.[7] Nursing workload also correlates with the incidence of nosocomial infections, especially pneumonia. ICU architecture must accommodate the isolation of infected patients.

Various Types of Nosocomial Infection

Nonspecific nosocomial infections similar to those observed in any medical or surgical ICU may appear after cardiac surgery. Pneumonia, septicemia, catheter-related sepsis, or urinary infections occur commonly, with the exact incidence dependent on the ICU. Nosocomial infections specific to cardiac surgery appear at the site of sternotomy or on the lower limbs (saphenous graft). Superficial wound infections are the most common. Sternitis, mediastinitis, and/or endocarditis are rare at this stage.

NONSPECIFIC NOSOCOMIAL INFECTIONS

Bronchopneumonia
Nosocomial pneumonia occurs in 4 to 5.6 percent of cardiac surgical patients in the early postoperative period.[1] The incidence is lower after cardiac surgery compared to the medical ICUs, primarily because patients are rapidly extubated, usually within 24 hours of the surgical procedure. However, these infections are severe with a 10 to 50 percent mortality, depending on the patient's pre-existing medical state. Gram-negative bacilli are the most frequent pathogens with two species, Enterobacteriaceae and *Pseudomonas aeruginosa,* observed in 50 to 70 percent of cases. *Staphylococcus aureus* is also frequent (20 to 50 percent) and multibacterial infections may be present.

Most often, the responsible pathogen comes from the patient's endogenous flora, but they can also be transmitted by hospital staff members. Antimicrobial prophylaxis, intubation, and surgery all contribute to the rapid alteration of the normal endogenous oropharyngeal flora and favor colonization with gram-negative bacilli.[8] Alkalinization of the gastric pH by H_2-histamine antagonists[9] or transient postoperative ileus favors gastric colonization by gram-negative bacilli. The pathogenesis of nosocomial pneumonia is intimately associated with micro- or macroaspiration of oropharyngeal and gastric contents.

Diagnosis of nosocomial pneumonia is often difficult. Purulent secretions are frequent after prolonged intubation; pulmonary infiltrates can be due to cardiogenic pulmonary edema or to adult respiratory distress syndrome (ARDS). Clinical pathologic studies have demonstrated that the classic criteria, such as fever, leukocytosis, purulent bronchial secretions, and radiologic infiltrates, are observed in the absence of pneumonia. The diagnostic value of microbiologic procedures is difficult to assess. Simple tracheal aspirations do not allow differentiation between colonization and infection. The use of protected specimen brush (PSB) combined with bronchoalveolar lavage (BAL) via fiberoptic bronchoscopy offers good diagnostic value, with respective bacterial significance at 10^3 CFU/ml for PSB and 10^5 CFU $\cdot$ ml^{-1} for BAL. However, PSB can induce hemoptysis and/or pneumothorax and is dangerous in patients with coagulation abnormalities. Adverse effects of BAL are well known: blood-gas alterations, fever, and sepsislike systemic symptoms. Blind bronchial sampling obtained by protected mini-bronchoalveolar lavage was recently shown to have a good diagnostic value.[8,10,11] Bacteriologic sampling via fine-needle or surgical biopsy specimens has a low specific diagnostic value and carries significant risk.

Antibiotic therapy with rapid bactericidal activity and good bronchopulmonary diffusion should be directed against gram-nega-tive bacilli and *Staphylococcus* because multi-resistant pathogens, such as *Serratia, Pseudomonas,* and *Acinetobacter,* are often encountered. The first-line antibiotic should be a β-lactam, such as ureidopenicillin, or a third-generation cephalosporin (ceftriaxone, ceftazidime) or imipenem, plus aminoglycosides or fluoroquinolones. The addition of β-lactamase inhibitors can be useful against hospital-acquired pathogens. Vancomycin is used against methicillin-resistant staphylococci, unless oxacillin is effective. Synergistic bitherapy is preferred to monotherapy, since it has a larger antimicrobial spectrum and prevents the emergence of resistant strains.[8,12] Aerosol or endotracheal administration of antibiotics (colimycin, aminoglycosides), while still controversial, can be used in addition to systemic therapy. Treatment should be no less than 15 days and may be maintained for longer periods in cases of associated septicemia.

Nosocomial bronchopneumonia can be prevented by the use of endotracheal tubes with low pressure and large volume cuffs, which lower bacterial microaspiration. Endotracheal and oropharyngeal sample aspirations should be performed as atraumatically as possible with observation of strict asepsis. Ventilator circuits must be changed every 48 hours when a heated humidifier is used, or less frequently if an antimicrobial filter is in use. The use of sucralfate, rather than H_2-histamine antagonists, for the prophylaxis of a stress ulcer induces less gastric bacterial colonization and is associated with a lower incidence of nosocomial pneumonia.[9] Benefit from selective digestive tract decontamination remains controversial.[13]

Urinary Infections

The incidence of urinary infections varies from 1.6 to 6.9 percent[1] according to the duration of bladder catheterization. Uropathogenic gram-negative bacilli are the most frequently encountered pathogens (*Escherichia coli, Proteus,* and *P. aeruginosa*). Enterococci are also frequently observed. Outbreaks due to multiresistant pathogens with prior colonization of the digestive tract (e.g., *Klebsiella pneumoniae* with an extended-spectrum β-lactamase) can also be observed. *Candida* spp. can be responsible for urinary tract infections in patients with prolonged bladder catheterization or on multiple antibiotic regimens. Urinary tract infection is diagnosed in patients with urinary catheters when leukocyturia is above 20 to 25 leukocytes · mm^{-2}. Bacteriuria without leukocyturia reveals urinary tract colonization but does not confirm the presence of infection. Associated bacteremia, pyelonephritis, or prostatitis are diagnosed by clinical examination, blood cultures, and a prostatic ultrasound examination if necessary. Antibiotic therapy is maintained for 7 to 10 days in females and for a longer period in males to avoid the risk of a partially treated prostatitis.

For simple urinary tract infections, directed monotherapy is sufficient. Quinolones have the advantage of good tissue diffusion, especially within the prostate. Bitherapy, including the use of an aminoglycoside initially, is mandatory in septicemia from urinary tract origin, or prostatitis. Therapy should continue for at least 21 days. Aminoglycosides are highly beneficial due to their rapid bactericidal activity and renal excretion.

Asymptomatic bacteriuria need not be treated. The single exception to this maxim occurs when the urinary catheter is changed while the patient is on antibiotics. Prevention of urinary infections relies first and foremost on asepsis, and secondarily on decreasing the duration of bladder catheterization. The use of a continuous system between the bladder catheter and the collecting bag is beneficial.

Vascular Catheter Infection,
Bacteriemia, and Septicemia
Bacteriemia and septicemia occur with an incidence of 1 to 3 percent.[1] Infections from indwelling vascular catheters must be differentiated from septicemia resulting from hematogenous bacterial seeding.

The incidence of vascular catheter-related sepsis, especially from Swan-Ganz catheters, following cardiac surgery is low, as most catheters are left in place for short time periods. Peripheral intravenous catheters rarely induce systemic infections. There are three potential sources[14] for catheter colonization and catheter-related sepsis: (1) skin and cutaneous flora at the site of insertion; (2) contamination of the catheter hub by handling; and (3) hematogenous seeding of the catheter from a distant focus (e.g., lung, gastrointestinal, or urinary tract). This pathophysiology explains the observed pathogens. Staphylococci, especially those that are coagulase negative, are the most frequent organisms isolated. Gram-negative bacilli, such as Enterobacteriaceae (*Klebsiella* spp., *Enterobacter* spp., *E. coli*), are acquired within the hospital environment. The incidence of *Acinetobacter* spp. is increasing.[15] These bacteria are often phage infected with the so-called "extended-spectrum" β-lactamases that result in resistance to multiple antibiotics. Infections due to *Candida* spp. are encountered rarely in the early postoperative period.

Catheter-related septicemia is diagnosed only after all other sources of infection are eliminated (i.e., pneumonia, wound, or urinary tract infections). Systemic infection is commonly caused by organisms native to the skin flora of patients with vascular catheters. It is suggested by the presence of a local (catheter exit-site) infection with the same organism as in the blood cultures. Cultures must be performed both on peripheral blood and on the catheter tip. Catheter-related sepsis is present when blood cultures via the catheter demonstrate at least a 10-fold increase above the colony count of peripheral blood.[14,16] The diagnosis is retrospectively confirmed by a colony count after catheter removal, using either the Maki semiquantitative technique (with a positive level at 15 colony forming units [CFU]) or the more sensitive Cleri quantitative technique (with a positive level at 10^3 organisms · ml^{-1}).

Both antibiotic therapy and catheter removal are mandatory for the treatment of catheter-related septicemia; otherwise, there is major risk of relapse, as manifested by an increase in mortality or endocarditis despite antibiotic therapy.[15] Within 48 hours of treatment, fever and sepsis should disappear, and blood cultures should become negative. Antibiotic therapy is continued for 7 to 10 days and for up to 15 days when *S. aureus* is the responsible pathogen. Despite effective treatment, endocarditis or septic thrombophlebitis may develop. Prolonged therapy is required and additional surgical procedures may be necessary to eradicate the infectious source.

Results of preventive measures against vascular catheter-related sepsis are highly variable.[14] Routine replacement of central catheters every 3 to 5 days does not prevent infection. Exchanging catheters over a guidewire increases the risk of septicemia.[17] Femoral sites for catheter insertion should be avoided,[16] except for placement of intra-aortic balloon counterpulsation. Internal jugular catheters are more likely to become infected than subclavian ones, although the incidence with either technique is less than 1 percent.[14,16]

Triple-lumen catheters are associated with higher rates of infection and their use should be restricted to patients in whom a single-lumen catheter is insufficient. Antiseptic solution for skin decontamination may influence the rate of catheter-related bacteremia and a chlorhexidine solution is preferred to povidone-iodine.[18] Dry gauze dressings are better than the more expensive transparent plastic dressings, which lead to higher microbial counts at the insertion site.[14] The best intervals for changing intravenous lines and dressings (i.e., every 24 or 72 hours) are not yet elucidated[14,16]; however, 48 hours seems to be the most reasonable.

Bacteremia and septicemia can also occur after hematogenous seeding from infected sites such as the lungs, the urinary tract, or the operative site. Bacterial translocation from the digestive tract is less frequent. Diag-nosis of septicemia requires at least five to six positive blood cultures, whereas a single positive blood culture alone suggests bacterial contamination of the culture medium (this is particularly true with coagulase-negative staphylococci).

Septicemia can lead to septic shock, resulting in further deterioration of the patient's early postoperative hemodynamic status. Double or even triple initial antibiotic therapy with rapid bactericidal activity and good tissue diffusion is mandatory.

Empiric treatment is chosen according to knowledge of the infectious focus and local epidemiology. New penicillins, third-generation or extended-spectrum cephalosporins are used in association with aminoglycosides (low-cost gentamycin or less nephrotoxic amikacin). First-line vancomycin is used when staphylococci are suspected, as most are methicillin-resistant. Surgical treatment may be necessary at the primary infectious site. If the diagnosis of septicemia is made, antibiotics must be continued for at least 21 to 28 days to avoid early endocarditis.

Other Infections

Unilateral or bilateral sinusitis is a classic complication after prolonged nasotracheal intubation, but it is also associated with nasogastric tubes and orotracheal intubation. Such infections are favored by the absence of adequate sinus ventilation. Gram-negative bacilli or staphylococci are the most frequent pathogens. Symptoms are initially absent, but purulent secretions from the nostrils are observed as the infection becomes manifest. In the absence of an early diagnosis, sinusitis can induce the suspected bacteremia or septicemia. Early diagnosis requires a thoughtful physical examination with attention to the differential diagnosis. Confirmation of source is obtained with radiographs or preferably a CT scan. Sinus puncture and drainage permit identification of the responsible organisms, which are treated via sinus irrigation and lavage with antibiotics; nevertheless, systemic antibiotic therapy should be added.

Infections originating from the digestive tract should be suspected in every septic patient. Low splanchnic blood flow with mesenteric ischemia occurs in the absence of any peripheral symptomatology or objective criteria of low cardiac output. Bacteremia or septicemia results from bacterial translocation from an altered mucosal gut barrier. Acalculous cholecystitis, aseptic at first, promotes microbial proliferation through cholestasis. Enterobacteriaceae and enterococci are the most frequent pathogens, but anaerobic organisms can be present. Subtle clinical symptoms can be misleading, and right upper quadrant tenderness may be absent in sedated patients. Also, classic symptoms of hepatic cholestasis are not always present. Ultrasound examination demonstrates an enlarged gallbladder with wall thickening or pericholecystic fluid (i.e., sludge without stones). Vesicular gangrene can appear in severe or overwhelming infections. The treatment of choice is an emergency cholecystectomy plus systemic antibiotic coverage. First choice is a combination of amoxicillin and clavulanic acid or a new-generation penicillin, such as piperacillin, with an aminoglycoside.

SPECIFIC NOSOCOMIAL INFECTIONS

Specific nosocomial infections include all infections at the operative site (i.e., the sternum and the leg wounds). Cutaneous flora are the main source of contamination. Early endocarditis is also considered a nosocomial infection, regardless of the type of surgical procedure; however, it is rarely observed within the first postoperative week.

Leg Wound Infections

Surgical wound infections at saphenous vein harvest sites occur with a 4 to 6 percent incidence after coronary artery bypass graft (CABG) surgery.[1,19] The observed microorganisms are mainly staphylococci (with an increasing frequency of methicillin resistant *S. epidermidis*) and streptococci. Gram-negative bacilli can also be responsible (particularly *Klebsiella* spp.[20]) and are often multire-sistant to antibiotics. Diagnosis is easy since the febrile patient complains of a painful inflammatory wound with localized swelling. Purulent or culture-positive fluid discharge can be obtained from a dehiscent or closed incision. Treatment relies on directed antibiotic therapy plus local wound care. Surgical wound debridement of necrotic tissues may be necessary in rare instances.[20]

Sternal and Mediastinal Infections

Sternitis and mediastinitis are the most serious infectious complications following CABG surgery with an incidence of 1 to 6 percent.[21–23] Mediastinitis-related mortality remains elevated and may reach 25 percent.[22] Both infections usually occur 15 days after surgery, but they can also be observed as early as 4 days after sternotomy. Early diagnosis carries a grave prognosis, since the anterior mediastinal space is not yet obliterated. Risk factors for mediastinitis include male gender, obesity, diabetes, re-exploration of the mediastinum in the case of excessive bleeding or tamponade, and low cardiac output syndrome.[23–25] Hospitalization prior to surgery favors the selection of cutaneous flora resistant to antimicrobial prophylaxis. Patients undergoing bilateral internal mammary artery grafts are at high risk of developing mediastinitis, as this division of arterial flow impairs sternal vascularization and local response to infection. Staphyloccocci are the most frequent responsible pathogens,[23,24] with an increased incidence of coagulase-negative staphylococci. Gram-negative bacilli are also frequent offenders, and there are scattered reports of *Legionella* and *Aspergillus fumigatus* as pathogens.

In the early postoperative period, the diagnosis is obvious in a patient with fever, marked leukocytosis, and a painful and inflammatory wound associated with frank dehiscence and purulent drainage; however, sternal signs are often missing. Bacterial cultures are obtained from chest tube drainage or temporary pacing electrodes. Needle aspiration of the anterior mediastinal space has great diagnostic value but is often difficult to obtain. Septicemia and early endocarditis are rare complications at this stage. A thoracic CT scan allows visualization of retrosternal fluid collections, but differentiation between purulent or blood collections is difficult in the early postoperative period.

Both medical and surgical treatment should be combined. Intravenous antibiotic therapy is continued for a duration of 21 days and is continued orally for several months. Double or triple empiric therapy must be active against staphylococci and gram-negative bacilli. Vancomycin is used despite its low bactericidal activity because most staphylococci are methicillin resistant. Third-generation cephalosporins or ureidopenicillins should be combined with an aminoglycoside or a fluoroquinolone. Surgical re-exploration allows for necrotic tissue debridement and drainage of the purulent collections. Mediastinal tubes are placed to perform irrigation with a dilute solution of povidone-iodine for 7 to 10 days with daily fluid cultures. The irrigation should be stopped within 10 days to avoid the appearance of a suprainfection. Failure of this method requires the use of other surgical techniques (which can be performed as first-line procedures),[21] such as thoracic pedicle transposition of omentum,[26,27] or total excision of the sternum and obliteration of the dead space with muscular flaps.[26,27]

Prevention of sternitis and mediastinitis relies on antimicrobial prophylaxis (as described further on), recognition, and avoidance of predisposing factors to infection and adequate skin preparation. Hair removal should be performed with minimal trauma and as close to the time of incision as possible. Use of a depilatory agent is limited because of its allergic effects, but shaving may favor infections via cutaneous excoriations. Screening for *S. aureus* within the nares or on the sternum before the operation could allow for elimination of a carrier state[28] but is possibly associated with much higher costs (i.e., delayed surgery).

Early Endocardititis

Early endocarditis is rare, and in our experience occurs in less than 0.5 percent of patients within the first postoperative week. The bacterial contamination that causes endocarditis occurs either after endocardial disruption from cardiac surgery itself or after invasive procedures such as urinary or intravenous catheterization.[29] Catheter infection, mediastinitis, and/or septicemia can also lead to endocarditis, especially after cardiac valvular procedures. *Staphylococcus,* particularly *S. epidermidis,* is almost always the responsible pathogen in early endocarditis. Gram-negative bacilli are less frequently observed. The presence of *Enterococcus* would suggest that sepsis originates from the digestive or urogenital tract. Sustained positive blood cultures despite directed antibiotic therapy (in the absence of other infectious sites) strongly suggests the diagnosis of endocarditis. Abnormal cardiac murmurs are often delayed; thus, a two-dimensional ultrasound examination is mandatory: prosthetic valvular dehiscence is easily diagnosed; vegetations can be evidenced in advanced endocarditis but are difficult to distinguish from intracavitary thrombus. An accelerated rate of deterioration is heralded by the onset of cardiac failure, septic shock, and neurologic or peripheral septic emboli.

Bactericidal and synergistic double or triple antibiotic therapy should be continued for at least 5 to 6 weeks. In the case of methicillin-resistant *Staphylococcus,* vancomycin must be associated with antibiotics with good intracardiac penetration, such as fucidic acid, fosfomicin, or rifampicin; however, bacterial mutation and resistance may develop under fosfomicin and rifampicin. Sustained infection with hemodynamic instability or septic emboli necessitates surgery. In case of *Staphylococcus*-related endocarditis, surgical treatment is mandatory because mortality is very high with antibiotics alone.[30] All infected cardiac tissue is excised and valvular replacement performed. The increased risk of sustained infection of the new prosthetic valve has led to the use of aortic and mitral homografts or the performance of a Carpentier mitral valvuloplasty, with excellent short- and long-term results.[31,32]

Early Postoperative Infections After Transplantation

The early postoperative period is the highest risk period for life-threatening infection because of the high initial immunosuppression and precarious pretransplant physiologic state. Infectious complications, however, are similar to those observed in any postoperative cardiac patient. They are most often due to nosocomial organisms, but the outcome is worse than in nontransplant patients. Gram-negative septicemia can induce a mortality rate of 20 to 50 percent. Opportunistic infections are rare during the early period, although recurrence of Herpes simplex infections may occur on postoperative day 8 or 10. Other early postoperative infections can be transmitted by the graft organ. Diagnosis of infection can be difficult with misleading clinical or biologic symptoms because of high steroid doses. Careful daily review of routine cultures from all sites, including peripheral blood, all indwelling catheters or drainage tubes, and bacterial analysis of protected distal bronchial specimen, is important for early detection of infections. All chest tubes and intravenous catheters should be systematically cultured when removed.

HEART TRANSPLANTATION

Infections after heart transplantation are similar to those observed in non-transplant cardiac surgical patients. The most frequently observed infections are sternitis, mediastinitis, pulmonary infections, septicemia, and urinary infections.

Mediastinitis
Infections at the surgical site occur in 2 to 8 percent of heart transplant recipients.[33] *Staphylococcus* is the most frequent pathogen, with an increasing incidence of *S. epidermidis.* Other common organisms are gram-negative bacilli, such as *Enterobacter cloacae, Serratia marcescens,* and *Pseudomonas.* Clinical symptoms are often missing, and diagnosis is frequently established by systematic cultures of all drains and chest tubes. CT-guided needle aspirations may be helpful in difficult cases. Guidelines for antibiotic therapy are similar to those followed in nontransplant patients. Surgical therapy is based on primary debridement and secondary closure with muscle flaps at about 10 days.[11]

Pneumonia
Pneumonia is the most frequent infection in heart transplant recipients, with a 20 to 40 percent mortality.[33,34] The responsible pathogens for nosocomial pneumonia are similar to those described above in nontransplant patients. Although rarely observed, *Aspergillus* and *Candida* spp. may cause a rapidly progressive pneumonia. Classic diagnostic procedures are used with routine microbiologic follow-up. CT scans are much better than radiographs at detecting basilar pneumonias, small areas of nodular infiltration, and fluid collections in the pleural space.

HEART-LUNG TRANSPLANTATION

Infection is responsible for 40 to 70 percent of early postoperative deaths after heart-lung transplantation.[35] The thorax and lungs are the major sites of infections. Prolongation of the donor's endotracheal intubation (prior to harvest) favors upper airway bacterial colonization and pulmonary parenchymal contamination. Surgical factors also enhance the risk of infection via tracheal opening, bleeding, and hematomas. Potential damage of the recurrent laryngeal nerve is responsible for many cases of postextubation aspiration pneumonia. Lung ischemia, denervation, and interruption of lymphatic drainage[18] alter lung defense mechanisms against infections.[35] Decreased vascularization at the site of tracheal or bronchial sutures is associated with fragile healing and at times leakage, which favors mediastinal or pleural infections. Improved surgical techniques, delayed introduction of steroids, and careful selection of transplant recipients may lower the incidence of these dramatic complications.

Pneumonia

The incidence of pneumonia can reach 35 to 42 percent after heart-lung transplantation.[35] Clinical and radiologic manifestations are similar to those observed in nontransplant patients. However, in heart-lung transplant recipients, pneumonia can be difficult to distinguish from acute rejection within the first 10 postoperative days, and both may coexist. Fever, hypoxemia, and radiologic abnormalities are nonspecific but transbronchial biopsies are useful in the differential diagnosis.

Apart from the classic risk factors, pneumonia may result from bronchial stenosis induced by ischemia or discongruence at the anastomotic site. The treatment of stenosis may require the placement of an endobronchial prosthesis. Most pneumonias are bacterial in origin, with 75 percent induced by gram-negative bacilli. *Pseudomonas* spp. are often multiresistant, especially in patients with cystic fibrosis, who have already received several courses of antibiotics prior to transplantation. Knowledge of the patient's pretransplant microbial flora is essential for directed perioperative antibiotic therapy.

Fungal organisms can also be responsible for severe pneumonia. Clinical and radiologic aspects are nonspecific, and serologic diagnosis is of no help. Therefore, fiberoptic bronchoscopy with BAL will confirm the presence of fungal infection and allow their identification: *Candida* spp. or *Aspergillus* spp. *Candida albicans* pneumonia is treated by fluconazol (200 to 400 mg · day^{-1} IV) or amphotericin B. *Aspergillus* is the most feared pathogen and is routinely fatal after heart-lung transplantation.[36] Infection may result either from pretransplant contamination (which is difficult to eradicate) or from massive environmental contamination during the perioperative period. Radiologic cavitary or infiltrative lesions are typical of pulmonary aspergillosis. *Aspergillus* infection rapidly disseminates to other organs, especially the

brain. Medical treatment relies on parenteral amphotericin B with the administration of progressively increased doses in order to limit its nephotoxicity. Liposomal amphotericin B has a lower toxicity, which permits higher daily doses, offering great therapeutic success, and is the preferred method of administration. The use of itraconazole is limited by its oral administration and its pharmacologic interference with cyclosporine; it is not available in the United States. Surgical treatment may be required for abscess excision.

Mediastinitis

The frequency of mediastinitis can reach 13 to 22 percent after heart-lung transplantation.[35] Among the various responsible microorganisms, *Staphylococcus* and gram-negative bacilli (*P. aeruginosa*) are frequent, as well as disseminated *Candida* and *Aspergillus* infections.[35] The lungs are the most frequent primary site of infection. Anastomotic dehiscence induces mediastinal contamination through either a direct or hematogenous route. Despite the delayed introduction of steroids, diagnosis is difficult. Mediastinal infection at this early postoperative stage often involves the pleural spaces. Surgical treatment is extremely difficult, as the procedure entails a second look at the tracheal anastomosis, repair of any dehiscence, and subsequent protection of the anastomotic site by omentopexy or muscular flaps. The prognosis is dismal with a mortality rate of 60 to 80 percent.[35]

Pyothorax

Most of the time, pyothorax is secondary to suprainfection of intrapleural hematomas. It can also result from tracheal or bronchial dehiscence, with a fatal outcome in most cases.

Antibiotic Prophylaxis

Antimicrobial prophylaxis is the subject of great controversy in cardiac surgery. However, it significantly reduces the incidence of early postoperative surgical infections, from

9 to 54 percent in placebo groups to 0 to 6.7 percent in treated patients.[37] Prophylaxis was established in order to lower the risk of endocarditis and wound infection after valve replacement surgery. Antibiotics effective against the cutaneous flora, which may contaminate the surgical wound, must reach the tissues before contamination occurs. Therefore, prophylactic antibiotic therapy must be administered within 2 hours prior to incision.[38] Staphylococci are the most frequent pathogens responsible for surgical infections, particularly *S. epidermidis,* which is often resistant to both methicillin and most cephalosporins.

CHOICE OF ANTIBIOTICS

First- and second-generation cephalosporins have been used for years because they appear to be more potent than antistaphylococcal penicillins.[37] However, the comparative efficacy of cefazolin to cefamandole or cefuroxime has given conflicting results.[1,37,39] In vitro, cefazolin binds more strongly to serum proteins than do the second-generation cephalosporins and has an increased susceptibility to bacterial β-lactamases. These differences have little clinical consequence. The efficacy of cefamandole and cefuroxime is similar.[37]

Vancomycin has long been prescribed in patients allergic to the β-lactam antibiotics and the increasing number of methicillin-resistant staphylococci are increasing its use.[1,40] Vancomycin induces hypotension or the "red man syndrome" if infused too rapidly (less than 30 minutes). The incidence of vancomycin-resistant gram-positive cocci has increased dramatically in the United States. Therefore, routine use of vancomycin should be restricted. Vancomycin is exclusively active against gram-positive cocci. Thus, depending on the local epidemiologic environment, antimicrobial prophylaxis may require additional antibiotic coverage against gram-negative bacilli.

In summary, routine antimicrobial prophylaxis by either cefazolin or a second-generation cephalosporin is sufficient in most cases. However, vancomycin is recommended to reduce the risk of endocarditis caused by resistant staphylococci in the following special cases: (1) high endemic rates of methicillin-resistant staphylococci; (2) high risk of cutaneous colonization with cephalosporin resistant gram-positive cocci; (3) prosthetic valve replacement[1]; and (4) early postoperative reintervention and repeat valve surgery.

ANTIMICROBIAL PROPHYLAXIS ADMINISTRATION

The duration of antimicrobial prophylaxis is still controversial, with no significant difference between short (one dose or less than 2 days) and long (3 days or greater) prophylaxis regimens[37] (Table 11-2). Antimicrobial prophylaxis is commonly continued for 48 hours after cardiac surgery or until chest

Table 11-2. Recommended Dosages for Antimicrobial Prophylaxis

Antibiotic	Anesthetic Induction	CPB	If Surgery >4 h	Postoperatively
Cefazolin (IVD)	1 g		+1 g	1 g·6 h^{-1}
Cefamandole (IVD)	2 g		+2 g	2 g·6 h^{-1}
Cefuroxime (IVD)	1.5 g			1.5 g·8 h^{-1}
Vancomycin (60-min infusion)	15 mg·kg^{-1} or 1 g	±7.5–10 mg/kg		15 mg·kg^{-1} or 1 g bid (according to renal function)

Abbreviations: CPB, cardiopulmonary bypass; IVD, intravenous directly.

tubes are removed. Doses vary according to antibiotic pharmacokinetics on CPB and its minimal inhibitory concentration. Vancomycin is prescribed in accordance with previous recommendations,[41] but recent studies[1,42] demonstrate that a second perioperative prophylactic dose is not necessary after completion of CPB.

SPECIFIC ANTIMICROBIAL PROPHYLAXIS

Endocarditis

In cases of surgical reoperation for early or late endocarditis, antibiotic therapy against the responsible pathogen(s) is, of course, continued and vancomycin is added empirically to cover the infectious risk of reoperation.

When surgery is performed within the first few months after the septicemic phase of endocarditis, vancomycin in association with previously prescribed antibiotics is necessary for prophylactic coverage. All antibiotics, including vancomycin, are continued until results of the valve cultures are available. Antibiotic therapy is stopped if valve cultures are negative; however, if they are still positive, antibiotics should be continued for 4 to 6 weeks.

Heart and Lung Transplatation

Antimicrobial prophylaxis in heart transplant recipients is generally achieved with cefazolin or cefamandole. However, local epidemiology has led several transplant teams to prescribe third-generation cephalosporins instead.

In heart-lung transplant recipients, antimicrobial prophylaxis is directed against pulmonary infections. The common regimen uses a third-generation cephalosporin[35] with vancomycin. Both heart and heart-lung transplant recipients should systematically receive oral amphotericin B. *Aspergillosis* prophylaxis would logically include either low-dose intravenous liposomal (adjusted to serum creatinine) or nebulized or aerosolized amphotericin B.

INFECTIOUS AGENTS TRANSMITTED BY BLOOD TRANSFUSIONS AND BY TRANSPLANTED ORGANS

In the early postoperative period, bacterial or protozoal infections directly caused by transfusions can lead to significant morbidity. Viral diseases transmitted by transfusions at this stage give rise to carrier or latent states with long incubation periods. Despite better selection[43] and current laboratory testing of heterologous blood donors (Table 11-2), zero infectious risk has not yet been achieved. Therefore, safer transfusion strategies using autologous blood products, single or pedigreed heterologous blood products, plus additional testing and procedures are recommended.

Autologous blood products are strongly recommended and their use has increased from 1 percent in 1986 to 10 percent in 1992.[44] Single donor blood products reduce donor exposure. Apharesis fresh frozen plasma is a 500-ml product collected from a single donor that contains the same amount of clotting factors as three 200-ml units of fresh frozen plasma obtained from whole blood. Single-donor platelets represent 60 percent of platelet usage and will eventually replace random platelets.

Repeat donation from the same donor decreases the incidence of positive viral markers, with a 100-fold decrease in anti-Hbc antibodies between first-time donors and donors making their eighth donation. Removal of leukocytes from blood products with special high-grade leukocyte filters virtually eliminates cytomegalovirus (CMV) transmission, regardless of serologic CMV status.[45,46] Substitution of blood products at risk of infectious disease transmission with lower or nonrisk agents is advantageous. Thus, cryoprecipitate is no longer acceptable as a source of factor VIII because newer factor VIII concentrates do not transmit human immunodeficiency virus (HIV), hepatitis B, or hepatitis C.

Recombinant human erythropoietin (rhEPO) increases erythropoiesis.[47] In some specific indications, rhEPO can be used in conjunction with autologous blood predonation (ABP) 3 weeks prior to surgery to reduce postoperative use of heterologous blood products.[48] Safety of solvent/detergent (S/D) treated-plasma with regard to HBV, HCV, and HIV transmission is better than fresh frozen plasma with comparable clinical efficacy in treating coagulation factor deficits.[49]

Viral Infections in the Early Postoperative Period

The risk of viral infection in the early postoperative period can be eliminated by avoiding blood transfusions or giving autologous blood, autotransfusions, and/or reinfusion of shed blood. Heterologous blood transfusions should be limited to strict necessity. The use of fresh frozen plasma should be restricted to severe intravascular coagulopathy or severe hemorrhaging, with a resultant dilutional effect on all clotting factors. Heterologous blood components carry in unavoidable viral risk. Current estimates of the risk of transfusion-transmitted infection are uncertain, since they continue to change and vary in different countries and within communities. In 1992, the annual risk of U.S. viral infections associated with approximately 16 million transfusions was estimated as 32 for HBV, 16,000 for HCV, and 160 for HIV.[50]

HEPATITIS B

Despite routine testing of heterologous donated blood for HBsAg and anti-HBc antibodies, the transmission of HBV, delta agent, and HCV is still possible in the case of a latent carrier state.

Washing of red blood cells does not eliminate the risk of HBV transmission. The approximate risk of hepatitis B per unit of transfused heterologous blood products in developed countries is 0.0002 percent.[51,52] The frequency of transfusion transmission of the hepatitis B virus (on the basis of surveillance studies and the efficiency of laboratory tests) is estimated to be 1 in 50,000 per recipient or about 1 in 200,000 per unit.[52] The mean incubation period was found to be 36 days (from 30 to 150 days). After hepatitis B exposure, HBsAg with HBV-DNA, DNA polymerase and HBeAg appear first in the incubation period, followed by anti-HBc. In acute clinical hepatitis B, at the onset of symptoms HBsAg reaches a peak. It decreases during convalescence and then disappears in 90 percent of patients one week to several months later. However, acute clinical hepatitis B can be fulminant in 1 to 3 percent of cases and chronic hepatitis develops in 5 to 10 percent of patients who will die later from cirrhosis or hepatocellular carcinoma.[53] Therefore, after heterologous blood transfusions, careful biologic monitoring of alanine transferase (ALT) levels, HBsAg, and anti-HBc antibodies is recommended.

The only effective measure against early postoperative hepatitis B is preoperative vaccination. Two types of vaccine are available and proved to be safe: one taken from the plasma of HBs carrier and the other a synthesized recombinant DNA product. Protective antibodies appear in 80 to 97 percent of subjects who receive the full immunization course. Cardiac failure may decrease the immune response rate. Thus, double doses or monthly injections until appearance of antibodies may be necessary in heart transplant candidates.

HEPATITIS DELTA VIRUS

The delta agent is a low-molecular-weight defective RNA virus coated with HBsAg. HDV is found in only HBsAg-positive subjects, with a prevalence rate of 3.8 percent.[54] Simultaneous infection by HBV and HDV in a previously healthy subject is usually followed by disappearance of serum markers for both viruses, although fulminant hepatitis or a more severe acute course is possible. Superinfection of HBsAg carriers with HDV is linked to a chronic course of delta infection in 70 to 90 percent of cases and a more severe underlying chronic hepatitis.[55] In HDV infection, the delta antigen is present in the liver and serum; viral RNA and anti-HDV can also be found in the serum. In the postoperative period, the same preventive measures against HDV as against hepatitis B are recommended, although there is no vaccine for HDV.

NON-A, NON-B HEPATITIS AND HEPATITIS C

The term non-A, non-B hepatitis (NANBH) was given in 1988 to cases of hepatitis in which hepatitis A, B, and D virus, as well as CMV, Epstein-Barr virus (EBV), and hepatotoxic substances were not present. Two forms of NANBH were then identified: HEV and HCV viral infections. In HEV infection, the enteric or epidemic form of NANBH, clinical symptoms are similar to those of hepatitis A, with the exception of a very high mortality rate during pregnancy and a lower rate of secondary transmission. No parenteral transmission of HEV infection has been reported. In HCV infections, the parenteral form of NANBH, diagnosis is established 2 to 26 weeks after transfusion, when characteristic fluctuation of ALT levels appears both in the acute and in the chronic phases.

HCV was identified by Choo[56] in 1989. This single-strand RNA virus belongs to the Flaviviridae virus family. Polymerase chain reaction (PCR) permits detection of HCV virus, which can appear as soon as 2 weeks following factor VIII administration.[57] The incidence of post-transfusion hepatitis C has decreased markedly since the implementation of donor screening for surrogate markers of NANBH and for antibodies to HCV. With the addition of screening for antibodies to HCV (0.03 percent per unit) in May 1990, the risk is now 0.57 percent per patient.[58] The risk of seroconversion was strongly associated with the volume of blood transfused, but not with the use of particular components. Hepatitis C incubation varies from 30 to 150 days, 90 percent of patients are anicteric during the acute phase. Evolution toward chronicity occurs in 50 to 60 percent of cases. Thus, strict limitation of heterologous blood transfusions is recommended with careful biologic and serologic monitoring of post-transfusion transaminase levels and anti-HCV antibodies.

HEPATITIS A VIRUS

Hepatitis A virus is transmitted by the fecal-oral route and causes only transient viremia without a carrier state. To our knowledge, no case of post-transfusion hepatitis A has been reported after cardiac surgery. However, it is theoretically possible that hepatitis A could be observed in the postoperative period, since the patient may be in the early stages of incubation immediately prior to surgery.

HUMAN IMMUNODEFICIENCY VIRUSES

HIV-1 and HIV-2

The causative virus of acquired immunodeficiency syndrome (AIDS) was originally described as lymphadenopathy-associated virus (LAV) by Montagnier and subsequently as HTLV-III by Gallo. HIV-I belongs to the Lentivirianae subfamily. HIV-2, a second distinct retrovirus, later isolated from West African patients, is also lymphotropic, cytotoxic, and neurotropic.

HIV has been transmitted by whole blood, cellular components, plasma, and clotting factor concentrates. HIV transmission rates through heterologous transfusions are steadily decreasing in developed countries through anti-HIV screening (anti-HIV-1, HIV-1 Ag, anti-HIV-2, and implementation of donor self-exclusion procedure); however, there is still a substantial risk.[59] Analysis of infectivity of the last seronegative blood donation from donors who subsequently seroconverted has shown that the infectious window period for HIV is about 45 days. HIV is transmissible by transplanted organs in heart and heart-lung transplant recipients.[60] In a pre- and postoperative study of cardiac surgery from 1985 to 1989, 4,163 adults who received 36,282 transfusions of blood components with an observed risk of HIV-1 transmission of 0.003 percent per unit.[61] The risk of AIDS and the incubation period before the development of AIDS are related to the donor's clinical course and the number of transfusions.

For the first few days after infection, no HIV markers are detectable in blood. Then, for a period of several weeks, viremia follows and HIV and p24 antigen can be detected in the serum. During this period, about one-third of patients develop an acute, flulike, or mononucleosislike syndrome. Two to 4 months after sexually transmitted infection and 1 to 2 months after transfusion-transmitted infection, a wide range of antibodies to the structural env, gag, and pol viral proteins develops. As soon as anti-p24 develops, p24 antigenemia disappears. However, antigenemia reappears in the late stage of AIDS and may reappear intermittently during the asymptomatic phase of infection, which can last more than 10 years. Symptomatic AIDS develops when CD4 helper cells have almost completely disappeared, leading to collapse of the immune system.

Therefore, HIV blood screening and restricted use of heterologous blood transfusions are necessary to decrease further the risk of HIV transmission. In heterologous blood-transfused recipients, serum sampling for HIV-1 and HIV-2 antibodies should be performed before discharge from the ICU. Presence of anti-HIV antibodies requires confirmation of infection by Western blot analysis.

HTLV-I and HTLV-II
Human T-cell leukemia virus type I (HTLV-I) was the first human retrovirus described and was later found to be a variant of the adult T-cell leukemia/lymphoma virus.[62] HTLV-I has been associated with tropical spastic paraparesis (TSP), polymyositis, and Kaposi sarcoma. HTLV-I and -II are lymphotropic and neurotropic retroviruses, belonging to the oncovirus family. They induce T-lymphocytes (mainly CD4+) polyclonal proliferation both in vitro and in vivo by trans activation of the cellular genes involved in growth control via the tax gene.

Transmission mainly occurs by sexual contact and breast feeding, but the virus is transmissible by transfusions.[63] Antibodies are usually detectable 14 to 30 days after transfusion. Time lag between transfusion and TSP varies from 18 weeks to 8 years. In two heart transplant recipients infected after transfusion, one seroconverted within weeks and developed TSP.[65]

Routine screening of blood donations for HTLV antibodies in the United States began in December 1988, and infection rates of 1 in 60,000 or less were estimated. By March 1990, only 0.04 percent of donations were repeatedly reactive, and 0.01 percent were confirmed as anti-HTLV-I positive.[59,65] The HTLV-I screening test in current use may not have optimal sensitivity to detect HTLV-II infection in donors. The licensed enzyme-linked immunosorbent assay (ELISA) test used by most blood banks derives its antigens from the lysate of an anti-HTLV-I cell culture and contains no antigen specific for HTLV-II. Although an estimated homology exists between the p24 antigens of HTLV-I and HTLV-II genomes, the homology with other core, polymerase, and envelope antigens is considerable less, suggesting that the present assay may be somewhat insensitive in detecting HTLV-I infected donors. HTLV-II is common in some groups of intravenous drug users, and most infected individuals are asymptomatic. The pathogenic potential of HTLV-II is not fully defined.[65]

CYTOMEGALOVIRUS

CMV is the agent most frequently transmitted by transfusions.[66] This double-strand DNA herpes virus is cell associated but is also found free in secretions and plasma. CMV has a direct cytopathic effect that leads to neutropenia, depressed cellular immunity, and increased susceptibility to simultaneous bacterial, fungal, and protozoal infections. CMV causes both an acute clinical and subclinical infection, as well as a chronic subclinical infection with shedding in saliva or urine. It remains latent in a large proportion of infected subjects. The presence of anti-CMV antibodies before surgery does not prevent recurrent infection, which includes both reactivation or reinfection by other strains. Primary infection is generally more severe than recurrent infection, diagnosed by a four-fold increase in the antibody titre or the presence of IgM anti-CMV antibodies. In the postoperative period, CMV antibodies may come from transfused blood; therefore, diagnosis relies on viral antigen detection using rapid viral culture or PCP.

The prevalence of CMV antibodies varies from 30 to 80 percent in developed countries. It has been estimated that 3 to 12 percent of blood units have the potential to transmit CMV.[67] Donors with IgM anti-CMV antibodies seem more likely to transmit CMV than others.

The consequence of transfusion-transmitted CMV infection depends largely on recipient factors. In immunocompetent subjects receiving heterologous transfusion, 30 percent of anti-CMV-negative patients develop infection.[68] In addition, some anti-CMV-positive patients develop recurrent infection. Almost all cases are asymptomatic, and less than 10 percent present as a mononucleosis-like syndrome, referred to as the post-transfusion syndrome. Spontaneously resolving fever, exanthema, hepatosplenomegaly, and enlarged lymph nodes occur within 3 to 6 weeks after transfusion. The presence of atypical circulating lymphocytes due to post-transfusion CMV infection should be distinguished from a response to allogeneic lymphocytes.

In transplant recipients or other immunosuppressed patients, CMV causes severe disease; primary infection can be fatal.[69] Clinical symptoms usually appear 2 months after transplantation but may occur as early as 10 days after the graft. Infection may be asymptomatic and is diagnosed only retrospectively by serologic follow-up. Three clinical forms can be distinguished: an isolated aseptic viral syndrome, a localized involvement of one organ, and a disseminated form with plurivisceral lesions: pneumonia, hepatitis, diges-

tive tract lesions, pancreatitis, or meningoencephalitis. Leukopenia with lymphopenia is common and can be associated with thrombocytopenia. CMV pneumonia is the most frequent manifestation in heart and heart-lung transplant recipients, with isolated cough, hypoxemia, and diffuse radiologic interstitial infiltrates (although focal or nodular lesions can be observed).[70,71] Bronchoalveolar lavage via fiberoptic bronchoscopy permits detection of CMV as well as any associated bacterial, fungal, or parasitic infections. Graft rejection and CMV infection can be associated.

CMV hepatitis increases transaminase or alaline phosphatase levels. High mortality rates are the norm: from 22 to 25 percent in symptomatic patients, to 66 percent in patients with pulmonary involvement following heart-lung transplantation. The treatment of choice is ganciclovir,[72,73] which inhibits DNA polymerase synthesis via intracellular kinase phosphoralation. Ganciclovir is given at an initial dose of $5 \text{ mg} \cdot \text{kg}^{-1}$ IV bid for 15 to 21 days, with doses adjusted for renal function. Viral resistance is rare. Because of the severity and dramatically poor outcome of CMV pneumonia in immunosuppressed transplant recipients, anti-CMV globulins can be added to ganciclovir; however, the benefit of this therapy is uncertain. Foscarnet, another inhibitor of DNA viral synthesis, is active against all types of herpes virus, including CMV. Its use, at daily doses of $200 \text{ mg} \cdot \text{kg}^{-1}$ for 14 to 21 days, is limited by its intrinsic nephrotoxicity, especially in the early postoperative period.

Prevention of CMV in the early postoperative period is mandatory for heart and heart-lung transplant recipients. In seronegative recipients, main sources of infection are donor-positive transplanted organs or blood products. If both donor and recipient are CMV negative, blood transfusions appear to be the major source of disease (although this is demonstrated in very few controlled studies).[74] Infection can be prevented by the use of CMV-negative packed cells and platelets.

Red blood cells alone, frozen deglycerolized red cells, or filtered white blood cell-depleted red cells can be transfused, since they have not been shown to transmit CMV. This measure appears to decrease the incidence of CMV disease from 71 to 34 percent.[76]

In CMV-negative heart or heart-lung transplant recipients transplanted with CMV-positive organs, prophylactic administration of specific hyperimmune IgG seems to reduce the severity of the disease.[69] Recent studies have demonstrated that prophylactic ganciclovir administered at a dose of 5 mg · kg^{-1} · day^{-1} IV for 15 to 21 days in the post-transplant period effectively decreases the incidence and severity of the disease in CMV-negative heart or heart-lung transplant recipients.[75] Acyclovir, which is commonly used against herpes and varicella-zoster virus (VZV), can also be used to prevent CMV but may not be as effective.[76]

EPSTEIN-BARR VIRUS

EBV, like CMV, is a herpes virus and is endemic throughout the world. Although EBV can cause symptomatic mononucleosis, it is most commonly asymptomatic with a consequent latent infection. More than 90 percent of blood donors have neutralizing anti-EBV antibodies, coexisting with latent EBV in peripheral blood B-lymphocytes and lymph nodes. Post-transfusion EBV infection is rare and symptomatic infection uncommon. To our knowledge, EBV infection has never been observed in the early postoperative period after cardiac surgery. Of five patients initially free of EBV and transfused, four produced high antibody levels that persisted for several months. Two of the four had concomitant CMV infection, and only one developed a mononucleosis syndrome with heterophile antibodies.[77] Post-transfusion mononucleosis is rarely seen in anti-EBV-negative immunocompetent patients. In reported cases, the incubation period in recipients was 21 to 30 days. Post-transfusion EBV infections contribute to the late development of lymphomas in transplant recipients.

OTHER HERPES VIRUSES

Herpes Simplex and Herpes Varicella Zoster
HSV and VZV have never been shown to be transmitted by blood transfusions. Viremia only occurs during primary infections.

HHV-6
HHV-6, a newly characterized human herpes virus, originally named human B-lymphotropic virus, is cytopathic for selected T-cell lines. HHV-6 seems to be ubiquitous, with a prevalence of 60 to 90 percent and can be transmitted by blood or organ transplantation. Its reactivation may occur within a few months after surgery in immunosupressed patients.

SERUM PARVOVIRUS-LIKE OR B19 VIRUS

Serum parvovirus-like (SPL) virus is a very small single-strand virus rarely transmitted by blood transfusion but more frequently by factor VIII concentrates. The extremely high concentrations (10^{12} virus particles · unit^{-1}) achieved in plasma make B19 resistant to several inactivation procedures used for plasma products. Antibodies to B19 are found in 25 percent of blood donors. B19 virus is the viral agent of Fifth's disease and can cause arthritus and purpura.[78]

Other Infections Transmitted by Blood Transfusions

Nonviral infections acquired by transfusions are rare; in the United States they are estimated at less than 1 per million units[44,79] transfused.

BACTERIAL INFECTIONS WITH IMMEDIATE REACTIONS

Shock following the injection of bacteria is presumably due to bacterial toxins, although an immune reaction between naturally occurring antibodies and bacteria may also produce grave consequences. Fever, chills, vomiting, tachycardia, and hypotension often occur during transfusions but may develop within a few hours. Transfusion of contaminated blood may produce immediate collapse, followed by profound shock and hyperpyrexia. Hemorrhagic phenomena due to DIC are common. The overall mortality rate is 26 percent.

The incidence of fatalities due to contaminated transfusions has increased in recent years and is attributed to storage of platelets at 20° to 24°C. The bacterial contaminant depends largely on the type of blood component. Red cells are contaminated mainly by *P. fluorescens, P. putida,* and *Yersinia enterocolitica.*[80] Transfusion of blood from donors with subclinical *Yersinia bacteremia,* a gram-negative aerobic rod, may cause fatal septicemia, especially in immunosuppressed patients. Eighteen cases were reported to the FDA from April 1987 to February 1991, with seven fatal outcomes. Platelet concentrates stored at 20° to 24°C may cause fatal sepsis when contaminated with any of several gram-negative or -positive organisms, such as staphlococci, streptococci, *Serratia* sp., flavobacteria, and salmonellae.

Cryoprecipitates and fresh frozen plasma can be contaminated with *P. cepacia* and *P. aeruginosa* during thawing in contaminated water baths. Investigations following the suspected transfusion of infected blood products include both culture of any remaining products from the same donor as well as culture of the recipient. A negative donor product culture excludes the possibility that it was heavily infected at the time of transfusion. Following a positive culture in the recipient, the origin of contamination cannot be identified with certainty. The blood may have been contaminated prior to, during, or after transfusion, or upon culture sampling. Bacteria originating from skin flora, such as *S. epidermidis, Micrococcus* spp., *Sarcina* spp., and diphtheroids, may gain entrance to the blood pack during donation. Bacteria from the environment, such as *Pseudomonas* and *Flavobacterium,* may gain entrance to blood components during collection or processing in open systems.

BACTERIAL INFECTIONS WITH DELAYED MANIFESTATIONS

Treponema pallidum

Transfused *Treponema pallidum,* responsible for syphilis, has an incubation period from 4 weeks to 4.5 months. All transfused units in the United States (as of 1992) are routinely screened for the following infectious agents:

1. ABO/Th
2. Syphilis
3. HBsAg
4. ALT
5. Anti-HIV-1
6. Anti-HBc
7. Anti-HTLV-I and -II
8. Anti-HCV
9. HIV1 Ag
10. Anti-HIV-2

Brucella abortus

Brucella abortus is known to survive for several months in stored blood, with few reports of blood transfusion-transmitted symptomatic infection. However, transfusion-induced brucellosis has never been reported in the United States.

Borellia burgdorferi

Although no cases of transmitted *Borellia burgdorferi,* the tick-borne spirochete responsible for Lyme disease, have been reported so far, blood transmission is theoretically possible.

Rickettsia rickettsii

Rickettsia rickettsii transmitted by blood transfusions has been reported.[81]

PARASITIC INFECTION ACQUIRED BY BLOOD TRANSFUSIONS

Malaria

Malaria can be transmitted by any blood component and usually responds to conventional drug therapy. The incubation period depends on the number and strain of transfused plasmodia. It varies between 1 week and 1 month with *P. falciparum* and may reach many months with *P. malariae.* The diagnosis relies on *Plasmodium* detection within the recipient's blood. Latent infection can be detected by indirect fluorescence antibody test or ELISA.

Toxoplasma gondii

Toxoplasma gondii is responsible for toxoplasmosis. It is rarely transmitted by blood transfusions. However, infection can be transmitted at the time of cardiac transplantation, and latent parasitic cysts in the transplant can produce severe myocarditis in the recipient. In seronegative transplant recipients, prophylaxis of toxoplasmosis is mandatory when the donor is seropositive; the use of sulfadoxine plus pyrimethamine is recommended.

Other Parasites

Other parasites, such as *Trypanosoma crusi* responsible for Chagas disease, *Babesia microti,* a tick-borne protozoan limited to the northern East Coast, Wisconsin, and Minnesota, or *Leishmaniasis* can be exceptionally transmitted by blood transfusions.

BLOOD TRANSFUSIONS AND MODULATION OF IMMUNE FUNCTION

Febrile adverse immune reactions may be caused by interaction between leukocytes, platelets, or plasma proteins and alloantibodies directed against them after transfusions, with consequent complement activation and liberation of vasoactive substances. The destruction of transfused leukocytes may be associated with fever, presumably because of the release of endogenous pyrogens, such as interleukin-1 (IL1), interferon, and tumor necrosis factor (TNF). When a patient develops flushing of the face or fever, this suggests complement activation with subsequent release of vasoactive substances. The cause of this type of reaction is extremely difficult to determine, as either no alloantibodies are detected or the patient has more than one type of alloantibody.

Reactions Due to Leukocyte Antibodies

Since 1954, when Dausset first suggested that leukocyte alloantibodies might cause transfusion reactions, a causal role for leukocytes in transfusion reactions with anti-HLA, -B, and -C antibodies has been established. Fever due to leucocyte alloantibodies usually occurs within 30 minutes of starting transfusion, but flushing may appear within 5 minutes if high titers of leukoagglutinins are present. Fibrinolysis can also be associated with severe febrile reactions. Granulocytes and perhaps monocytes play an important role in these febrile transfusion reactions since they react with anti-HLA as well as with granulocyte- and monocyte-specific alloantibodies. Their subtraction (by passing blood through leukocyte filters) suppresses reactions in most patients who were previously febrile during transfusions.

Transfusion-Induced Graft-Versus-Host Disease

Graft-versus-host disease appears when, following successful engraftment of allogeneic lymphocytes on their precursors, the foreign HLA-incompatible cells attack host tissues. Severe erythema multiform-like skin rash develops over the entire body approximately 10 days after the operation, followed by fever, diarrhea, jaundice, transaminemia, pancytopenia, and marrow aplasia. A few cases of transfusion-associated acute GVHD after cardiac surgery were recently reported in Japan, with an associated mortality rate as high as 90 percent. The calculated incidence in Japan is 1 in 659 cases.[82,83] GVHD after transfusions may occur in nonimmunocompromised patients when the donor is homozygous for one of the recipient's haplotypes or in previously immunosuppressed patients.

REFERENCES

1. Maki DG, Bohn MJ, Stolt SM et al: Comparative study of cefazoline, cefamandole, and vancomycin for surgical prophylaxis in cardiac

and vascular operations. J Thorac Cardiovasc Surg 104:1423–34, 1992

2. Orita H, Shimanuki T, Fukasawa M et al: A clinical study of postoperative infections following open heart surgery occurrence and microbiological findings in 782 cases. Surg Today 22:207–12, 1992

3. Body JI, Pickering NJ, Fink GB, Behr E: Altered lymphocyte subsets during cardiopulmonary bypass. Am J Clin Pathol 86:626–8, 1987

4. Pien FD, Ho HWL, Furgusson DJG: Fever and infection after cardiac operation. Ann Thorac Surg 33:382–4, 1982

5. Voss A, Leick CA, Torremorell Y et al: Handwashing agent use a possible marker for nosocomial infections, abstract 59. Presented at the Thirty-third ICAAC symposium, New Orleans, 1993

6. Freeman J: Prevention of nosocomial infections by locations of sinks for handwashing adjacent to the bedside, abstract 60. Presented at the Thirty-third ICAAC symposium, New Orleans, 1993

7. Sokalski SJ, Jewell MA, Asmus-Shillington AC et al: An outbreak of *Serratia marcescens* in 14 adult cardiac surgical patients associated with 12 lead electrocardiogram bulbs. Arch Intern Med 152:841–4, 1992

8. Torres A, Elbiary M, Rodriguez-Rosin R: Nosocomial pneumonia current opinion. Infect Dis 6:167–70, 1993

9. Cook DJ, Laine LA, Goyatt GH, Raffin TA: Nosocomial pneumonia and the role of the gastric pH: a meta-analysis. Chest 100:7–13, 1991

10. Papazian L, Gonin F, Saux P et al: Low sensitivity of protected specimen brush in the diagnosis of nosocomial bronchopneumonia in mechanically ventilated patients, abstract 856. Presented at the Thirty-third ICAAC symposium, New Orleans, 1993

11. Rouby JJ, Martin de Lassale EM, Poete P et al: Nosocomial bronchopneumonia in the critically ill. Am Rev Respir Dis 146:1059–66, 1992

12. Pennington JC: Hospital-acquired pneumonia. p. 321 In Wenzel R (ed): Prevention and Control of Nosocomial Infections. Williams & Wilkins, Baltimore, 1987

13. Craven DE: Use of selective decontamination of the digestive tract: is the light at the end of the tunnel red or green? Ann Intern Med 117:609–11, 1992

14. Raad II, Bodey GP: Infectious complications of indwelling vascular catheters. Clin Infect Dis 15:197–210, 1992

15. Jansen B: Vascular catheter-related infection: etiology and prevention. Curr Opin Infect Dis 6:526–31, 1993

16. Johnson A, Oppenthein BA: Vascular catheter-related sepsis: diagnosis and prevention. J Hosp Infect 20:67–78, 1992

17. Cobb DK, High KP, Sawyer RG et al: A controlled trial of scheduled replacement of central venous and pulmonary-artery catheters. N Engl J Med 8:1062–8, 1992

18. Maki DG, Ringer M, Alvarado CJ: Prospective randomized trial of povidone-iodine, alcohol and dilorhexidine for prevention of infection associated with central venous and arterial catheters. Lancet 338:339–43, 1991

19. Moreles E, Herwaldt L, Embrey R et al: The epidemiology of saphenous vein harvest site wound infections after cardiothoracic surgery, abstract 64. Presented at the Thirty-third ICAAC symposium, New Orleans, 1993

20. Rode H, Brown RA, Millar AJW: Surgical skin and soft tissue infections. Curr Opin Infect Dis 6:683–90, 1993

21. Serry C, Bleck PC, Javid H et al: Sternal wound complications: managements and results. J Thorac Cardiovasc Surg 80:861–7, 1980

22. Newman LS, Szczukowski LC et al: Suppurative mediastinitis after open heart surgery. A case control study of risk factors. Chest 94:546–53, 1988

23. Culliford AT, Cunningham JN, Zeff RH et al: Sternal and costochrondral infections following open heart surgery. J Thorac Cardiovasc Surg 72:714–26, 1976

24. Grossi EA, Culliford AT, Kreiger KH et al: A survey of 77 major infectious complications of median sternotomy: a review of 7,949 consecutive operative procedures. Ann Thorac Surg 40:214–23, 1985

25. Hudec M, Domanig E, Hiertz H et al: Risk factors for severe bacterial infections after valve replacement and aortocoronary bypass operations. Analysis of 246 cases by logistic regression. Ann Thorac Surg 40:224–8, 1985

26. Lee AB, Schimert G, Shatkin S: Total excision of the sternum and thoracic pedicle transposition of the greater omentum; useful strata-

gems in managing severe mediastinal infection following open heart surgery. Surgery 8: 433–6, 1976

27. Hellman AA, Lammermeier DE, Cooley DA: Management of the complicated sternotomy incision: results of omentopexy with primary skin closure. Tex Heart Inst J 16:11–4, 1989

28. Morales E, Herwaldt L, Embrey R et al: The epidemiology of spanenous vein harvest site wound infections after cardiothoracic surgery, abstract 1446. Presented at the Thirty-third ICAAC symposium, New Orleans, 1993

29. Fdezguerrero M, Verdejo C, Gorgolas M, Azofra J: Nosocomial endocarditis: evidence of an emerging problem, abstract 1306. Presented at the Thirty-third ICAAC symposium, New Orleans, 1993

30. Wolff M, Witchitz S, Chastang CL: Prostetic valve endocarditis: prognostic factors and outcome, abstract 13605. Presented at the Thirty-third ICAAC symposium, New Orleans, 1993

31. Dreyfus G, Seffaf A, Jebara VA et al: Valve repair in acute endocarditis. Ann Thorac Surg 49:706–13, 1990

32. Acar C, Farge A, Ramsheyi A et al: Mitral valve replacement using a cryopreserved mitral homograft. Ann Thorac Surg 57:746–8, 1994

33. Gentry LO, Zeluff BJ: Diagnosis and treatment of infection in cardiac transplant patients. Surg Clin North Am 66:459–65, 1986

34. Horn JE, Bartlett JG: Infectious complications following heart transplantation. p. 220. In Baumgartner WA, Reitz BA, Achuff SC (eds): Heart and Heart-Lung Transplantation. WB Saunders, Philadelphia, 1990

35. Dauber JH, Paradis IL, Dummer JS: Infectious complications in pulmonary allograft recipients. Clin Chest Med 11:291–308, 1990

36. Musial CE, Cockerill FR, Roberts GD: Fungal infections of the immunocompromised host: clinical and laboratory aspects. Clin Microbiol Rev 10:349–64, 1988

37. Kreter B, Woods M: Antibiotic prophylaxis for cardiothoracic operations. Meta-analysis of thirty years of clinical trials. J Thorac Cardiovasc Surg 104:590–9, 1992

38. Classen DC, Evans RS, Pestotnik SL et al: The timing of prophylactic administration of antibiotics and the risk of surgical wound infection. N Engl J Med 326:281–6, 1992

39. Doebbeling B, Pfaller M, Kuhns K et al: Cardi-

ovascular surgery prophylaxis: a randomized controlled comparison of cefazolin and cefuroxime. J Thorac Cardiovasc Surg 99:981–9, 1990

40. Woods M, Tillman D: Antibiotic prophylaxis in cardiothoracic surgery 1990: results of a third survey. Hosp Pharm 27:404–7, 1992

41. Farber BF, Karchmer ALU, Buckley MJ, Moellering RC: Vancomycin prophylaxis in cardiac operations: determination of an optimal dosage regimen. J Thorac Cardiovasc Surg 85:933–40, 1983

42. Martin C, Alaya M, Viviand X et al: Penetration of vancomycin into mediastinal and cardiac tissues in human, abstract 166. Presented at the Thirty-third ICAAC symposium, 33rd New Orleans, 1993

43. Dodd RY: The risk of transfusion transmitted infection. N Engl J Med 327:419–20, 1992

44. National Blood Resource Education Program Expert Panel: The use of autologous blood. JAMA 263:414–7, 1990

45. Andreu G: Role of leukocyte depletion in the prevention of transfusion-induced cytomegalovirus infection. Semin Hematol, suppl 5. 28: 26–31, 1991

46. De Graan-Hetzen YCE, Gratama JW, Mudde GC et al: Prevention of primary cytomegalovirus infection in patients with hematologic malignancies by intensive white cell depletion of blood products. Transfusion 29:757–60, 1990

47. Goodnough LT, Rudnick S, Price TH et al: Increased preoperative collection of autologous blood with recombinant huam erythropoietin therapy. N Engl J Med 321:1163–8, 1989

48. Kyo S, Omoto R, Hirashima K et al: Effect of recombinant erythropoietin on reduction of homologous blood transfusion in open heart surgery. A Japanese multi-center study. Circulation, suppl II. 86:413–8, 1992

49. Horowitz B, Bonomo R, Prince AM et al: Solvent/detergent-treated plasma: a virus-inactivated source substitute for fresh frozen plasma. Blood 79:826–31, 1992

50. Horowitz B, Prince AM, Rywkin S et al: Preparation and characterization of virus sterilized blood components. Symposium sur la sécurité transfusionnelle. Actualité. In Actuar, 20: 49–52, 1992

51. Hoofnagle JH: Posttransfusion hepatitis B. Transfusion 30:384–6, 1990

52. US Public Health Service Inter-agency guide-

line for screening donors of blood, plasma, organs, tissues and semen for evidence of hepatitis B and hepatitis C. MMWR, RR-4. 40:1–17, 1991

53. Wright TL, Lau JYN: Clinical aspects of hepatitis B virus infection. Lancet 342:1340–4, 1993

54. Centers for Disease Control. Delta hepatitis—Massachussets. MMWR 33:493–4, 1984

55. Monjardino JP, Saldanha JA: Delta hepatitis. The disease and the virus. Br Med Bull 46: 399–407, 1990

56. Choo QL, Kuo G, Weiner AJ et al: Isolation of a cDNA clone derived from a blood-borne non-A, non-B viral hepatitis genome. Science 244: 359–61, 1989

57. Garson JA, Ring C, Tuke P, Tedder RS: Enhanced detection by PCR of hepatitis C virus RNA, letter Lancet 2:878–9, 1990

58. Donahue JG, Munoz A, Ness PM et al: The declining risk of post transfusion hepatitis C virus infection. N Engl J Med 327:369–73, 1992

59. Cohen ND, Munoz A, Reitz BA et al: Transmission of retroviruses by transfusion of screened blood in patients undergoing cardiac surgery. N Engl J Med 320:1172–6, 1989

60. Schwarz A, Offermann G, Keller F et al: The effect of cyclosporine on the progression of human immunodeficiency virus type 1 infection transmitted by transplantation—data on 4 cases and review of the literature. Transplantation 55:95–103, 1993

61. Nelson KE, Donahue JG, Munoz A et al: Transmission of retroviruses from seronegative donors by transfusion during cardiac surgery. Ann Intern Med 117:554–9, 1992

62. Yoshida M, Miyoshi I, Hinuma Y: Isolation and characterization of retrovirus from cell lines of human adult T-cell leukemia and its implication in the disease. Proc Natl Acad Sci USA 79:2031–5, 1982

63. Yamaguchi K: Human T-lymphotrophic virus type I in Japan. Lancet 343:213–5, 1994

64. Gout O, Baulac M, Gessain A et al: Rapid development of myelopathy after HTLV1 infection acquired by transfusion during cardiac transplantation. N Engl J Med 322:383–8, 1990

65. Hjelle B, Mills R, Mertz G, Swenson S: Transmission of HTLV2 via blood transfusion. Vox Sang 59:119–22, 1990

66. Zaia JA: Epidemiology and pathogenesis of cytomegalovirus disease. Semin Hematol, suppl I. 27:5–10, 1990

67. Tegmeier GE: Posttransfusion cytomegalovirus infections. Arch Pathol Lab Med 113: 236–45, 1989

68. Domart Y, Trouillet JL, Fagon JY et al: Incidence and morbidity of cytomegalovirus infection in patients with mediastinitis following cardiac surgery. Chest 97:18–22, 1990

69. Freeman R, Gould FK, McMaster A: Management of cytomegalovirus antibody negative patients undergoing heart transplantation. J Clin Pathol 43:373–6, 1990

70. Anderson DJ, Jordan MC: Viral pneumonia in recipients of solid organ transplants. Semin Respir Infect 5:38–49, 1990

71. Dauber JH, Paradis IL, Dummer JS: Infectious complications in pulmonary allograft recipients. Clin Chest Med 11:291–308, 1990

72. Faulds D, Heel RC: Ganciclovir: a review of its antiviral activity pharmokinetic properties and therapeutic efficacy in cytomegalovirus infections. Drugs 39:597–638, 1990

73. Duncan SR, Cook DJ: Survival of ganciclovir-treated heart transplant recipients with cytomegalovirus pneumonitis. Transplantation 52: 910–3, 1991

74. Sayers MH, Anderson KC, Goodnough LT et al: Reducing the risk of transfusion-transmitted cytomegalovirus infection. Ann Intern Med 116:55–62, 1992

75. Merigan TC, Renglud DG, Keay S et al: A controlled trial of Ganciclovir to prevent cytomegalovirus disease after heart transplantation. N Engl J Med 326:1182–6, 1992

76. Balfour HH Jr, Chace BA, Stapleton JT et al: A randomized placebo-controlled trial of oral acyclovir for the prevention of cytomegalovirus disease in recipients of renal allograft. N Engl J Med 320:1381–7, 1989

77. Gerber P, Walsh JH, Rosenblum EN, Purcell RH: Association of EBV virus infection with the post perfusion syndrome. Lancet 1:593–5, 1969

78. William HD et al: Transmission of human parvovirus B19 by coagulation factor concentrates. Vox Sang 58:177–81, 1990

79. Goldman M, Blajchman MA: Blood product associated bacterial sepsis. Transfus Med Rev 5:73–83, 1991

80. Tipple MA, Bland LA, Murphy JJ et al: Sepsis associated with transfusion of red cells con-

taminated with *Yersinia enterocolitica*. Transfusion 30:207–13, 1990

81. Wells GM, Woodward TE, Fiset P, Hornick RB: Rocky mountain spotted fever caused by blood transfusion. JAMA 239:2763–5, 1978

82. Sakakibara T, Ida T, Mannouji E et al: Post-transfusion graft-versus-host disease following open heart surgery. Report of six cases. J Cardiovasc Surg 30:687–91, 1989

83. Juji T, Takahashi K, Shibata Y, Ide H et al: Post-transfusion graft-versus-host disease in immunocompetent patients after cardiac surgery in Japan. N Engl J Med 321:56–7, 1989

84. Altemeier WA, Burke JF, Pruirt BA Jr, Sandusky WR: Definitions and classifications of surgical infections p. 28. In Altemeier WA (ed): Manual on Control of Infection in Surgical Patients. 2nd Ed. JB Lippincott, Philadelphia, 1984

12

Neurologic Assessment and Outcome

Carin Hagberg
James Berry
Jeffrey Katz

During many forms of open heart surgery, the normal circulation to the brain undergoes various temporary changes that have either short-lived (common) or prolonged (uncommon) detrimental effects on normal neurologic function. In some circumstances (e.g., hypothermic circulatory arrest), the circulation to the brain is interrupted completely. It is not surprising that the literature contains numerous studies, reports, and anecdotes documenting a range of neurologic sequelae following cardiac surgery. These changes vary from minor and temporary to gross central nervous system (CNS) dysfunction that is permanent.

Over the past three decades, the performance of coronary artery bypass graft (CABG) surgery has become a routine procedure. As in most cardiac surgical procedures, CABG depends on the successful assumption of the heart's normal pump function by a machine. The pump-oxygenator is able to both pump and oxygenate the blood, allowing the surgeon to work in a quiescent environment.

Heart-lung machines (regardless of the method used to oxygenate) add their own special set of complicating factors that affect neurologic perfusion and function.

It is of major import that the sine qua non of anesthesiologists is to depress neurologic function temporarily in order to render patients insensate to pain, discomfort, or awareness during surgery. It is reasonable to assume that the various drugs and techniques used to achieve these goals can and do, in some cases, have lasting effects on neurologic function. Some of the temporary neurologic impairment is expected and regarded as a "necessary evil" accompanying general anesthesia. However, much of this impairment is unexpected and, even though temporary, causes considerable anxiety for patients and family members.

It is our obligation to search continually for causes, influential factors, and techniques that we might minimize, eliminate, or at least control these neurologic sequelae. This chapter attempts to present our current level of knowledge regarding these issues, offer an up-to-date summary on the types of neurologic injury observed in cardiac surgery, describe how we can make accurate diagnoses, and formulate the latest treatment regimens. Furthermore, this chapter discusses the factors that affect CNS perfusion and how best to monitor patients to prevent lapses in perfusion. Finally, we present a current but brief discussion on the subject of brain protection during cardiac surgery.

SCOPE OF THE PROBLEM

Each year approximately one-quarter of a million people undergo CABG surgery in the United States. An additional 50,000 per year require valve replacement. In a prospective study conducted in 1987, Shaw and associates[1] found that 4.8 percent of patients undergoing CABG had evidence of stroke (312 patients). In this same study, 78 patients (25 percent) had postoperative ophthalmologic abnormalities, including areas of retinal infarction in 54 (17 percent). In all, 191 patients (61 percent) had neurologic or neuropsychiatric complications. If these statistics are applied to the general population undergoing CABG surgery in the United States, approximately 150,000 patients will suffer a neurologic complication.

Slogoff et al.[2] presented in 1982 evidence that neuropsychiatric complications were more than twice as likely following "open ventricle" procedures such as valve replacements. Indeed, Shaw's study[1] found a 100 percent incidence of retinal microvascular occlusion during cardiopulmonary bypass (CPB) when bubble oxygenators were used. While these data could raise considerable alarm, there is great variability in the incidence as reported by different investigators.

Clearly, in those studies in which thorough preoperative and postoperative evaluations are performed, the incidences are higher.

This is probably related to improved detection of subtle changes when compared to the preoperative evaluation.[1-3] Additionally, many pathophysiologic changes do not have detectable clinical correlates, and clinicians might be underestimating the incidence of injury on this basis. Henricksen[4] measured regional cerebral blood flow (rCBF) in 37 patients before and after open heart surgery and found a general reduction of 15 to 20 percent during and after surgery. None of these patients had obvious postoperative deficits. The reduction in rCBF correlated with advanced age, duration of bypass, and low perfusion pressure[2,5] during bypass. It is widely accepted today that increased age,[2] open ventricle surgery,[2] pre-existing cerebrovascular disease,[2,6] and increased duration of bypass[2,4] are all factors that raise the incidence of neurologic dysfunction.

Pragmatism might lead the observer to conclude that if the majority of complications are either subclinical or temporary and the patient leaves the hospital intact, these complications are irrelevant and can be largely ignored. However, length of stay (both in the intensive care unit and in the hospital) and expensive therapeutic techniques (i.e., days on a ventilator, days on intravenous infusions, requirements for assist devices, and the need for expensive investigations) have become critical issues in evaluating outcome. The difference in cost between a 1-week stay and a 3-week stay with complications is considerable.

In a very pertinent study from 1989, Weintraub et al.[7] were able to demonstrate that patients with neurologic complications after CABG had two and one-half to three times the length of stay in the hospital. As the conservative management of coronary occlusive disease improves, it is likely that age and the presence of ancillary medical problems will either negatively impact the number of patients coming to CABG or, conversely, ensure that those patients undergoing CABG are at high risk of neurologic sequelae.

FACTORS AFFECTING CENTRAL NERVOUS SYSTEM PERFUSION DURING CARDIOPULMONARY ANESTHESIA

Cerebral Physiology

Cerebral blood flow (CBF) is normally 45 to 50 ml $\cdot$ 100 g^{-1} $\cdot$ min^{-1}, and cerebral oxygen consumption (CMRO$_2$) is 3 ml $\cdot$ 100 g^{-1} $\cdot$ min^{-1}. In normal individuals, a critical reduction in CBF occurs when mean blood pressure falls below 40 mmHg.[5] Although the primary determinant of CBF in the normal individual is usually cerebral metabolism (flow-metabolism coupling), CBF and oxygen delivery are influenced by an extraordinary variety of interacting factors, including blood pressure, central venous pressure (CVP), intracranial pressure (ICP), cardiac output (CO), PCO$_2$, pH, PO$_2$, hemoglobin (Hb) concentration, hematocrit (Hct), blood viscosity, vasoactive compounds (endogenous and exogenous), temperature, cerebral metabolic rate (CMR), and direct innervation of the cerebral vessels.[8] The coupling of CBF to metabolism allows a balance between local nutrient supply and metabolic demands of the brain; ischemia occurs when there is an imbalance. It is very difficult to determine or predict at what point ischemia occurs because of the multiple interacting factors mentioned.

Autoregulation is a term used by several investigators describing the hemodynamic regulation of flow in response to changes in perfusion pressure aside from flow-to-metabolism coupling.[9] Research on CBF autoregulation in the patient undergoing cardiac surgery is extremely important, since there is much discussion in the literature of absolute ischemic flow thresholds. Hypoperfusion and ischemia may result from either focal, regional, or global ischemia, yet the metabolic consequences of reduced CBF are similar. Both the degree and duration of an ischemic flow reduction determine the possible development of cerebral infarction.[10] During CPB, anesthesia and moderate hypothermia combine to reduce CMRO$_2$ markedly to 10 to 30 percent of normal. However, the changes in CBF associated with hypothermic perfusion depend on which of the two acid-base management strategies are currently employed.

Pathophysiology

CNS complications following cardiac surgery have been attributed to many risk factors, several of which remain controversial. These risk factors may be categorized as those related to the patient, surgical procedure, extracorporeal circuit, or management of bypass[11] (Table 12-1). Although there are certain inherent neurologic risks associated with CPB and cardiac surgery, the factors listed in Table 12-1 add to them.[12]

The incidence of neurologic complications after CABG increases markedly with age and is disproportionate to the risk of cardiac complications.[13] Older patients may have more

Table 12-1. Possible Determinants of Neurologic Outcome Following Cardiopulmonary Bypass

Patient selection
Elderly
Prior neurologic disease
Aortic atherosclerosis
Left ventricular thrombosis or dysfunction
Individual patient tolerance
Surgical procedure
Open (valve/aneurysm) versus closed (CABG)
Aortic cannulae placement
Extracoporeal circuit
Membrane oxygenation
Arterial filtration
Pulsatile flow
CPB duration >2 hours
Bypass management
Blood-gas management
Hypotension
Hypothermia
Hemodilution
Glucose

Abbreviations: CABG, coronary artery bypass graft; CPB, cardiopulmonary bypass.

extensive peripheral vascular disease, placing them at higher risk not only of macroembolism during CABG,[2,14,15] but also of a decrease in regional cerebral perfusion.[16–18]

Slogoff et al.[2] reported in 1982 that patients older than 60 years suffered 4.5 times the neurologic complications as those below age 60. Although these investigators offered no explanation for the relationship between age and neurologic dysfunction, they noted that, with increasing age, cerebral response to both extrinsic and intrinsic stimuli is altered independent of any cerebrovascular disease and that subclinical cerebrovascular disease is probably age related. In a more recent prospective study by Tuman et al.,[19] the incidence of postoperative neurologic deficits was significantly greater in patients over 75 years of age. When compared to those patients aged 65 to 74 years, the incidence was twice as high and in patients under 65 years of age it was nine times higher. Since the average age of patients undergoing cardiac surgery is increasing, the risk of major neurologic complications is expected to rise concomitantly.

Prior neurologic symptoms, including stroke and transient ischemic attacks (TIAs) appear to increase the risk of neurologic dysfunction significantly following cardiac surgery.[20–22] Patients who are neurologically symptomatic may be more susceptible to cerebral ischemia secondary to more severe cerebral atherosclerosis, impaired cerebral autoregulation, and poor collateral perfusion.[23] Asymptomatic carotid artery disease, on the other hand, does not increase the likelihood of the development of acute neurologic complications in patients undergoing cardiac surgery.[24–27] This is consistent with data in noncardiac surgical patients.[28]

Management of patients with carotid atherosclerosis who must undergo a procedure requiring CPB is often problematic. In general, the presence of a symptomatic carotid bruit requires evaluation by ultrasound imaging of the carotid artery, and possibly cerebral arteriography. If severe stenosis is demonstrated (i.e., when lumen area is reduced by more than 70 percent or diameter is reduced by more than 50 percent), carotid endarterectomy (CEA), either before or during cardiac surgery, may be necessary. It is unreasonable to dictate a uniform approach for those patients with both carotid and coronary occlusive disease. The approach must take into account both the risks (potential hazards of a staged versus a combined surgical approach) and benefits (one operation versus two), as well as the severity of the disease in either system.[29]

The timing of CEA and CABG is controversial. It makes good sense that patients experiencing both TIAs and unstable angina should undergo simultaneous CEA and CABG, whereas in patients with active TIAs and stable angina, CEA (possibly under regional anesthesia) before CABG is recommended. Also, in a patient with an asymptomatic carotid artery lesion and unstable angina, CABG before CEA is recommended.[13] It is generally agreed that there is little benefit in subjecting patients with an asymptomatic carotid bruit to prophylactic CEA.[21,29–35]

By contrast, in patients who are symptomatic, the decision must be as to which approach, combined versus staged, would be best individualized to the patient. One must also consider whether the carotid disease is unilateral or bilateral. Patients with unilateral carotid disease and coronary artery disease experience a similar incidence of completed stroke when managed by either staged or combined procedures. The incidence of stroke in these patients is similar to the incidence of stroke in a large series of CABG patients.[30] Both Hertzer et al.[36] and Mehigan et al.[37] concluded that the staged approach is reserved for patients with severe carotid occlusive disease (especially when bilateral) and less severe coronary artery disease. In a more recent and intensive review of combined CEA/CABG, Rizzo et al.[38] found it to be a very useful procedure for those with extensive atherosclerosis (59 percent had bilateral carotid stenosis) with benefits including long-term protection from ipsilateral stroke, the avoidance of subsequent hospitalization, and the imposition of additional anesthetic periods during which the patient is at high risk of either perioperative stroke or myocardial infarction. However, the combined procedure involves the performance of CEA, followed immediately by CABG, which requires anticoagulation and possibly perioperative hypotension; thus, it has been slow to gain widespread acceptance.

The Patient

Another possible determinant of neurologic outcome following CPB is the status of the patient's ascending aorta, which usually must be cannulated, cross-clamped and manipulated during the procedure. During any of these maneuvers, cholesterol or calcific plaque debris may become dislodged and act as emboli.[39,40] Presumably, aortic atherosclerosis increases the risk of neurologic injury. This premise is based on the rate of cerebral embolization during instrumentation of the aorta and the onset of bypass.[24] Since aortic manipulation is necessary in both open (valve, aneurysm) and closed (CABG) cardiac procedures, the risk of particulate embolization in these types of procedures should be similar, except for the additional risk of embolized valve fragments and air. Severe atherosclerosis of the ascending aorta (present in at least 84 percent of cardiac surgery patients) is possibly the major mechanism of focal stroke and thus CNS morbidity.[23,41]

Transcranial Doppler studies recently demonstrated frequent cerebral embolization during cannulation of the ascending aorta and with the initiation of bypass.[42] Clinical recognition of atherosclerosis in the ascending aorta before cannulation is difficult, which has led to the use of intraoperative ultrasonography (for a full discussion, see Ch. 14). Barzilai et al.[43] demonstrated the efficacy of aortic ultrasonography, in which its use resulted in altered surgical strategy in 12 to 25 percent of patients. Alterations included changes in sites of cannulation, cross-clamping, proximal anastomosis, cardioplegia insertion, resection of the ascending aorta during profound hypothermic circulatory arrest, as well as alternate surgical approaches.[13] The implicit assumption is that these alterations might reduce the incidence of intraoperative emboli. Various centers have begun to use intraoperative ultrasonography to identify and avoid atheromatous sections of the ascending aorta.[42] Transesophageal echocardiography (TEE) has also been able to demonstrate atherosclerotic changes in the aorta during cardiac surgery but has not been widely used to date for this purpose.[13]

Recent studies are examining the relationship of left ventricular performance to neurologic dysfunction following cardiac surgery.[1,23,25,44] All studies agree that if preoperative ventricular function is poor, the incidence of neurologic complications increases.

The literature is almost evenly divided regarding the incidence of neurologic deficits when comparing open versus closed cardiac procedures.[2,45–47] Open chamber procedures including valve replacement or repair, ventricular aneurysm resection, or closure of a septal defect theoretically have a higher incidence of neurologic injury because of embolization of valve fragments, clot, and intraventricular air once ejection has resumed.[24] Slogoff et al.[44] found that open chamber procedures carried twice the incidence of both transient and persistent dysfunction when compared to closed chamber procedures. By contrast, Topal et al.[48] found that the severity of neurologic outcome was indistinguishable despite a greater incidence and severity of intracardiac bubbles in valve replacement patients as compared to CABG patients. In a large retrospective study performed by Kuroda et al.[49] comparing CABG and AVR, the major factors affecting CNS complications after surgery were pre-existing cerebrovascular disease and CPB time, rather than the difference in these two procedures per se.

Cardiopulmonary Bypass Circuit

Efforts to decrease the risk of neurologic complications during cardiac surgery assume that various technical or physiologic details of CPB are important determinants of neurologic outcome. Thus, changes in the components of the CPB circuit itself including membrane rather than bubble-oxygenators and microfilters in both the arterial pump line and cardiotomy return have been implemented. These measures would have little impact on direct embolization from the surgical field but might reduce air and particulate microemboli from possible circuit sources.[50–52] It is unlikely that even the most current bypass device is capable of eliminating all embolic events. Furthermore, the evidence that there is a reduction in the actual incidence of neurologic dysfunction following equipment changes is equivocal.

Blauth et al.[53] investigated the incidence of retinal microvascular lesions (consistent with microvascular occlusion) in patients undergoing CABG using either a bubble or membrane oxygenator. They detected a trend toward more severe retinal microvascular lesions and neurophysical deficits in the bubble-oxygenator group. High flow rates, low-reservoir volumes, or high gas flows can increase bubble release with bubble oxygenators. The cause appears to be related to the blood-gas interface and, since the membrane oxygenator has no such interface, it is less embologenic.[54]

Regardless of which system is chosen (bubble or membrane), the most crucial factor in reducing emboli to the patient appears to be the use of microfilters in the arterial pump line and cardiotomy return. Muraoka et al.[55] demonstrated fewer abnormalities on postoperative computed tomography (CT) scans in patients with a 20-μm pore filter in comparison to a 40-μm pore filter. Elevated levels of brain-specific enzymes, such as creatine phosphokinase-BB, were demonstrated in patients undergoing open heart surgery[56–58] and prevented with the use of an arterial filter in dogs.[59] Others have suggested that arterial filtration can reduce neurologic and neuropsychological dysfunction following cardiac surgery.[47,60] The benefits of arterial line filtration have been confirmed in several reports using Doppler or TEE detection of reduced quantities of microemboli[61–65] or improved patient scores on neuropsychological tests following CPB.[66] The use of arterial and cardiotomy filtration is now virtually routine in the United States, and its use is increasing.

Whether pulsatile versus nonpulsatile flow provides advantages in preserving cerebral function is a controversial issue. There are various methods of producing pulsatile flow, but the two most common are the newer roller pumps that are able to rotate at varying speeds and partial CPB with the use of an intra-aortic balloon pump (IABP).[67] Theoretical advantages of pulsatile flow include improved renal function and enhanced lymph flow.[68–70] Some data suggest improvement in neurologic outcome with pulsatile flow,[71–76] although most clinical studies have failed to show any significant clinical differences between the two techniques.[21,77–80] In any event, the controversy over the two techniques needs further clarification and is likely to continue.

Increasing bypass duration, especially greater than 2 hours, may also be important in determining neurologic outcome following cardiac surgery. Again, the literature is divided as to whether there is a relationship between duration of perfusion and the incidence of neurologic deficits. Gardner et al.[16] found that the risk of perioperative stroke was three times greater if the duration of CPB exceeded 120 minutes. Among the possible explanations for this finding include prolonged duration may reflect a greater degree of difficulty in the operation and a higher likelihood of particulate embolization, and microaggregates in the perfusion may increase in size with prolonged bypass duration.[2] On the other hand, recent studies have not demonstrated an association between bypass duration and neurologic or neuropsychological outcome.[45,81,82]

Bypass Management

What represents optimal management of $PaCO_2$ for patients undergoing hypothermic CPB has been the subject of numerous studies and has long been debated. For decades, physiologists and clinicians alike have attempted to define normal levels of $PaCO_2$ and pH under hypothermic conditions. Theoretical concerns principally involve the effect of CO_2 on CBF: hypocarbia results in cerebral hypoperfusion, whereas hypercarbia increases CBF and may predispose patients to cerebral microembolism.[83] Two approaches have been advocated (Table 12-2).

The pH-stat strategy maintains a pH near 7.4, as the patient's body temperature varies by the addition of CO_2 to the pump. Since CO_2 solubility in plasma is greater with hypothermia, pH-stat management produces relative hypercarbia and acidemia as compared to α-stat management. Using this form of management, autoregulation is abolished and CBF becomes pressure dependent, thus allowing a further excess of CBF over metabolic requirements, so-called "luxury perfusion." Such unregulated CBF may either cause a "steal" phenomenon or increase microemboli to the brain.[4,84,85]

The α-stat method of acid-base management is a more recent strategy that appears to be more popular.[86] In contrast to the pH-stat strategy, it maintains a constant $PaCO_2$ of 40 mmHg and pH of 7.4 at 37°C, regardless of body temperature. In addition, it is associated with maintained CO_2 responsiveness and intact cerebral autoregulation. Luxury perfusion of the brain also occurs with this method, since the reduction of oxygen delivery attributable to hypothermia is less than the reduction of the brain's metabolic needs.[84,87] α-Stat management is criticized because of the possibility of critical CBF limitations. Measurements of cerebral venous oxygen saturation are less than 70 percent in one-third of cases.[88]

Whether blood-gas management influences neurologic or neuropsychological outcome in patients undergoing CPB or deep hypothermic circulatory arrest remains to be seen. Prough et al.[11] suggest that resolution of this matter will require correlation of neuropsychological endpoints with measured circulatory and metabolic changes in individual patients in these settings. Bashein et al.[89] failed to demonstrate any correlation between the two strategies and postoperative neurologic outcome, although it is unlikely that this study alone will settle the issue.

Blood pressure is another factor that may affect neurologic outcome. Early studies regarding outcome and mean arterial pressure (MAP) during CPB indicated a higher incidence of cerebral complications in patients with "low" arterial pressures and that in order

Table 12-2.   Different Approaches to Blood-Gas Management in Cardiopulmonary Bypass

	pH-Stat	α-Stat
pH	Respiratory alkalosis (7.5)	Normal (7.4)
$PaCO_2$	Relative hypercarbia	Normal (40 mmHg)
Temperature correction	Corrected at 28°C	Uncorrected at 37°C
Relationship of cerebral metabolic rate and metabolism	Uncoupled	Coupled
Autoregulation	Impaired	Intact
Luxury perfusion	Yes; intracerebral steal	Yes
Hypothetical concern	Increased proportion of embolic debris to the brain, rather than systemic circulation	Critical hypoperfusion in selected patients

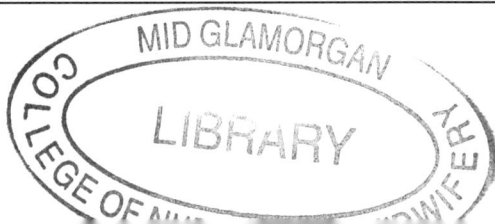

to prevent cerebral dysfunction, a MAP greater than 50 mmHg should be maintained.[50,90] Perfusion pressure during CPB is related to the composition of the pump prime and the resulting hematocrit. Low perfusion pressure may not necessarily reflect low perfusion flow but rather only acutely reduced perfusate viscosity.[45,91]

Stockard et al.[50] were the first to suggest an association between hypotension and an increased incidence or severity of cerebral injury. Several recent studies, on the other hand, have not found an association between MAP during CPB and neurologic outcome.[45,84,92,93] The discrepancy may be related to the fact that early studies used pH-stat blood-gas management, whereas the more recent work has used α-stat management during CPB. Studies are lacking that correlate actual measurements of CBF and cerebral outcome or that determine whether patients managed at low versus high perfusion pressures are at higher risk of neuropsychological deficits. Individual differences in patient tolerance to bypass make it difficult to define safe thresholds universally for either flow or pressure.

Many of the studies concerning adequacy of perfusion pressure were performed in conjunction with hypothermia.[94] Murkin et al.[84] found CBF to be independent of an MAP of 30 to 100 mmHg during hypothermic bypass. Feddersen et al.[95] found that cerebral metabolism was maintained by increased oxygen extraction when CBF decreased at MAPs of up to 30 mmHg during hypothermic bypass. These findings are consistent with additional studies[45,92] that support the concept that, in the absence of cerebrovascular disease, CBF is adequately maintained during hypothermic bypass with cerebral perfusion pressure as low as 35 to 40 mmHg.

This may not be the case during normothermic bypass. Since there has been a recent trend in cardiac surgery toward normothermic bypass in combination with warm retrograde cardioplegia, additional outcome studies are indicated to assess the effect of temperature during CPB on neurologic and neuropsychological function. If the predominant mechanisms of neurologic injury are confined to time intervals when the brain is warm (i.e., outside of CPB), outcome studies comparing hypothermic versus normothermic CPB techniques should be equivocal.[24] Indeed, in a recent study, Wong et al.[96] showed that CNS dysfunction, as assessed by psychomotor and memory testing, is comparable between normothermic and hypothermic techniques.

Hemodilution is employed during CPB for several reasons. It reduces the need for donor blood utilization, compensates for hypothermia-induced increases in blood viscosity, and finally may improve tissue oxygen delivery. Several studies demonstrate that cerebral oxygen supply and demand relationships are well preserved at 27°C with hematocrits in the mid-20s.[97,98] The manner in which viscosity and hematocrit-related changes in arterial oxygen content interact with perfusion pressure is unknown.[2,29]

Hemodilution may improve perfusion in areas of low flow (i.e., those subject to cerebral ischemia) possibly leading to improvements in neurologic outcome. Although a minimum acceptable hematocrit has yet to be defined, hematocrits less than 30 percent following CPB induce cerebral vasodilation and increase oxygen extraction in order to maintain cerebral oxygen delivery.[99] Areas of cerebral ischemia might be compromised at low hematocrits, since they have limited vasodilatory or oxygen extraction reserve.

Shaw et al.[1] found that acute neurologic and neuropsychological outcome was significantly worse in patients whose hematocrit was reduced to the greatest extent. Theoretically, blood with hematocrits of 15 to 20 percent carry sufficient oxygen to maintain CNS function (if fully saturated), and lower values may be safe if CBF can increase to compensate for the reduced oxygen content.

Protocols that employ predetermined flows or pressures to achieve adequate cerebral perfusion and that fail to make allowance for impediments to cerebral flow are dangerous. Higher pressures may be required in those patients with carotid occlusive disease or cases in which hematocrits of less than 20 percent are expected. In addition, an assessment of cerebral function such as electroencephalographic (EEG) monitoring may be warranted in such situations.[29]

Glucose management during CPB is also a controversial subject. Hyperglycemia is common during CPB and is usually ignored. Many clinicians make the assumption that hyperglycemia can be protective, since it may provide added metabolic substrate even in the presence of reduced O_2 delivery.[29] Several studies, however, demonstrate an association between hyperglycemia and worsened neurologic outcome.[100,101]

The basis for this concern is that hyperglycemia provides more glucose for anaerobic metabolism to occur, resulting in the development of increased intracellular acidosis. This acidosis, in turn, initiates a cascade of secondary processes that result in permanent neurologic injury.[102] Other studies challenge the doctrine that hyperglycemia is deleterious.

Metz and Keats[103] reported that aggravation of hyperglycemia using a glucose-containing priming solution did not increase postoperative neurologic injury and had the beneficial effect of reducing intraoperative fluid requirements as well as improving perioperative fluid balance. There are no prospective outcome studies that demonstrate a detrimental effect of hyperglycemia during cardiac surgery. Even in the setting of acute stroke, no definitive recommendations have been made concerning the use of glucose or glucose-lowering therapies at this time.[104] Although hypoglycemia can be dangerous and should be avoided, many centers do avoid administration of glucose-containing solutions in the intravenous fluids of the CPB patient during cardiac surgery.

MONITORING OF CEREBRAL FUNCTION

Several methods of evaluating cerebral injury are becoming more and more sophisticated with time. Thus far, only a few techniques can be employed during cardiac surgery in a manner that may have an immediate impact on the procedure.

During cardiac surgery, CBF can be measured by using externally placed scintillation or γ detectors and radioactive xenon-133. Although application of these techniques to patients undergoing CPB has improved our understanding of factors influencing CBF, often this information is not obtained in a timely enough fashion to allow for corrective action in individual cases.

The most recent development in CBF measurement has included tomographic methods that are three-dimensional. Nonradioactive stable xenon (sXe) CT uses approximately 30 percent inhaled concentrations of radiodense xenon gas along with rapid sequential CT scanning.[105] Although CT scanners are accessible and can give quantitive measurements of CBF, their routine use for this purpose is limited because of possible anesthetic side effects, significant radiation exposure, and cost.

CT scanning is more commonly used when a new and persistent focal neurologic defect is identified postoperatively in order to locate an extracranial mass legion or vascular anomaly. A newly ischemic area may appear normal for hours to days[106]; therefore, a negative CT scan in this period does not exclude the diagnosis of stroke.

Magnetic resonance imaging (MRI) uses paramagnetic tracers that can be excited in a magnetic field. Clinical investigations of cerebral transit time (and thus indirectly CBF and CBV) are possible with the use of standard intravascular MRI contrast agents and rapid sampling.[107] Many cardiac surgery patients develop postoperative MRI abnormalities characteristic of cerebral ischemia even in the absence of corresponding focal neurologic deficits, so that unless MRI is routinely performed, the abnormality may go undiagnosed. The use of both pre- and postoperative MRI evaluations can provide an excellent resource for research data. Because of its resolution and ability to correlate CBF with structural information, MRI may become the "gold standard" for CBF measurement.

Intraoperative EEG monitoring can be of value during cardiac surgery, although its routine use is debatable. At the present time, the EEG provides the only reliable technique for neurologic evaluation of the anesthetized patient and offers the potential for corrective action in the clinical setting. Problems with electrical interference and the need for additional personnel to interpret the massive quantity of data have limited the widespread use of the multichannel EEG. Technologic advances have made EEG monitoring more convenient to use and interpret, permitting the collection of useful data during cardiac surgery. EEG abnormalities can occur as a consequence of several reasons, including embolism (gaseous or particulate), hypoxia, aortic dissection at the cannulation site, reduced perfusion pressure or flow, and impaired venous drainage.[13] Nevertheless, there are significant limitations to EEG monitoring, and it has yet to be determined in large clinical trials whether it can improve patient outcome.

Evoked potentials have been employed at some centers to monitor cerebral function during cardiac surgery. They represent computer averaging of the brain's electrical response to repetitive external stimuli. Its use is limited because access to certain areas of the brain is limited and it is technically demanding.[11]

Ultrasonic devices, including transcranial, transesophageal, and Doppler flow, as well as echo machines are becoming very popular as monitors during cardiac surgery. These noninvasive techniques offer promise in the elucidation of mechanisms and evaluation of interventions related to adverse neurologic and neuropsychological outcome as mentioned earlier in regard to assessment of the aorta. Transcranial Doppler signals are directed through the temporal bone, which enables continuous measurement of flow velocity in the middle temporal artery, providing a qualititative gauge of cerebral perfusion.

Newer Doppler equipment that will be able to separate gaseous from particulate emboli and quantite embolic events should be extremely useful. Intraoperative TEE is also a sensitive method for the detection of intravascular as well as intraventricular bubbles, especially during open chamber procedures[108,109] (see Ch. 14). Although precise quantification of the amount of retained air is not possible using TEE, the qualitative estimates obtained may be clinically useful, specifically with regard to assessment of air removal techniques during open chamber procedures.

As mentioned previously, Blauth et al.[53,110] used intraoperative retinal fluorescein angiography in an investigation designed to assess the superiority of membrane oxygenators. The retina provides an in vivo window to the microcirculatory bed within the CNS. Fluorescein enhances small retinal vessels that are not normally distinguishable because of the red reflex of the optic fundus. Blauth and colleagues observed retinal microvascular occlusions in 100 percent of patients undergoing CPB with a bubble-oxygenator and significantly fewer lesions with the use of a membrane oxygenator. These investigators demonstrated that the extent of retinal ischemic lesions can be quantified by digital image analysis, which in turn can be applied to comparative studies of perfusion equipment and techniques.

Technology similar to that used in pulse oximetry is being developed to monitor cerebral oxygenation. Near-infrared spectroscopy provides a continuous noninvasive measure of cerebral hemoglobin oxygen saturation that may explain and help prevent neurologic complications. The cerebral oximeters consist of a single probe placed on the forehead that measures the ratio of oxyhemoblobin and deoxyhemoglobin in the brain. Near-infrared light penetrates the tissues to a few centimeters depth and, thus, the measurements are taken from the brain. Cerebral oximetry is under investigation and evaluation. Although its applications have not been delineated, it is hoped that it will have a place in monitoring patients at high risk of cerebral hypoperfusion.

NEUROLOGIC FUNCTION AND DYSFUNCTION

Mechanism of Injury

The neurologic insults seen after CPB are presumably referable to alterations in CBF or distribution, with resultant ischemia. Ischemic insults can be classified as global, focal, or secondary (Table 12-3).

Global cerebral hypoperfusion, although certainly a catastrophic complication of CPB, is relatively uncommon and is usually related to obvious problems with equipment or technique. There are reports claiming global CNS dysfunction after otherwise routine CPB procedures,[50,111] however, numerous studies of CBF during CPB have demonstrated favorable hemodynamic factors. Using temperature-uncorrected measurement of $PaCO_2$, coupling of CBF and cerebral oxygen utilization were found to be preserved within the normal range of perfusion pressures during

Table 12-3. Cerebral Events After Cardiopulmonary Bypass

Ischemic insults
  Global
    Hypoperfusion
    Massive embolization
    Vascular occlusion
  Focal
    Embolization
      Atheroma
      Valvular calcification
      Thrombi
      Air
      Fat
      Platelet aggregates
      Fibrin
      Plastic fragments (from CPB circuit)
    Regional hypoperfusion due to
      Atherosclerotic disease
      Abnormal vascular anatomy
  Secondary
    Cerebral edema

CPB.[84] Cerebral autoregulation is also preserved under the same "α-stat" management of PaCO2.[4,77,84,85]

A large clinical study concluded that decreased perfusion was not related to postoperative neurologic impairment.[23] Another large, prospective study concluded that there was no relationship between MAP during CPB and neurologic outcome.[83] In a series of 504 adult patients studied by Slogoff,[44] the correlation between perfusion pressure and flow with signs of cerebral or renal hypoperfusion found no relationship between low pressure (or flow) during CPB and new onset of renal or CNS impairment. These investigators concluded that episodes of circulatory failure occurring before or after CPB were the major cause of postoperative renal and CNS dysfunction.[46]

Hypoperfusion is an unavoidable component of procedures involving controlled circulatory arrest during CPB. Although performed under deep hypothermia (as low as 15° to 20°C), experimental evidence shows that prolonged circulatory arrest exposes the brain to a significant ischemic insult.[112–114] This will produce clinical signs of diffuse hypoxic or ischemic brain injury ranging from prolonged awakening and subtle neuropsychiatric changes to coma, seizure activity, and myoclonus.

Global hypoperfusion can also be produced by massive embolization of thrombus, atheroma, or gas. Such macroembolization can be the result of aortic cannulation, disruption of valvular deposits, or post-bypass ejection of ventricular air or thrombus.[1] Catastrophic air embolization may also occur as a result of defects in the integrity of the CPB circuit. These patients will suffer both the immediate and delayed consequences of cerebral ischemia, depending on the severity of the insult and on whether immediate recognition and treatment were possible. In these patients where gross air embolization is suspected, immediate hyperbaric oxygen therapy may be life-saving.

Focal hypoperfusion is, by far, the most common mechanism of brain injury during and after CPB. A pathologic study of the brains of 206 patients who died after CPB demonstrated evidence of fibrin or platelet microemboli in 7 to 20 percent of cases. Fat emboli were detected in 32 to 78 percent of cases, while control brains showed 10 to 30 percent. Microemboli, along with perivascular hemorrhage and neuronal necrosis, represented a triad of findings representative of post-bypass cerebral injury.[115] Other animal studies have demonstrated profuse production of microemboli by traditional bubble oxygenators, correlating with a reduction of CBF and cerebral oxygen metabolism. These findings are ameliorated significantly by the use of arterial filters in the CPB circuit.[116]

Now that membrane oxygenators and arterial filters are in routine use in many institutions, pump-associated sources of microemboli should not be a major factor in post-bypass cerebral ischemia. However, the potential for embolization of atheroma, thrombus, or air associated with aortic cannulation, surgical manipulation, or post-bypass cardiac activity remains a significant technical problem in cardiac surgery.

Secondary cerebral ischemia is an unusual phenomenon during or after CPB. Ischemic insults classified as "secondary" would be those due to hypoperfusion following cerebral edema and secondary increases in intracranial pressure. Cerebral edema may result from primary ischemia (usually requiring a large infarct to be clinically significant) or from electrolyte abnormalities (hyponatremia with associated decrease in intravascular osmolarity).

So far, only a few factors have been associated positively with less than optimal neurologic outcome after CPB. These include prolonged bypass times, open chamber procedures, increased age, and, possibly, profound and prolonged hypotension.[50,93]

Neurologic Assessment of Postoperative Patients

One of the most difficult aspects of post-bypass care is the early recognition of an adverse neurologic event. Emergence from the

Table 12-4. Common Neurologic Abnormalities After Anesthesia

Cranial nerves
  Pupillary light response depressed or absent
  Lid reflex depressed
  Eye opening difficult
Spinal reflexes
  Hyperreflexia
    Biceps
    Quadriceps
  Clonus (sustained and unsustained) ankle
  Babinski
Generalized
  Decerebrate posturing
  Myoclonus
  Opisthotonos
  Increased muscle tone
  Shivering
  Seizures
  Extrapyramidal reactions

effects of anesthesia after cardiac surgery complicates and delays careful neurologic assessment. Even after noncardiac surgery, emergence times are highly variable, and delayed arousal is more commonly due to residual anesthetic effects than to neurologic injury.[117] Three to 9 percent of general surgical patients may be "unarousable" after up to 90 minutes of recovery.[117,118]

Another confounding factor is that neurologically intact patients may exhibit abnormal reflexes during emergence from anesthesia (Table 12-4). Areflexia in cranial nerves and peripheral hyperreflexia are common in the early emergence phase and, even in fully awake patients, reflex abnormalities may persist.[119,120] This is most common following inhalation-based anesthetics, although it can occur following any technique.[119]

There are reflex abnormalities not attributable to drug effects. They include the snout, grasp, palmomental, and Hoffman reflexes. Much emphasis has been placed on the appearance of these "primitive reflexes" as signs of diffuse cortical injury.[21,121] Although nonspecific and present in some normal patients,[122] they are associated with an increased incidence of cerebral dysfunction.[123]

Early neurologic examination must, of necessity, be focused on gross evaluation of motor function, responsiveness, and reflexes. Even in the presence of abnormal reflexes, asymmetry should be sought as an early indicator of focal dysfunction.

There are significant obstacles to cooperation in the postoperative cardiac patient; the effects of physical limitations inherent in modern surgical and intensive care intervention must be considered during neurologic evaluation (Table 12-5). Residual pharmacologic effects are often invoked as a limitation to early postoperative assessment. Although patient responses vary, it should be possible to perform a limited assessment on most cardiac patients within 1 hour of the end of surgery.

Although a few centers attempt to awaken fully and extubate patients at the completion of surgery, cardiac patients will usually remain artificially ventilated for a number of hours.[124-126] Postoperative analgesia is usually provided with opiate agonists such as fentanyl or morphine. The analgesic properties of these agents also provide some control of airway reflexes stimulated by the presence of an endotracheal tube. Unconsciousness may effectively be extended well into recovery by either administering sedative or hypnotic agents early in the recovery period or by using long-acting agents near the end of the surgical procedure. This procedure will inevitably delay the neurologic assessment of the patient. Is should not be necessary to routinely delay the return of consciousness to

achieve the immediate goals of postoperative recovery (hemodynamic stability and freedom from pain, agitation, or other stressors) (see Ch. 15).

Patient cooperation with neurologic assessment is essential for a complete examination. Numerous physical factors may limit the patient's ability to respond appropriately. These include surgical drains and dressings, as well as monitoring catheters, wires, and respiratory equipment. Tracheal intubation limits the patient's ability to provide verbal responses although, in an awake patient, notes written by the patient provide strong evidence of intact cognitive and motor skills.

The initial screening neurologic assessment should be performed as soon as the patient is able to respond to command. Earlier assessment is usually limited to pain-elicited responses such as avoidance or posturing; in the presence of significant opiate levels, these responses (or lack of responses) are not reliable. Level of consciousness, gross motor responses, and yes or no responses to simple questioning are sufficient at an early stage to verify that no catastrophic CNS damage has occurred.

Failure of a patient to arouse sufficiently to allow even gross neurologic evaluation should prompt an active search for etiologic factors. Anesthetic effects should be reversed if possible; drug interaction that would slow the elimination of anesthetic agents should be considered. Benzodiazepine and neuromuscular blocking drugs will produce prolonged unresponsiveness; both are amenable to reversal and should be the first consideration in the unresponsive patient. Opiate antagonists are more problematic. Significant morbidity may accompany the indiscriminate use of naloxone[127] and residual opiates are rarely the primary cause of postoperative coma.

Hypothermia must be sought and treated. Temperatures below 34°C are associated with changes in mental state, including obtundation, hyporeflexia, stupor, and coma.[128] CBF decreases due to increased vascular re-

Table 12-5. Obstacles to Postoperative Neurologic Assessment

Drug effects
    Somnolence
    Poor cooperation
    Inattentiveness
Physical factors
    Intubation
    IV tubing
    Monitors
    Surgical apparatus (e.g., drains, tubes)
Pain

sistance[129] will aggravate any preexisting ischemic insult.

The patient's medical history should be reviewed for any evidence of cerebrovascular disease, bleeding diathesis or malignancy. Undiagnosed cerebral tumors have been discovered after unexpected changes in mental state following cardiac surgery. One dramatic example is the case of a patient with an undiagnosed pituitary adenoma presenting with obtundation and right-sided cranial nerve palsies after CPB. CT of the brain revealed infarction of the pituitary tumor, a diagnosis of pituitary apoplexy following CPB was reported (one of eight cases in the literature).[130-133] It is postulated that abnormalities in the blood supply to neoplasia render them more susceptible to hypoperfusion and ischemia during CPB, as well as to the (more common) spontaneous infarction.[134-136]

In summary, the neurologic course of the patient after CPB is impacted by the ability of the intensivist to recognize quickly and treat any evidence of global or focal cerebral hypoperfusion. It is imperative that emergence from anesthesia not be delayed in order to assess and intervene expediently, should any CNS dysfunction be apparent.

Neurologic Assessment

After apparently full recovery from the acute effects of anesthesia and surgery, subtle defects in cognitive function may become detectable in patients subjected to CPB. These abnormalities may be transient or persistent but are quantifiable by neuropsychological tools. A number of different intellectual and cognitive domains may be assessed with specific examinations. Many of these require the dedicated presence of a trained psychologist. More detailed information about the correlation of clinical states and ischemic events (e.g., the correlation of an affective depression with a left anterior watershed infarcts)[137] is becoming available. A detailed assessment of the methodologic issues in

neuropsychological testing is available in the work of Murkin and Martzke.[138]

In many of the series reviewed, the deficit in cognitive function was most obvious from 7 days to 7 months postoperatively, with a relative return to baseline at 1 to 2 years after cardiac surgery.[45,133,139] However, one study showed an increasing difference at the 5-year follow-up.[139] It is becoming clear that the neurologic deficits and the cognitive disability seen after CPB have distinct differences in time course and resolution.[140] This implies a different pathophysiology and mechanism of injury between the two entities. It is hoped that further clinical study will elucidate the mechanisms of CPB-associated cognitive deficits.

CONCLUSION

The effect of CPB on the CNS is a subject that has received a great deal of attention in both past and recent literature. While there remains considerable debate concerning specific CPB techniques as they relate to the patient's neurologic outcome, research and education should increase our understanding of this topic and further reduce levels of morbidity and mortality. Much progress has been made by paying attention to all the possible determinants of neurologic dysfunction and should continue with the use of the more advanced modalities of CNS monitoring. Further outcome studies are necessary that carefully define neurologic and neuropsychological endpoints with measured cerebral, circulatory, and metabolic changes during CPB.

REFERENCES

1. Shaw PJ, Bates D, Cartlidge NEF et al: Neurologic and neuropsychological morbidity following major surgery: comparison of coronary artery bypass and peripheral vascular surgery. Stroke 18:700–7, 1987
2. Slogoff S, Girgis KZ, Keats AS: Etiologic factors in neuropsychiatric complications asso-

ciated with cardiopulmonary bypass. Anesth Analg 61:903–11, 1982

3. Nussmeier NA, Arlund C, Slogoff S: Neuropsychiatric complications after cardiopulmonary bypass: cerebral protection by a barbiturate. Anesthesiology 64:165–70, 1986

4. Henriksen L: Brain luxury perfusion during cardiopulmonary bypass in humans: a study of the cerebral blood flow response to changes in CO_2, O_2, and blood pressure. J Cereb Blood Flow Metab 6:366–78, 1986

5. Shapiro HM: Anesthesia effects on cerebral blood flow, cerebral metabolism, and the electroencephalogram. p. 795. In Miller RD (ed): Anesthesia Churchill Livingstone New York, 1981

6. Artchner MM, McRae LP: Carotid occlusive disease as a risk factor in major cardiovascular surgery. Arch Surg 117:1086, 1982

7. Weintraub WS, Jones EL, Craver J et al: Determinants of prolonged length of hospital stay after coronary bypass surgery. Circulation 80:276–84, 1989

8. Purves MJ: Do vasomotor nerves significantly regulate cerebral blood flow? Circulation 43:487–93, 1978

9. Young WL: Cerebral blood flow: when should we be concerned? p. 132. Presented at the IARS, 1994 Review Course Lectures, Sixty-eight Clinical and Scientific Congress. International Anesthetic Research Society, Orlando, FL, March 5–9, 1994

10. Jones TH, Morawetz RB, Crowell RM et al: Thresholds of focal cerebral ischemia in awake monkeys. J Neurosurg 54:773–82, 1981

11. Prough DS, Rogers AT, Johnston WE: Cardiopulmonary bypass and the brain. p. 6. Presented at the IARS, 1992 Review Course Lecture, Sixty-sixth Congress, San Francisco, March 13–17, 1992

12. Crosby G: Impaired central nervous system function. p. 356. In Berum of JA, Saidman LJ (eds): Anesthesia and Perioperative Complications. CV Mosby, St. Louis, 1991

13. Mills SA: Cerebral complications of cardiopulmonary bypass. In Wechsler AS (ed): Systemic Effects of Cardiopulmonary Bypass. Am J Surg, Presented by The Medical College of Virginia, Virginia Commonwealth University, Office of Medical Education, New York, 1993

14. Martin WRW, Hashimoto SA: Stroke in coronary bypass surgery. Can J Neurol Sci 9: 21–6, 1982

15. Parker FB, Marvasti MA, Bove EL: Neurologic complications following coronary artery bypass: the role of atherosclerotic emboli. Thorac Cardiovasc Surg 33:207–9, 1985

16. Gardner TJ, Homeffer PJ, Manolio TA et al: Stroke following coronary artery bypass grafting: a ten-year study. Ann Thorac Surg 40:574–81, 1985

17. Fuse K, Makuuchi H: Early and late results of coronary artery bypass grafting in the elderly. Jpn Circ J 52:460–5, 1988

18. Coffey CE, Massey EW, Roberts KB et al: Natural history of cerebral complications of coronary artery bypass graft surgery. Neurology 33:1416–21, 1983

19. Tuman KJ, McCarthy RJ, Najafi H, Ivankovich AD: Differential effects of advanced age on neurologic and cardiac risks of coronary artery operations. J Thorac Cardiovasc Surg 104:1510–7, 1992

20. Barnes RW: Asymptomatic carotid disease in patients. undergoing major cardiovascular operations: can prophylactic endarterectomy be justified? Ann Thorac Surg, suppl. 42: S36–40, 1986

21. Shaw PJ, Bates D, Cartlidge NE et al: An analysis of factors predisposing to neurological injury in patients undergoing coronary bypass. Q J Med 72:633–46, 1989

22. Gardner TJ, Horneffer PJ, Manolio TA et al: Major stroke after coronary artery bypass surgery: changing magnitude of the problem. J Vasc Surg 3:684–7, 1986

23. Hindman BJ: Neurologic complications of cardiac anesthesia and surgery. p. 1. Presented at the ASA Annual Refresher Course Lectures, Washington, DC, 155:October 9–13, 193

24. Turnipseed WD, Berkoff HA, Belzer FO: Postoperative stroke in cardiac and peripheral vascular disease. Ann Surg 192:365–7, 1980

25. Barnes RW, Liebman PR, Marzalek PB et al: The natural history of asymptomatic carotid disease in patients undergoing cardiovascular surgery. Surgery 90:1075–81, 1981

26. Ivey TD, Strandness E, Williams DB et al: Management of patients with carotid bruit undergoing cardiopulmonary bypass. J Thorac Cardiovasc Surg 87:183, 1984

27. Harrison MJG, Schneidau A, Ho R et al: Cere-

brovascular disease and functional outcome after coronary artery bypass surgery. Stroke 20:235–7, 1989

28. Ropper AH, Wechsler LR, Wilson LS: Carotid bruit and risk of stroke in elective surgery. N Engl J Med 307:1388, 1982

29. Todd MM, Drummond JC: Cereral protection during cardiac surgery. p. 551. In Kaplan JA (ed): Cardiac Anesthesia. Vol. 2: Cardiovascular Pharmacology. Grune & Stratton, New York, 1983

30. Reed GI III, Singer DE, Picard EH et al: Stroke following coronary-artery bypass surgery: a case-control estimate of the risk from carotid bruits. N Engl J Med 319:1246–50, 1988

31. Schultz RD, Sterpetti AV, Feldhaus RJ: Early and late results in patients with carotid disease undergoing myocardial revascularization. Ann Thorac Surg 45:603–9, 1988

32. Brener BJ, Brief DK, Alpert J et al: The risk of stroke in patients with asymptomatic carotid stenosis undergoing cardiac surgery: a follow-up study. J Vasc Surg 5:269–79, 1987

33. Furlan AJ, Craciun AR: Risk of stroke during coronary artery bypass graft surgery in patients with internal carotid artery disease documented by angiography. Stroke 16:797–9, 1985

34. Gravlee GP, Cordell AR, Graham JE et al: Coronary revascularization in patients with bilateral internal carotid occlusions. J Thorac Cardiovasc Surg 90:921–5, 1985

35. von Reutem G-M, Hetzel A, Birnbaum D et al: Transcranial Doppler ultrasonography during cardiopulmonary bypass in patients with severe carotid stenosis or occlusion. Stroke 19:674–80, 1988

36. Hertzer NR, Loop FD, Taylor PC et al: Staged and combined surgical approach to simultaneous carotid and coronary vascular disease. Surgery 84:803–11, 1978

37. Mehigan JT, Buch WS, Pipkin RD et al: A planned approach to coexistent cerebrovascular disease in coronary artery bypass candidates. Arch Surg 112:1403–9, 1977

38. Rizzo RJ, Whittemore AD, Couper GS et al: Combined carotid and coronary revascularisation: the preferred approach to the severe vasculopath. Ann Thorac Surg 54:1099–1109, 1992

39. Tobler HG, Edwards JE: Frequency and loca-

tion of atherosclerotic plaques in the ascending aorta. J Thorac Cardiovasc Surg 96:304–6, 1988

40. Wareing TH, Davila-Roman VG, Barzilai B et al: Management of the severely atherosclerotic ascending aorta during cardiac operations. J Thorac Cardiovasc Surg 103:453–62, 1992

41. Mills NL, Everson CT: Atherosclerosis of the ascending aorta and coronary artery bypass. J Thorac Cardiovasc Surg 102:546–53, 1991

42. Pugsley W, Klinger L, Paschalis C et al: Microemboli and cerebral impairment during cardiac surgery. Vasc Surg 24:34–43, 1990

43. Barzilai B, Marshall WG Jr, Saffitz JE, Kouchoukos N: Avoidance of the ascending aorta. Circulation 80:1275–9, 1989

44. Slogoff S, Reul GJ, Keats AS et al: Role of perfusion pressure and flow in major organ dysfunction after cardiopulmonary bypass. Ann Thorac Surg 50:911–8, 1990

45. Aberg T, Kihlgren M: cerebral protection during open-heart surgery. Thorax 32:525–33, 1977

46. Savageau JA, Stanton BA, Jenkins CD, Klein MD: Neuropsychological dysfunction following elective cardiac operation. I. Early assessment. J Thorac Cardiovasc Surg 84:585–94, 1982

47. Townes BD, Bashein G, Hornbein TF et al: Neurobehavioral outcomes in cardiac operations: a prospective controlled study. J Thorac Cardiovasc Surg 98:774–82, 1989

48. Topol EJ, Humphrey LS, Borkon AM et al: Value of intraoperative left ventricular microbubbles detected by transesophageal two-dimensional echocardiography in predicting neurologic outcome after cardiac operations. Am J Cardiol 56:773–5, 1985

49. Kuroda Y, Uchimoto R, Kaieda R et al: Central nervous system complications after cardiac surgery: a comparison between coronary artery bypass grafting and valve surgery. Anesth Analg 76:222–7, 1993

50. Stockard JJ, Bickford RG, Schauble JF: Pressure-dependent cerebral ischemia during cardiopulmonary bypass. Neurology 23:521–9, 1973

51. Solis RT, Noon GP, Beall AC et al: Particulate microembolism during cardiac operation. Ann Thorac Surg 17:332–44, 1974

52. Clark RE, Dietz DR, Miller JG: Continuous

detection of microemboli during cardiopulmonary bypass in animals and man. Circulation, suppl III. 54:74–8, 1976

53. Blauth CI, Smith PL, Arnold JV et al: Influence of oxygenator type on the prevalence and extent of microembolic retinal ischemia during cardiopulmonary bypass. Assessment by digital image analysis. J Thorac Cardiovasc Surg 99:61–9, 1990

54. Wright JS, Fisk GC, Torda TA et al: Some advantages of the membrane oxygenator for open-heart surgery. J Thorac Cardiovasc Surg 69:884–90, 1975

55. Muraoka R, Yokota M, Aoshima M: Subclinical changes in brain morphology following cardiac operations as reflected by computed tomographic scans of the brain. J Thorac Cardiovasc Surg 81:364–9, 1981

56. Aberg T, Ronquist G, Tyden H et al: Release of adenylate kinase into cerebrospinal fluid during open-heart surgery and its relation to postoperative intellectual function. Lancet 1:1139–42, 1982

57. Lundar T, Stokke O: Total creatine kinase activity in cerebrospinal fluid as an indicator of brain damage during open-heart surgery. Scand J Thorac Cardiovasc Surg 17:157–61, 1983

58. Aberg T, Ronquist G, Tyden H et al: Adverse effects on the brain in cardiac operations as assessed by biochemical, psychometric, and radiologic methods. J Thorac Cardiovasc Surg 87:99–105, 1984

59. Taylor KM, Devlin BJ, Mittra SM et al: Assessment of cerebral damage during open-heart surgery; a new experimental model. Scand J Thorac Cardiovasc Surg 14:197–203, 1980

60. Carlson RG, Lande AJ, Landis B et al: The Lande-Edwards membrane oxygenator during heart surgery. Oxygen transfer, microemboli counts, and Bender-Gestalt visual motor test scores. J Thorac Cardiovasc Surg 66:894–905, 1973

61. Smith PLC: Interventions to reduce cerebral injury during cardiac surgery—introduction and the effect of oxygenator type. Perfusion 4:139–45, 1989

62. Meloni L, Abbruzzese PA, Cardu G et al: Detection of microbubbles released by oxygenators during cardiopulmonary bypass by intraoperative transesophageal echocardiograph. Am J Cardiol 66:511–4, 1990

63. Sellman M, Ivert T, Stensved P et al: Doppler ultrasound estimation of microbubbles in the arterial line during extracorporeal circulation. Perfusion 5:23–32, 1990

64. Griffin S, Pugsley W, Treasure T: Microembolism during cardiopulmonary bypass: a comparison of bubble oxygenator with arterial line filter and membrane oxygenator alone. Perfusion 6:99–103, 1991

65. Abbruzzese PA, Meloni L, Cardu G et al: Role of arterial filters in the prevention of systemic embolization by microbubbles released by oxygenators, letter. Am J Cardiol 67:911–2, 1991

66. Treasure T: Interventions to reduce cerebral injury during cardiac surgery—the effect of arterial line filtration. Perfusion 4:147–62, 1989

67. Nussmeier NA, Mills AM: Complications related to cardiopulmonary bypass. p. 284. In Benum of JL, Saidman LJ (eds): Anesthesia and Perioperative Complications. Mosby-Year Book, St. Louis, MO, 1992

68. Wilkins H, Regelson W, Hoffmeister FS: The physiologic importance of pulsatile blood flow. N Engl J Med 267:443–6, 1962

69. Sanderson JM, Wright G, Sims FW: Brain damage in dogs immediately following pulsatile and non-pulsatile blood flows in extracorporeal circulation. Thorax 27:275–86, 1972

70. Mavroudis C: To pulse or not to pulse. Ann Thorac Surg, 25:259–71, 1978

71. Wright G, Sanderson JM: Brain damage and mortality in dogs following pulsatile and non-pulsatile blood flows in extracorporeal circulation. Thorax 27:738–47, 1972

72. Matsumoto T, Wolferth CC, Perlman MH: Effects of pulsatile and non-pulsatile perfusion upon cerebral and conjunctival microcirculation in dogs. Ann Surg 37:61–4, 1971

73. Geha A, Salaymeh MT, Abe T et al: Effects of pulsatile cardiopulmonary bypass on cerebral metabolism. J Surg Res 12:381–7, 1972

74. Taylor KM, Wright GS, Bain WH et al: Comparative studies of pulsatile and non-pulsatile flow during cardiopulmonary bypass. III. Response of anterior pituitary gland to thyrotropin-releasing hormone. J Thorac Cardiovasc Surg 75:579–84, 1978

75. Williams GD, Seifen AB, Lawson NW et al:

Pulsatile perfusion versus conventional high-flow non-pulsatile perfusion for rapid core cooling and rewarming of infants for circulatory arrest in cardiac operation. J Thorac Cardiovasc Surg 78:667–77, 1979

76. Mori A, Sono J, Nakashima M et al: Application of pulsatile cardiopulmonary bypass for profound hypothermia in cardiac surgery. Jpn Circ J 45:315–22, 1981

77. Govier AV, Reves JG, McKay RD et al: Factors and their influence on regional cerebral blood flow during nonpulsatile cardiopulmonary bypass. Ann Thorac Surg 38:592–600, 1984

78. Kritikou PE, Branthwaite MA: Significance of changes in cerebral electrical activity at onset of cardiopulmonary bypass. Thorax 32: 534–8, 1977

79. Hindman BJ, Dexter F, Ruy KH et al: Pulsatile versus nonpulsatile cardiopulmonary bypass. Anesthesiology 80:1137–47, 1994

80. Henze T, Stephan H, Sonntag H: Cerebral dysfunction following extracorporeal circulation for aortocoronary bypass surgery: no differences in neuropsychological outcome after pulsatile versus non-pulsatile flow. Thorac Cardiovasc Surg 38:65–8, 1990

81. Townes BD, Bashein G, Hombein TF et al: Neurobehavioral outcomes in cardiac operations: a prospective controlled study. J Thorac Cardiovasc Surg 98:774–82, 1989

82. Fish KJ, Helms KN, Samquist FH et al: A prospective randomized study of the effects of prostacyclin on neuropsychological dysfunction after coronary artery surgery. J Thorac Cardiovasc Surg 93:609–15, 1987

83. Crosby G: Cardiac surgery and cardiopulmonary bypass. p. 62. In Barash PG, Deutsch S, Tinker J (eds): Central Nervous System Dysfunction in the Perioperative Period: Causes and Solutions. Vol. 20. American Society of Anesthesiologists. JB Lippincott, Philadelphia, 1992

84. Murkin JM, Farrar JK, Tweed WA et al: Cerebral autoregulation and flow/metabolism coupling during cardiopulmonary bypass: the influence of $PaCO_2$. Anesth Analg 66: 825–32, 1987

85. Rogers AT, Stump DA, Gravlee GP et al: Response of cerebral blood flow to phenylephrine infusion during hypothermic cardiopulmonary bypass: influence of $PaCO_2$

management. Anesthesiology 69:547–51, 1988

86. Groom RC, Hill AG, Akl BF et al: Pediatric perfusion surgery. Proc Am Acad Cardiovasc Perfusion 11:78–84, 1990

87. Murkin JM: Cerebral hyperfusion during cardiopulmonary bypass: the influence of $PaCO_2$. p. 47–66. In Hilberman M (ed): Brain Injury and Protection During Heart Surgery. Martinus Nijhoff, Boston, 1988

88. Prough DS, Stump DA, Troost BT: $PaCO_2$ management during cardiopulmonary bypass: intriguing physiologic rationale, convincing clinical data, evolving hypothesis? Anesthesiology 72:3–6, 1990

89. Bashein G, Tawnes BD, Nessly ML et al: A randomized study of carbon dioxide management during hypothermic cardiopulmonary bypass. Anesthesiology 72:7–15, 1990

90. Tufo HM, Osfeld AM, Shekelle R: Central nervous system dysfunction following open heart surgery. JAMA 212:1333–40, 1970

91. Gordon RJ, Ravin M, Rawitscher RE et al: Changes in arterial pressure, viscosity, and resistance during cardiopulmonary bypass. J Thorac Cardiovasc Surg 69:552–61, 1975

92. Ellis RJ, Wisniewski A, Potts R et al: Reduction of flow rate and arterial pressure at moderate hypothermia does not result in cerebral dysfunction. J Thorac Cardiovasc Surg 79: 173–80, 1980

93. Kolkka R, Hilberman M: Neurologic dysfunction following cardiac operation with low-flow, low-pressure cardiopulmonary bypass. J Thorac Cardiovasc Surg 79:432–7, 1980

94. Carlsson C, Hagerdal M, Siesjo BK: Protective effect of hypothermia in cerebral oxygen deficiency caused by arterial hypoxia. Anesthesiology 44:27–35, 1976

95. Feddersen K, Aren C, Nilsson NJ et al: Cerebral blood flow and metabolism during cardiopulmonary bypass with special reference to effects of hypotension induced by prostacyclin. Ann Thorac Surg 41:395–400, 1986

96. Wong BI, McLean RF, Naylor CD et al: Central-nervous-system dysfunction after warm or hypothermic cardiopulmonary bypass. Lancet 339:1383–4, 1992

97. Croughwell ND, Frasco P, Blumenthal JA et al: Warming during cardiopulmonary bypass is associated with jugular bulb desaturation. Ann Thorac Surg 53:827–32, 1992

98. Hindman BJ et al: Brain blood flow and metabolism do not decrease at stable brain temperature during cardiopulmonary bypass in rabbits. Anesthesiology 77:342–50, 1992

99. Maruyama M et al: The effects of extreme hemodilutions on the autoregulation of cerebral blood flow, electroencephalogram and cerebral metabolic rate of oxygen in the dog. Stroke 16:675–9, 1985

100. Pulsinelli WA, Waldman S, Rawlinson D, Plum F: Moderate hyperglycemia augments ischemic brain damage: a neuropathologic study in the rat. Neurology 32:1239–46, 1982

101. Nedergaard M: Transient focal ischemia in hyperglycemic rats is associated with increased cerebral infarction. Brain Res 408: 79–85, 1987

102. Siesjo BK, Bengtsson F: Calcium fluxes, calcium antagonists, and calcium-related pathology in brain ischemia, hypoglycemia, and spreading depression: a unifying hypothesis. J Cereb Blood Flow Metab 9:127–40, 1989

103. Metz S, Keats AS: Benefits of a glucose-containing priming solution for cardiopulmonary bypass. Anesth Analg 72:428–34, 1991

104. Helgason CM: Blood glucose and stroke. Stroke 19:1049–53, 1988

105. Breuer AC, Hanson MR, Furlan AJ et al: Central nervous system complications of myocardial revascularization a prospective analysis of 400 patients. Stroke 11:1135, 1980

106. Davis O, Kobrine A: Computed tomography. In Youmans JR (ed): Neurological Surgery. WB Saunders, Philadelphia, 1982

107. Sontaniemi KA, Juolasmaa A, Hokkanen ET: Neuropsychological outcome after open heart surgery. Arch Neurol 38:2–8, 1981

108. Spencer MP, Thomas GI, Nicholls SC, Sauvage LR: Detection of middle cerebral artery emboli during carotid endarterectomy using Doppler ultrasonography. Stroke 21:415–23, 1990

109. Diehl JT, Ramos D, Dougherty F et al: Intraoperative, two-dimensional echocardiography-guided removal of retained intracardiac air. Ann Thorac Surg 43:674–5, 1987

110. Blauth CI, Arnold JV, Schulenberg WE et al: Cerebral microembolism during cardiopulmonary bypass. Retinal microvascular studies in vivo with fluorescein angiography. J Thorac Cardiovasc Surg 95:668–76, 1988

111. Henriksen L: Evidence suggestive of diffuse brain damage following cardiac operations. Lancet 1:816, 1984

112. Fisk GC, Wright JS, Hicks RG et al: The influence of duration of circulatory arrest at 20°C on cerebral changes. Anaesth Intensive Care 4:126–34, 1976

113. Treasure T, Naftel DC, Conger KA et al: The effect of hypothermic circulatory arrest time on cerebral function, morphology, and biochemistry: an experimental study. J Thorac Cardiovasc Surg 86:761–70, 1983

114. Molina JE, Einzig S, Mastri AR et al: Brain damage in profound hypothermia: perfusion versus circulatory arrest. J Thorac Cardiovasc Surg 87:596–604, 1984

115. Aguilar MJ, Gerbode F, Hill JD: Neuropathologic complications of cardiac surgery. J Thorac Cardiovasc Surg 61:676–85, 1971

116. Brennan RW, Patterson RH, Kessler J: Cerebral blood flow and metabolism during cardiopulmonary bypass: evidence of microembolic encephalopathy. Neurology 21:665–72, 1971

117. Zelcer J, Wells DG: Anaesthetic-related recovery room complications. Anaesth Intensive Care 15:168–74, 1987

118. Forrest JB, Cahalan MK, Rehder K et al: Multicenter study of general anesthesia. II. Results. Anesthesiology 72:262–8, 1990

119. Rosenberg H, Clofine R, Bialik O: Neurologic changes during awakening from anesthesia. Anesthesiology 54:125–30, 1981

120. Solimon MG, Gillies DM: Muscular hyperactivity after general anesthesia. Can Anaesth Soc J 19:529–35, 1972

121. Strenge H, Lindner V, Paulsen G et al: Early neurological abnormalities following coronary artery bypass surgery. A prospective study. Eur Arch Psychiatr Neurol Sci 239: 277–81, 1990

122. de Noordhout AM, Delwaide PJ: The palmomental reflex in Parkinson's disease. Arch Neurol 45:425–7, 1988

123. Whittle IR, Douglas-Miller J: Clinical usefulness of the palmomental reflex. Med J Aust 146:137–9, 1987

124. Prakash O, Jonson B, Meij S et al: Criteria for early extubation after intra-cardiac surgery in adults. Anesth Analg 56:703–8, 1977

125. Quasha AL, Loeber N, Feeley TW et al: Postoperative respiratory care: a controlled trial of early and late extubation following coro-

nary-artery bypass grafting. Anesthesiology 52:135–41, 1980

126. Lichtenthal PR, Wade LD, Niemyski PR, Shapiro BA: Respiratory management after cardiac surgery with inhalation anesthesia. Crit Care Med 11:603–5, 1983

127. Andree RA: Sudden death following naloxone administration. Anesth Analg 59:782–4, 1980

128. Kaplan RF: Hypothermia/hyperthermia in complications during anesthesia, p. 121. In Gravenstein N (ed): JB Lippincott, Philadelphia, 1991

129. Ward MP, Milledge JS, West JB: High Altitude Medicine and Physiology, Chapman Hall Medical, London, 1989

130. Cooper DM, Bazaral MG, Furlan AJ et al: Pituitary apoplexy: a complication of cardiac surgery. Ann Thorac Surg 41:547–50, 1986

131. Peck V, Lieberman A, Pinto R, Culliford A: Pituitary apoplexy following open-heart surgery. NY State J Med 80:641–3, 1980

132. Slavin ML, Budabin M: Pituitary apoplexy associated with cardiac surgery. Am J Ophthalmol 98:291–6, 1984

133. Absalom M, Rogers KH, Moulton RJ, Mazer

CD: Pituitary apoplexy after coronary artery surgery. Anesth Analg 76:648–9, 1993

134. Reid RL, Quigley ME, Yen SSC: Pituitary apoplexy: a review. Arch Neurol 42:712–9, 1985

135. Rovit RL, Rein JM: Pituitary apoplexy: a review and reappraisal. J Neurosurg 37:280–8, 1972

136. Cardoso ER, Peterson EW: Pituitary apoplexy: a review. Neurosurgery 14:363–73, 1984

137. Robinson RG, Kubos KL, Starr LB et al: Mood disorders in stroke patients. Importance of location of lesion. Brain 107:81–93, 1984

138. Murkin JM, Martzke JS: Central nervous system dysfunction after cardiopulmonary bypass. p. 1225. In Kaplan JA (ed): Cardiac Anesthesia. WB Saunders, Philadelphia, 1993

139. Sotaniemi KA, Mononen H, Hokkenen TE: Long-term cerebral outcome after open-heart surgery: a five-year neuropsychological follow-up study. Stroke 17:410–6, 1986

140. Murkin JM, Martzke JS, Buchan AM et al: Cognitive and neurological function after coronary artery surgery: a prospective study. Anesth Analg 74:S215, 1992

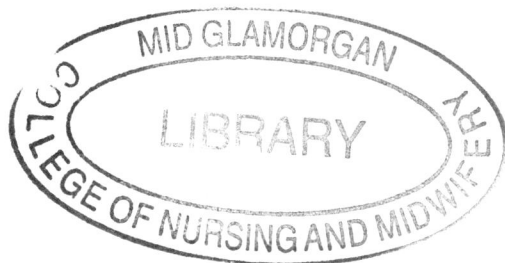

13

Dysrhythmias Following Open Heart Surgery

Nicholas Deutsch
Gerald V. Naccarelli

Cardiac dysrhythmias occur commonly after cardiac surgery. These dysrhythmias can be a significant source of cardiac morbidity and mortality. This chapter reviews the incidence, diagnosis, and management of dysrhythmias occurring after cardiac surgery.

INCIDENCE OF DYSRHYTHMIAS

Dysrhythmias are a frequent problem in the postoperative period following open heart surgery. Sustained supraventricular dysrhythmias are more common than sustained ventricular dysrhythmias. The reported incidence of dysrhythmias varies according to the method of recording the electrocardiogram (ECG) and the definition of dysrhythmia used. The reported incidence of postoperative dysrhythmias has changed little during the past 15 years despite improvements in surgical technique. Following coronary artery bypass graft (CABG) surgery, the reported incidence of sustained supraventricular dysrhythmias varies from 11 to 40 per-

cent, with most studies reporting an incidence of close to 30 percent. Following valve replacement, the incidence of supraventricular dysrhythmias may approach 60 percent. The most common dysrhythmias following open heart surgery is atrial fibrillation, followed by atrial flutter and paroxysmal supraventricular tachycardia (PSVT), and lastly, junctional rhythms.[1-8] The peak incidence of supraventricular dysrhythmias is usually on day 2 postoperatively.[8-12] Elderly patients and patients in whom β-blockers had been discontinued perioperatively appear to be at greater risk of atrial dysrhythmias postoperatively. However, there was no correlation of postoperative atrial dysrhythmias with a number of other factors, including pre-existing hypertension, previous myocardial infarction, unstable angina, poor left ventricular function, extent of coronary artery disease, or gender.[13-15] Therefore, it is difficult to predict which patients will develop atrial fibrillation postoperatively.

Ventricular ectopy and even complex ventricular ectopy are seen commonly following open heart surgery. Fortunately, the inci-

243

dence of sustained ventricular tachycardia or of ventricular fibrillation is rare.[16] Sustained ventricular dysrhythmias are often associated with intraoperative myocardial infarction or poor ventricular function and are a significant cause of late-occurring morbidity and mortality in patients with poor ventricular function. There is no apparent correlation between multiple risk factors, including extent of disease or complexity of surgery, and the incidence of postoperative ventricular dysrhythmias.[16,17]

DIAGNOSIS OF DYSRHYTHMIAS

The differentiation between atrial or ventricular dysrhythmias is usually simple; however, wide QRS complex beats may be either of ventricular origin or supraventricular with aberrant conduction. A history of coronary artery disease and myocardial infarction favors a ventricular origin for the tachycardia. Left axis deviation, QRS duration greater than 140 ms, concordance of the QRS complex in the precordial leads, and atrioventricular (AV) dissociation suggest a ventricular origin for the dysrhythmia. Although AV dissociation is diagnostic of ventricular tachycardia, a one-to-one ventricular-to-atrial relationship does not exclude ventricular tachycardia, since many patients will have retrograde conduction from the ventricle to the atrium. In addition, ventricular tachycardia more frequently has a right bundle-branch block configuration, a monophasis R-wave in V_1 or a R-S or Q wave in V_6, while supraventricular tachycardia with aberrancy more typically has a RSR' (triphasic) "rabbit ear" configuration in V_1.[18] In those cases in which the diagnosis of the dysrhythmia is unclear, the temporary atrial pacing wiring can be used to help diagnose the dysrhythmia, since it gives a large-amplitude recording of the atrial activity. Using an ECG monitor, the right and left arm leads are connected to the atrial pacing wires and the rest of the leads are connected in a standard fashion. Lead I,

which records between right and left arm, give a bipolar atrial ECG. Leads II and III give unipolar ECGs, since the recordings are between the right and left arms, respectively, and the left leg.

The response of a tachycardia to vagal maneuvers or intravenous drugs may also be useful in the differential diagnosis of wide-complex tachycardias. Termination of the tachycardia with vagal maneuvers, intravenous adenosine, verapamil, or diltiazem suggests re-entrant supraventricular tachycardia, using the AV junction as part of the circuit (AV nodal re-entrant or AV re-entrant tachycardia). If these maneuvers cause AV block (i.e., more P-waves than QRS complexes), the tachycardia is atrial in origin (such as ectopic atrial tachycardia or atrial flutter). Termination of the tachycardia with intravenous lidocaine suggests the tachycardia is ventricular in origin. Intravenous verapamil should never be used in the differential diagnosis of wide-QRS complex tachycardia, since the negative inotropic effects of verapamil may cause cardiovascular collapse, given that most wide-complex tachycardias are ventricular and that patients with ventricular tachycardia usually have depressed ventricular function.

MANAGEMENT OF DYSRHYTHMIAS

In general, the principles of antidysrhythmic management in the post-bypass patient are similar to those in other patients, but there may be different reversible precipitating factors. The actual management of postoperative dysrhythmias depends on the hemodynamic consequences of the dysrhythmias and on the likelihood that the dysrhythmia will degenerate to a more serious dysrhythmia. Dysrhythmias in the postoperative phase are very common, and in most cases no specific etiology can be found. Nonetheless, a dysrhythmia may be the first sign of a serious physiologic or pharmacologic derangement. One should always consider myocardial ischemia, hypoxia, hypo/hypercarbia, acidosis, electrolyte imbalance, "light anesthesia," and drug interactions or overdose.

Dysrhythmia Prophylaxis

Atrial and ventricular ectopy occur quite frequently in the postoperative period. The ectopy is usually very well tolerated hemodynamically. In the past, many textbooks recommended treating ventricular ectopic activity that occurred at a rate greater than 5 beats · min^{-1} or was multifocal or was "R-on-T." The prophylaxis was recommended in order to prevent these dysrhythmias from degenerating to ventricular fibrillation. There are no direct data from postoperative cardiac patients to determine whether prophylaxis of ventricular ectopy is beneficial. The only data from which we can extrapolate are those obtained from patients with acute myocardial infarction (AMI). Lidocaine prophylaxis has been shown to reduce the incidence of ventricular fibrillation with AMI. However, recent studies have shown that lidocaine administered prophylactically in the presence of an uncomplicated AMI will actually increase the mortality rate and is therefore no longer recommended.[19] In addition, the value of warning dysrhythmias, such as frequent or multiform premature beats, R-on-T phenomenon, and repetitive couplets or salvos, has recently been reassessed. Many reports have shown that ventricular fibrillation occurs without warning in most patients and that frequent and complex ventricular premature beats occur commonly in patients who never develop ventricular fibrillation.[20-22] Therefore, the authors recommend that in the postoperative cardiac patient, lidocaine should be reserved for patients who have sustained or symptomatic ventricular dysrhythmias, as has been suggested for patients with AMI.[23,24] Since atrial fibrillation is the most common sustained arrhythmia in the postoperative period, a number of trials with different drugs have been tried to prevent the

onset of postoperative atrial fibrillation. Most patients tolerate atrial dysrhythmias quite well. In addition, atrial fibrillation rarely lasts more than a few days in patients without a prior history of atrial fibillation.[1,2,6,7,9,11,13,25] Atrial fibrillation in the postoperative setting rarely causes embolic events.[9,26] However, patients with poor ventricular function may depend heavily on the atrial contribution to ventricular filling, and patients with prosthetic valves tend to tolerate tachydysrhythmias poorly. In addition, a recent study reported that the average hospital stay was 3 days longer in patients who developed atrial fibrillation after CABG surgery and that the development of atrial fibrillation increased the hospital bill by approximately $8,000.[27] A number of different studies have examined the role of digoxin, β-blockers, and verapamil for prophylaxis against atrial fibrillation. In two recent meta-analyses combining a number of previous studies that have examined the use of digoxin, β-blockers, and verapamil, it was found that β-blockers when used alone, or even more impressively when used in combination with digitalis, can prevent the development of atrial fibrillation after CABG surgery.[28,29] β-Blocker therapy when used alone decreased the incidence of sustained supraventricular dysrhythmias from 20.2 percent in the control groups to 9.8 percent in the β-blocker groups in 1,418 patients; when β-blocker therapy was combined with digoxin, the incidence of supraventricular dysrhythmias dropped to 2.2 percent compared to 29.4 percent in the control groups in 292 patients.[29] Prophylactic trials with digoxin or verapamil alone were unsuccessful.

DYSRHYTHMIA THERAPY

This section presents the treatment of cardiac dysrhythmias in an algorithm format, similar to that used in advanced cardiac life support (ACLS).[19] Algorithms provide summary information applicable to a broad range of patients. By necessity, algorithms are simplified and treatment must be individualized to the given patient. Our algorithms assume that the dysrhythmia occurs during the perioperative period when the patient has an intravenous line and is being continuously monitored with a blood pressure cuff, ECG, and pulse oximeter. Adequate oxygenation and ventilation is essential for all therapeutic regimens. A key decision in the treatment of the patient is whether the patient is stable. With an awake patient, the signs of instability are depressed consciousness, chest pain, and shortness of breath. With an anesthetized patient, we arbitrarily define a rhythm disorder as unstable if the rhythm is causing hypotension (greater than 30 percent below baseline), myocardial ischemia, or pulmonary edema. Cardioversion is the treatment of choice for tachydysrhythmias in hemodynamically unstable patients. It is our bias to be aggressive about cardioverting patients if they are still anesthetized after the operation for rhythm disturbances, even when they are not hemodynamically unstable. Electrical cardioversion offers the advantage of immediate restoration of sinus rhythm, and the distinction between supraventricular and ventricular dysrhythmias is less important than when medical management is used. Cardiac enzymes and myocardial scintigraphy are usually normal after cardioversion, even though ST elevation may occur. Dysrhythmias with synchronized cardioversion are usually transient. Ventricular fibrillation following cardioversion, although possible, is extremely rare and can be readily treated with defibrillation. In patients with permanent pacemakers, careful consideration must be given to defibrillation, since defibrillation may damage the pacemaker. The defibrillation paddles should be placed away from the pacemaker generator.

Tachycardia Treatment Algorithm

An algorithm for treatment of tachycardia is presented in Figure 13-1. Tachycardia is defined as a heart rate greater than 100 beats · min^{-1} in an adult. The clinician must evalu-

ate the type of tachycardia, whether a given tachycardia is causing the patient to be unstable, and the underlying etiology of the tachycardia.

The underlying cause of the tachycardia should be treated, and the differential diagnosis includes inadequate analgesia/sedation, hypoxia, hypercarbia, myocardial ischemia, pulmonary embolus, electrolyte abnormalities, toxic effects of medications (particularly epinephrine), hypovolemia, and malignant hyperthermia. In addition, if the rhythm is not sinus tachycardia and the patient is unstable, cardioversion is recommended (sinus tachycardia should not be cardioverted). While cardioversion is being prepared, appropriate medications based on the underlying rhythm may be administered (see below for a discussion of stable ventricular tachycardia). The standard sequence of energy levels recommended for cardioversion is 100, 200, 300, and then 360 joules (J), with the exception of atrial flutter and PSVT, which often respond to 50 J, and polymorphic ventricular tachycardia, which should be treated as for ventricular fibrillation. In general, we favor higher-energy cardioversion, since low-energy cardioversion may be ineffective, requiring several more shocks and in rare cases can be prodysrhythmic.[30] Cardioversion should be synchronized. If one is unable to synchronize the shock, the defibrillation mode should be used. Medical therapy for tachycardias is based on the underlying rhythm. The goals of therapy in patients with supraventricular dysrhythmias are twofold. The first is to slow the ventricular response rate with agents that slow conduction through the AV node. Second, an attempt may be made to convert the patient to normal sinus rhythm. The clinician should be able to distinguish between five categories of rhythm disturbances: (1) atrial origin tachycardias, such as atrial fibrillation, atrial flutter, multifocal atrial tachycardia, and intra-atrial tachycardia; (2) PSVT using the AV junction (e.g., AV nodal re-entrant and AV re-entrant tachycardia); (3) ventricular tachycardia; (4) wide-complex tachycardia of un-

```
┌─────────────────────────────────────────────────┐
│ • Assess vital signs, oxygenation, ventilation   │
│ • Assess possible etiologies                      │
└─────────────────────────────────────────────────┘
                        │
                        ▼
         ┌──────────────────────────┐  Yes  ┌────────────────────────────┐
         │                          │ ────▶ │ Prepare for cardioversion   │
         │   Unstable, symptomatic  │       │ May give trial of medication│
         │                          │       │ or pacing based on rhythm   │
         └──────────────────────────┘       └────────────────────────────┘
```

| Atrial fibrillation Atrial flutter | PSVT | Wide-complex tachycardia Uncertain type | Ventricular tachycardia |

No / No / No / No

| Consider the following: β-Blockers Verapamil Diltiazem Digoxin Procainamide Overdrive pacing (A-flutter) | Vagal maneuvers | Vagal maneuvers | |

| | Adenosine x2 | Lidocaine x2 | Lidocaine x2 |

| | Verapamil x2 Diltiazem | Adenosine x2 | |

| | Procainamide | | Procainamide |

Ineffective

| | Consider rate-control drugs | | Bretylium |

| | | | IV amiodarone |

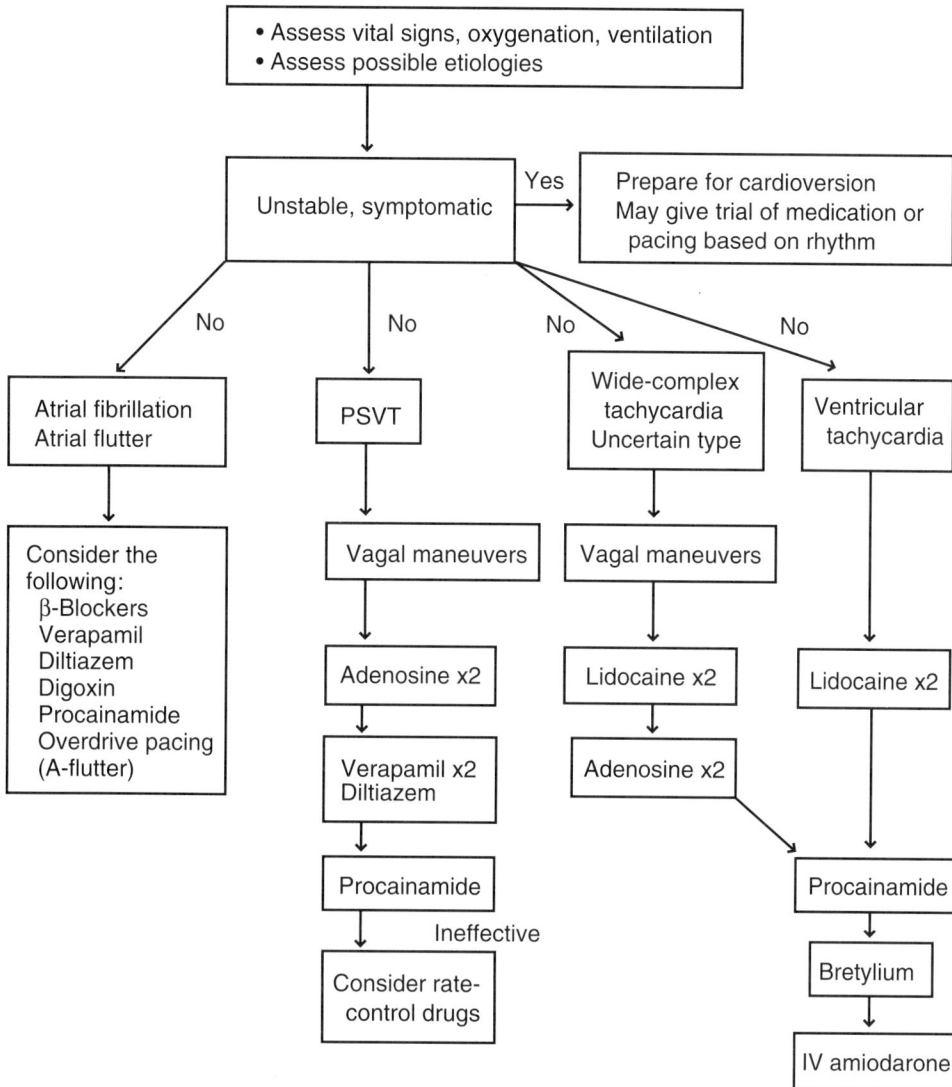

Fig. 13-1. Medical algorithm for treating tachycardia. The algorithm is simplified and must be individualized to the given patient.

certain type; and (5) ventricular fibrillation or pulseless ventricular tachycardia.

TACHYCARDIAS OF ATRIAL ORIGIN

With tachycardias of atrial origin, such as atrial fibrillation and flutter (Figs. 13-2 and 13-3), the first priority should be to slow the ventricular response. For rate control, β-blockers (e.g., esmolol, metoprolol, and propranolol) and calcium channel blockers (e.g., diltiazem and verapamil) are good choices. Calcium channel blockers are the drugs of choice in patients with bronchospastic disease. Intravenous β- and calcium channel blockers may reduce the ventricular response by 25 to 35 percent within 3 to 7 minutes of administration. In patients with severely impaired ventricular function, cardioversion may be the preferred treatment, even if hypotension is not present. Pa-

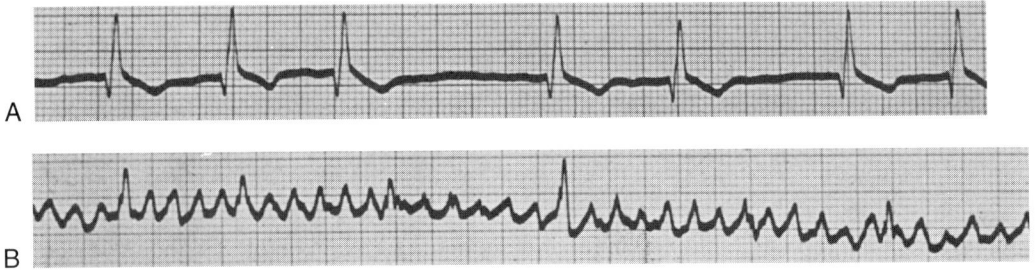

Fig. 13-2. Examples of atrial fibrillation with a slow ventricular response. **(A)** The fibrillatory waves are not apparent, but the rhythm is irregular, and there are no obvious P-waves. **(B)** The fibrillatory waves are coarse.

tients with atrial fibrillation of more than a few days' duration should receive anticoagulation prior to cardioversion because of the risk of systemic embolization of intra-atrial thrombi. Digoxin has been a traditional favorite for the treatment of atrial fibrillation or flutter. However, the use of digoxin for the acute onset of atrial fibrillation or flutter is seldom, if ever, indicated.[31] The primary mechanism by which digoxin slows the ventricular rate is by increasing vagal tone, but is ineffective in slowing conduction through the AV node in a clinical setting associated with enhanced sympathetic tone. The perioperative clinical situations in which one would consider using digoxin are usually associated with enhanced sympathetic tone. In addition, rate control with digoxin may take hours to days. Concomitant use of β- or calcium-channel blockers, though, may be of help. Rapid overdrive pacing with the atrial epicardial

pacing wires also can be effective treatment for atrial flutter. Atrial flutter has been divided into types I and II.[32] Type I atrial flutter has a flutter rate of 240 to 340 beats $\cdot$ min^{-1} and responds to rapid overdrive pacing. Rapid overdrive atrial pacing should be performed at 120 to 130 percent of the intrinsic atrial rate for 10 to 30 seconds.

PSVT

Vagal maneuvers increase vagal tone and may break an episode of PSVT (Fig. 13-4). Many vagal maneuvers are possible, but the most practical intraoperatively is the use of carotid sinus massage or pressure on the eyeballs. If the patient is at risk of carotid disease, carotid sinus massage should be avoided. Adenosine is considered the drug of choice for PSVT. Adenosine is as effective as calcium channel blockers but is considered safer because of its very brief half-life. The elimination half-life is 1 to 6 seconds. It

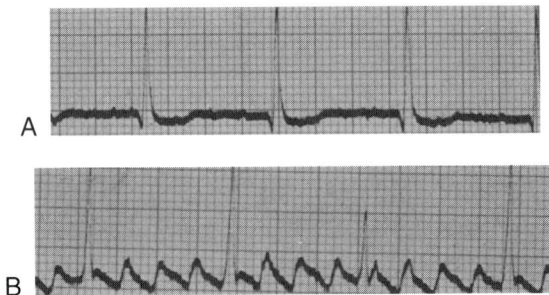

Fig. 13-3. Example of atrial flutter. **(A)** In lead I, the flutter waves are not apparent. **(B)** Examination of another lead shows that the flutter waves are apparent at a rate of approximately 300 beat $\cdot$ min^{-1} conducted to the ventricle in a 4:1 ratio.

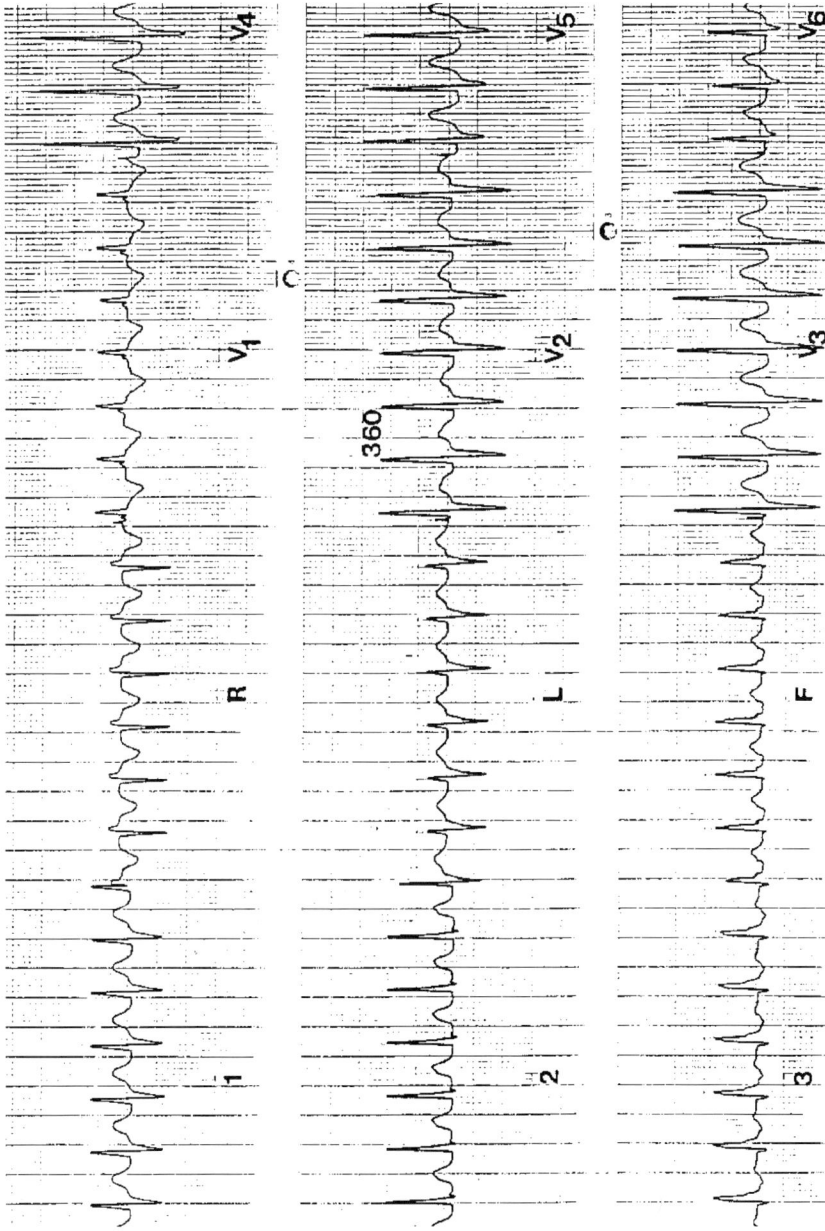

Fig. 13-4. Example of paroxysmal supraventricular tachycardia (PSVT). The ventricular rate is approximately 150 beats · min^{-1}.

249

should be noted that methylxanthines are antagonists competitive with adenosine and that therapeutic concentrations of theophylline block the effect of adenosine. Adenosine should be administered intravenously with good flow and as centrally as available, since its success depends on achieving a high peak plasma concentration; adenosine (6 mg) should be administered by rapid IV push and, if unsuccessful, a second dose (12 mg) should be given 1 to 2 minutes later. PSVT may recur in up to 50 percent of cases.[33] The rate of recurrence of PSVT after verapamil treatment is slightly lower.[34] A recommended sequence of agents for persistent PSVT is adenosine twice and, if the blood pressure has not dropped, verapamil twice. Verapamil should be given with extreme caution in patients receiving β-blockers or with impaired ventricular function. The recommended dose of verapamil is 2.5 to 5 mg given slowly over 2 minutes. If PSVT persists or recurs, a second dose of 5 to 10 mg may be given in 15 minutes. Diltiazem is an alternative calcium channel blocker that probably has less negative inotropic effect and equal efficacy to adenosine or verapamil.[35] The dose of intravenous diltiazem is 0.25 mg $\cdot$ kg^{-1} over 2 minutes, followed 15 minutes later by 0.35 mg $\cdot$ kg^{-1} if the first dose was tolerated but ineffective.

STABLE VENTRICULAR TACHYCARDIA

For ventricular tachycardia that is clinically stable, lidocaine is the drug of choice (Fig. 13-5). The initial bolus dose is 1 to 1.5 mg $\cdot$ kg^{-1}, followed by a second dose of 0.5 to 0.75 mg $\cdot$ kg^{-1} 5 to 10 minutes later, if needed. A lidocaine infusion of 2 to 4 mg $\cdot$ min^{-1} can then be started if the initial lidocaine terminated the ventricular tachycardia. Second- and third-line therapies for ventricular tachycardia is procainamide and bretylium. Procainamide should be infused at a maximum of 30 mg $\cdot$ min^{-1} to a maximum dose of 17 mg $\cdot$ kg^{-1}. The endpoints of procainamide therapy are suppression of the dysrhythmia, hypotension, or more than 50 percent widening of the QRS complex. If procainamide suppresses the ventricular tachycardia, a continuous infusion at 1 to 4 mg $\cdot$ min^{-1} should be begun. Bretylium should be loaded with a dose of 5 to 10 mg $\cdot$ kg^{-1} over 10 minutes; if it suppresses the ventricular tachycardia, a continuous infusion at 1 to 2 mg $\cdot$ min^{-1} should be started. Intravenous amiodarone may be used in refractory patients. The exception to the above treatment recommendation is for torsades de pointes. For torsade de pointes, overdrive pacing is the treatment of choice. This can be accomplished with epicardial, transcutaneous, or transvenous pacing. Isoproterenol (2 to 10 μg $\cdot$ min^{-1}) can also be used to increase the ventricular rate, to break the dysrhythmia. Magnesium sulfate in a dose of 1 to 2 g IV over 1 to 2 minutes can abolish runs of torsade and should be given as front-line treatment. Defibrillation should be used for unstable torsade. In addition, correction of reversible causes of a prolonged QT interval should be made in a timely fashion.

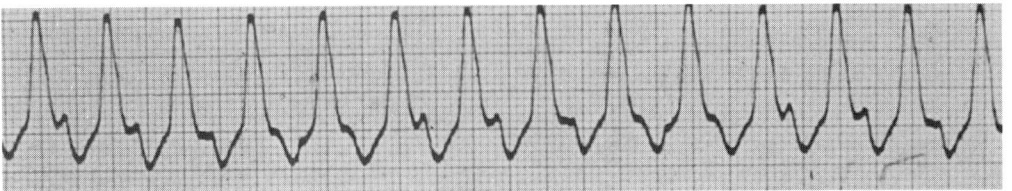

Fig. 13-5. Example of ventricular tachycardia at a rate of approximately 150 beats $\cdot$ min^{-1}. Note the wide-complex QRS complexes and AV dissociation.

WIDE-COMPLEX TACHYCARDIA OF UNCERTAIN TYPE

The distinction between ventricular tachycardia and wide-complex RSVT with aberrant conduction is difficult in the perioperative setting. If the tachycardia complex appears wide, it should be treated initially as for ventricular tachycardia, unless it is known for certain that the rhythm is PSVT. Clinicians should not use hemodynamic or ECG criteria in the acute setting to attempt to distinguish between ventricular tachycardia and wide-complex PSVT. In addition, if the rhythm is hemodynamically unstable, the patient should be electrically cardioverted. The initial drug therapy should be with lidocaine as for ventricular tachycardia. Procainamide is also an acceptable choice, but takes longer to act. If the tachycardia persists after lidocaine treatment, adenosine should be given, since adenosine produces little harm in patients with ventricular tachycardia, as its half-life is so short and converts many cases of wide-complex PSVT. Verapamil should not be given to a patient with wide-complex ventricular tachycardia, unless it is known for certain that the rhythm is PSVT. Verapamil given to patients with Wolff-Parkinson-White syndrome or ventricular tachycardia may be lethal.

VENTRICULAR FIBRILLATION OR PULSELESS VENTRICULAR TACHYCARDIA

An algorithm for treatment is presented in Figure 13-6. When ventricular fibrillation or ventricular tachycardia is recognized on the monitor, the first maneuver should be to determine whether a pulse is present. If a pulse is present, the diagnosis of ventricular fibrillation is erroneous due to ECG artifact, or the patient has pulsatile ventricular tachycardia and should be treated with the tachycardia algorithm. If there is not a palpable pulse, defibrillation should be performed as quickly as possible. Three shocks should be delivered consecutively, if needed: 200, 200 to 300, and 360 J. The sequence of shocks should not

be interrupted for pulse checks, to perform cardiopulmonary resuscitation (CPR), or to administer medications if the monitor shows persistent ventricular tachycardia/ventricular fibrillation (VF/VT). If a non-VT/VF rhythm appears on the monitor, the defibrillator paddles should be removed from the chest and a pulse should be sought. If VT/VF persist after three countershocks, CPR should be continued along with intubation, if it has not already been done. Epinephrine (1 mg) every 3 to 5 minutes remains the drug of choice for cardiac arrest. If 30 to 60 seconds after drug administration VT/VF persists, the use of either bretylium or lidocaine is recommended at this point. Human clinical trials have failed to show a clear clinical superiority of lidocaine over bretylium. The initial dose of lidocaine is 1.5 mg $\cdot$ kg^{-1} IV push, which can be followed in 3 to 5 minutes by an additional 1.5 mg $\cdot$ kg^{-1}. Additional doses of 0.5 mg $\cdot$ kg^{-1} may be given every 8 to 10 minutes. Upon return of spontaneous circulation, a continuous infusion at 2 to 4 mg $\cdot$ min^{-1} should be started. Bretylium tosylate at a dose of 5 mg $\cdot$ kg^{-1} is administered as an IV bolus and can be repeated at a dose of 10 mg $\cdot$ kg^{-1} every 5 minutes for a total dose of 30 to 35 mg $\cdot$ kg^{-1}.

OTHER THERAPIES

Sodium bicarbonate therapy should be individualized to the particular clinical scenario. Bicarbonate therapy is not indicated in a hypoxic cardiac arrest with lactic acidosis, since there is not a bicarbonate deficit and buffering the arterial pH may actually worsen the intracellular acidosis. Abnormal magnesium or potassium levels may lead to persistent VT/VF. Hyperkalemia can be treated with CaCl$_2$ (4 mg $\cdot$ kg^{-1}) or insulin and glucose. Hypokalemia should be treated with intravenous potassium chloride (20 to 40 mEq IV over 0.5 hours). Low magnesium should be treated with magnesium sulfate 1 to 2 g IV over 1 to 2 minutes. Procainamide at a dose of 30 mg $\cdot$ min^{-1} IV is also a treatment option in refractory VF/VT, up to a total of 17 mg $\cdot$

```
┌─────────────────────────────────┐
│ Assess oxygenation and vital signs │
│ Perform CPR                      │
└─────────────────────────────────┘
                │
                ▼
                                    ──→ Successful
┌─────────────────────────────┐  ⟨
│ Defibrillate x3 if needed   │  
└─────────────────────────────┘    ──→ Different arrhythmia
                │
          Unsuccessful
                │
                ▼
        ┌──────────────┐
        │ Continue CPR │
        └──────────────┘
                │
                ▼
    ┌──────────────────────────┐
    │ Epinephrine 1 mg q3–5 min │
    └──────────────────────────┘
                │
                ▼
          ┌──────────────┐
          │ Defibrillate │
          └──────────────┘
                │
                ▼
    ┌──────────────────────────────┐
    │ Consider lidocaine x2,        │
    │   bretylium, magnesium sulfate │
    └──────────────────────────────┘
                │
                ▼
          ┌──────────────┐
          │ Defibrillate │
          └──────────────┘
                │
                ▼
    ┌──────────────────────────────┐
    │ Consider procainamide, bicarbonate, │
    │   IV amiodarone                │
    └──────────────────────────────┘
                │
                ▼
          ┌──────────────┐
          │ Defibrillate │
          └──────────────┘
```

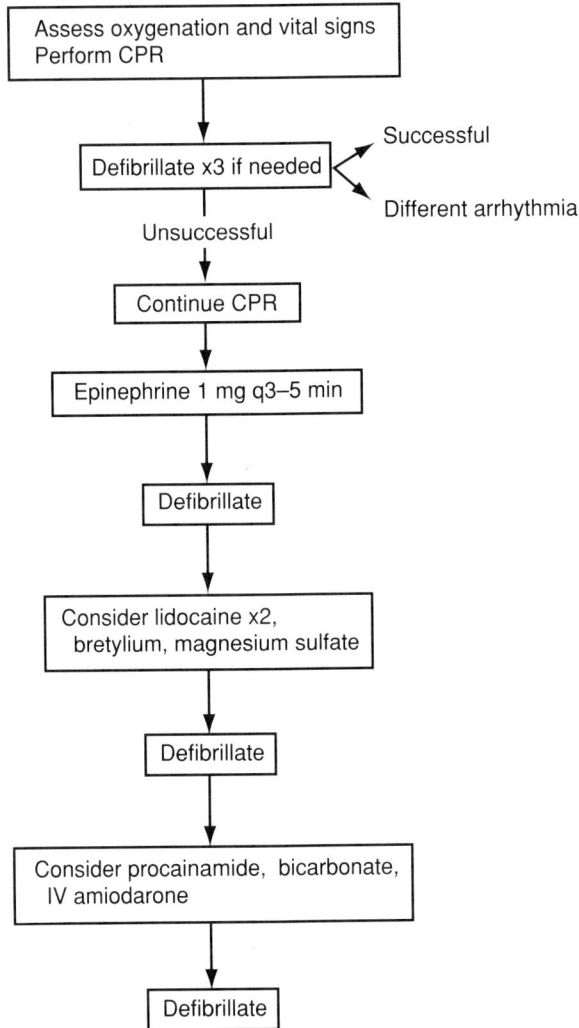

Fig. 13-6. Treatment algorithm for unstable ventricular tachycardia or ventricular fibrillation.

kg^{-1}. Intravenous amiodarone may be lifesaving in patients refractory to the above treatment plans.

Bradycardia Treatment Algorithm

Bradycardia has traditionally been defined as a heart rate of less than 60 beats · min^{-1} in an adult. However, in the postoperative cardiac patient, a higher heart rate is often desired. A search for the cause of the bradycardia is mandatory. The differential diagnosis of hypoxia, myocardial ischemia, hyperkalemia, severe acidosis, hypothermia, drug overdose, or increased parasympathetic tone should be considered. The clinical decision is whether a given heart rate is causing serious problems (hypotension or decreased cardiac output) in that patient. In patients who are hemodynamically stable, observation is the best option, whether in the intensive care unit or on telemetry. Discontinuation or reduction of drugs that may cause bradycardia should be considered. If no readily reversible cause for the bradycardia is apparent (e.g., hypoxia), in symptomatic patients pacing with the epicardial atrial or ventricular pacing wires is appropriate. If the epicardial pacing wires are absent or nonfunctional, an appropriate intervention sequence for symptomatic bradycardia is atropine (0.5 to 1 mg IV), transcutaneous pacing, dopamine (5 to 20 $\mu g \cdot kg^{-1} \cdot min^{-1}$) and epinephrine (2 to 10 $\mu g \cdot min^{-1}$). While increasing the heart rate, isoproterenol causes increased myocardial oxygen consumption and peripheral vasodilation and should be used with caution.

Pulseless Electrical Activity Algorithm

Pulseless electrical activity (PEA) is defined as the absence of a pulse and the presence of a rhythm other than ventricular tachycardia or ventricular fibrillation and includes electromechanical dissociation, pseudo-electromechanical dissociation, idioventricular rhythms, ventricular escape rhythms, bradyasystolic rhythms, and post-defibrillation idioventricular rhythms. Severe hypovolemia is a common cause of PEA, as well as cardiac tamponade, tension pneumothorax, and massive pulmonary embolism. Hyperkalemia, acidosis, massive acute myocardial infarction, and drug overdose with anesthetics, digitalis, β-blockers, and calcium-channel blockers can cause PEA. Therapy should be directed toward correcting the specific clinical state. Nonspecific drug therapies are epinephrine and atropine in the presence of bradycardia.

Asystole Treatment Algorithm

With asystole, CPR should be continued, and the diagnosis should be confirmed in more than one ECG lead. The treatment of choice is pacing (using the epicardial pacing wires), atropine, and epinephrine. The differential diagnosis of hypoxia, hyperkalemia, hypokalemia, severe acidosis, hypothermia, drug overdose, or increased parasympathetic tone should be considered. Succinylcholine

administration can cause bradycardia or transient asystole, particularly in pediatric patients or after repeated doses. Succinylcholine-induced asystole usually readily responds to chest compressions and atropine. Routine defibrillation of asystole is discouraged since electric shocks increase parasympathetic tone and may decrease the likelihood of spontaneous cardiac activity.

ADDITIONAL CLINICAL CONSIDERATIONS

Late-Occurring Dysrhythmias and Long-term Therapy for Dysrhythmias

In patients who develop postoperative supraventricular dysrhythmias, the risk of dysrhythmia recurrence after hospital discharge appears to be low. In most cases, prophylactic agents are administered for 1 to 2 months after hospital discharge and then discontinued. Patients with supraventricular dysrhythmias occurring late after bypass surgery should be treated similarly to patients developing these dysrhythmias in other settings. Patients who develop sustained ventricular dysrhythmias 48 hours or more after the operation and in whom no reversible precipitating factor can be identified are candidates for programmed electrical stimulation-guided therapy.[36]

High-Dose Epinephrine

The standard dose of epinephrine recommended in ACLS protocols is 1 mg for adults. Recent interest has focused on the use of higher doses of epinephrine. In prospective randomized trials of more than 2,400 adult patients in both in-hospital and out-of-hospital cardiac arrest, increased rates of return of spontaneous circulation with higher-dose epinephrine (5 to 10 mg for adults) were demonstrated, but there was no statistically significant improvement in hospital discharge rate compared to standard 1-mg-dose epinephrine. Importantly, the studies failed to demonstrate any adverse effects of higher-dose epinephrine. These studies involved patients with unwitnessed cardiac arrests, and the use of epinephrine represented efforts to resuscitate patients with a very poor chance of survival.[19] It is our opinion that high-dose epinephrine (5 to 10 mg) is appropriate for intraoperative cardiac arrests when the initial standard 1-mg dose of epinephrine has failed.

Magnesium Therapy

There has been considerable interest recently in the use of magnesium for the management of dysrhythmias. Magnesium deficiency is correlated with cardiac dysrhythmias. In cases of known or suspected hypomagnesemia with refractory VT/VF, magnesium should be administered. A recent study of cardiac surgical patients found that nearly 20 percent of patients were hypomagnesemic preinduction, that figure increased to 70 percent after bypass. The patients who were hypomagnesemic had nearly a threefold increased rate of dysrhythmias.[37]

SUMMARY

Dysrhythmias are a common problem during the postoperative period. Fortunately, most dysrhythmias are atrial, which the majority of patients tolerate well. Dysrhythmias that are symptomatic need to be treated aggressively. This chapter outlines treatment strategies. One of the most important principles in dysrhythmia treatment is that one should never merely treat the dysrhythmia but should also search for any untoward physiologic or pharmacologic event that may be causing the dysrhythmia.

REFERENCES

1. Mohr R, Smolinsky A, Goor DA: Prevention of supraventricular tachyarrhythmia with low-dose propranolol after coronary artery bypass. J Thorac Cardiovasc Surg 81:840, 1981

2. Matangi MF, Neutze JM, Graham IC et al: Arrhythmia prophylaxis after aorta-coronary bypass: the effect of minidose propranolol. J Thorac Cardiovasc Surg 89:439, 1985

3. Johnson LW, Dickenstein RA, Freuhan CT et al: Prophylactic digitalization for coronary artery bypass surgery. Circulation 53:819, 1976

4. Parker FB Jr, Greiner-Hayes C, Bove EL et al: Supraventricular arrhythmias following coronary artery bypass: the effect of postoperative digitalis. J Thorac Cardiovasc Surg 86:594, 1983

5. Stephenson LW, MacVaugh H, Tomasello DN, Josephson ME: Propanolol for prevention of postoperative cardiac arrhythmias: a randomized study. Ann Thorac Surg 29:113, 1980

6. Mills SA, Poole GV Jr, Breyer RH et al: Digoxin and propanolol for the prophylaxis of dysrhythmias after coronary artery bypass grafting. Circulation, suppl II. 68:222, 1983

7. Vecht RJ, Nicolaides EP, Ikweuke JK et al: Incidence and prevention of supraventricular tachyarrhythmias after coronary artery bypass surgery. Int J Cardiol 13:124, 1986

8. Rabino MD, Dreifus S, Likoff W: Cardiac Arrhythmias following intracardiac surgery. Am J Cardiol 7:681, 1981

9. Tyras DH, Stothert JC, Kaiser GC et al: Supraventricular tachyarrhythmias after myocardial revascularization: a randomized trial of prophylactic digitalization. J Thorac Cardiovasc Surg 77:31, 1979

10. Silverman NA, Wright R, Lewvitsky S: Efficacy of low-dose propranolol in preventing postoperative supraventricular tachyarrhythmias. Ann Surg 196:194, 1982

11. Angelini P, Feldman MJ, Lutschanowski R et al: Cardiac arrhythmias during and after heart surgery: diagnosis and management. Prog Cardiovasc Dis 16:469, 1974

12. Smith EEJ, Shore DF, Munro JJ et al: Oral Verapamil fails to prevent supraventricular tachycardia following coronary artery surgery. Int J Cardiol 9:37, 1985

13. White HD, Antman GM, Glynn MA et al: Efficacy and safety of timolol for prevention of supraventricular tachyarrhythmias after coronary artery bypass surgery. Circulation 70: 479, 1984

14. Leitch JW, Thompson D, Baird DK, Harris P: The importance of age as a predictor of atrial fibrillation and atrial flutter after coronary ar-

tery bypass grafting. J Thorac Cardiovasc Surg 100:338, 1990

15. Fuller JA, Adams GC, Buxton B et al: Atrial fibillation after coronary artery bypass grafting. J Thorac Cardiovasc Surg 97:821, 1989

16. Rubin DA, Nieminski KE, Monteferrante JC et al: Ventricular arrhythmias after coronary artery bypass surgery: incidence, risk factors, and long-term prognosis. J Am Coll Cardiol 6: 307, 1985

17. Michelson EL, Morganroth J, MacVaugh H: Postoperative arrhythmias after coronary and cardiac valvular surgery detected by long-term electrographic monitoring. Am Heart J 97:442, 1979

18. Wellens HJ, Bar FWH, Lie KL: The value of the electrocardiograms in the differential diagnosis of a tachycardia with a widened QRS complex. Am J Med 64:27, 1978

19. Emergency Cardiac Care Committee. Guidelines for Cardiopulmonary Resuscitation and Emergency Cardiac Care. JAMA 268:2171, 1992

20. Weinberg B, Zipes D: Strategies to manage the post-MI patient with ventricular arrhythmias. Clin Cardiol 12:86, 1989

21. Lee KJ, Wellens HJJ, Dorsnar E, Durrer D: Observations on patients with primary ventricular fibrillation complication acute myocardial infarction. Br Heart J 38:415, 1976

22. El-Sherif N, Myerburg RJ, Scherlag BJ et al: Electrocardiographic antecedents of primary ventricular fibrillation. Value of the R-on-T phenomenon in myocardial infarction. Br Heart J 38:415, 1976

23. Wyse DG, Kellen J, Rademaker AW: Prophylactic versus selective lidocaine for early ventricular arrhythmias of myocardial infarction. J Am Coll Cardiol 12:507, 1988

24. Hine LK, Laird N, Hewitt P, Chalmers, TC: Meta-analytic evidence against prophylactic use of lidocaine in acute myocardial infarction. Arch Intern Med 149:2694, 1989

25. Waldo AL, Henthorn RW, Epstein AE et al: Diagnosis and treatment of arrhythmias during and following open heart surgery. Med Clin North Am 68:1163, 1974

26. Taylor GJ, Malik SA, Colliver JA et al: Usefulness of atrial fibrillation as a predictor of stroke after isolated coronary artery bypass grafting. Am J Cardiol 60:905, 1987

27. Kowey PR, Stonowski A, Schnoor E et al: Impact of atrial fibrillation on duration of hospital stay and cost of coronary artery surgery. Clin Res 40:365A, 1992

28. Andrews TC, Reimold SC, Berlin JA et al: Prevention of supraventricular arrhythmias after coronary artery bypass surgery. Circulation 84:236, 1991

29. Kowey PR, Taylor JE, Rials SJ et al: Meta-analysis of the effectiveness of prophylactic drug therapy in preventing supraventricular arrhythmia early after coronary artery bypass grafting. Am J Cardiol 69:963, 1992

30. Rinkenberger RL, Naccarelli GV: Evaluation and treatment of narrow complex tachycardias. Crit Care Clin 5:569–97, 1989

31. Ewy GA: Urgent parental digoxin therapy: a requiem. J Am Coll Cardiol 15:1248–9, 1990

32. Well JL, Maclean WAH, James TN et al: Characterization of atrial flutter. Studies in man after open heart surgery using fixed atrial electrodes. Circulation 60:665, 1979

33. Cairns CB, Niemann JT: Intravenous adenosine in the emergency department management of paroxysmal supraventricular tachycardia. Ann Emerg Med 20:717, 1991

34. DiMarco JP, Miles W, Akhtar M et al: Adenosine for paroxysmal supraventricular tachycardia: dose ranging and comparison with verapamil: assessment in placebo-controlled, multicenter trials: the Adenosine for PSVT Study Group. Ann Intern Med 113:513, 1990

35. Salerno DM, Diaz VC, Kleiger RE et al: Efficacy and safety of intravenous diltiazem for treatment of atrial fibrillation and atrial flutter. Am J Cardiol 63:1046, 1989

36. Rinkenberger RL, Naccarelli GV: Evaluation and acute treatment of wide-complex tachycardias. Crit Care Clin 5:599, 1989

37. Aglio LS, Stanford CG, Maddi R et al: Hypomagnesia is common following cardiac surgery. J Cardiothorac Vasc Anesth 5:201, 1991

14

Transesophageal Echocardiography and Cardiac Critical Care

David T. Porembka

Transesophageal echocardiography (TEE) is the ideal diagnostic modality for the critical care physician.[1-8] In cardiac intensive care patients, the etiology of acute hemodynamic instability may be difficult to delineate because of the limitations of existing technology, (that is, for pulmonary arterial catheterization, incomplete information often results from pulmonary artery occlusion pressure, or for transthoracic echocardiography [TTE], a limited acoustic window often results in nondiagnostic data). In such cases, TEE provides immediate valuable information on the etiology. This facilitates lifesaving therapeutic medical and surgical interventions, while avoiding unnecessary surgical procedures (e.g., re-exploration and evacuation of a fictitious pericardial tamponade) or the transportation of critically ill patients for further diagnostic procedures (e.g., angiography for an aortic dissection). This chapter discusses the benefits of echocardiography in the cardiac intensive care unit (ICU) with an emphasis on TEE and its use in ventricular performance; pericardial effusion and cardiac tamponade; valvular heart disease; native and prosthetic valves (including complications); aortic pathology; dissection, debris, thrombus, and traumatic injury; endocarditis and associated abscesses; intracardiac mass; intracardiac shunts; congenital and acquired patent foramen ovale (PFO); and pulmonary embolism (PE).[1-8]

INDICATIONS

TEE provides instantaneous and global knowledge of the patient's ventricular performance: both left and right ventricles, systolic and diastolic function, end-systolic and end-diastolic volume, physiologic and/or mechanical compression from pericardial effusion or tamponade (possibly loculated), and complications of cardiac injury (i.e., ischemia, infarction, or myocardial contusion via the detection of regional wall motion abnormalities [RWMA]). A dynamic left ventricular outflow tract obstruction (systolic anterior motion of the anterior leaflet of the mitral valve) or iatrogenic mitral stenosis, following placement of a Carpentier's mitral valve ring, as the cause of postoperative hypotension may be visualized by TEE in a patient in whom shock and pulmonary edema develop, following myocardial infarction, the diagnosis of a ruptured papillary muscle, chordae tendineae, or ventricular septal defect is rapidly assessed with TEE. The function and integrity of cardiac valves (native or prosthetic) may be visualizable perioperatively only with TEE. The source for cerebral embolism, either intracardiac (i.e., thrombi in the atrial appendage) or aortic (for mobile pedunculated thrombi) is easily diagnosed by TEE. The prompt identification of an acute aortic dissection or traumatic injury and associated findings may be lifesaving. TEE is of proven value in these critical situations and should be the first diagnostic tool used.

In patients with suspected endocarditis, TTE may be equivocal or nondiagnostic (this is particularly true in those with a prosthetic valve). TEE is then used for the identification of the vegetation(s) and associated abscesses. TTE can usually evaluate atrial or septal defects; however, in situations such as penetrating cardiac trauma, small, multiple, or irregular defects may only be characterized by the use of TEE. PFO is another possible indication for TEE because of the increased sensitivity compared to TTE. This "normal" anatomic finding may be the harbinger for paradoxic embolism or hypoxia. In patients who are hypotensive and/or hypoxic, the TEE assessment may identify characteristic echocardiographic findings consistent with an acute pulmonary embolism. Finally, TEE may be of value in patients with small intracardiac masses or tumors where TTE is limited.[9-19]

CONTRAINDICATIONS

TEE is contraindicated in patients with esophageal pathology, including history of esophageal surgery (including total gastric resection), neoplasm, strictures, diverticulum, esophagitis, systemic sclerosis, trau-

matic penetrating injury, or fistulae. Dysphagia, odynophagia, recent chest wall radiation, and upper gastrointestinal bleeding are only relative contraindications. If esophageal disease is suspected, a gastroenterologist should be consulted. If the patient's airway is not protected (i.e., by use of an endotracheal tube), the "elective" patient should be fasting (nothing per os [NPO]) for 6 to 8 hours prior to the procedure.[9-19] Patients at high risk of aspiration of gastric contents should receive prophylaxis (i.e., H_2-antagonist and nonparticulate antacids) prior to the procedure. Pregnant patients have undergone TEE procedures without any difficulties, but judicious sedation is required in these individuals.[20] If large dosages of sedative medications (midazolam and/or fentanyl) are required, the airway must be adequately protected prior to the procedure.

COMPLICATIONS

Even though the TEE procedure is considered semi-invasive and is used in patients with known cardiac disease who are critically ill, it is quite safe. In a large multicenter investigation of 10,419 TEE examinations, consisting primarily of conscious patients, only one death was associated with the procedure.[21] This patient succumbed to hematemesis due to an unsuspected lung carcinoma that eroded into the esophagus. In this study, and in a related Mayo Clinic study, the incidence of major complications were 0.18 to 0.5 percent. Some of the other complications included dysrhythmias, laryngospasm, transient hemodynamic aberrations (hypotension or hypertension), congestive heart failure, bronchospasm, laryngospasm, hypoxia, and temporary vocal chord dysfunction.[22] Mechanical complications such as transtracheal placement, bronchial obstruction, and aortic compression were more common in children.[23-25] Mechanical malfunction of the TEE probe (i.e., buckling of the distal tip) was described in four patients (the only sign was resistance during manipulation

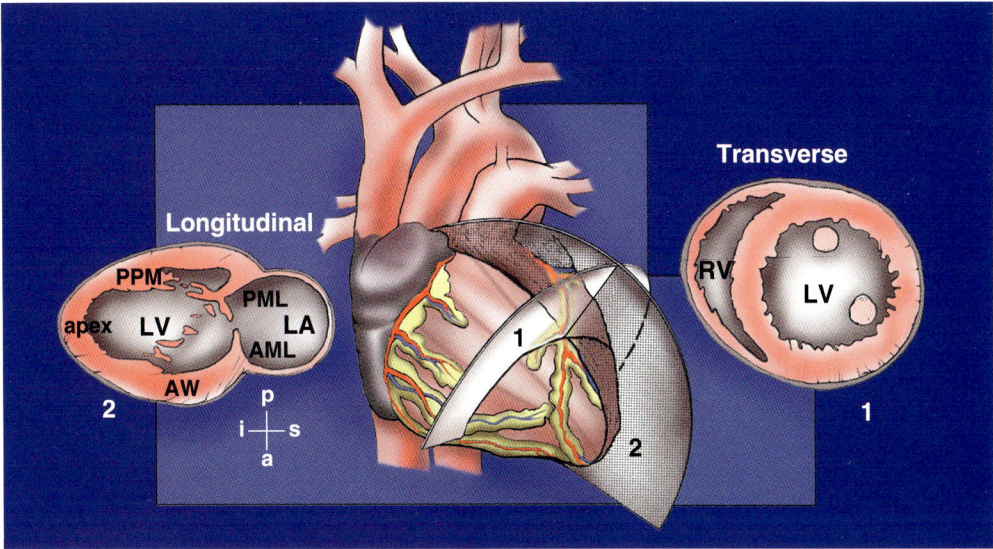

Plate 14-1. Transgastric view. Longitudinal and transverse imaging with transesophageal echocardiography. A, anterior; AML, anterior mitral leaflet; AW, anterior wall; I, inferior; LA, left atrium; LV, left ventricle; P, posterior; PML, posterior mitral leaflet; RV, right ventricle; S, superior. (From Porembka DT, Stein K, Bierman M, Masciangelo T: Transesophageal echocardiography in critical care. In Ayres S, Grenvik A, Holbrook P, Shoemaker W (eds): Textbook of Critical Care. 3rd Ed. WB Saunders, Philadelphia, 1995, with permission.)

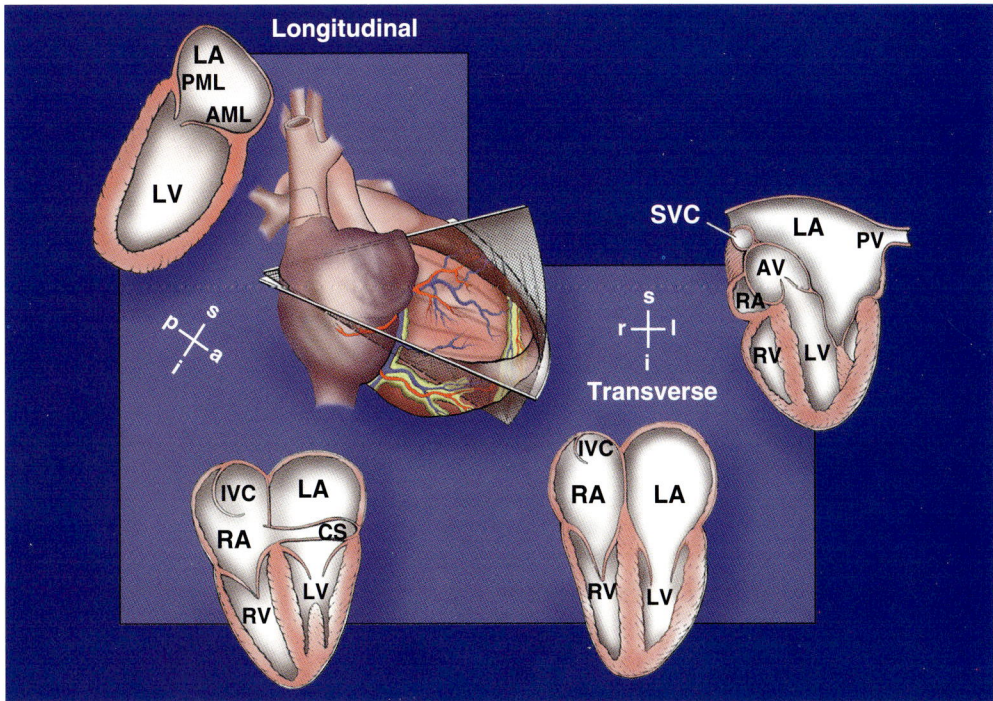

Plate 14-2. Midesophageal view. Longitudinal and transverse imaging with transesophageal echocardiography. LA, left atrium; LV, left ventricle; RA, right atrium; RV, right ventricle; AML, anterior mitral leaflet; PML, posterior mitral leaflet; CS, coronary sinus; PV, pulmonary vein; S, superior; I, inferior; A, anterior; P, posterior; IVC, inferior vena cava; SVC, superior vena cava. (From Porembka DT, Stein K, Bierman M, Masciangelo T: Transesophageal echocardiography in critical care. In Ayres S, Grenvik A, Holbrook P, Shoemaker W (eds): Textbook of Critical Care. 3rd Ed. WB Saunders, Philadelphia, 1995, with permission.)

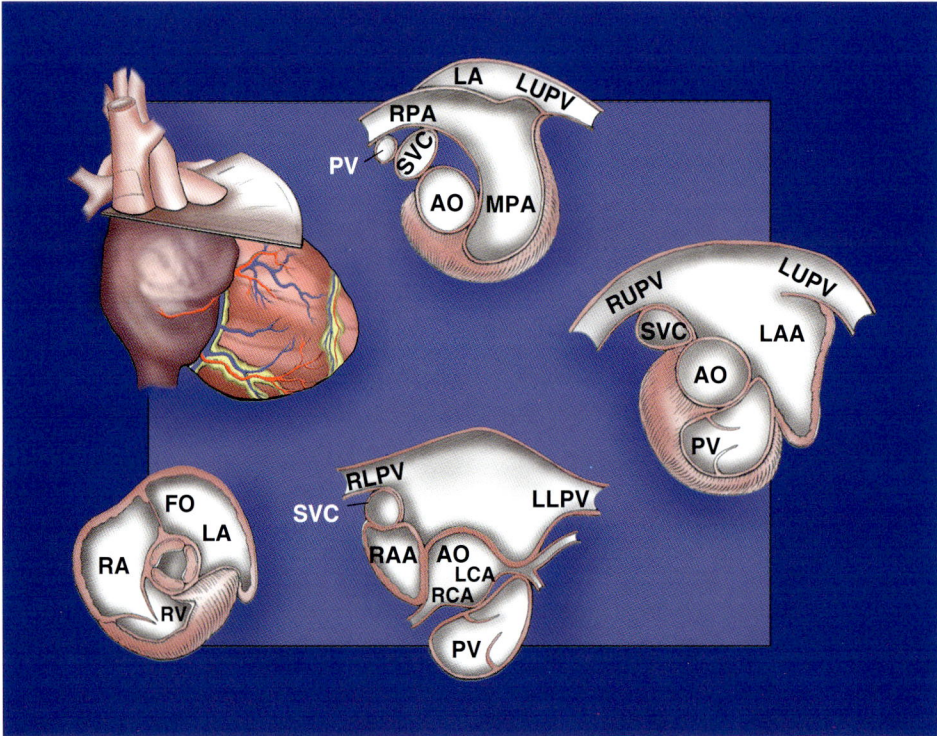

Plate 14-3. Base of the heart. Transverse imaging with transesophageal echocardiography. AO, aorta; LA, left atrium; LAA, left atrial appendage; LLPV, left lower pulmonary vein; LUPV, left upper pulmonary vein; FO, fossa ovalis; LCA, left coronary artery; MPA, main pulmonary artery; PV, pulmonary vein; RA, right atrium; RAA, right atrial appendage; RCA, right coronary artery; RLPV, right lower pulmonary vein; RPA, right pulmonary artery; RUPV, right upper pulmonary vein; RV, right ventricle; SVC, superior vena cava. (From Porembka DT, Stein K, Bierman M, Masciangelo T: Transesophageal echocardiography in critical care. In Ayres S, Grenvik A, Holbrook P, Shoemaker W (eds): Textbook of Critical Care. 3rd Ed. WB Saunders, Philadelphia, 1995, with permission.)

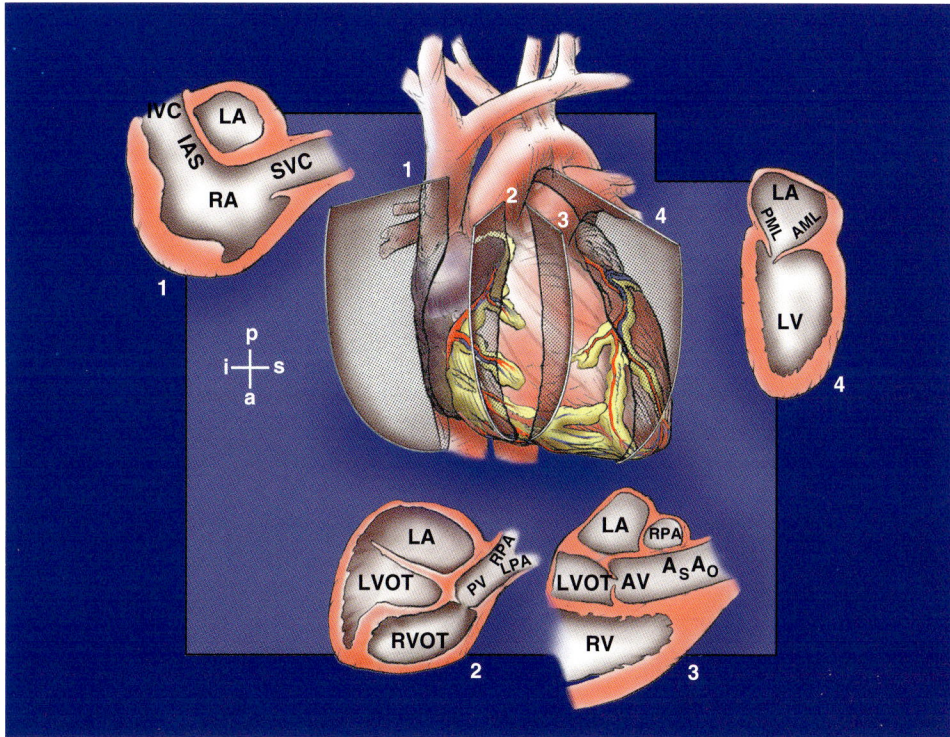

Plate 14-4. Base of the heart. Longitudinal views with transesophageal echocardiography. AML, anterior mitral valve leaflet; A_SA_O, ascending aorta; AV, aortic valve; IAS, interatrial septum; IVC, inferior vena cava; LA, left atrium; LPA, left pulmonary artery; LV, left ventricle; LVOT, left ventricle outflow tract; PML, posterior mitral valve leaflet; PV, pulmonary valve; RA, right atrium; RPA, right pulmonary artery; RV, right ventricle; RVOT, right ventricular outflow tract; SVC, superior vena cava. (From Porembka DT, Stein K, Bierman M, Masciangelo T: Transesophageal Echocardiography in Critical Care. In Ayres S, Grenvik A, Holbrook P, Shoemaker W (eds): Textbook of Critical Care. 3rd Ed. WB Saunders, Philadelphia, 1995, with permission.)

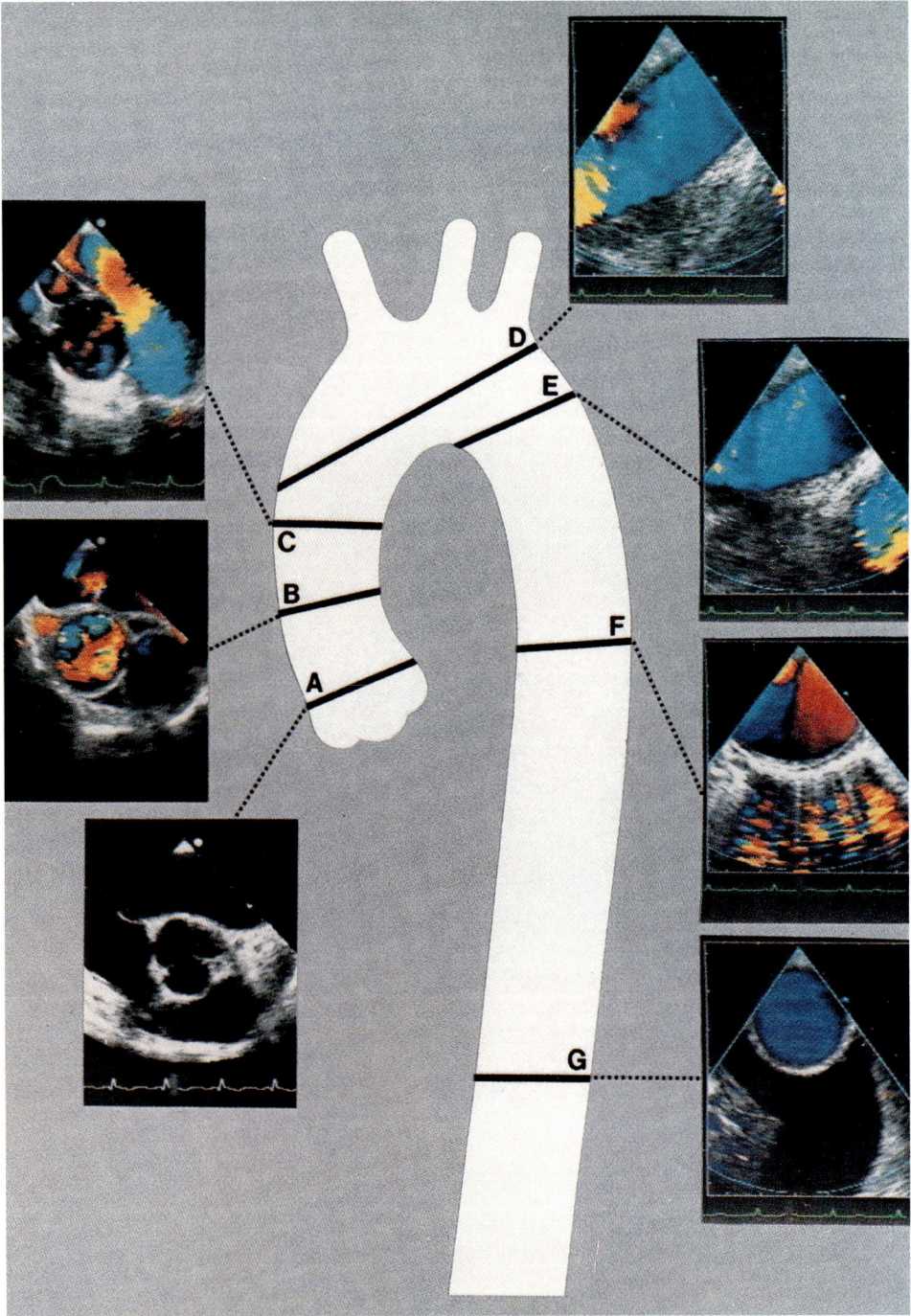

Plate 14-5. Thoracic aorta. Sequential transverse imaging of the ascending, arch, and descending thoracic aorta of normal anatomy with color-flow Doppler echocardiography. (Courtesy of Chandrasekaran K, Likoff Cardiovascular Institute, Hahnemann University Hospital, Philadelphia, PA.)

of the probe).[26] Two esophageal perforations were reported: one not specified and the other a Mallory-Weiss tear diagnosed in the cardiac ICU.[27] Despite this high benefit-to-risk ratio, experienced operators should be present, keeping in mind that no procedure is benign.

ANATOMIC IMAGES

TTE images are limited, particularly after a cardiothoracic surgical operation, because of the interference of dressings, tapes, and chest thoracostomy tubes. Obese patients with chronic obstructive pulmonary disease (COPD) or subcutaneous emphysema will have limited acoustic windows with TTE. The major advantage with TEE is the ability to image the heart and adjacent structures from a retrocardiac position free from the lung parenchyma and intervening chest wall. Detailed anatomic descriptions are given elsewhere (Refs. 11, 13, 14, 18, 19), but in this text a brief portrayal is presented. Transverse TEE imaging allows superior visualization of the mitral valve apparatus for mitral regurgitation of both native and prosthetic valves where there is acoustic attenuation with TTE. Only TEE can examine the left atrial appendage for thrombus. Most of the thoracic aorta is seen with the single-plane transverse view, but the addition of longitudinal imaging increases the visualization of the aorta even when it is ectatic. The other advantage of longitudinal planes is the improved characterization of the atrial septum, aortic valve, right ventricular outflow tracts, proximal pulmonary artery and the pulmonary valve, apical region of the left ventricle, and mitral valve leaflets, as well as any regurgitant jets present. The only limited views we have experienced are in patients with mediastinal emphysema (three cases).

There are three major transverse views: basal short-axis, four-chamber, and short-axis view of the left ventricle. Corresponding longitudinal views are at the mid-esophageal and transgastric regions (Plates 14-1 to 14-4). The majority of the thoracic aorta is visualized by both transverse and longitudinal imaging; however, the superior portion of the ascending aorta and the aortic arch can be poorly visualized or can return false-positive results (echoes) (Plate 14-5). Omniplanar imaging can scan a continuum of the images presented in this context. There are standard accepted transverse views; however, the orientation of the longitudinal views vary depending on institutional practice standards.[11,13,14,18,19]

VENTRICULAR PERFORMANCE

Global Function

One of the major benefits of TEE is the rapidity with which the diagnosis can be established. As a clinician responds to the lability of a patient's systemic blood pressure, TEE may be crucial. Global systolic function (ejection fraction) is usually evaluated first in the directed TEE examination. Systolic index or fraction and fractional shortening are also inspected to evaluate global function. While these indices may be helpful in the stable or outpatient setting, they are exquisitely load-dependent (i.e., preload, afterload) measures of ventricular performance. Thus, these measures are supplanted in the ICU environment with other global systolic functions, such as M-mode, two-dimensional, and Doppler echocardiography.

The most common means of measuring qualitative or quantitative systolic function and volume assessment is with two-dimensional echocardiography. Areas and volume are easily assessed with TEE by the visualization of the ventricles from the short-gastric and foreshortened views. Generally, the end-diastolic area at the midpapillary region correlates approximately 87 percent with actual left ventricular volumes.[28]

Konstadt et al.[29] showed a good approximation between the volume assessments obtained with TEE and thermodilution cardiac output. Beaupre and colleagues[30] compared the stroke volume obtained with thermodilution to the fractional short-axis changes of TEE and described an excellent correlation (91 percent). In their study, as expected, there was only a 23 percent interdependence of the pulmonary occlusion pressure and end-diastolic short-axis change. When compared with nuclear techniques, TEE results were favorable.[31,32] In a similar study, but using radionuclide angiography, TEE volume estimates were excellent (r = 0.92).[33]

Volume interpretation can be crucial in the care of the critically ill. Can TEE be used for the estimation of volume depletion (hypovolemia)? In the pediatric population, Reich et al.[33] found an 80 percent rate of concordance between ventricular dimensional changes and blood withdrawal or reinfusion. In a similar study (adult) conducted by Cheung and colleagues,[34] the left ventricular determinants of preload (TEE) correlated well with the blood pressure in patients with either normal or abnormal left ventricular function during graded hypovolemia. This correlation was readily apparent with only a 2.5 percent estimated blood volume deficit.

Different results were seen in a study by Van Daele et al.,[35] in which patients underwent acute hypervolemic hemodilution. Initially there was an increase in stroke volume and end-diastolic area, but with progressive hemodilution the end-systolic area decreased.

Systolic cavitary obliteration is considered an early echocardiographic sign of hypovolemia and generally precedes peripheral hemodynamic aberrations.[36] This systolic obliteration is also noticeable in patients with hyperdynamic states (e.g., liver failure, systemic inflammatory response syndrome, pancreatitis, trauma, and poisons that interfere with the cytochrome or electron transport systems) who are euvolemic and adequately resuscitated. If these patients become hypovolemic, not only will systolic cavitary obliteration occur, but some patients may exhibit left ventricular outflow tract obstruction from systolic anterior motion (SAM) of the anterior mitral valve leaflet.

End-diastolic area is also useful in estimating the degree of hypovolemia. A decrease in this area to less then $5.5 \text{ cm}^2 \cdot \text{m}^{-2}$ is commonly associated with hypovolemia. However, this demarcation is not reliable in patients in whom actual hypovolemia may coexist with severe depressions in contractility and a resultant dilatory response by the ventricle. These state-dependent interactions are among the more obvious limitations with TEE. For example, these discrepancies are readily apparent in patients with acute lung injury and myocardial dysfunction.

The adequacy of measured preload is a daily controversy in the critically ill, particularly in those patients with adult respiratory distress syndrome (ARDS). In patients requiring high levels of positive end-expiratory pressure (PEEP), the estimation of ventricular volumes is enhanced with TEE. Not only are volume (dimensions) evaluable, but common intracardiac interactions that depress cardiac output (i.e., enlarged right atrium and abnormal atrial septal motion with bulging fossa ovalis, right ventricular dilation and global dysfunction with septal shift, and decreased ventricular indices) may be serially evaluated during the course of illness and therapy. Schuster and Jardin's investigations demonstrate much of the interplay involved in acute lung injury.[37,38] In a recent evaluation of patients undergoing pressure-controlled inverse ratio ventilation, TEE was used for hemodynamic appraisal. The hemodynamic effects were not different whether pressure-controlled or volume-controlled ventilation with a deceleration flow pattern was used.[39] There is ample evidence that the application of TEE will assist the physician in managing patients in whom significant left and right heart interactions occur.

The inherent difficulties with qualitative assessment of preload and myocardial performance echocardiographically stimulated the development of computer-enhanced imaging. Cine-loop digitization has greatly refined the accuracy of visual assessment of ventricular volume and function. Acoustic quantification (AQ) is also a useful methodology for quantifying ventricular volume and performance. Excellent results were depicted in Cahalan's study when the method of AQ was compared with thermodilution cardiac output.[40] A recent investigation that compares AQ with the conductance method for ventricular volume assessment, an experimental "gold standard" for ventricular performance and volume measurements, found a high correlation (0.93).[41] Three-dimensional reconstruction of the heart is the next obvious step.[42–49]

Regional Function

Identification of the high-risk patient with ischemic heart disease remains a major hurdle for the clinician. In many cases these patients are physiologically and symptomatically "silent." Standard electrocardiographic (ECG) technology is limited by the following patient conditions: left ventricular hypertrophy, intraventricular conduction delay, paced rhythm, drug effect (e.g., digitalis), lead positioning, and patient movement or agitation. Echocardiography may be the ideal diagnostic tool with which to establish the diagnosis as extrapolations from animal and angioplasty studies appear to indicate.[50,51] Once perfusion is interrupted, the earliest signs of myocardial ischemia, in decreasing order of sensitivity, are as follows: systolic wall thickening, impaired ventricular relaxation, RWMA, global compliance alterations, ST-segment changes, and finally, angina.[52]

When the TEE probe is positioned to view the left ventricle at the mid-papillary region, ischemic segments or RWMA are easily detectable with echocardiography.[52,53] There is an excellent temporal relationship between the onset of myocardial ischemia (total or marginal occlusion) and development of a RWMA.[54] Only when there is complete occlusion of coronary arterial inflow will ECG and echocardiographic techniques correlate in the detection of ischemia[54] (Fig. 14-1). To improve the characterization of the RWMA, various "semiquantitative" scoring systems are available (e.g., a proposed wall motion index

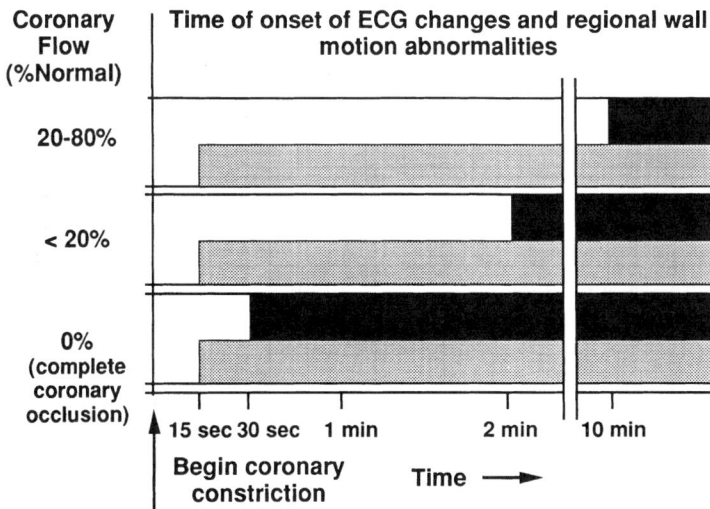

Fig. 14-1. Temporary relationship of regional wall motion abnormalities and ECG readings indicative of myocardial ischemia with varied coronary artery blood flow. Black bars represent ECG changes (ST depression/elevation); gray bars, regional wall motion abnormalities (hypokinesia, akinesia, dyskinesia). (Modified from Clements and de Bruijn,[315] with permission.)

representing 16 segments of the left ventricle developed by the American Society of Echocardiography).

Numerous investigations have shown superior efficacy of echocardiography for the detection of myocardial ischemia as compared to the ECG.[53,55-58] Smith et al.[53] evaluated these two techniques in cardiac and vascular patients. These investigators found that 48 percent of patients had new RWMAs, while in only six patients were coincidental ST-segment changes noted. In comparison, patients with identifiable ST-segment changes all had RWMAs.[53]

A small study by Leung et al.[59] compared ECG with TEE in 50 patients; these workers reported the following detection rates of myocardial ischemia: pre-bypass, 20 percent (TEE) versus 7 percent (ECG); post-bypass, 36 percent (TEE) versus 25 percent (ECG); and ICU 25 percent (TEE) versus 16 percent (ECG). Forty-four of their 50 patients developed RWMA. Of all the patients with ECG-identifiable ischemia, only 18 percent had concurrent echocardiographic findings. Additionally, the presence of a RWMA was characterized as a marker for an adverse event. As expected, most of these patients had normal hemodynamics when a RWMA was occurring.[59-61] Although some patient populations (e.g., vascular patients) may not benefit broadly from a TEE for elucidating RWMA, their ischemic presentation may be severe global dysfunction, which *is* best managed with TEE.[56]

Various sensitivities and specificities for the echocardiographic identification of myocardial ischemia are reported because not all RWMA are of an ischemic nature. Intrinsic causes include paced rhythms, aberrant ventricular contractions or conduction abnormalities, prior tissue fibrosis, and mechanical shifting of cardiac structures. Extrinsic situations that produce RWMAs include tethering of adjacent segments, iatrogenic and physiologic constraints, and regional alterations in afterload. It is typical for one or more of these conditions to occur in the intensive care patient. Critical evaluation of the patient's disease state is crucial. The question that must be addressed is whether the patient is exhibiting myocardial ischemia or an intrinsic/extrinsic condition. Coordination of all the information from the patient leads to the diagnosis.

Analyses of RWMA and ejection fraction is subjective. Deutsch et al.[62] evaluated the variability of visual interpretation of RWMA during cardiac surgery. In this study the left ventricle was represented by six segments; four grades of wall motion were used: normal, hypokinetic, akinetic, and dyskinetic. On two separate interpretations, only 5 percent of the 480 segments reviewed were recorded differently by the same observer. However, different observers noted disparate results in 9 percent of segments and in 39 percent of patients. The grade difference was very small—less than one grade in all cases.[62] In Saada's investigation, ejection fraction was correctly identified in 49 percent of cases and volume changes accurately estimated in 62 percent of cases.[63] Similar results were seen in Doer's series.[64] As expected, gross changes are easily detected, but subtle alterations are invariably missed (58 percent).[65]

In spite of these limitations, stress echocardiography is approaching nuclear techniques in its efficacy for the evaluation of ischemic heart disease.[66-79] In Marwick's study, the sensitivity for the diagnosis of ischemia was essentially equivalent (72 percent) to sestamibi scintigraphy (76 percent).[73] Interestingly, though, perfusion imaging offers a lower specificity for ischemic detection than echocardiography. To estimate the area of myocardium at risk during stress and the location or extent of coronary artery disease, dobutamine stress echocardiography is increasing in use.[75] In Baer's study, the agreement between dobutamine stress echocardiography and fluorine-18 flurodeoxyglucose positron emission tomography was 90 percent. The positive and negative predictive accuracy for dobutamine echocardiography was 81 percent and 97 percent, respectively.[77] Thus, stress echocardiography has become a viable alternative to the more expensive, less mobile, and cumbersome nuclear techniques.

Improvements in probe technology and computer manipulation of images, as well as the addition of contrast agents, will definitely increase the sensitivity as well as the specificity of echocardiography for the diagnosis of myocardial ischemia. Contrast agents (e.g., sonicated albumin) are being investigated for the assessment of myocardial protection (antegrade and retrograde cardioplegia) and the quality of the distal anastomosis.[80,81] The use of these agents enhances our understanding of the mechanisms involved in incomplete myocardial protection (i.e., aortic regurgitation and right-to-left shunt).[82] Eventually echocardiography with contrast agents may be useful in the ICU setting to assist the intensivist and/or cardiologist in the evaluation of myocardial perfusion and associated defects.

Diastolic Function

One of the many benefits of echocardiography is the ability to assess diastolic function. Existing technology (i.e., pulmonary artery catheter) and the information recovered are often misleading and stand in contradistinction to the actual pathology of the patient. Diastolic dysfunction is a common event in the critically ill patient.

Predictably, TEE will visualize the pulmonary veins for evaluating the flow patterns. Examination of transmitral and pulmonary venous flow patterns are helpful in clarifiying suspected discrepancies between patient pathology and pulmonary artery data (Plate 14-6). Commonly, the pulmonary vein flow signal is depicted by four phases: (1) systolic flow due to ventricular contractions with drop of the mitral annulus toward the apex; (2) diastolic inflow secondary to the opening of the mitral valve; (3) retrograde flow secondary to atrial contraction; and (4) systolic inflow due to atrial relaxation. Normal profiles have been described.[83-87]

In dilated hearts, systolic peak flow will decrease, while the diastolic component decreases both in hypertrophied and in dilated hearts.[88] Overall, the second component of the pulmonary flow pattern (i.e., systole) is influenced by systolic function (i.e., contraction), while the diastolic phase and atrial systole are affected by impaired diastolic function (i.e., relaxation), which is similar to the factors that affect the transmitral velocities.[89,90]

Transmitral velocities are helpful when analyzing diastolic function. This velocity represents two distinct filling waves that coalesce to form the instantaneous relationship between left ventricular and atrial pressures (Fig. 14-2). The E wave heralds the onset of rapid filling early in diastole, while the A wave represents the onset of atrial contraction. Normally, the A wave is smaller than the E wave.

Alterations in the E to A wave ratio occur frequently and are the result of varied loading conditions or impaired ventricular function. When the ratio approaches 1.0, it is indicative of impaired ventricular relaxation, which commonly occurs in patients with systemic and pulmonary hypertension, myocardial injury, ischemia or cardiomyopathy, and left ventricular hypertrophy.

A second prototypical pattern is the result of restrictive inflow (i.e., an (increased E-to-A ratio). Typically this occurs in patients with impaired systolic function and increased left atrial or ventricular end-diastolic volume. A normal pattern, however, is not reliably indicative of normal physiology. This pattern is dependent on the underlying pathophysiology, age, sampling technique, and heart rate.[91]

In an attempt to examine these various flow patterns, various loading conditions were simulated in an animal model.[91] During volume loading, the pericardium had a restraining effect on the left and right ventricular filling over an extensive range of physio-

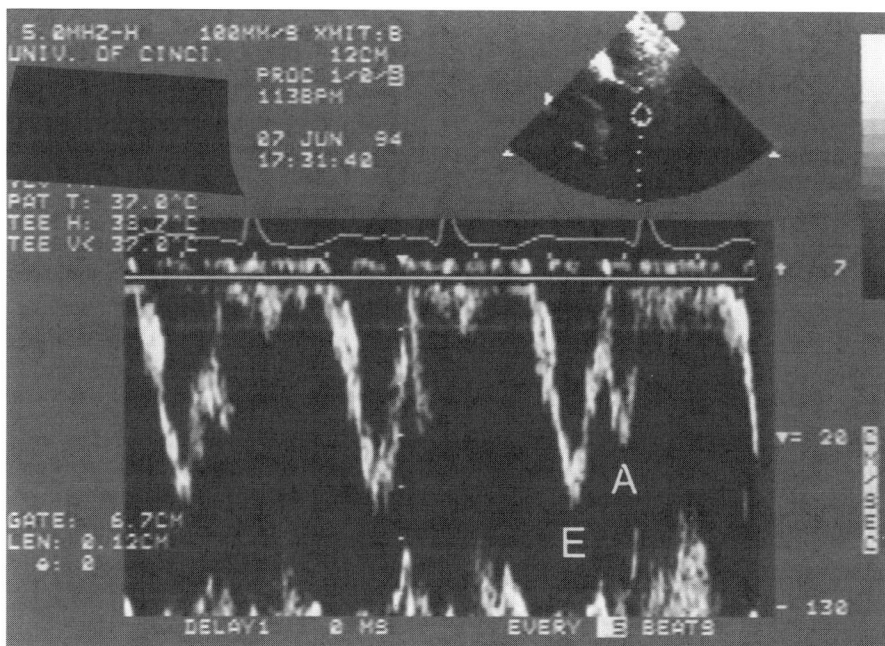

Fig. 14-2. Mitral inflow velocities. Transverse foreshortened long-axis view of the left ventricle with pulsed-wave echocardiography sampling just proximal with left juxtaposition to the apposition of the mitral valve leaflets. A, late diastolic filling; E, early diastolic filling.

logic volumes and pressures; thus, a pericardectomy would be expected to have a noticeable effect on flow patterns.[91]

The effect of PEEP, which alters both loading conditions and ventricular compliance, was studied over several levels. There was a significant reduction in the total mitral-time integral and velocity-time integral of the E wave. At a level of 15 cm H_2O pressure, the ratio of E-to-A wave dramatically decreased.[92]

It has been proposed that either the E-to-A ratio of the transmitral inflow velocities or the pattern of pulmonary venous inflow characteristics may be used for an estimation of left ventricular filling.[92–95] There are limited data to substantiate an inverse relationship between high left atrial pressure and the systolic component of the pulmonary venous flow pattern.[95] However, in patients with impaired left ventricular dysfunction, this correlation does not occur. Unfortunately, this is the usual experience in critically ill patients (e.g., those with the systemic inflammatory

response syndrome [SIRS]). The authors recently evaluated the correlation of pulmonary venous flow patterns with pulmonary artery occlusion pressure in patients with SIRS and acute lung injury and found discouraging results.[96,97]

Pericardial Effusion and Cardiac Tamponade

It is not atypical in the cardiac ICU to evaluate a patient with suspected cardiac tamponade. Pericardial effusions that are clinically "silent" occur in approximately 56 percent of postcardiac surgical patients, while a cardiac tamponade occurs in 1.0 to 2.5 percent of patients. Identifying a patient who is developing cardiac tamponade is lifesaving, since the patient's outcome is directly related to its prompt decompression.[98–100]

An intact pericardium has a constraining effect during the development of a pericardial effusion, limiting the dilation of the cardiac chambers.[101,102] While the intravascular volume (preload) remains constant and the pressure (volume) increases in the pericardium, the absolute transmural pressure will decrease until the pericardial pressure exceeds the intracavitary pressure, at which point the myocardial wall will move inward.

The compensatory rise in venous pressure is insufficient, and as right ventricular diastolic and pericardial pressures rise toward the left ventricular diastolic pressure, there results a decrease in the systemic arterial pressure (hypotension). In this sequence of events, the pressure/volume curve of the pericardium is equal to, or steeper than, that of the ventricles. This results in an emphasis shift in cardiac filling from a ventricular compliance to a pericardial compliance curve.[101,102]

In a patient with a pericardial effusion, comprehensive echocardiographic examinations should be performed. Most effusions are seen with TTE, the primary imaging plane being the parasternal long-axis view of the left ventricle. When TTE is technically inadequate, a TEE examination should be performed expeditiously, if clinically feasible.

Once pulsus paradoxus (an exaggeration of the normal inspiratory decline in aortic pressure) intervenes, the echocardiographic signs of cardiac tamponade are present. These characteristic findings are inversion of the right atrial and ventricular free wall (due to the reversal of the transmural pressure gradient), compression of the right atrium and ventricle at high intrapericardial pressure, and exaggerated respiratory variation of the mitral and tricuspid inflow velocities[103-105] (Fig. 14-3).

Right ventricular diastolic collapse or inversion is the most characteristic echocardiographic sign seen in a tamponade situation. During diastole, after the opening of the mitral valve, a persistent inward or posterior motion of the right ventricular free wall appears as a localized concavity. This is the consequence of pericardial pressures higher than the intracavitary pressures. In the supine patient, this occurs in the proximal infundibulum and in the right ventricular free wall.

Clinically, there appears to be no consistent relationship between the duration or extent of inversion and the severity of tampon-

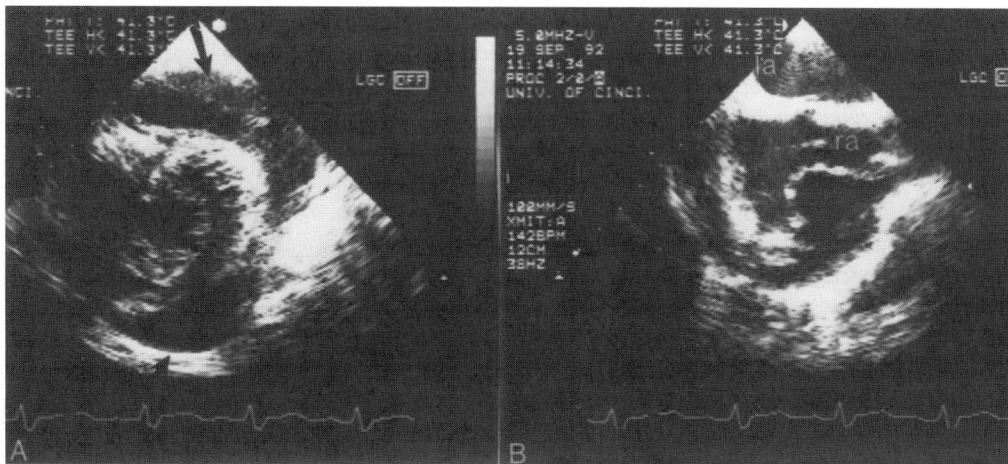

Fig. 14-3. Cardiac tamponade. **(A)** Transverse view of the left ventricle at the midpapillary region reveals large anterior and posterior pericardial effusions with decreased left ventricular dimensions. **(B)** Corresponding transverse biatrial view of the same patient reveals inward movement of the right atrial free wall in diastole. la, left atrium; ra, right atrium.

ade. Once the critical pericardial volume of fluid is reached, right ventricular diastolic inversion occurs. At this point, the cardiac output decreases (21 percent), but mean systemic arterial pressure is maintained. In other words, right ventricular diastolic collapse occurs after the rise in venous and intrapericardial pressures, but prior to the clinical presentation of tamponade. In extreme cases, right ventricular diastolic collapse persists throughout diastole, and the right ventricular cavity is essentially obliterated.[106]

Typically, in critically ill cardiac patients myocardial performance is depressed, while the adequacy of preload is uncertain. The extent of right ventricular diastolic collapse is affected by all the following factors contributing to the patient's hemodynamic state: chamber compliance, pre-existing left or right ventricular dysfunction, and right ventricular preload.[107–110] In a canine model, volume replacement reduces the magnitude of right ventricular collapse, presumably by increasing the ventricular transmural pressure differential.[111]

Similarly, the extent of the right ventricular diastolic collapse will be delayed or reduced in patients who have pre-existing pulmonary artery hypertension or an acute elevation of pulmonary arterial pressure.[109] These delayed echocardiographic findings are also seen consistently in patients with acute left ventricular pressure overload. Hoit et al.[101] have shown that the presence or absence of an intact pericardium has an effect on right ventricular diastolic collapse and the filling of both ventricles over a wide range of volumes and pressures. At equivalent left ventricular end-diastolic volumes, a pericardiectomy alters the pressure-to-volume relationships and ventricular filling more on the right side than on the left. At equivalent intrapericardial pressures, the transmural pressure gradient affects the chamber stiffness and ventricular shape on the right more than the left.

The sensitivity of right ventricular diastolic collapse as an indicator of tamponade is rela-tively good in medical patients. In surgical patients the sensitivities are lower (48 to 77 percent).[103] The discrepancies reported in these sensitivities are the result of using clinical or echocardiographic definitions of cardiac tamponade. If cardiac tamponade is defined clinically as a decrease in systemic arterial pressure with pulsus paradoxus, right ventricular diastolic collapse is not specific. If, however, right ventricular diastolic collapse is an identifiable marker, this sign is highly specific.

This matter is even more controversial in patients who have an acute lung injury requiring high levels of PEEP. Increasing PEEP increases the extent of the right ventricular collapse as the transmission of the airway pressure to the central circulation increases. This allows a previously insignificant pericardial effusion to become echocardiographically significant in spite of a minimal decrease in arterial pressure.

Another possible indicator of cardiac tamponade is right atrial inversion or compression.[104,105] Normally, during systole and diastole, the configuration of the atrial free wall is rounded because of the positive-pressure gradient. With the reversal of this gradient, the atrial free wall moves inward, particularly during late diastole. As the volume of tamponade increases the pericardial pressure rises, and this inward movement continues through systole. During the progression of tamponade, right atrial inversion occurs prior to right ventricular inversion. At high intrapericardial pressures, collapse of both right atrium and ventricle occurs. The systemic pressure is usually declining when this is visualized. Right atrial inversion is uniformly a sensitive sign for cardiac tamponade, while the specificity is 82 percent. The sensitivity and specificity increase to 94 percent and 100 percent, respectively, when the duration of right atrial collapse extends through one-third of the cardiac cycle.[104]

M-mode echocardiography assists in the timing and extent of cardiac tamponade. The M-mode findings include a decreased mitral valve opening during inspiration, diminished E-to-A slope, and decreased excursion of the anterior leaflet. Ventricular dimensions will vary during the respiratory phase in an interdependent manner because during inspiration there is decreased flow to the left heart with an associated increase in right heart filling.[112]

During complete examination of a patient with presumed tamponade, Doppler echocardiography is a useful addition. Normally, during inspiration, mitral inflow velocity decreases (10 percent), while tricuspid inflow velocity increases (17 percent). These characteristics are associated with a slight decrease in aortic pressure and with an increase in flow in the pulmonary artery. As expected in the progression of cardiac tamponade, these flow relationships remain the same but increase in magnitude. The transtricuspid flow increases by as much as 80 percent, while transmitral velocities decrease approximately 40 percent. Prior to pericardiocentesis, Appleton and colleagues[113] noted that the peak A-wave and peak E-wave velocities decreased by 25 percent and 43 percent, respectively, while the corresponding transtricuspid velocities increased by 58 percent and 85 percent.

One of the benefits of TEE and a limitation of TTE is the ability to detect a loculated effusion or regional tamponade. This type of tamponade can occur late in the postoperative course of the cardiac surgical patient or of a patient with blunt or penetrating cardiothoracic trauma. Initially there is a diagnostic dilemma.[114,115] The patient is hemodynamically compromised without the classic finding of equalization of all the diastolic pressures and pulsus paradoxus. Not infrequently TTE misdiagnoses this malady. A localized hematoma can compress the right or left atrium without affecting the normal function of the remaining cardiac chambers. Several reports have shown the usefulness of TEE in these patients.[103] Because of the increased imaging capabilities of TEE, the clinician may be able to delineate other potential causes of

hypotension, such as hematomas (loculated tamponade) compressing the venae cava or the pulmonary veins.

VALVULAR HEART DISEASE

Native Valvular Disease

STENOSIS

Echocardiography has made a major impact in patients with valvular heart disease. TEE is more than complementary to the transthoracic approach. The ability to examine (or, in the vernacular, interrogate) the mitral valve apparatus, adjacent structures, integrity and function of the atrial septum, thrombus formation in the appendages, and identification of spontaneous echo contrast is greatly enhanced by TEE.

The mitral valve can be visualized in either the midesophageal or gastric planes, where assessment of stenosis can be completed by using either the continuity equation, planimetry, deceleration time, or pressure half-time (for an explanation of these techniques, please read on). Mitral valvular stenosis (primarily as a result of rheumatic heart disease) causes a diminished orifice with obstruction to inflow. The leaflets are thickened, immobile, calcified, and deformed with fusion of the subvalvular apparatus and commissures. The etiology of stenosis is rarely congenital. Hemodynamic assessment of the mitral valve is attained by directing (or, in the vernacular, steering) a continuous-wave Doppler at the inflow jet within the left ventricle. A pressure gradient is derived by application of the Bernoulli equation: maximal pressure gradient approximates four times the square of the maximal inflow velocity.

The pressure half-time method or rate of decline of the diastolic pressure gradient allows one to derive an average area. This is rooted in the premise that as the severity of stenosis increases, the diastolic pressure gradient is maintained longer and there is prolongation of the early diastolic signal[116]:

Mitral valve area (MVA) = 220/pressure half-time

The continuity equation assumes that the inflow volume transversing the mitral annulus is comparable to the left ventricular stroke volume. This equation is represented by

$$MVA = SV/TVIm$$

where TVIm is the time velocity integral of mitral inflow. MVA is also estimated by the annular cross-sectional method, where

$$MVA = \frac{(\text{aortic annular cross-sectional area}) \cdot \text{TVI aorta}}{TVIm}$$

Finally, the last method for area assessment may be done by simple planimetry.[9,10,19]

Although TTE can roughly estimate the severity of mitral stenosis, TEE with biplanar or omniplanar imaging improves the accuracy of this assessment dramatically.[117] Possible complications of the disease process are easily assessed by TEE (i.e., atrial thrombus). TEE is especially useful for patients undergoing mitral valvuloplasty. Complications from this intervention can be detected with TEE, including leaflet tear, significant residual mitral insufficiency, and interatrial shunting.

The same techniques can be applied to patients who have aortic stenosis (acquired rheumatic, degenerative, and atherosclerotic and congenital bicuspid valves). The accuracy of the assessment by TEE is limited in this disease process, especially when there is coexisting severe calcification of the leaflets. The use of the transgastric approach (analogous to the transgastric parasternal long-axis view in TTE) enhances the ability of the clinician to interrogate the aortic valve and left ventricular outflow tract. Planimetry of the aortic valve is possible in most patients, but the results often overestimate severity if a true short-axis view of the valve is not obtained.[118] With the transgastric approach (longitudinal view), pressure gradients are evaluated with continuous-wave Doppler (modified Bernoulli equation) or by application of the continuity equation.[119] As the role of TEE expands, it may be beneficial for the evaluation of the patient who has undergone an aortic valvuloplasty.[120]

REGURGITATION

Of all the valvular disorders evaluable by TEE, mitral regurgitation has received the greatest attention. The role of TEE assumes paramount importance if, following an examination, surgery is altered and the patient's outcome improved. A prospective study (154 cardiac valves) found that the decision regarding surgical approach was changed in 27 percent of patients solely on the information obtained by TEE (mitral valve cases were altered in 40 percent).[121] Sheikh's investigation noted that angiographically derived information was discordant with TEE data in 46 percent of cases, with the TEE data being more accurate.[122] A similar result was encountered in Stewart's study.[123] The ability of TEE to assess the quality of surgical repair or replacement as well as postoperative ventricular function provides the clinician with valuable insight into the patient's potential outcome.

TEE provides information regarding mitral valve anatomy, integrity, and residual ventricular dysfunction not completely appreciated with TTE. However, as more investigations report the benefits of TEE, the more we will understand its limitations. During evaluation of regurgitant lesions, the clinician must remain cognizant of the technical and physiologic considerations that affect the regurgitant jet. Alterations in loading conditions on the atrium as well as contractility influence the size of the regurgitant jet. This is especially typical of the ICU patient, in whom numerous and complex interactions result either from the disease state itself or from iatrogenic causes (e.g., inotropes, PEEP). Accurate decisions are possible only after total appreciation of the disease process and comprehension of the principles of echocardiography.[9,10,19,124]

With color Doppler, mitral regurgitation is visualized as a multicolored mosaic pattern

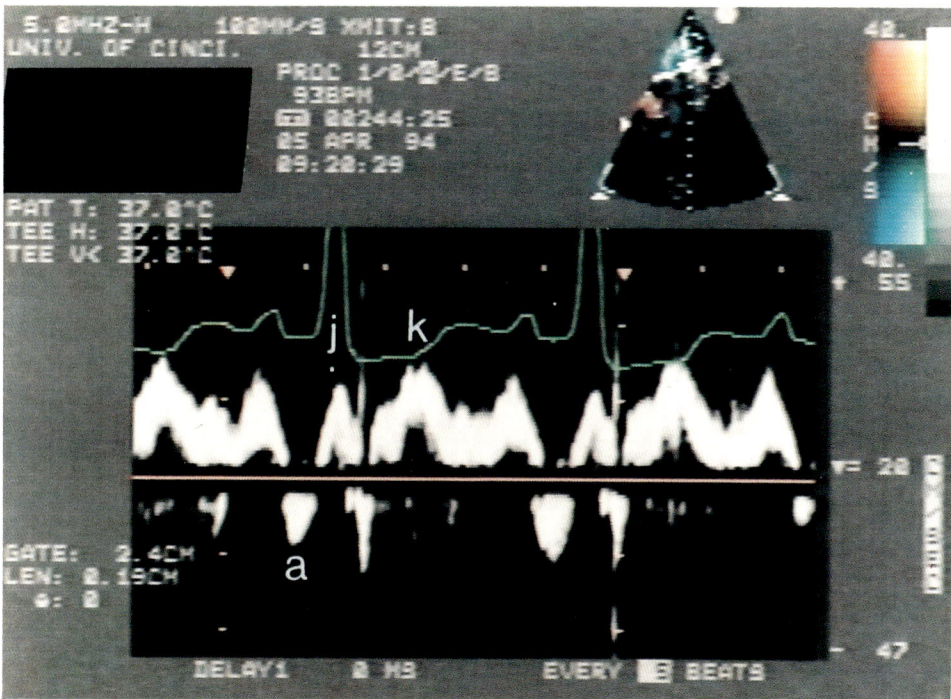

Plate 14-6. Pulmonary venous flow. The plate shows a representative normal pulmonary venous flow pattern with pulsed-wave Doppler echocardiography (top right) and an example of a typical flow pattern characterized by severe mitral regurgitation. a, atrial contraction; j, systolic phase; k, diastolic phase.

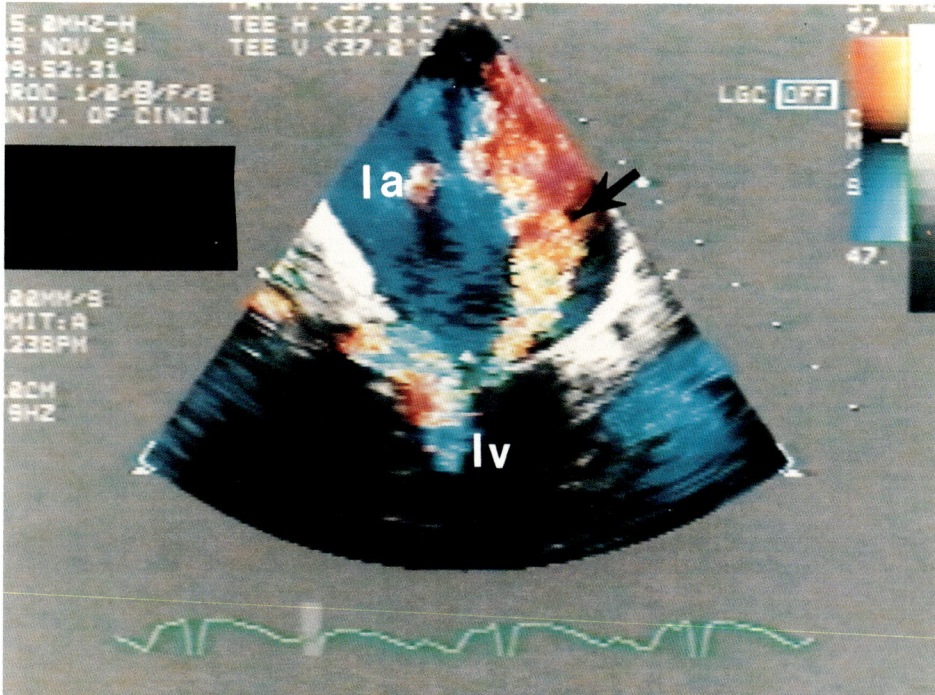

Plate 14-7. Mitral regurgitation. Transverse view revealing a posterior-lateral eccentric jet in the left atrium. la, left atrium; lv, left ventricle.

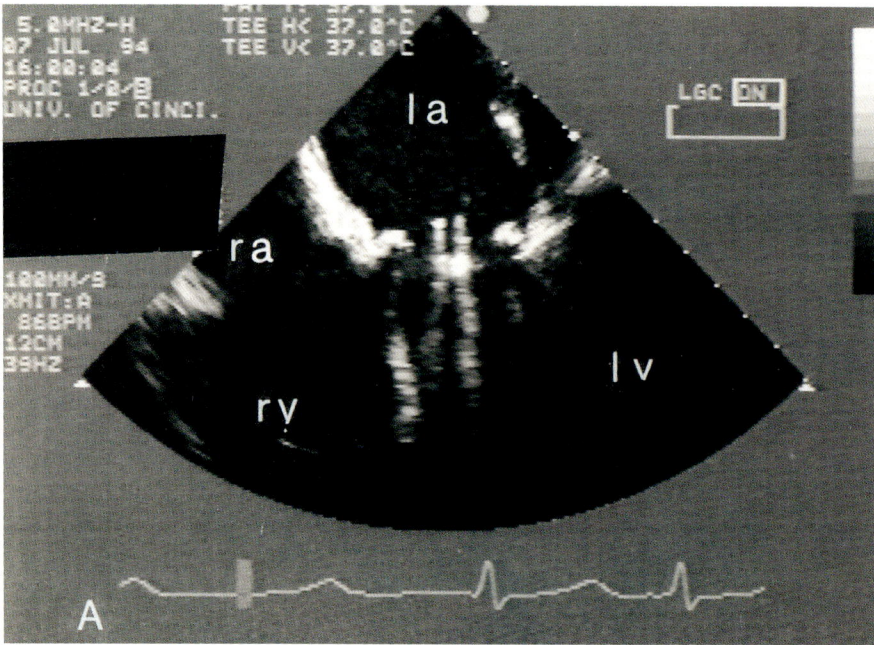

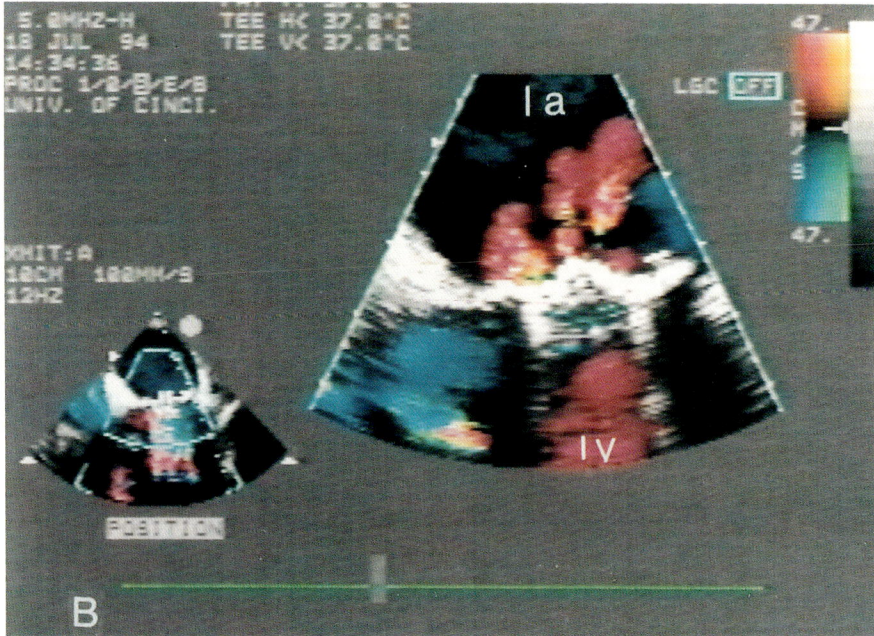

Plate 14-8. Prosthetic cardiac valves. **(A)** A transverse view of the St. Jude valve in the mitral position. **(B)** Three characteristic flamelike jets into the left atrium typical of the St. Jude valve. la, left atrium; lv, left ventricle; ra, right atrium; rv, right ventricle.

within the left atrium during systole.[9,10,19,125–127] The direction and location of the jet are readily apparent with TEE. Eccentric jets are usually the result of a posterior overriding, flail, or prolapsing leaflets or of the presence of a mass or vegetation (Plate 14-7). Centrally positioned jets within the left atrium are often the result of myocardial ischemia or of a concentric disease process of the leaflets (i.e., a patient with rheumatic disease or annular dilation).[9,10,19,127]

Several principles apply when estimating the severity of the mitral regurgitant lesion: proximal flow convergence, diameter of the jet at the orifice, and the area of the jet combined with an assessment of pulmonary venous flow patterns. The simplest method is the area estimation, where the maximal jet cross-sectional area is measured and averaged in both transverse and longitudinal imaging planes. Results are comparable with either TTE or TEE.[128,129] However, it is not unusual to detect regurgitation only with TEE.[128]

The area method is especially limited when the jet is eccentric (the area is less than the physiologic severity) and overestimation of the area is usually the case.[129–131] When comparing angiography to TEE, Castello and Kamp and their coworkers[127,132] have found favorable results. In Kamp's study, sensitivity and specificity were 96 percent and 44 percent, respectively. When the TEE areas were segmented and confirmed to the maximal high-flow mosaic areas (less than 3.0 cm and greater than 6.0 cm), sensitivities increased to 96 percent and 91 percent, respectively.[132] Biplanar averaging of the mosaic areas also improved accuracy and resulted in the following functional definitions: trivial mitral regurgitation less than 1.5 cm^2, mild mitral regurgitation 1.5 to 4.0 cm^2, moderate mitral regurgitation 4.0 to 7.0 cm^2, and severe mitral regurgitation greater than 7.0 cm^2.[133]

In addition to the area assessment, alterations in pulmonary venous flow pattern assist one in the determination of the lesion's severity.[134–136] As the severity of mitral regurgita-

tion increases, the systolic velocity integral and peak systolic velocity decrease, while the corresponding diastolic velocity integral and peak diastolic velocity increase. In patients with clinically significant (i.e., severe) regurgitation, the diastolic component reverses. The reported sensitivity and specificity for this pattern are 90 percent and 100 percent, respectively.[134] In patients with eccentric jets, the corresponding pulmonary vein must be interrogated.[137] In Lai's investigation, systolic reversal was an excellent marker of grade 3 or 4 (97 percent) angiographic regurgitation, while an area greater than 6.0 cm^2 alone was a lesser indicator.[136]

Discrepancies always occur when evaluating the severity of mitral regurgitation. Other methods should be used to corroborate preliminary findings. The principle of flow acceleration proximal to a narrowed or regurgitant orifice is one option. This method is characterized by a series of proximal (to the orifice) colored rings that are produced as the signal "aliases"* with increasing velocity. Each ring represents an isovelocity area, in which all points equidistant to the center of the orifice are equivalent in velocity. Using the continuity equation, the flow through the orifice must equal flow proximal to the orifice. Regurgitant flow is then calculated by the velocity at which aliasing occurs, represented by the proximal isovelocity surface area.[9,10,19] This method shows an excellent correlation ($r = 0.93$) with angiography.[138–141] Assessing the diameter of the jet at the orifice is another method that is gaining accep-

---

*Aliasing can be thought of as having too slow a movie camera. If the image you are capturing is moving within a confined space faster than your camera's ability to image, the image may appear to move in a direction opposite to its true direction. This phenomenon is most easily examined by watching an old black and white western where the wheels of the wagon appear to be spinning backward. Thus, as the velocity of the red cells increases beyond the computer's sampling rate, they appear to the computer to be slowing down, not speeding up. The color assigned to them is similarly incorrect and is said to alias, or to "wrap-around."

tance.[142–144] Pulsed or continuous-wave Dopplers are also useful in calculating the regurgitant velocities in mitral insufficiency.[134,145]

Aortic regurgitation is assessed by examining the jet width at the orifice of the valve and contrasting that dimension with the diameter of the left ventricular outflow tract.[146,147] Using this ratio, four grades of aortic regurgitation are proposed: grade I (mild), 0.25; grade II (moderate), 0.25 to 0.46; grade III (moderately severe), 0.47 to 0.64; and grade IV (severe), greater than 0.65.[147] Pulsed Doppler examination of aortic flow or measurement of the aortic regurgitant orifice is available by using the continuity equation.[148,149] Continuous-wave Doppler may be used for estimating severity of aortic regurgitation by evaluating the rate of decline of the aortic regurgitant velocity—the pressure half-time method.[150] As expected, assessment of eccentric jets may underestimate actual severity.

Prosthetic Valvular Disease

Many times TTE can give adequate information about the patient with a native valvular disorder. However, if there is either a biologic or mechanical prosthetic device, TTE is quite limited (owing to acoustic shadowing and artifacts), while TEE retains the ability to examine the integrity and function of these devices. This is commonly the case with prosthetic devices in the mitral position. Pathologic conditions involving these devices vary from regurgitation (located in the perivalvular, or transvalvular, position and resulting from thickening or calcification, leaflet perforation, tear or dishiscence, and mechanical complications such as thrombosis, pannus, or disk variance), stenosis (thrombosis, degenerative, pannus ingrowth), endocarditis (vegetations, fistula, and valve ring abscess), pseudoaneurysm, and hematoma.

Besides the anatomic characterization of these complications, spectral or color Doppler provides assessment of forward-flow hemodynamics. Continuous-wave Doppler allows the clinician to measure prosthetic valve gradients. The combination of continuous-wave and pulsed-wave Doppler is useful for the estimation of affected orifice areas, while color flow imaging provides a velocity map of flow through the prothesis.[9,10,19] TEE color flow imaging (biplanar or omniplanar) is particularly useful for the detection of the closing volume of the mitral valve prosthesis. In a prospective clinical evaluation of prosthetic devices with TEE, normal regurgitation was detected uniformly, while periprosthetic leaks were appreciated in 31 percent of cases, spontaneous echo contrast in 21 percent of cases, and obstruction in one patient.[165]

Appreciation of what is "normal" is crucial in the evaluation of these patients. For instance, a classic "normal" pattern for a St. Jude valve would have three flamelike jets into the left atrium, while a tilting disk prosthesis exhibits small holosystolic jets (Plate 14-8). (A Starr-Edwards valve has a single systolic regurgitant jet, and the Medtronic Hall device has a jet area quantitatively larger but qualitatively similar to that exhibited by the St. Jude valve.[151–162] Taams and colleagues[163] are attempting to classify the appearance of normal versus pathologic jets in patients with a prosthetic device. They characterize these jets by length, width, direction, and color with Doppler echocardiography.[163]

Multiple comparisons document the inferiority of TTE when compared to TEE. Khandheria and colleagues[152] noted that TEE identified abnormalities in 48 percent of the patients with a normal TTE examination, with 92 percent of the TEE results established at surgery. Daniel et al.[157] reported that TEE examinations resulted in a detection rate of 9 percent for perivalvular mitral regurgitation compared to 24 percent for TEE. Two other studies compared TEE to angiography; and TEE correctly identified the jet in most patients (92 percent), while TTE underestimated the actual severity.[153,164]

With the current trend toward valvuloplasties or repairs, TEE is increasingly effective in the evaluation of these patients. For example, following placement of a mitral Carpen-

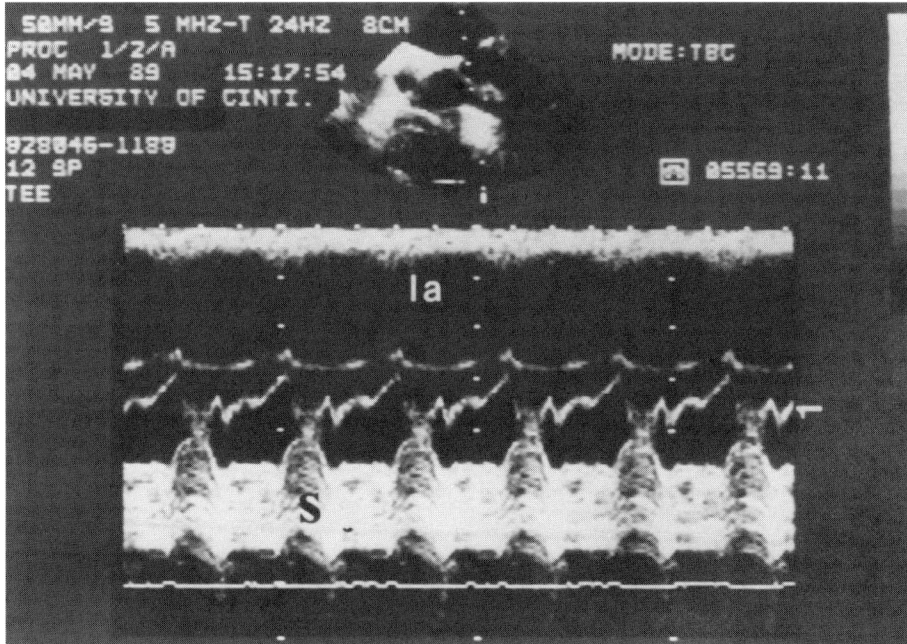

Fig. 14-4. Systolic anterior motion (SAM) of mitral valve. Patient was in shock following Carpenter's ring placement. Systolic anterior motion of anterior leaflet of the mitral valve with M-mode echocardiography reveals systolic anterior motion of the anterior leaflet of the mitral valve, SAM, and outflow tract obstruction. la, left atrium; S, septum.

tier ring, patients may exhibit a dynamic outflow tract obstruction accentuated by hypovolemia. The typical pattern seen is SAM of the anterior leaflet of the mitral valve with turbulence in the left ventricular outflow tract (Fig. 14-4). Augmentation of intraventricular volume may not alleviate this problem and surgical correction may be needed.[166] Patients who undergo myomectomy should have a TEE examination at surgery, to search for potential complications (e.g., SAM, residual obstruction, ventricular septal defects, and sustained pressure gradients).[167,168]

AORTIC PATHOLOGY

Aortic Dissection

TEE is a proven diagnostic tool for the critical care physician in the assessment of an acute aortic dissection, traumatic tear, or transection.[113–115,169–177]

The morbidity and mortality for aortic dissection are considerable. The 3-year mortality remains at 29 percent and 21 percent for distal and proximal aortic dissections, respectively.[175] Unappreciated and/or unrecognized acute aortic dissection has a very high mortality. Development of two-dimensional echocardiography circumvented the inherent limitations of M-mode echocardiography.[176] The sensitivity of TTE in various studies was 70 to 80 percent, primarily as a result of the limited acoustic windows.[9,10] TEE provides most, if not all, of the clinical information necessary for the identification of an acute aortic dissection.[19]

The characteristic findings of an acute aortic dissection are identification of a small true lumen, large false lumen, intimal flap with typical undulating motion, visualization of entry site(s), communication between the lumens, accentuation of flow into the true lumen, and thrombus or visualization of spon-

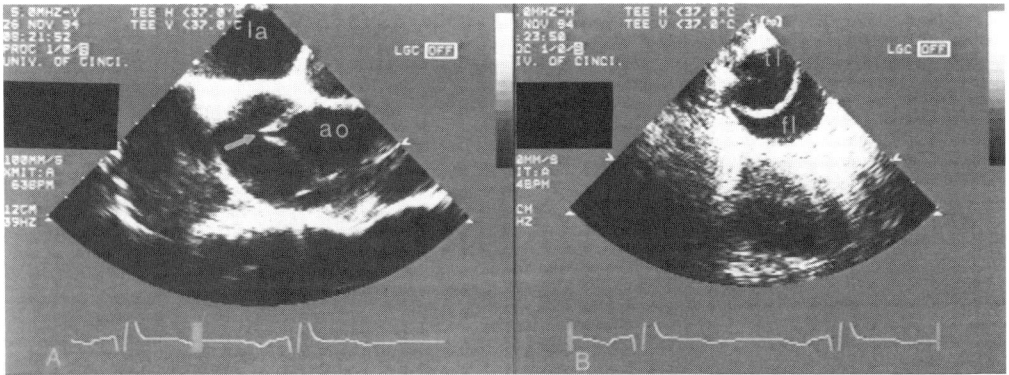

Fig. 14-5. Aortic dissection, transverse view. **(A)** Proximal ascending aorta (ao). **(B)** Descending thoracic. Arrow indicates intimal tear. la, left atrium; fl, false lumen; tl, true lumen.

taneous echo contrast (indicative of rouloux formation of red blood cells) in the false lumen (Fig. 14-5). The TEE examination can also identify the presence, severity, and etiology of aortic insufficiency. Additional information, such as involvement of the coronary arteries, presence of a pericardial effusion, and assessment of ventricular function, may be obtained during the examination.[9,10]

In the European Cooperative Study, Erbel et al.[169] published remarkable results with TEE compared to "standard" diagnostic methods of computed tomography (CT) scanning and angiography. Eighty-two of 164 patients with dissection had independently proven diagnoses by necropsy, angiography, surgery, or CT scan. The sensitivity and specificity of TEE (transverse planar imaging only) were 99 percent and 98 percent, respectively, with a positive predictive value of 98 percent, as compared to sensitivity and specificity of angiography (88 percent and 94 percent) and CT (83 percent and 100 percent). In their study, 17 patients underwent a surgical procedure from the information obtained only by TEE, and in all these patients the diagnosis was confirmed at surgery.[169]

To assist in the diagnosis of aortic dissection, color-flow or spectral Doppler is used. At the entry site there is generally identification of turbulent flow. A unidirectional jet suggests the presence of more than one intimal tear (i.e., one entry, one exit), while bidirectional jets are useful in determining true versus false lumens. Flow to the true lumen occurs in diastole, while flow to the false lumen occurs in systole. Utilization of TEE and color flow Doppler echocardiography in two studies correctly identified all cases of a dissecting aortic aneurysm (entry site and intimal flap).[171,177] This compared to a detection rate of 42 percent by conventional modalities.

In a separate study, Ballal and colleagues[170] appropriately identified aortic dissection in 33 of 34 patients (sensitivity 97 percent and specificity 100 percent). CT scanning correctly characterized aortic dissection in 67 percent of these patients and misclassified the type of dissection in 33 percent of the patients. TEE also correctly detected extent of the dissection in 29 of the patients (corroborated at surgery). In seven of the 34 (21 percent) patients (all of whom had proximal aortic dissections), TEE provided information on the involvement of the coronary arteries. In six of these seven patients, the intimal flap extended into the ostium and lumen of the coronary artery, which are indications for emergency surgery. Other indications for surgery include pericardial tamponade and aortic regurgitation, as a result of symmetric dilation of the root, incomplete central cusp coaptation, asymmetric cusp association resulting in diastolic flail, or prolapse of one of the aortic cusps.

TEE with color flow Doppler echocardiography was also recently compared to magnetic resonance imaging (MRI) for the diagnosis of an acute aortic dissection.[172,173] The sensitivities for TEE and MRI were 100 percent; however, the specificities were 100 percent for MRI and 68.2 percent for TEE. As expected, there was good correlation between the two techniques in detecting pericardial effusions, aortic insufficiency, and entry site.

A later investigation from the same group evaluated CT, MRI, TTE, and TEE.[173] The sensitivities of TTE, CT, MRI, and TEE were 59.3 percent, 93.8 percent, 98.3 percent, and 97.7 percent, respectively. The corresponding specificities were 76.9 percent, 87.1 percent, 97.8 percent, and 83.0 percent respectively.

The false-positive results with TEE were the consequence of inaccurate visualization due to artifacts within an ectatic aorta with circumferential mural plaque formation and significant calcification.[173] Biplanar imaging with color flow Doppler echocardiography, which was not initiated in the two preceding investigations, would undoubtedly increase the specificity in the diagnosis of aortic dissection because of its increased imaging capabilities.[174,175] The most noticeable advantage of TEE in critically ill patients is bedside evaluation of the aorta, rather than evaluation that requires transporting them to a distant MRI or CT suite.

Kearney and colleagues[184] identified 69 patients with suspected thoracic aortic injury and compared TEE and angiography with regard to diagnostic accuracy. These investigators identified seven patients with aortic injury with TEE while only four of these patients had concurrent positive findings with angiography. Angiograms produced one false-positive and two false-negative results. They reported that the sensitivity and specificity for TEE in their series was 100 percent.

Of particular importance in patients who sustain a traumatic chest injury is the identification of a mediastinal hematoma, which only TEE can diagnose.[185] Many patients undergo "unnecessary" angiography for a widened mediastinum seen on a chest radiograph. Le Bret et al.[186] performed TEE examinations in thoracic trauma patients. In their study the sensitivity was 100 percent and the specificity 75 percent. The TEE results were confirmed by either CT or surgical evaluation.

Le Bret and coworkers described several echocardiographic signs for a mediastinal hematoma: a double contour of the aortic wall, identification of the ultrasound signal between the visceral pleura and aortic wall, and an expanded distance between the aortic wall and the TEE probe (greater than 3 mm). The last of these signs appears to be the most diagnostically sensitive. One of the limitations in this study was the use of single plane TEE. If biplanar or omniplanar TEE imaging is used, the specificity should be higher. Undoubtedly, further TEE studies are required to evaluate the efficacy of biplanar or omniplanar imaging in these patients. As ultrasound technology evolves, intravascular echocardiography may be one of the diagnostic tools to evaluate either traumatic aortic injuries or aortic dissection(s).

Erbel and colleagues,[175] from the European Cooperative Study Group on Echocardiography, evaluated aortic dissection with TEE prospectively to determine the degree of communication between the true and false lumens and its impact on prognosis and management. Eight centers studied 168 patients with aortic dissection. The patients were classified according to the modified DeBakey criteria. Type I, II, and III aortic dissections were detected in 35 percent, 17 percent, and 48 percent of the patients, respectively. The preoperative mortality was 3 percent, 7 percent, and 2 percent (overall mortality of 6.8 percent), while the survival rates were 52 percent, 69 percent, and 70 percent, respectively.

The early utilization of TEE in these patients appeared to decrease the preoperative mortality rate. Fluid extravasation, periaortic effusion, mediastinal hematoma, pleural effusion, and pericardial tamponade were identified as risk factors (mortality of 52 percent). The open false lumen with a high communication was also appreciated as a potential risk factor. The rate of thrombus formation was inversely related to prognosis. This finding suggests that surgical closure reduces mortality from thrombus formation by reducing aortic wall stress.[176] The 12 percent incidence of noncommunicating aortic dissection (echocardiographically characterized as the absence of intimal flap movement, tears, and Doppler flow signals) is in accordance with previous anatomic studies.[178] Patients with this type of dissection have a lower mortality than occurs in those with a communication. This investigation demonstrates that TEE offers an excellent tool for the prognostic evaluation of aortic dissection in the perioperative and follow-up phases of medical care.[175]

Atypical aortic dissection is easily diagnosed by TEE and accounts for approximately 5 to 15 percent of all dissections. In these cases, there is no discernible intimal flap, but rather a thickened smooth aortic wall described as either crescenteric or eccentric in morphology.[179,180] The pathogenesis of atypical dissection is from spontaneous rupture of vasa vasorum or undiagnosed small intimal tears. False-negative angiograms are reported. This unrecognized aortic intramural hematoma may progress to a "classic" dissection or frank rupture that contributes to the high mortality noted in some series. The early identification of this malady by TEE may prevent mortality.[179-182]

TEE is also beneficial in excluding the diagnosis of aortic dissection. In Chan's study of 40 patients, TEE detected conditions that imitated a dissection in 55 percent.[183] Chan found minimal diltation of the aorta in 17 patients and myocardial ischemia in five patients. Two extrinsic masses were found juxtaposed to the aorta. One was a postoperative hematoma and the other a small cell carcinoma. Following blunt chest trauma, one patient with an intra-aortic thrombus was visualized.

The increased imaging capability of TEE combined with its expeditious and low-risk nature ensures that the information obtained in post-traumatic patients is often invaluable and life saving.[184,185] In addition to the appraisal of ventricular function and volume in these critically ill patients, the aorta can be assessed for an intimal injury, tear, or hematoma.

Aortic Aneurysms

The most common etiologies of thoracic aortic aneurysm are atherosclerosis from cystic medial degeneration related to Marfan syndrome or idiopathic. These conditions are initially appreciated on a chest radiograph as a widened mediastinum. The "gold standards" of CT and angiography have inherent limitations. Angiography allows relatively good spatial resolution of the aorta, as well as delineating involvement of the aneurysm with branch vessels, but it may not reveal the presence or the actual size of an aneurysm. CT imaging is obtained in transverse views and may not accurately assess a tortuous aorta because of obliquity of the views and cannot visualize fistula formation. TEE circumvents these limitations and evaluates most thoracic aneurysms, including such complications as fistulae, plaques, thrombus, and dissection.[187,188] In Taam's study, all thoracic aneurysms were identified with TEE, while many cases were missed by CT scanning.[189]

Aortic Debris and Thrombus

The recognition of atherosclerosis of the aorta as a potential source of morbidity and mortality has definitely increased since the development of TEE. Atherosclerosis usually involves the abdominal aorta, followed by descending aorta, aortic arch, and the ascending aorta.[190] Significant aortic atherosclerosis is an important marker for diffuse involvement of the cerebrovascular and coronary circulation.[190,191] Angiography has definite disadvantages because of an inability to delineate the aortic wall, the intimal surface, and/or mobile atheromatous material. There is also an associated risk of a systemic embolism during the procedure. TEE obviates all these limitations and has the capacity for high-quality high-resolution imaging of the aorta.

Uncomplicated atherosclerotic plaques may be visualized as either smooth, focal, or echodense structures. Extensive or complex plaques may be irregular, pedunculated, and/or mobile and associated with thrombi (Fig. 14-6). Karalis et al.[192] studied 556 patients and detected atherosclerotic aortic debris in 7 percent of patients. Uncharacteristically, atherosclerotic debris was confined to the arch and the descending aorta in 70 percent of patients, while the abdominal aorta was involved in only 30 percent of patients. Of particular importance, systemic embolism was greater in patients with freely mobile and pedunculated lesions (73 percent) than laminated immobile plaques (12 percent).

An intraoperative TEE evaluation of aortic atheromas as a risk factor for a stroke was investigated by Katz et al.[193] Protruding atheromas were identified in 18 percent of patients (n = 23) and were the only variable predictive of a stroke. Katz and colleagues suggested that placement of the aortic cannula was crucial in minimizing embolization and presumably a subsequent central event. In 183 patients with brain ischemia from an embolic source, TEE identified an extensive mobile aortic plaque in 4 percent of patients. The primary location of the plaque was the superior posterior aspect of the ascending aorta or transverse arch. This study suggests that TEE is uniquely capable of pinpointing the source when evaluating a patient with a central embolic event.[194]

Penetrating aortic atherosclerotic ulcers are also a potentially life-threatening problem if left unrecognized.[195] They occur in patients with diffuse atherosclerotic vascular disease and are typically located in the descending thoracic aorta or distal aortic arch. The ulceration of the atheromatous plaque disrupts the intima and either extends into the media, resulting in an intramural hematoma, or penetrates the media, resulting in a pseudoaneurysm. Perforation through the adventitia results in frank rupture. Meticulous TEE (biplanar or omniplanar) examination should be performed in these patients.

TEE has increased our awareness of aortic pathology and its possible consequences. Even as some answers are found, more ques-

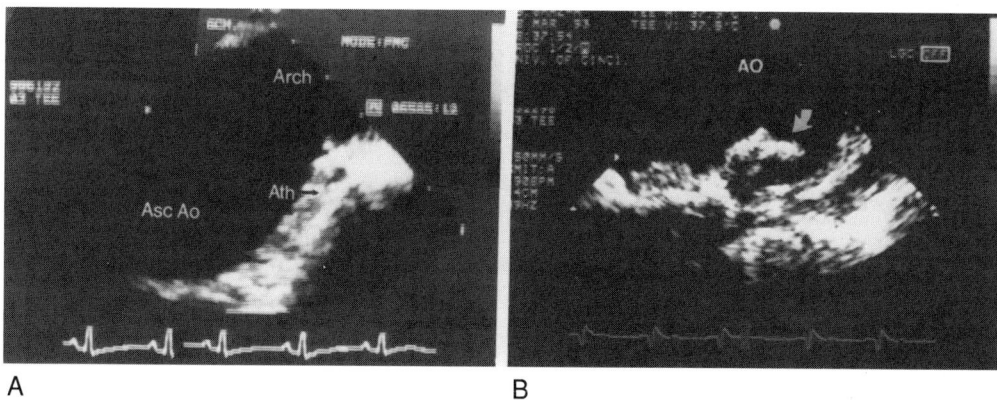

Fig. 14-6. Aortic debris, transverse views. **(A)** Ascending aorta (Asc Ao) reveals atheromatous debris (Ath). **(B)** Arch of the aorta shows large, pedunculated, free-flowing debris. Arch, proximal aortic arch; Ao, aorta.

tions are raised. What is the optimal management in patients with aortic pathology, particularly when the patient is asymptomatic? Should mobile and protruding aortic debris be surgically removed? Should cardiac angiography be averted in patients with extensive aortic debris and thrombi? How aggressive should clinicians be in the removal of these mobile harbingers of stroke or organ failure? Porembka et al.[196] and Tunnick et al.[197] reported several cases in which a thrombus was the etiology for patient morbidity. Surgical intervention proceeded promptly after identification of the thrombus with TEE. Coy et al.[198] and Rubin et al.[199] described situations in which aortic pathology was identified as the etiology for occult renal dysfunction and acute lower extremity ischemia.

Heparin-induced thrombocytopenia and thrombus formation is an unusual complication of heparin, but it can be life-threatening. Movsowitz and colleagues[196] identified a dilated aorta with two thrombi: one mobile laminated thrombus proximal to the subclavian artery and a second fixed thrombus approximately 10 cm distal to the subclavian artery. They were also able to follow the resolution of these thrombi once heparin was discontinued.

ENDOCARDITIS

Endocarditis offers numerous possibilities for complications. If the infectious process extends into either the valvular or perivalvular tissue, the ensuing destruction results in catastrophic embolic events. Echocardiography is a unique tool for delineating the extent of this process. TEE circumvents the inherent limitations of TTE, permitting early and accurate diagnosis of this malady. In the diagnostic scheme of patients with suspected infectious endocarditis, TEE is used when TTE is equivocal. In the intensive care setting, the classic signs and symptoms of infectious endocarditis are not always apparent, and the systemic inflammatory response syndrome may be the presenting condition. In these sit-

uations we routinely use TEE to assess the heart.[200,201]

The accuracy of echocardiography for the identification of infective endocarditis is dependent on both the method of visualization and the presence of positive bacterial cultures. The first published report of diagnostic accuracy with M-mode echocardiography was by Dillon et al.[204] in 1977; however, sensitivity estimates since that time vary considerably (14 to 75 percent).[202,203] The addition of two-dimensional echocardiography improves the diagnostic accuracy (41 to 78 percent), but 20 percent of cases result in inadequate imaging particularly in patients with prosthetic valves.[204] If in addition there were abnormal findings on TTE examination, the sensitivity rose to 80 to 90 percent.[204–216] Even with positive results, "lesions" occur that mimic a vegetation: papillary fibromas, myxomatous disease, retracted chordae, healed vegetations, disrupted prosthetic valves, and filamentous strands adjacent to prosthetic devices.

Typically, an abnormal finding is described as a vegetation or vegetation like mass attached to a valve leaflet, chord, or chamber wall with motion independent of adjacent structures and tissue consistency different from that of normal tissue. Lesions commonly associated with the endocarditis process include leaflet perforation, periprosthetic or annular echolucent spaces (abscesses), fistulae, chordal rupture, or sinus of Valsalva aneurysms.

The size of the vegetation clearly effects detection rate. With technically adequate TTE images, vegetations as small as 2.0 to 5.0 mm are detected in only 25 percent of cases. With lesions as large as 6.0 to 10.0 mm, the detection rate approaches 70 percent. Only when lesions are greater than 11.0 mm and are not associated with a prosthetic device will the detection rate approximate 100 percent.[208] Overall, the sensitivity of detection for endocarditis with TTE will vary from 60 to 70 percent.[206,207] If prosthetic devices that involve acoustic reflectance and shadow-

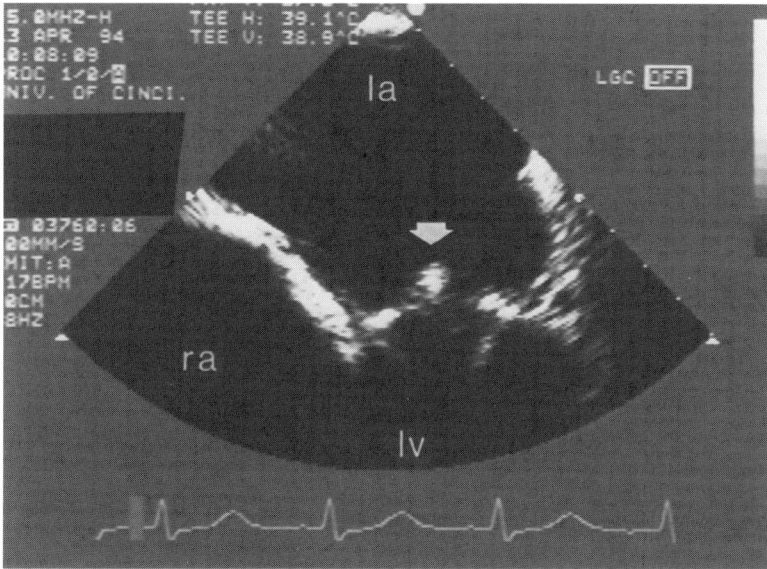

Fig. 14-7. Endocarditis: prosthetic valve, transverse view. Prosthetic mitral valve reveals a vegetation (*arrow*). This lesion was not visualized by transthoracic echocardiography. la, left atrium; lv, left ventricle; ra, right atrium.

ing are added, the sensitivity will decrease to 20 to 30 percent.[205,208,212]

The advent of TEE surmounted most of the technical and mechanical limitations associated with TTE. This is especially true in patients with prosthetic devices in the mitral position (Fig. 14-7) in whom the identification rate for TEE will approach 100 percent.[208,218–226]

Daniel et al.[205] were among the earliest investigators to demonstrate the efficacy of TEE in suspected endocarditis. Of 196 patients with the diagnosis of endocarditis, 20 percent had an inadequate TTE image, while there were 82 abnormal findings consistent with endocarditis. The detection rates for TEE and TTE were 94 percent and 40 percent, respectively.[205]

Other investigators have corroborated these results[206–225] Erbel's early results were more impressive, with TEE sensitivity and specificity of 100 percent and 98 percent, respectively; TTE sensitivity and specificity of 63 percent and 98 percent, respectively.[206] In Mugge's comparative series (TTE versus

TEE), the detection rate with TEE (90 percent) was considerably higher than with TTE (58 percent).[208] In Shively's prospective series, TEE was better suited for the interrogation of the aortic and mitral valves, while evaluation of the tricuspid valve was equivalent for both techniques.[223] There were comparable results in Birmingham's[220] and Shapiro's studies.[225] In Shapiro's study, the sensitivity of TEE for detection of the lesions was 97 percent, while the rate with TTE was only 68 percent.[225]

Embolism is a major complication in patients with infective endocarditis (Fig. 14-8). When the size of the vegetation exceeds 10 mm, the chance of an embolic event is quite high (47 percent). These adverse events occur more frequently when the vegetation is mobile (38 percent) as opposed to sessile (19 percent). In addition to size of the vegetation, other apparent independent predictors for embolic complications are the mitral valve location and the presence of spontaneous echo contrast.[208,227,228]

TEE is clearly superior to TTE for the

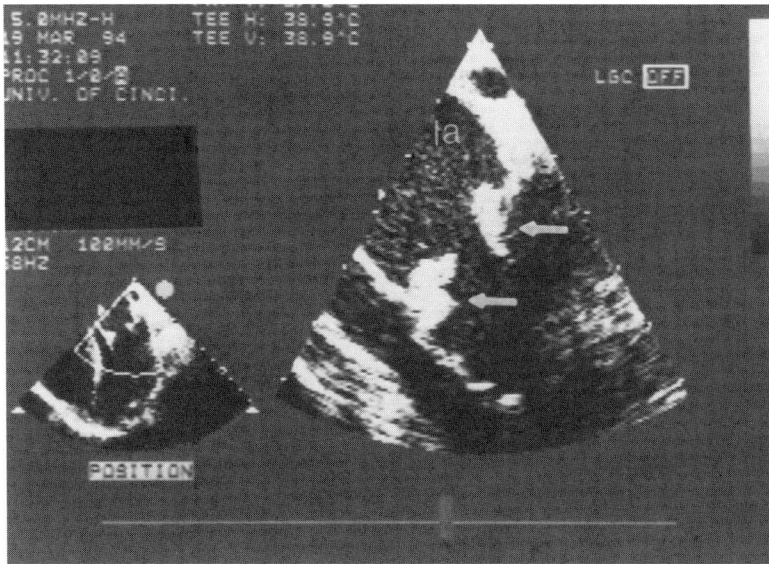

Fig. 14-8. Endocarditis: native valve in an elderly patient with a stroke. Transverse view (expanded) of the mitral valve apparatus reveals two large vegetations (with severe mitral regurgitation) (*arrows*) as the etiology of the embolic event. la, left atrium.

detection of abscesses, valvular and perivalvular destruction, aneurysms, and fistulae.[225,229–231] In confirmed abscesses, 87 percent were identified by TEE as compared to 28 percent for TTE.[229] In Shapiro's inquiry, periannular complications were reliably identified with TEE, but only occasionally with TTE.[225] For example, mitral insufficiency may be the result of valvular incompetence, perforation, or involvement of the subjacent mitral valve apparatus. Patients who experience unexplained congestive heart failure with mitral regurgitation as a component should undergo a TEE examination immediately.[230]

The use of biplanar and omniplanar imaging improves the diagnostic accuracy for endocarditis and its associated complications, particularly of the mitral, tricuspid, and pulmonic valves.[221,222,232] TEE is also useful in patients with clinical evidence of right-sided endocarditis and a negative TTE. A negative TEE does not exclude the possibility of endocarditis, however, particularly if the vegetation is exceedingly small or was previously embolized.[226] TEE is useful in the serial evaluation of patients following surgical intervention as well as patients who are not surgical candidates. As technology improves, the effectiveness of TEE as a powerful diagnostic instrument in the evaluation of critically ill patients will become evident.

INTRACARDIAC MASSES

TEE offers a major advance in the diagnostic evaluation of patients with unexplained central embolic events. In our experience, TEE is characteristically used in these patients to identify a potential embolic source. In addition to the aorta, masses (either thrombi or tumor) in the cardiac chambers (including the atrial appendages) may be the origin.

Lee et al.[233] performed TEE and TTE in patients after a transient ischemic attack or stroke and compared the detection rates for an intracardiac mass. An intracardiac abnormality was found in 46 percent of patients who had a negative TTE. The incriminating situations for TTE were atrial enlargement, atrial fibrillation, and thickening of the mitral valve. The contributing factors noted by TEE were left atrial or left atrial appendage thrombus, PFO, and the appearance of spontaneous contrast. Mobile filamentous strands were also visualized on the mitral valve in 22 percent of patients.

TTE is often of no value in the diagnosis of an intracardiac mass when the mass is small, in the atrial appendage, or associated with a prosthetic valve. TEE circumvents the prosthetic obfuscation by imaging posterior to the mechanical device.[234–240] Spontaneous echocardiographic contrast is invariably seen only with TEE Pearson et al.[234] detected the source of embolism with TEE in 57 percent of selected patients, as compared with a detection rate with TTE of only 15 percent. TEE predictably visualized spontaneous contrast, PFO, and atrial septal aneurysms. In patients without suspected cardiac disease, TEE identified either an isolated atrial aneurysm or an aneurysm associated with a PFO and had a diagnostic yield of 39 percent. In Pearson's investigation, the echocardiographic techniques were similar in the identification of an apical ventricular thrombus or mitral valve prolapse.

Atrial septal aneurysm and PFO are apparent risk factors in patients under 55 years of age who have sustained a cryptogenic stroke. Cabanes et al.[241] employed TEE in this patient subgroup and found that atrial septal aneurysms and PFO are significant risk factors for stroke development and are synergistic. The size of the atrial septal aneurysm was also a contributing factor if it exceeded 10 mm. The odds of having a stroke were approximately 33 percent greater in patients with these two maladies than in those without. While MRI is an ideal technique for the identification of an intracardiac masses, it may not be helpful if masses are highly mobile. This was apparent in Mera's study, in which an atrial septal aneurysm simulated a left atrial mass.[242]

Pop et al.[235] and colleagues[235] believe that

TEE should be one of the first diagnostic tests used in patients following a central nervous system event. Albers et al.[236] used TEE, TTE, carotid ultrasonography, and brain imaging in 145 consecutive patients with either a stroke or transient ischemic attack. With TEE such positive findings as left atrial thrombi, spontaneous contrast, atrial septal aneurysm, ventricular thrombus or aneurysm, myxomatous mitral valve, or interatrial shunt were detected in 46 percent of patients, compared to 8 percent with a TTE study. Lacunar syndromes were associated with atrial septal aneurysms, while interatrial shunts were prevalent in all stroke subtypes. Neither septal aneurysms nor interatrial shunts occurred in the patients with unexplained stroke. No definitive risk assessment with TEE could be made in Alber's study in a subgroup of patients with ipsilateral carotid stenosis because of the small numbers. Albers and colleagues[236] concluded that in patients with symptoms suggestive of an embolic stroke, the yield of TEE is substantial and can alter clinical management.

Atrial fibrillation occurs commonly in many types of patients, the critically ill. The role of TEE in documenting unsuspected atrial thrombi in these patients is growing. In Manning's inquiry (n = 119) the incidence of atrial or appendage thrombi was 13 percent by TEE.[243] These investigators suggested that cardioversion proceed, without prior oral anticoagulation, only in patients with no identifiable thrombus by TEE.

In addition to atrial fibrillation, other factors contribute to the development of a thrombus: mitral stenosis valve area of less than 1.5 cm^2, left atrial end-systolic area of greater than 30 cm^2, and formation of spontaneous echocardiographic contrast.[240] By evaluating the appendage velocities, Grimm et al.[244] found that organized atrial function returned in 80 percent of patients following cardioversion. Spontaneous echo contrast increased in 35 percent of patients, suggesting that atrial function is "stunned" and is predisposed to thrombus formation during this time. In two patients described by Salka et al.,[245] cerebral embolism occurred after elective cardioversion; however, there was no previous identification of left atrial thrombus or left atrial spontaneous contrast with TEE. More studies are required to identify the pathogenesis of clot formation after cardioversion for atrial fibrillation. The role of TEE with regard to anticoagulation management is uncertain; however, if may help in diagnosing patients who develop thrombi.[246]

Other masses may be identified with TEE, such as thrombi associated with central lines.[247] TEE is also useful in the identification of masses for biopsy or excision.[248] Faletra and colleagues[249] compared TEE, TTE, MRI, and CT for the evaluation of mediastinal masses. As expected, MRI and CT had excellent results. In comparison with TTE, TEE was more accurate in the identification of the mass, its structure, and its relationship to adjacent structures. Although CT and MRI are better diagnostic tools for mediastinal masses, TEE in the critically ill may uncover an unexpected mass that is contributing to patient morbidity.[250]

INTRACARDIAC SHUNTS

Patent Foramen Ovale

PFO is a well-described anatomic abnormality in necropsy studies, occurring in 25 to 35 percent of the population.[251,252] The incidence and size of the PFO are distributed by age. In Hagen's study, the overall incidence was 27.3 percent and chronologically decreased with age: first three decades, 34.3 percent; fourth to eighth decades, 25.4 percent; and ninth and tenth decades, 20.2 percent. The size of the PFO increased with age: a mean of 3.4 mm in the first decade, increasing to a mean of 5.8 mm in the tenth decade, the overall mean was 4.9 mm with a range of 1.0 to 19 mm[252] (Fig. 14-9).

Alber's study revealed that control subjects had an incidence of interatrial shunts of approximately 20 percent.[253] Is this interatrial shunt (presumably a PFO), a harbinger for a stroke or transient ischemic event? Does a PFO play a role in the pathogenesis of a cerebral infarct in patients with no apparent deep venous thromboses? Is a PFO a passageway for paradoxic embolism? Is a PFO the conduit for a large right-to-left shunt resulting in relative or refractory hypoxia? It appears that there is an association with interatrial shunts and atrial septal aneurysms that increases the potential for cerebral embolic incidents.

Several pathophysiologic characteristics augment flow across a PFO: acidemia, hypoxemia, and pre-existing or acute elevations in right ventricular pressures, (usually volumes associated with an increase in right atrial pressure). Normally, the interatrial septum protrudes slightly into the right atrium. In the abnormal physiologic state described earlier, the septum will bulge into the left atrium. Paradoxic movement of the septum also occurs at end-diastole. In patients with mitral stenosis (i.e., left atrial diltation), the septum will elongate and protrude more into the right atrium, irrespective of diastole or systole. In acute volume overload of the left atrium, the septum will protrude at end-systole, while at end-diastole the shape will be normal, flat, or convexed to the left.[254]

Echocardiography (TTE or TEE) is a unique tool for the identification of a PFO. However, when TTE studies are inconclusive, TEE is ideal for the evaluation of septal motion, orientation, and anatomic characterization.[255] Contrast echocardiography is a standard technique for detecting an intracardiac shunt. The incidence of PFO varies among several series because of the variable diagnostic classification or definition.[256]

The diagnosis of PFO is also affected by operator-dependent and technical limitations. If the amount of agitated saline is insufficient to opacify the right atrium, absorption of the microbubbles will occur, and the diagnosis of PFO is unappreciated. In contrast, the diagnosis is ensured in patients with impaired right ventricular function because of the decreased transit time and reconcentra-

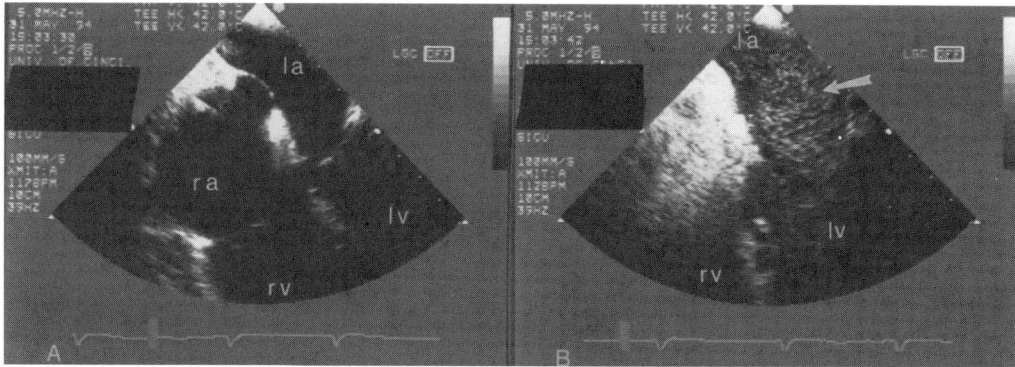

Fig. 14-9. Patent foramen ovale and paradoxical embolism, transverse views. **(A)** Chamber view reveals a large right atrium (ra) and bulging fossa ovalis. **(B)** Corresponding transverse view with agitated saline as a contrast agent (early injection), shows multiple microbubbles in left atrium (la), indicative of a large right-to-left shunt. lv, left ventricle; rv, right ventricle.

tion of the agitated saline. Provocative maneuvers such as a cough or Valsalva maneuver will augment the interatrial pressure differential, allowing for improved characterization of the PFO. Prior to the administration of the agitated saline, there must be optimal adjustment of the signal gain, gray-scale compression controls, and transmitted ultrasound power. Adjustment of the depth of field will permit maximal visualization of the atria and interatrial septum.[257]

Preceding TEE, TTE was considered the noninvasive method of choice for the diagnosis of PFO.[258-262] The detection rate for PFO with TTE varied at 5 to 18 percent. After the augmentation maneuvers described above, the rate increased to 10 to 24 percent.[263-266] The detection rate for PFO with TEE under similar circumstances was 8 to 44 percent without augmentation and 22 to 63 percent following augmentation.[266-271] Lechat et al.[263] found that the diagnosis of PFO was more prevalent in patients with a stroke (40 percent) than in those without (10 percent).

In a comparable study of 238 patients, Hausmann and colleagues[264] investigated the prevalence of PFO with TTE and TEE. They stratified their patients into three groups: group A, transient cerebral ischemic attacks or peripheral embolic events with a history of otherwise unexplained ischemic stroke; group B, history of similar circumstances explained by other cardiac irregularities; and group C, no embolic episodes. The overall detection rates with contrast TEE and Doppler echocardiography were 21 percent and 19 percent, respectively. When the two echocardiographic techniques (TEE and TTE) were compared, the results diverged for the detection of PFO. In the individual groups the detection rates for TEE were 22 percent, 21 percent, and 22 percent, respectively. On the other hand, contrast-TTE detected only 8 percent of all patients. When the groups were subdivided by age (less than 40 years or greater than or equal to 40 years) and an unexplained ischemic stroke, the PFO prevalence by TEE was 50 percent.[264]

A subsequent study concluded that cryptogenic stroke occurred more regularly (21 percent) when contrast agent was detected in the left atrium than when it was not (0 percent).[272] To demonstrate further the increased sensitivity of TEE for the diagnosis of PFO, Chen et al.[266] corroborated their results with the "gold standard" of either cardiac catheterization or surgical exploration. In their study of 32 patients, the detection rate for TTE was only 25 percent during spontaneous respiration and 38 percent during Valsalva maneuver. The corresponding detection rate by TEE was 44 percent and 63 percent, respectively. In this study only one patient with a positive TEE could not be confirmed by cardiac catheterization from the placement of a probe through the fossa ovalis.

There appears to be an association between paradoxic embolism via a PFO and deep venous thrombosis. Stollberger and colleagues[256] examined 264 patients with a suspected embolic event and detected a PFO in 19 percent. Of these patients, 84 percent had a cerebral event and 16 percent had peripheral limb ischemia. Venous thrombosis of the calf or popliteal veins was established in 59 percent of patients with a documented PFO. Should all patients at high risk of the development of deep venous thrombosis have contrast echocardiography performed to identify a possible PFO?

Another result of an open PFO is hypoxia. In patients who develop acute right heart failure, the normal left and right pressure differential across the interatrial septum may reverse, resulting in hypoxia. Additionally, iatrogenic conditions such as PEEP and high mean airway pressures may aggravate this pressure differential. Until these conditions diminish, the pressure in the right atrium will continue to exceed that of the left atrium and result in a persistent physiologic shunt. This clinical scenario is not unusual and often occurs in patients with acute lung injury. Two case reports have documented PFO as a contributing factor to hypoxemia.[273,274] In one of the cases, after surgical closure of the interatrial shunt, oxygenation improved from a PaO_2 of 40 to 400 mmHg at an FiO_2 value of 1.0. Unfortunately, there is no prospective investigation evaluating the efficacy of surgical correction of PFO in these critically ill patients.

Other Septal Defects

Other intracardiac shunts, such as atrial septal defects (ASD) and ventricular septal defects (VSD), may be assessed by TEE. TTE is often the initial diagnostic tool for the visualization of the intracardiac shunt. In asymptomatic patients, these shunts are detected when echocardiography is performed for other reasons. Right ventricular diltation or hypertrophy (evidence of right ventricular overload) should prompt the clinician to search for the existence of an ASD.

Multiple views are obtained when evaluating the atrial septum. The ostium primum ASD is easily detected, but secundum defects are more difficult secondary to echo dropout and shadowing. With TTE, the subcostal four-chamber view is superior to the apical four-chamber view. If an ASD is detected, there commences a search for associated abnormalities (i.e., a cleft mitral valve, aortic regurgitation, VSD, or an aberrant attachment of the septal leaflet of the mitral valve).

Imaging with TTE in intensive care patients is often limited and inconclusive. TEE overcomes these limitations and reliably evaluates the atrial septal anatomy and function.[270,275–278] Sinus venosus defects, although an extremely rare occurrence in the adult population, are easily appreciated with TEE.[279] Other modalities that are of value in the search for an ASD include Doppler and color flow imaging.[280–282] A comparative study of detection rates for ASD revealed a sensitivity for TEE of 93 percent as compared to a sensitivity with TTE of 57 percent. A positive right atrial echo contrast study detected the ASD in 93 percent of patients by TEE, while the detection rate for TTE was only 58 percent.[283]

VSDs occur in three regions: the inlet septum, the trabecular septum, and the infundibular septum. The accuracy of detection depends on both location and size. Multiple views are required because of the potential complexity of this lesion. The sensitivity for detection with two-dimensional echocardiography decreases from inlet defects (100 percent) to perimembranous defects (80 to 90 percent) to trabecular defects (50 percent).[284] The advent of Doppler echocardiography and color flow imaging enhanced detection.[285,286]

Parasternal long-axis and short-axis views are the best for visualization of perimembranous lesions. The apical four-chamber view allows for greater visualization of inlet and trabecular ventricular defects. Most of large VSDs are detectable by TEE. Smaller defects and defects located at the perimembranous portion of the septum may not be appreciated with TEE. Zotz and colleagues[287] evaluated a variety of echocardiographic techniques for the detection of VSD following a ventricular infarction. Multiple TTE views found a VSD in 12 of 17 patients, confirmed by necropsy, surgery, or cardiac catheterization. The use of color Doppler echocardiography with TTE detected a rupture in 15 patients. TEE located the defect in six of nine patients. With the addition of Doppler and contrast echocardiography, all the ventricular septal ruptures were discovered by TEE.[287]

Acquired Intracardiac Shunts

As the incidence of penetrating cardiac trauma continues to increase simultaneously with the imaging capabilities of TEE, the role of TEE will undoubtedly extend to this patient population. At some time during the perioperative phase of these patients, dependent on the specific clinical situation a TEE examination is necessary. Patients who are severely hypotensive will require standard resuscitative interventions first, as hypovolemia and cardiac tamponade are the clinician's initial concerns. A standard TTE examination does not reveal a large pericardial effusion. After surgical decompression of the pericardial fluid, TEE may detect inimical residual lesions that were not be appreciated by TTE.

Porembka et al.[288] reported turbulence, as evidenced by color flow echocardiography, in the ascending aorta as an initial sign for a residual lesion. Further TTE examinations failed to detect the lesion, while serial TEE examinations did locate an expanding lesion. This prompted surgical intervention and de-

finitive repair of an aortic right ventricular defect. As depicted in this case, only close scrutiny and serial examinations lead to the diagnosis. Indeed, small, irregular wounds are not easily diagnosed with angiography or TTE.[288,289]

In a recent case report, McIntyre at al.[290] described the benefit of TEE in the assessment of a patient sustaining a gunshot wound to the chest. TTE and angiography identified the retained bullet near the root of the ascending aorta; however, definitive description of extent of injury was only appreciated by TEE, which located the bullet within the aortic wall. Similar benefits of TEE were also seen in a case described by LiMandri et al.[291] Traumatic aortic lesions are only accessible by TEE in the early phases of these dynamic clinical circumstances.[292] The value of TEE is clearly seen in a patient in whom TEE revealed a VSD postoperatively, while other techniques were limited.[293]

These case descriptions reflect the value of TEE in critically ill patients. Skoularigis and colleagues[294] investigated the role of TEE in the initial phase of postoperative care of patients sustaining penetrating stab wounds to the heart. Forty-three consecutive patients who survived a penetrating cardiac wound were evaluated for this study. All patients underwent surgical exploration of the injury and repair of the superficial myocardial wound. In nine patients, residual intracardiac defects were noted by TTE. Four of these patients had multiple lesions. A biplanar TEE was performed in those patients in whom a lesion was identified by TTE. TTE missed two lesions: a significant tricuspid regurgitation and perforation of the septal leaflet of the tricuspid valve. In this same patient subset, only TEE was able to identify perforation of the anterior leaflet of the mitral valve in two patents, perforation of the aortic valve, and an aortic right ventricular fistulae.

PULMONARY EMBOLISM

In critically ill patients, the definitive diagnosis may not be available with the use of existing technology. We have experienced

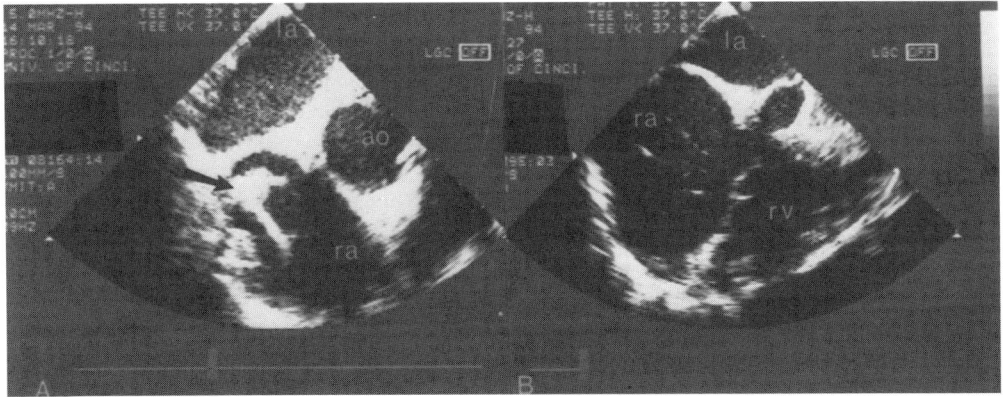

Fig. 14-10. Pulmonary embolism, transverse views. An elderly patient after recent surgery developed acute hypotension and hypoxemia. **(A)** Thrombus (in transit, *arrow*) identified in the right atrium (ra). **(B)** Corresponding view of the right atrium (ra) reveals a large right atrium and the interatrial septum bulging into the left atrium (la), indicative of a pressure overload situation. ao, ascending aorta; rv, right ventricle.

the benefit of TEE in many patients who are hypoxic and hypotensive (Fig. 14-10). In several patients, we suspected a possible PE because of the circumstances surrounding the case. Generally, these patients are too unstable to undergo a pulmonary angiogram to make the definitive diagnosis. However, TEE was performed in these patients and the echocardiographic hemodynamic characteristics indicative of PE found. Thrombus was also detected in three of the patients.

The diagnosis of PE whether massive or submassive, is the third most common cardiovascular disease, after following acute ischemic disorders and stroke.[295,296] Pulmonary embolism and its progenitor, deep venous thrombosis, may be difficult to diagnose in the critically ill because of many complex and confounding disease processes. In spite of major clinical advances, there are still 50,000 deaths from PE every year. Depending on the necropsy study, the rate of underdiagnosis may be as high as 84 percent, while overdiagnosis may be between 32 to 62 percent.[295,296] Clinical suspicion is the key in the initiation and guidance of diagnostic inquiries.

The clinical consequences from a PE de-

pend on the extent of flow obstruction in the pulmonary artery, release of vasoactive substances, and the premorbid cardiopulmonary state. In patients without pre-existing cardiac disease, physiologic relevance occurs when obstruction exceeds 25 percent of the normally compliant pulmonary vascular bed. As a result, right ventricular and pulmonary artery pressures will rise, although it is uncommon for the systolic pulmonary pressure to exceed 40 mmHg even when there is 50 percent obstruction. As a consequence of this right ventricular pressure overload, the right ventricle becomes dilated and hypokinetic, resulting in tricuspid regurgitation. With further increases in right ventricular afterload, right ventricular size increases and displaces the interventricular septum into the left ventricle. Right ventricular failure occurs as a consequence of decreased left ventricular output and subsequent deterioration in coronary blood flow.[297]

The classic echocardiographic findings in PE are dilated hypokinetic right ventricle, abnormal septal position and paradoxic systolic motion, increased ratio of right ventricular to left ventricular dimensions, dilated main or proximal branches of the pulmonary artery, and reduced left ventricular dimensions. There may be significant tricuspid and pulmonic regurgitation with increased velocities by Doppler echocardiography. Obviously, the anatomic identification of thrombotic material is diagnostic.

Similar hemodynamic findings have been found by other investigators.[298-304] In 14 cases of massive PE, an echocardiographic study detected all the aforementioned characteristic echocardiographic findings.[303] During the acute event, left ventricular function was preserved in spite of reduced dimensions. The right-sided volume indices were increased (end-systolic dimensions 12.3 $\pm$ 3.4 cm^2 · m^{-2} and end-diastolic dimensions 15.4 $\pm$ cm^2 · m^{-2}) and associated with interventricular septal flattening. In 64 percent of cases there was mild to moderate tricuspid insufficiency.[303] In another study (n = 105) by Kasper and colleagues,[304] TTE examination demonstrated a dilated right ventricle (75 percent), abnormal septal motion (44 percent), decreased left ventricular dimensions (42 percent), dilated pulmonary artery (77 percent), and a decreased EF slope of the mitral valve (50 percent). Thrombi were identified in 30 patients: superior vena cava (n = 1), innominate vein (n = 1), right atrium (n = 1), right ventricle (n = 3), and right pulmonary artery (n = 11).

In addition to the geometric considerations that occur during a PE, the clinician may evaluate the extent of tricuspid and/or pulmonary insufficiencies with Doppler echocardiography. The quantification of regurgitation has been validated with TTE but has yet to be substantiated with TEE.

The pressure gradient across an orifice is estimated by the simplified Bernoulli equation $\Delta P = 4(V^2)$, where V is the peak flow velocity within the orifice. Thus the peak pressure gradient across the tricuspid valve is four times the square of the maximal tricuspid regurgitant velocity (in meters · second^{-1}). This should equal the difference between the peak right ventricular systolic pressure and pressure within the atrium.

These results were confirmed by Currie et al.[305] during cardiac catheterization. Similar results are obtained during interrogation of the maximal flow velocity within the regurgitant jet of the pulmonic valve. At end-diastole, flow velocity in the pulmonary insufficiency jet is determined by the difference between the right ventricular and the pulmonary arterial end-diastolic pressures.[306] Thus, one can estimate this gradient and any pressure associated with it.

As the utilization of TEE increases in the ICU, the benefit of TEE will prove its clinical worth as a powerful diagnostic tool. We recently used TEE to make a diagnosis in a patient who became hypoxic and hypotensive following an elective total knee replacement. Other than the time course of the development of the symptoms, the provisional diagnosis was a PE. During the resuscitative phase, in which the patient was too unstable for a definitive pulmonary angiogram, TEE revealed both geometric and hemodynamic echocardiographic findings consistent with the diagnosis of PE. The anatomic identification of a thrombus located in the proximal left pulmonary artery was later confirmed by pulmonary angiogram. Other similar cases are being described with the use of TEE.[307-314] Hunter et al.[308] detected a large thrombus in the right atrium and ventricle that was not appreciated with TTE. Thrombi have even been located in the superior vena cava and pulmonary vein with TEE.[310,312] The routine postoperative evaluation of all lung transplants at UCLA Medical Center includes a TEE examination to evaluate the flow and anatomic characteristics of the pulmonary vascular anastomoses (John P. Williams, personal communication).

REFERENCES

1. Pearson, AC, Castello R, Labovitz AJ et al: Safety and utility of transesophageal echocardiography in the critically ill patient. Am Heart J 119:1083, 1990
2. Porembka DT, Hoit BD: Transesophageal

echocardiography in the intensive care patient. Crit Care Med 19:826, 1991

3. Oh JK, Seward JB, Khandheria BK et al: Transesophageal echocardiography in critically ill patients. Am J Cardiol 66:1492, 1990

4. Foster E, Schiller NB: The role of transesophageal echocardiography in critical care: USCF experience. J Am Soc Echocardiogr 5:368, 1992

5. Wolfe LT, Rossi A, Ritter SB: Transesophageal echocardiography in infants and children: use and importance in the cardiac intensive care unit. J Am Soc Echocardiogr 6:286, 1993

6. Hwang J, Shyu K, Chen J et al: Usefulness of transesophageal echocardiography in the treatment of critically ill patients. Chest 104:861, 1993

7. Khoury AF, Afridi I, Quinones MA et al: Transesophageal echocardiography in critically ill patients: feasibilty, safety, and impact on management. Am Heart J 127:1363, 1994

8. Porembka DT: Transesophageal echocardiography in the critically ill. pp. 296–346. In Critical Care: State of the Art. Vol. 15. Williams & Wilkins, Baltimore, 1995

9. Feigenbaum H: Echocardiography. 5th Ed. Lea & Febiger, Philadelphia, 1994

10. Weyman AE: Principles and Practice of Echocardiography. 2nd Ed. Lea & Febiger, Philadelphia, 1994

11. Erbel R, Khandheria BK, Brennecke R et al. (eds): Transesophageal, a New Window to the Heart. Springer-Verlag, Heidelberg, 1989

12. Popp RL: Medical progress: echocardiography review articlcs. II. N Engl J Med 323:165, 1990

13. Seward JB, Khandheria BK, Edwards WD et al: Biplanar transesophageal echocardiography: anatomic correlations, image orientation, and clinical applications. Mayo Clin Proc 65:1193, 1990

14. Bansal RC, Shakudo M, Shah PM et al: Biplane transesophageal echocardiography: technique, image orientation, and preliminary experience in 131 patients. J Am Soc Echocardiogr 3:348, 1990

15. Bansal RC and Shah PM: Current Problems in Cardiology, Transesophageal Echocardiography. Vol. XV. CV Mosby–Year Book, 1990

16. Khandheria BK, Seward JB, Tajik AJ: Transesophageal echocardiography. In Braunwald E (ed): Transesophageal Echocardiography. Heart Disease. A Textbook of Cardiovascular Medicine. 3rd Ed. Suppl 12. WB Saunders, Philadelphia, 1991

17. Missri J (ed): Transesophageal Echocardiography: Clinical and Intraoperative Applications. Churchill Livingstone, New York, 1993

18. Schiller NB, Foster E, Redberg RF (eds): Transesophageal Echocardiography, Cardiology Clinics. Vol. 11, No. 3. WB Saunders, Philadelphia, 1993

19. Freeman WK, Seward JB, Khandheria BK, Tajik AJ (eds): Transesophageal Echocardiography. Little, Brown, Boston, 1994

20. Stoddard MF, Longaker RA, Vuocolo LM et al: Transesophageal echocardiography in the pregnant patient. Am Heart J 124:785, 1992

21. Daniel WG, Kasper W, Erbel R: Safety of transesophageal echocardiography: a multicenter survey of 10,419 examinations. Circulation 83:817, 1991

22. Khandheria BK, Oh J: Transesophageal echocardiography: state-of-the-art and future directions. Am J Cardiol 69:61H, 1992

23. Fagan LF Jr, Weiss R, Castello R et al: Transtracheal placement and imaging with a transesophageal echocardiographic probe. Am J Cardiol 67:909, 1991

24. Gilbert TB, Panico FG, McGill WA et al: Bronchial obstruction by transesophageal echocardiography probe in a pediatric cardiac patient. Anesth Analg 74:156, 1992

25. Lunn RJ, Oliver WC Jr, Hagler DJ et al: Aortic compression by transesophagel echocardiographic probe in infants and children undergoing cardiac surgery. Anesthesiology 77:587, 1992

26. Kronzon I, Cziner DG, Katz ES et al: Buckling of the tip of the transesophageal echocardiography probe: a potentially dangerous technical malfunction. J Am Soc Echocardiogr 5:176, 1992

27. Dewhirst WE, Stragand JJ, Fleming BM: Mallory-Weiss tear complicating intraoperative transesophageal echocardiography in a patient undergoing aortic valve replacement. Anesthesiology 73:777, 1990

28. Rankin JS, McHale PA, Arentzen CE et al: Three-dimensional dynamic geometry of the left ventricle in the conscious dog. Circ Res 39:304, 1976

29. Konstadt SN, Thys D, Mindich BP et al: Validation of quantitative intraoperative transesophageal echocardiography. Anesthesiology 65:418, 1986

30. Beaupre PN, Cahalan MK, Kremer PF et al: Does pulmonary artery occlusion pressure adequately reflect left ventricular filing during anesthesia and surgery? Anesthesiology 59:A3, 1988

31. Urbanowicz JH, Shaaban J, Cohen NH et al: Comparison of transesophageal echocardiographic and scintigraphic estimates of left ventricular end-diastolic volume index and ejection fraction in patients following coronary artery bypass grafting. Anesthesiology 72:607, 1990

32. Clements FM, Harpole DH, Quill T et al: Estimation of left ventricular volume and ejection fraction by two-dimensional transesophageal echocardiography: comparison of short axis imaging and simultaneous radionuclide angiography. Br J Anaesth 64:331, 1990

33. Reich DL, Konstadt SN, Nejat M et al: Intraoperative transesophageal echocardiography for the detection of cardiac preload changes induced by transfusion and phlebotomy in pediatric patients. Anesthesiology 79:10, 1993

34. Cheung AT, Savino JS, Weiss SJ et al: Echocardiographic and hemodynamic indexes of left ventricular preload in patients with normal and abnormal ventricular function. Anesthesiology 81:376, 1994

35. Van Daele ME, Trouwborst A, Woerkens LC et al: Transesophageal echocardiographic monitoring of preoperative hypervolumic hemodilution. Anesthesiology 81:602, 1994

36. Leung JM, Levine EH: left ventricular end-systolic cavity obliteration as an estimate of intraoperative hypovolemia. Anesthesiology 81:1102, 1994

37. Schuster S, Erbel R, Weilemann LS et al: Hemodynamics during PEEP ventilation in patients with severe left ventricular failure studied by transesophageal echocardiography. Chest 97:1181, 1990

38. Jardin F, Brun-Ney D, Hardy A et al: Combined thermodilution and two-dimensional echocardiographic evaluation of right ventricular function during respiratory support with PEEP. Chest 99:162, 1991

39. Porembka D, Hoit B, McMannis K et al: Correlation of pulmonary artery occlusion pressure with pulmonary venous flow pattern by transesophageal echocardiography. Crit Care Med 21:S268, 1993

40. Cahalan MK, Ionescu P, Melton HE et al: Automated real-time analysis of intraoperative transesophageal echocardiograms. Anesthesiology 78:477, 1993

41. Katz WE, Mandarino WA, Gorcsan J et al: Noninvasive pressure-volume relations to evaluate left ventricular function during dobutamine infusion. J Am Soc Echocardiogr 7:S38, 1994

42. Martin RW, Bashein G: Measurement of stroke volume with three-dimensional transesophageal ultrasonic scanning: comparison with thermodilution measurement. Anesthesiology 70:470, 1989

43. Martin RW, Bashein G, Detmer PR et al: Ventricular volume measurement from a multiplanar transesophageal ultrasonic imaging system: an in vitro study. IEEE Trans Biomed Eng 37:442, 1990

44. Roelandt JRTC, Thomson IR, Vletter WB et al: Multiplane transesophageal echocardiography: latest evolution in an imaging revolution. J Am Soc Echocardiogr 5:361, 1992

45. Kuroda T, Kinter TM, Seward JB et al: Accuracy of three-dimensional volume measurement using biplane transesophageal echocardiographic probe: in vitro experiment. J Am Soc Echocardiogr 4:475, 1991

46. Roelandt JRT, Cate F, Vletter WB et al: Ultrasonic dynamic three-dimensional visualization of the heart with a multiplane transesophageal imaging transducer. J Am Soc Echocardiogr 7:217, 1994

47. Belohlavek M, Foley DA, Gerber TC et al: Three- and four-dimensional cardiovascular ultrasound imaging: a new era for echocardiography. Mayo Clin Proc 68:221, 1993

48. Bashein G, Sheehan FH, Nessly ML et al: Three-dimensional transesophageal echocardiography for depiction of regional left-ventricular performance: initial results and future directions. Int J Cardi Imaging 9:121, 1993

49. Gorcsan J, Mandarino WA, Denault AY et al: Measurement of changes in left ventricular volume throughout the cardiac cycle: comparison of transesophageal echocardiographic automated border detection with

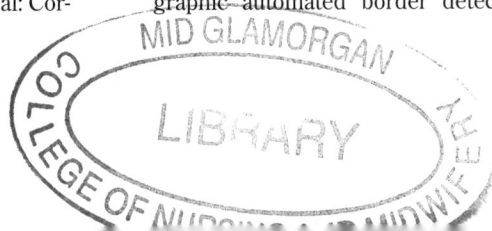

conductance catheter techniques. J Am Soc Echocardiogr 7:S38, 1994

50. Tennant R, Wiggers C: The effect of coronary occlusion on myocardial contraction. Am J Physiol 112:351, 1935

51. Alam M, Khaja F, Brymer J et al: Echocardiographic evaluation of the left ventricle during coronary artery angioplasty. Am J Cardiol 57:20, 1986

52. Beaupre DN, Kremer PF, Cahalan MK et al: Intraoperative detection of changes in left ventricular segmental wall motion by transesophageal two-dimensional echocardiography. Am Heart J 107:1021, 1984

53. Smith JS, Cahalan MK, Benefiel DJ et al: Intraoperative detection of myocardial ischemia in high-risk patients: electrocardiography versus two-dimensional transesophageal echocardiography. Circulation 72:1015, 1985

54. Vatner SF: Correlation between acute reductions in myocardial blood flow and function in conscious dogs. Circ Res 47:201, 1980

55. Rozien MF, Beaupre PN, Alper RA et al: Monitoring with two-dimensional transesophageal echocardiography. J Vasc Surg 1:300, 1984

56. London MJ, Tubau MG, Wong E et al: The "natural history" of segmental wall motion abnormalities in patients undergoing noncardiac surgery. Anesthesiology 73:644, 1990

57. Ellis JE, Shah MN, Briller JE et al: A comparison of methods for the detection of myocardial ischemia during noncardiac surgery: automated ST-segment analysis systems, electrocardiography, and transesophageal echocardiography. Anesth Analg 75:764, 1992

58. Atkov OY, Akchurin RS, Tkachuk M et al: Intraoperative transesophageal echocardiography for detection of myocardial ischemia. Herz 6:372, 1993

59. Leung JM, O'Kelly B, Browner WS et al: Prognostic importance of post-bypass regional wall motion abnormalities in patients undergoing coronary artery bypass graft surgery. Anesthesiology 71:16, 1989

60. Van Daele M, Sutherland GR, Mitchell MM et al: Do changes in pulmonary capillary wedge adequately reflect myocardial ischemia during anesthesia? A correlative preoperative hemodynamic, electrocardiographic, and transesophageal echocardiographic study. Circulation 81:865, 1990

61. Leung JM, O'Kelly BF, Mangano DT: Relationship of regional wall motion abnormalities to hemodynamic indices of myocardial oxygen supply and demand in patients undergoing CABG surgery. Anesthesiology 73:802, 1990

62. Deutsch HJ, Curtius JM, Leischik R et al: Reproducibility of assessment of left ventricular function using intraoperative transesophageal echocardiography. Thorac Cardiovasc Surg 41:54, 1993

63. Saada M, Cahalan MK, Lee E et al: Real time evaluation of echocardiograms. Anesthesiology 71:344, 1989

64. Doer HK, Quinones MA, Zoghbi WA et al: Accurate determination of left ventricular ejection fraction by transesophageal echocardiography with a nonvolumetric method. J Am Soc Echocardiogr 6:476, 1993

65. Berquist BD, Lemon KW, Bellows WH et al: Real-time determination of ejection fraction by transesophageal echocardiography: how accurate are "eyeball" estimates? Anesthesiology 79:A69, 1993

66. Armstrong WF, O'Donnell J, Dillon JC et al: Complementary value of two-dimensional exercise echocardiography to routine treadmill exercise testing. Ann Intern Med 105:829, 1986

67. Lambertz H, Kreis A, Trumper H et al: Simultaneous transesophageal atrial pacing and transesophageal two-dimensional: a new method of stress echocardiography. J Am Coll Cardiol 16:1143, 1990

68. Zabalgoitia M, Gandhi DK, Abi-Mansour P et al: Transesophageal stress echocardiography: detection of coronary artery disease in patients with normal resting left ventricular contractility. Am Heart J 122:1456, 1991

69. Berthe C, Pierard LA, Hiemaux M et al: Predicting the extent and location of coronary artery disease in acute myocardial infarction by echocardiography during dobutamine infusion. Am J Cardiol 58:1167, 1986

70. Sawada SG, Segar DS, Brown SE et al: Dobutamine stress echocardiography for evaluation of coronary disease. Circulation 80:II-66, 1989

71. Picano E, Lattanzi F, Masini M et al: Comparison of the high-dose dipyridamole-echocar-

diography test and exercise two-dimensional echocardiography for diagnosis of coronary artery disease. Am J Cardiol 59:539, 1987

72. Bolognese L, Sarasso G, Aralda D et al: High dose dipyridamole echocardiography early after uncomplicated acute myocardial infarction: correlation with exercise testing and coronary angiography. J Am Coll Cardiol 14: 357, 1989

73. Marwick T, D'hondt A, Baudhuin T et al: Optimal use of dobutamine stress for the detection and evaluation of coronary artery disease: combination with echocardiography or scintigraphy, or both? J Am Coll Cardiol 22: 159, 1993

74. Forster T, McNeill AJ, Salustri A et al: Simultaneous dobutamine stress echocardiography and technetium-99m isonitrile single-photon emission computed tomography in patients with suspected coronary artery disease. J Am Coll Cardiol 21:1591, 1993

75. Takeuchi M, Araki M, Nakasima Y et al: Comparison of dobutamine stress echocardiography and stress thallium-201 single-photon emission computed tomography for detecting coronary disease. J Am Soc Echocardiogr 6:593, 1993

76. Panza JA, Laurienzo JM, Curiel RV et al: Transesophageal dobutamine stress echocardiography for evaluation of patients with coronary artery disease. J Am Coll Cardiol 24:1260, 1994

77. Baer FM, Voth E, Deutsch HJ et al: Assessment of viable myocardium by dobutamine transesophageal echocardiography and comparison with Fluorine-18 Fluorodexyglucose positron emission tomography. J Am Coll Cardiol 24:343, 1994

78. Roger VL, Pellikka PA, Oh JK et al: Stress echocardiography. Part I. Exercise echocardiography: techniques, implementation, clinical applications, and correlations. Mayo Clin Proc 70:5, 1995

79. Pellika PA, Roger VL, Oh JK et al: Stress echocardiography. Part II. Dobutamine stress echocardiography: techniques, implementation, clinical applications, and correlations. Mayo Clin Proc 70:16, 1995

80. Aronson S, Lee BK, Wiencek JG et al: Assessment of myocardial perfusion during CABG surgery with two-dimensional transesopha-geal contrast echocardiography. Anesthesiology 75:433, 1991

81. Nanda NC, Schlied R (eds): Advances in Echo Imaging Using Contrast Enhancement. Kluwer Academic, Dordrecht, the Netherlands, 1993

82. Voci P, Bilotta F, Caretta Q et al: Mechanisms of incomplete cardioplegia distribution during coronary artery surgery. Anesthesiology 79:904, 1993

83. Appleton CP, Gonzalez MS, Basnight MA et al: Relationship of left atrial pressure and pulmonary venous flow velocities: importance of baseline mitral and pulmonary venous flow velocity patterns studied in lightly sedated dogs. J Am Soc Echocardiogr 7:264, 1994

84. Castello R, Pearson AC, Lenzen P et al: Evaluation of pulmonary venous flow by transesophageal echocardiography in subjects with a normal heart: comparison with transesophageal echocardiography. J Am Coll Cardiol 18:65, 1991

85. Meijburg HWJ, Visser CA, Westerhof PW et al: Normal pulmonary venous flow characteristics as assessed by transesophageal pulsed Doppler echocardiography. J Am Soc Echocardiogr 5:558, 1992

86. Bartzokis T, Lee R, Yeoh TK et al: Transesophageal echo-Doppler echocardiographic assessment of pulmonary venous flow patterns. J Am Soc Echocardiogr 4:457, 1991

87. Akamatsu S, Terazawa E, Kagawa K et al: Transesophageal Doppler echocardiographic assessment of pulmonary venous flow pattern in subjects without cardiovascular disease. Intl J Card Imaging 9:195, 1993

88. Iuchi A, Oki T, Ogawa S et al: Evaluation of pulmonary venous flow pattern in hypertrophied and dilated hearts: a new study with transesophageal pulsed Doppler echocardiography. J Cardiol 21:75, 1991

89. Appleton CP, Hatle LA, Popp RL: Relation of transmittal flow velocity patterns to left ventricular diastolic function: new insights from a combined hemodynamic and Doppler echocardiographic study. J Am Coll Cardiol 12:426, 1988

90. Pearson AC, Gudipati CV, Labovitz AJ: Effects of aging on left ventricular structure and function. Am Heart J 121:871, 1991

91. Lavine SJ: Left ventricular diastolic function in idiopathic cardiomyopathy: Doppler he-

modynamic correlations. Echocardiography 8:151, 1991

92. Hoffmann R, Lambertz H, Jutten H et al: Mitral and pulmonary venous flow under influence of positive end-expiratory pressure ventilation analyzed by transesophageal pulsed Doppler echocardiography. Am J Cardiol 68: 697, 1991

93. Nishimura RA, Abel MD, Hatle LK et al: Relation of pulmonary vein velocities by transesophageal Doppler echocardiography: effect of different loading conditions. Circulation 81:1488, 1990

94. Kuecherer HF, Kusumoto F, Muhiudeen IA et al: Pulmonary venous flow patterns by transesophageal pulsed Doppler echocardiography: relation to parameters of left ventricular systolic and diastolic function. Am Heart J 122:1683, 1991

95. Kuecherer HF, Muhiudeen IA, Kusumoto FM et al: Estimation of mean left atrial pressure from transesophageal pulsed Doppler echocardiography of pulmonary venous flow. Circulation 82:1127, 1990

96. Hoit BD, Shao Y, Gabel M et al: Influence of myocardial contractile dysfunction on the pattern of pulmonary venous flow. Circulation 84:369, 1991

97. Hoit BD, Shao Y, Gabel M et al: Influence of loading conditions and contractile state on pulmonary venous flow. Circulation 86:651, 1992

98. Stevenson LW, Childs J, Laks H et al: Incidence and significance of early pericardial effusion after cardiac surgery. Am J Cardiol 54: 848, 1984

99. Kochar GS, Jacobs LE, Kotler MN: Right atrial compression in postoperative cardiac patients: detection by transesophageal echocardiography. J Am Coll Cardiol 16:511, 1990

100. Shoebrechts B, Herregods MC, Van de Werf F et al: Usefulness of transesophageal echocardiography in patients with hemodynamic deterioration late after cardiac surgery. Chest 104:1631, 1993

101. Hoit BD, Dalton N, Bhargava V et al: Pericardial influences on right and left ventricular filling dynamics. Circ Res 68:197, 1991

102. Glantz SA, Misbach GA, Moores WY et al: The pericardium substantially affects the left ventricular diastolic pressure-volume relationship in the dog. Circ Res 42:433, 1978

103. Kronzon I, Cohen ML, Winer HE: Diastolic atrial compression: a sensitive echocardiographic sign of cardiac tamponade. J Am Coll Cardiol 2:770, 1983

104. Gillam LD, Guyer DE, Gibson TC et al: Hydrodynamic compression of right atrium: a new echocardiographic sign of cardiac tamponade. Circulation 68:294, 1983

105. Singh S, Wann LS, Schuchard GH et al: Right ventricular and right atrial collapse in patients with cardiac tamponade: a combined echocardiographic and hemodynamic study. Circulation 70:966, 1984

106. Leimgruber PP, Klopfenstein S, Wann LS et al: The hemodynamic derangement associated with right ventricular diastolic collapse in cardiac tamponade: an experimental echocardiographic study. Circulation 68:612, 1983

107. Cogswell TL, Bernath GA, Wann LS et al: Effects of intravascular volume state on the value of pulsus paradoxus and right ventricular diastolic collapse in predicting cardiac tamponade. Circulation 72:1076, 1985

108. Klopfenstein HS, Cogswell TL, Bernath GA et al: Alterations in intravascular volume affect the relation between right ventricular diastolic collapse and the hemodynamic severity of cardiac tamponade. J Am Coll Cardiol 6:1057, 1985

109. Hoit BD, Gabel M, Fowler NO: Cardiac tamponade in left ventricular dysfunction. Circulation 82:1370, 1990

110. Labib SB, Udelson JE, Pandian NG et al: Echocardiography in low pressure cardiac tamponade. J Am Coll Cardiol 63:1156, 1989

111. Tunick PA, Nachamie M, Kronzon I: Reversal of echocardiographic signs of pericardial tamponade by transfusion. Am Heart J 119: 199, 1990

112. Torelli J, Marwick TYH, Salcedo EE: Left atrial tamponade: diagnosis by transesophageal echocardiography. J Am Soc Echocardiogr 4:413, 1991

113. Appleton CP, Hatle LK, Popp RL: Cardiac tamponade and pericardial effusion: respiratory variation in transvalvular flow velocities studied by Doppler echocardiography. J Am Coll Cardiol 11:1020, 1988

114. Berge KH, Lanier WL, Reeder GS: Occult cardiac tamponade detected by transesophageal echocardiography. Mayo Clin Proc 67: 667, 1992

115. Cujec B, Johnson D, Bharadwaj B: Cardiac tamponade by loculated pericardial hematoma following open heart surgery: diagnosis by transesophageal echocardiography. Can J Cardiol 7:37, 1991

116. Hatle L, Angelsen B, Tromsdal A: Noninvasive assessment of atrioventricular pressure half-time by Doppler ultrasound. Circulation 60:1096, 1979

117. Stoddard MF, Prince CR, Ammash NM et al: Two-dimensional transesophageal echocardiographic determination of mitral valve area inadult with mitral stenosis. Am Heart J 127: 1348, 1994

118. Stoddard MF, Arce J, Liddell NE et al: Two-dimensional transesophageal echocardiographic determination of aortic valve area in adults with aortic stenosis. Am Heart J 122: 1415, 1991

119. Bengur AR, Snider AR, Meliones JN et al: Doppler evaluation of aortic valve area in children with aortic stenosis. J Am Coll Cardiol 18:1499, 1991

120. Cyran SE, Kimball TR, Schwartz DC et al: Evaluation of balloon aortic valvuloplasty with transesophageal echocardiography. Am Heart J 115:460, 1988

121. Sheikh KH, deBruijn NP, Rankin JS et al: The utility of trasnesophageal echocardiography and Doppler color flow imaging in patients undergoing cardiac valve surgery. J Am Coll Cardiol 15:363, 1990

122. Sheikh KH, Bengtson JR, Rankin JS et al: Intraoperative transesophageal Doppler color flow imaging used to guide patient selection and operative treatment of ischemic mitral regurgitation. Circulation 84:594, 1991

123. Stewart WJ, Currie PJ, Salcedo EE et al: Intraoperative Doppler color flow mapping for decision-making in valve repair for mitral regurgitation. Techniques and results in 100 patients. Circulation 81:556, 1990

124. Stewart WJ, Currie PJ, Salcedo EE et al: Jet direction by color flow mapping accurately depicts the mechanism of mitral regurgitation. Circulation 78:434, 1988

125. Jacobs LE, Wertheimer JH, Kotler MN et al: Quantification of mitral regurgitation: a comparison of transesophageal echocardiography and contrast ventriculography. Echocardiography 9:145, 1992

126. Sadoshima J, Koyanagi S, Sugimachi M et al: Evaluation of the severity of mitral regurgitation by transesophageal Doppler flow echocardiography. Am Heart J 123:1245, 1992

127. Kamp O, Dijkstra JW, Huitnink H et al: Transesophageal color flow Doppler mapping in the assessment of native mitral valvular regurgitation: comparison with left ventricular angiography. J Am Soc Echocardiogr 4:598, 1991

128. Castello R, Fagan L, Lenzen P et al: Comparison of transthoracic and transesophageal echocardiography for assessment of left-sided valvular regurgitation. Am J Cardiol 68: 1677, 1991

129. Smith MD, Harrison MR, Pinton R et al: Regurgitant jet size by transesophageal compared with transthoracic Doppler color flow imaging. Circulation 83:79, 1991

130. Helmcke F, Nanda NC, Hsiung MC et al: Color Doppler assessment of mitral regurgitation with orthogonal planes. Circulation 75: 175, 1987

131. Cape EG, Yoganathan AP, Weyman AE et al: Adjacent solid boundaries alter the size of regurgitant jets on Doppler color flow maps. J Am Coll Cardiol 17:1094, 1991

132. Castello R, Lenzen P, Aguirre F et al: Quantification of mitral regurgitation by transesophageal echocardiography with color flow mapping: correlation with cardiac catherization. J Am Coll Cardiol 19:1516, 1992

133. Yoshida K, Yoshikawa J, Yamaura Y et al: Assessment of mitral regurgitation by biplane transesophageal color Doppler flow mapping. Circulation 82:1121, 1990

134. Castello R, Pearson AC, Lenzen P et al: Effect of mitral regurgitation on pulmonary venous velocities derived from transesophageal echocardiography color-guided pulsed Doppler imaging. J Am Coll Cardiol 17:1499, 1991

135. Klein AL, Stewart WJ, Bartlett J et al: Effects of mitral regurgitation on pulmonary venous flow and left atrial pressure: an intraoperative transesophageal echocardiographic study. J Am Coll Cardiol 20:1345, 1992

136. Lai L, Shyu K, Chen J et al: Usefulness of pulmonary venous flow pattern and maximal jet area detected by transesophageal echocardiography in assessing the severity of mitral regurgitation. Am J Cardiol 72:1310, 1993

137. Klein AI, Bailey AS, Cohen GI et al: Impor-

tance of sampling both pulmonary veins in grading mitral regurgitation by transesophageal echocardiography. J Am Soc Echocardiogr 6:115, 1993

138. Bargiggia GS, Tronconi L, Sahn DJ et al: A new method for quantitation of mitral regurgitation based on color flow Doppler imaging of flow convergence proximal to regurgitant orifice. Circulation 84:1481, 1991

139. Rivera JM, Vandervoort PM, Thoreau DH et al: Quantification of mitral regurgitation with the proximal flow convergence method: a clinical study. Am Heart J 134:1289, 1992

140. Chen C, Koschyk D, Brockhoff C et al: Non-invasive estimation of regurgitant flow rate and volume in patients with mitral regurgitation by Doppler color maping of accelerating flow field. J Am Coll Cardiol 21:374, 1993

141. Giesler M, Grossman G, Schmidt A et al: Color Doppler echocardiographic determination of mitral regurgitant flow from the proxiaml velocity profile of the flow convergence region. Am J Cardiol 85:1248, 1992

142. Tribouilly C, Shen WF, Quere JP et al: Assessment of severity of mitral regurgitation by measuring regurgitant jet width at its origin with transesophageal Doppler color flow imaging. Circulation 85:1248, 1992

143. Wang SS, Rubenstein JJ, Goldman M et al: A new Doppler-echo method to quantify regurgitant volume. J Am Soc Echocardiogr 5: 107, 1992

144. Enriquez-Sarano M, Bailey KR, Seward JB et al: Quantitative Doppler assessment of valvular regurgitation. Circulation 83:841, 1993

145. Tribouilloy C, Chen WF, Slama MA et al: Non-invasive measurement of the regurgitant fraction by pulsed Doppler echocardiography in isolated pure mitral regurgitation. Br Heart J 66:290, 1991

146. Dittrich HC, McCann HA, Walsh TP et al: Transesophageal echocardiography in the evaluation of prosthetic and native aortic valves. Am J Cardiol 66:758, 1990

147. Perry GJ, Helmcke F, Nanda JC et al: Evaluation of aortic insufficiency by Doppler color flow mapping. J Am Coll Cardiol 9:952, 1987

148. Tribouilloy C, Avinee P, Shen WF et al: End diastolic flow velocity just beneath the aortic isthmus assessed by pulsed Doppler echocardiography: a new predictor of aortic regurgitant fraction. Br Heart J 65:37, 1991

149. Nishimura RA, Vonk GD, Rumberger JA et al: Semiquantification of aortic regurgitation by different Doppler echocardiographic techniques and comparison with ultrafast computed tomography. Am Heart J 124:995, 1992

150. Labovitz AJ, Ferrara RP, Kem MJ et al: Quantitative evaluation of aortic insufficiency by continuous wave Doppler echocardiography. J Am Coll Cardiol 8:1341, 1986

151. Stoddard MF, Arce J, Liddell NE et al: Two-dimensional transesophageal echocardiographic determination of aortic valve area in adults with aortic stenosis. Am Heart J 122: 1415, 1991

152. Khandheria BK, Seward JB, Oh JK et al: Value and limitations of transesophageal echocardiography in assessment of mitral valve prosthesis. Circulation 83:1956, 1991

153. Nellessen U, Schnittger I, Appleton CP et al: Transesophageal two-dimensional echocardiography and color Doppler velocity mapping in the evaluation of cardiac valve prosthesis. Circulation 78:848, 1988

154. van den Brink RBA, Visser CA, Basart DCG et al: Comparison of transthoracic and transesophageal color flow Doppler imaging in patients with mechanical prosthesis in the mitral valve position. Am J Cardiol 63:1471, 1989

155. Alam M, Serwin JB, Rosman HS et al: Transesophageal color flow Doppler and echocardiographic features of normal and regurgitant St. Jude Medical prostheses in the mitral valve position. Am J Cardiol 66:871, 1990

156. Alam M, Serwin JB, Rosman IIS et al: Transesophageal echocardiographic features of normal and dysfunctioning bioprosthetic valves. Am Heart J 121:1149, 1991

157. Daniel LB, Grigg LE, Weisel RD et al: Comparison of transthoracic and transesophageal echocardiography in evaluating prosthetic or bioprosthetic valve dysfunction. Am J Cardiol 69:697, 1992

158. Lange HW, Olson JD, Pedersen WR et al: Transesophageal color Doppler echocardiography of the normal St. Jude Medical mitral valve prosthesis. Am Heart J 122:489, 1991

159. Hixson CS, Smith MD, Mattson MD et al: Comparison of transesophageal color flow Doppler imaging of normal mitral regurgitant jets in St. Jude Medical and medtronic

hall cardiac prosthesis. J Am Soc Echocardiogr 5:57, 1992

160. Herrea CJ, Chaudhry FA, DeFrino PF et al: Value and limitations of transesophageal echocardiography in evaluating prosthetic or bioprosthetic valve dysfunction. Am J Cardiol 69:697, 1992

161. Alton ME, Pasierski TJ, Orsinelli DA et al: Comparison of transthoracic and transesophageal echocardiography in evaluation of 47 Starr-Edwards prosthetic valves. J Am Coll Cardiol 20:1503, 1992

162. Daniel WG, Mugge A, Grote J et al: Comparison of transthoracic and transesophageal echocardiography for detection of abnormalities of prosthetic and bioprosthetic valves in the mitral and aortic positions. Am J Cardiol 71:210, 1993

163. Taams MA, Gussenhoven EJ, Cahalan MK et al: Transesophageal Doppler color flow imaging in the detection of native and Bjork-Shiley mitral valve regurgitation. J Am Coll Cardiol 13:95, 1989

164. Mohr-Kahaly S, Kupferwasser I, Erbel R et al: Regurgitant flow in apparently normal valve prosthesis: Improved detection and semiquantitative analysis by transesophageal two-dimensional color-coded Doppler echocardiography. J Am Soc Echocardiogr 3:187, 1990

165. Skudicky D, Skoularigis J, Essop MR et al: Prevalence and clinical significance of mild paraprosthetic ring leaks and left atrial spontaneous echo contrast detected on transesophageal echocardiography three months after isolated mitral valve replacement with a mechanical prosthesis. Am J Cardiol 72:848, 1993

166. Freeman WK, Schaff HV, Khandheria BJ et al: Intraoperative evaluation of mitral valve regurgitation and repair by transesophageal echocardiography: Incidence and significance of systoli anterior motion. J Am Coll Cardiol 20:599, 1992

167. Grigg LE, Wigle D, Williams WG et al: Transesophageal Doppler echocardiography in obstructive hypertrophic cardiomyopathy: clarification of pathophysiology and importance in intraoperative decision making. J Am Coll Cardiol 20:42, 1992

168. Stevenson JG, Sorensen GK, Gartman DM et al: Left ventricular outflow tract obstruction: an indication for intraoperative transesophageal echocardiography. J Am Soc Echocardiogr 6:525, 1993

169. Erbel R, Engberding R, Daniel W et al: Echocardiography in the diagnosis of aortic dissection. European Cooperative Study Group for Echocardiography. Lancet 1:457, 1989

170. Ballal RS, Nanda NC, Gatewood R et al: Usefulness of transesophageal echocardiography in assessment of aortic dissection. Circulation 84:1903, 1991

171. Hashimoto S, Kumada T, Osakada G et al: Assessment of transesophageal Doppler echocardiography in dissecting aortic aneurysm. J Am Coll Cardiol 14:1253, 1989

172. Nienaber CA, Spielmann RP, von Kodolitsch Y et al: Diagnosis of thoracic aortic dissection. Magnetic resonance imaging versus transesophageal echocardiography. Circulation 85:434, 1992

173. Nienaber CA, von Kodolitsch Y, Nicholas V et al: The diagnosis of thoracic aortic dissection by noninvasive imaging procedures. N Engl J Med 328:1, 1993

174. Roudaut RP, Marcaggi XL, Deville C et al: Value of transesophageal echocardiography combined with computed tomography for assessing repaired type A aortic dissection. Am J Cardiol 70:1468, 1992

175. Erbel R, Oelert H, Meyer J et al: Effect of medical and surgical therapy on aortic dissection evaluated by transesophageal echocardiography. Circulation 87:1604, 1993

176. Nanda NC, Gramiak R, Shah PM: Diagnosis of aortic root dissection by echocardiography. Circulation 48:506, 1973

177. Takamoto S, Omoto R: Visualization of thoracic dissecting aortic aneurysm by transesophageal Doppler color flow mapping. Herz 12:187, 1987

178. Hayashi K, Meaney TF, Zelch JV, Tarar R: Aortographic analysis of aortic dissection. AJR 122:769, 1974

179. Yamada T, Tada S, Harada J: Aortic dissection without intimal rupture: diagnosis with MR imaging and CT. Radiology 168:347, 1988

180. Wolff KA, Herold CJ, Tempany CM et al: Aortic dissection: atypical patterns seen at MR imaging. Radiology 181:489, 1991

181. Mohr-Kahaly S, Erbel R, Puth M et al: Aortic intramural hematoma visualized by transesophageal echocardiography. Follow-up

and prognostic implications. Circulation 84: II-128, 1991

182. Blackshear JL, Safford RE, Lane GE et al: Unruptured noncoronary sinus of Valsalva aneurysm: preoperative characterization by transesophageal echocardiography. J Am Soc Echocardiogr 4:485, 1991

183. Chan K-L: Impact of transesophageal echocardiography on the treatment of patients with aortic dissection. Chest 101:406, 1992

184. Kearney PA, Smith W, Johnson SB et al: Use of transesophageal echocardiography in the evaluation of traumatic aortic injury. J Trauma 34:696, 1993

185. Shapiro MJ, Yanofsky SD, Trapp J et al: Cardiovascular evaluation in blunt thoracic trauma using transesophageal echocardiography (TEE). J Trauma 31:835, 1991

186. Le Bret F, Ruel P, Rosier H et al: Diagnosis of traumatic mediastinal hematoma with transesophageal echocardiography. Chest 105:373, 1994

187. Taams MA, Gussenhoven WJ, Bos E et al: Saccular aneurysm of the transverse thoracic aorta detected by transesophageal echocardiography. Chest 93:436, 1988

188. Kamp O, Van Rossum AC, Torenbeek R: Transesophageal echocardiography and magnetic resonance imaging for the assessment of saccular aneurysm of the transverse thoracic aorta. Int J Cardiol 33:330, 1991

189. Taams MA, Gussenhoven WJ, Schippers LA et al: The value of transesophageal echocardiography for diagnosis of thoracic aorta pathology. Eur Heart J 9:1308, 1988

190. Tobler HG, Edwards JE: Frequency and location of atherosclerotic plaques in the ascending aorta. J Thorac Cardiovasc Surg 96:304, 1988

191. Fazio GP, Redbers RF, Winslow T et al: Transesophageal echocardiographically detected atherosclerotic aortic plaque is a marker for coronary artery disease. J Am Coll Cardiol 21:144, 1993

192. Karalis DG, Chandrasekaran K, Victor MF et al: Recognition and emboli potential of intraaortic atherosclerotic debris. J Am Coll Cardiol 17:73, 1991

193. Katz ES, Tunick PA, Rusinek H et al: Protruding aortic atheromas predict stroke in elderly patients undergoing cardiopulmonary bypass: experience with intraoperative trans-

esophageal echocardiography. J Am Coll Cardiol 20:70, 1992

194. Horowitz DR, Tuhrim S, Budd J et al: Aortic plaque in patients with brain ischemia: diagnosis by transesophageal echocardiography. Neurology 42:1602, 1992

195. Stanson AW, Kazmier FJ, Hoollier LH et al: Penetrating atherosclerotic ulcers of the thoracic aorta: natural history and clinicopathologic correlations. Ann Vasc Surg 1:15, 1986

196. Porembka DT, Johnson DJ, Fowl RJ et al: Descending thoracic aortic thrombus as a cause of multiple system organ failure: diagnosis by transesophageal echocardiography. Crit Care Med 20:1184, 1992

197. Tunick PA, Culliford AT, Lamparello PJ et al: Atheromatosis of the aortic arch as an occult source of multiple systemic emboli. Ann Intern Med 114:391, 1991

198. Coy KM, Maurer G, Goodman D et al: Transesophageal echocardiographic detection of aortic atheromatosis may provide clues to occult renal dysfunction in the elderly. Am Heart J 123:1684, 1992

199. Rubin BG, Barzilai B, Allen BT et al: Detection of the source of arterial emboli by transesophageal echocardiography: a case report. J Vasc Surg 15:573, 1992

200. Yvorchuk KJ, Chan K-L: Application of transthoracic and transesophageal echocardiography in the diagnosis and management of infective endocarditis. J Am Soc Echocardiogr 14:294, 1994

201. Khanderia BK: Suspected bacterial endocarditis: to TEE or not to TEE. J Am Coll Cardiol 21:222, 1993

202. Dillon LC, Feigenbaum H, Konecke LL et al: Echocardiographic manifestations of valvular vegetations. Am Heart J 86:698, 1973

203. Sheikh MU, Covarrubias EA, Ali N et al: M-mode echocardiographic observations during and after healing of active bacterial endocarditis limited to the mitral valve. Am Heart J 101:37, 1981

204. Gilbert BW, Haney RS, Crawford F et al: Two-dimensional echocardiographic assessment of vegetative endocarditis. Circulation 55:346, 1977

205. Daniel WG, Schroder E, Nonnast-Daniel B et al: Conventional and transesophageal echocardiography in the diagnosis of infec-

tive endocarditis. Eur Heart J, suppl J. 8:287, 1987

206. Erbel R, Rohmann S, Drexler M et al: Improved diagnostic value of echocardiography in patients with infective endocarditis by transesophageal approach. A prospective study. Eur Heart J 9:43, 1988

207. Klodas E, Edwards WD, Khanderia BK: Use of transesophageal echocardiography for improving detection of valvular vegetations in subacute bacterial endocarditis. J Am Soc Echocardiogr 2:386, 1989

208. Mugge A, Daniel WG, Frank G et al: Echocardiography in infective endocarditis: reassessment of prognostic implications of vegetation size determined by the transthoracic and transesophageal approach. J Am Coll Cardiol 14:631, 1989

209. Bardy G, Talano J, Reisberg B et al: Sensitivity and specificity of echocardiography in a high-risk population of patients for infective endocarditis: significance of vegetation size. J Cardiovasc Ultrasonogr 2:23, 1983

210. Come P, Isaacs R, Riley M: Diagnostic accuracy of M-mode echocardiography in active infective endocarditis and prognostic implications of ultrasound detectable vegetations. Am Heart J 103:839, 1982

211. Hickey A, Wolfers J, Wilcken D: Reliability and clinical relevance of detection of vegetations by echocardiography. Br Heart J 46: 624, 1981

212. Jaffe W, Morgan D, Pearlman A et al: Infective endocarditis, 1983–1988: echocardiographic findings and factors influencing morbidity and mortality. J Am Coll Cardiol 15: 1227, 1990

213. Markiewicz W, Peled B, Alroy G et al: Echocardiography in infective endocarditis: lack of specificity in patients with valvular pathology. Eur J Cardiol 10:247, 1979

214. Martin R, Meltzer R, Chia B et al: Clinical utility of two-dimensional echocardiography in infective endocarditis. Am J Cardiol 46: 379, 1980

215. Mintz G, Kotler M, Segal B et al: Comparison of two-dimensional and M-mode echocardiography in the evaluation of patients with infective endocarditis. Am J Cardiol 43:738, 1979

216. Scanlan JG, Seward JB, Tajik AJ: Valve ring abscess in infective endocarditis: visualiza-

tion with wide angle two dimensional echocardiography. Am J Cardiol 49:1794, 1982

217. Daniel WG, Schroeder E, Mugge A et al: Transesophageal echocardiography in infective endocarditis. Am J Card Imaging 2:78, 1988

218. Taams MA, Gussenhoven EJ, Bos E et al: Enhanced morphological diagnosis in endocarditis by transesophageal echocardiography. Br Heart J 63:109, 1990

219. Pedersen WR, Walker M, Olson JD et al: Value of transesophageal echocardiography as an adjunct to transthoracic echocardiography in evaluation of native and prosthetic valve endocarditis. Chest 100:351, 1991

220. Birmingham GD, Rahko PS, Ballantyne F III: Improved detection of infective endocarditis with transesophageal echocardiograpy. Am Heart J 123:774, 1992

221. Shapiro SM, Young E, Ginzton LE et al: Pulmonic valve endocarditis as an underdiagnosed disease: role of transesophageal echocardiography. J Am Soc Echocardiogr 5:48, 1992

222. Winslow T, Foster E, Schiller NB: Pulmonary valve endocarditis: improved diagnosis with biplane transesophageal echocardiography. J Am Soc Echocardiogr 5:206, 1992

223. Shively BK, Gurule FT, Roldan CA et al: Diagnostic value of transesophageal compared with transthoracic echocardiography in infective endocarditis. J Am Coll Cardiol 18: 391, 1991

224. San Roman JA, Vilacosta I, Zamorano JL: Transesophageal echocardiography in right-sided endocarditis. J Am Coll Cardiol 21: 1226, 1993

225. Shapiro SM, Young E, de Guzman S et al: Transesophageal echocardiography in diagnosis of infective endocarditis. Chest 105: 377, 1994

226. Sochowski RA, Chan K-L: Implication of negative results on a monoplane transesophageal echocardiographic study in patients with suspected infective endocarditis. J Am Coll Cardiol 21:216, 1993

227. Rohmann S, Erbel R, Gorge G et al: Clinical relevance of vegetations localization by transesophageal echocardiography in infective endocarditis. Eur Heart J 13:446, 1992

228. Rohmann S, Erbel R, Darius H et al: Spontaneous echo contrast imaging in infective en-

docarditis: a predictor of complications? Intl J Card Imaging 8:197, 1992

229. Daniel WG, Mugge A, Martin RP et al: Improvement in the diagnosis of abscesses associated with endocarditis by transesophageal echocardiography. N Engl J Med 324: 795, 1991

230. Karalis DG, Bansal RC, Hauck AJ et al: Transesophageal echocardiographic recognition of subaortic complications in aortic valve endocarditis. Clinical and surgical implications. Circulation 86:353, 1992

231. Bansal RC, Graham BM, Jutzy KR et al: Left ventricular outflow tract to left atrial communication secondary to rupture of mitral-aortic intervalvular fibrosa in infective endocarditis: diagnosis by transesophageal echocardiography and color flow imaging. J Am Coll Cardiol 15:499, 1990

232. Herrera CJ, Mehlman DJ, Harte RS et al: Comparison of transesophageal and transthoracic echocardiography for diagnosis of right-sided cardiac lesions. Am J Cardiol 21: 216, 1993

233. Lee RJ, Bartzokis T, Yeoh TK et al: Enhanced detection of intracardiac sources of cerebral emboli by transesophageal echocardiography. Stroke 22:734, 1991

234. Pearson AC, Labovitz AJ, Tatineni S et al: Superiority of transesophageal echocardiography in detecting cardiac source of embolism in patients with cerebral ischemia of uncertain etiology. J Am Coll Cardiol 17:66, 1991

235. Pop G, Sutherland GR, Koudstaal PJ et al: Transesophageal echocardiography in the detection of intracardiac embolic sources in patients with transient ischemic attacks. Stroke 21:560, 1990

236. Albers GW, Comess KA, DeRook FA et al: Transesophageal echocardiographic findings in stroke subtypes. Stroke 25:23, 1994

237. Aschenberg W, Schluter M, Kremer P et al: Transesophageal two-dimensional echocardiography for the detection of left atrial appendage thrombus. J Am Coll Cardiol 7:163, 1986

238. Kronzon I, Tunick PA, Colossman E et al: Transesophageal echocardiography to detect atrial clots in candidates for percutaneous transseptal mitral balloon valvuloplasty. J Am Coll Cardiol 16:1320, 1990

239. Hwang J, Kuan P, Lin S et al: Reappraisal by transesophageal echocardiography of the significance of left atrial thrombi in the prediction of systemic arterial embolization in rheumatic mitral valve disease. Am J Cardiol 70:769, 1992

240. Vigna C, de Rito V, Criconia GM et al: Left atrial thrombus and spontaneous echo-contrast in non anticoagulated mitral stenosis. Chest 103:348, 1993

241. Cabanes L, Mas JL, Cohen A et al: Atrial septal aneurysm and patent foramen ovale as risk factors for cryptogenic stroke in patients less than 55 years of age. Stroke 24:1865, 1993

242. Mera F, Patt J, Israel W, Dubin JD: Atrial septal aneurysm simulating a left atrial mass diagnosed by transesophageal echocardiography. Am Heart J 126:1224, 1993

243. Manning WJ, Silverman DI, Gordon SPF et al: Cardioversion from atrial fibrillation without prolonged anticoagulation with use of the transesophageal echocardiography to exclude the presence of atrial thrombi. N Engl J Med 328:750, 1993

244. Grimm RA, Stewart WJ, Maloney JD et al: Impact of electrical cardioversion for atrial fibrillation on left atrial appendage function and spontaneous echo contrast: characterization by simultaneous transesophageal echocardiography. J Am Coll Cardiol 22:1359, 1993

245. Salka S, Saeian K, Sagar KB et al: Cerebral thromboembolization after cardioversion of atrial fibrillation in patients without transesophageal echocardiographic findings of left atrial thrombus. Am Heart J 126:722, 1993

246. Hata JS, Ayres RW, Biller J et al: Impact of transesophageal echocardiography on the anticoagulation management of patients admitted with focal cerebral ischemia. Am J Cardiol 72:707, 1993

247. Cohen GI, Kein AL, Chan KL et al: Transesophageal echocardiographic diagnosis of right-sided cardiac masses in patients with central lines. Am J Cardiol 70:925, 1992

248. Starr SK, Pugh DM, O'Brien-Ladner A et al: Right atrial mass biopsy guided by transesophageal echocardiography. Chest 104: 969, 1993

249. Faletra F, Ravini M, Moreo A et al: Transesophageal echocardiography in the evalua-

tion of mediastinal masses. J Am Soc Echocardiogr 5:178, 1992

250. Ren WD, Nicolosi GL, Lestuzzi C et al: Role of transesophageal echocardiography in the evaluation of pulmonary venous obstruction by paracardic neoplastic masses. Am J Cardiol 70:1362, 1992

251. Patten BM: The closure of the foramen ovale. Am J Anat 48:19, 1931

252. Hagen PT, Scholtz DG, Edwards WD: Incidence and size of a patent foramen ovale during the first 10 decades of life: an autopsy study of 965 normal hearts. Mayo Clin Proc 59:17, 1984

253. Albers GW, Comess KA, DeRook FA et al: Transesophageal echocardiographic findings in stroke subtypes. Stroke 25:23, 1994

254. Tei C, Tanaka H, Kashima T et al: Real-time cross-sectional echocardiographic evaluation of the interatrial septum by right atrium-interatrial septum-left atrium direction of ultrasound beam. Circulation 60:539, 1979

255. Schwinger ME, Gindea AJ, Freedberg RS et al: The anatomy of the interatrial septum: a transesophageal echocardiographic study. Am Heart J 119:1401, 1990

256. Stollberger C, Schneider B, Abzieher F et al: Diagnosis of patent foramen ovale by transesophageal contrast echocardiography. Am J Cardiol 71:604, 1993

257. Suzuki Y, Kambara H, Kadota K et al: Detection and evaluation of tricuspid regurgitation using a real-time, two dimensional, color-coded, Doppler flow imaging system: comparison with contrast two-dimensional echocardiography and right ventriculography. Am J Cardiol 57:811, 1986

258. Kronik G, Mosslacher H: Positive contrast echocardiography in patients with patent foramen ovale and normal right heart hemodynamics. Am J Cardiol 49:1806, 1982

259. Lynch JJ, Schuchard GH, Gross CM, Wann LS: Prevalence of right-to-left atrial shunting in a healthy population: detection by Valsalva maneuver contrast echocardiography. Am J Cardiol 53:1478, 1984

260. Dubourg O, Bourdarias JP, Farcot JC et al: Contrast echocardiographic visualization of cough-induced right to left shunt through a patent foramen ovale. J Am Coll Cardiol 4:587, 1984

261. Strunk BL, Cheitlin MD, Stulbarg MS, Schiller NB: Right-to-left interatrial shunting through a patent foramen ovale despite normal intracardiac pressures. Am J Cardiol 60:413, 1987

262. Biller J, Johnson MR, Adams HP Jr et al: Further observations on cerebral or retinal ischemia in patients with right-left intracardiac shunts. Arch Neurol 44:740, 1987

263. Lechat PH, Mas JL, Lascault G et al: Prevalence of patent foramen ovale in patients with stroke. N Engl J Med 318:1148, 1988

264. Hausmann D, Mugge A, Becht I et al: Diagnosis of patent foramen ovale by transesophageal echocardiography and association with cerebral and peripheral embolic events. Am J Cardiol 70:668, 1992

265. Guggiari M, Lechat P, Garen-Colonne C et al: Early detection of patent foramen ovale by two-dimensional contrast echocardiography for prevention of paradoxical air embolism during sitting position. Anesth Analg 67:192, 1988

266. Chen WJ, Kuan P, Lien WP et al: Detection of patent foramen ovale by contrast transesophageal echocardiography. Chest 101:1515, 1992

267. Black S, Muzzi DA, Nishimura RA et al: Preoperative and intraoperative echocardiography to detect right-to-left shunt in patients undergoing neurosurgical procedures in the sitting position. Anesthesiology 72:436, 1990

268. Konstadt SN, Louie EK, Black S et al: Intraoperative detection of patent foramen ovale by transesophageal echocardiography. Anesthesiology 74:212, 1991

269. Porembka D, Valente J, Anderson G et al: Postoperative detection of patent foramen ovale by transesophageal echocardiography. Crit Care Med 21:S269, 1993

270. Siostrzonek P, Zangeneh M, Gossinger H et al: Comparison of transesophageal for detection of a patent foramen ovale. Am J Cardiol 68:1247, 1991

271. Louie EK, Konstadt SN, Rao TL et al: Transesophageal echocardiographic diagnosis of right to left shunting across the foramen ovale in adults with prior stroke. J Am Coll Cardiol 21:1231, 1993

272. Van Camp G, Schulze D, Cosyns B et al: Relation between patent foramen ovale and unexplained stroke. Am J Cardiol 71:596, 1993

273. Dewan NA, Gayasaddin M, Angelillo VA et

al: Persistent hypoxemia due to patent foramen ovale in a patient with adult respiratory
distress syndrome. Chest 89:611, 1986

274. DeSio JM, Goodnough SR, Hajduczok ZD:
The effect of positive end-expiratory presure
on right-to-left shunting at the atrial level as
documented by transesophageal echocardiography. Anesthesiology 77:1033, 1992

275. Mehta RH, Helmcke F, Nanda NC et al: Uses
and limitations of transthoracic echocardiography in the assessment of atrial septal defect
in the adult. Am J Cardiol 67:288, 1991

276. Mehta RH, Helmcke F, Nanda NC et al:
Transesophageal Doppler color flow map-
ping assessment of atrial septal defect. J Am
Coll Cardiol 16:1010, 1990

277. Hausmann D, Daniel WG, Mugge A et al:
Value of transesophageal for detection of dif-
ferent types of atrial septal defects in adults.
J Am Soc Echocardiogr 5:481, 1992

278. Morimoto K, Matsuzaki M, Tohma Y et al:
Diagnosis and quantitative evaluation of se-
cundum-type atrial septal defect by transesophageal Doppler echocardiography. Am
J Cardiol 66:85, 1990

279. Kronzon I, Tunick PA, Freedberg RS et al:
Transesophageal echocardiography is superior to transthoracic echocardiography in the
diagnosis of sinus venosus atrial septal defect. J Am Coll Cardiol 17:537, 1991

280. Shub C, Tajik AJ, Seward JB: Clinically "silent" atrial septal defect: diagnosis by two-
dimensional and Doppler echocardiography.
Am Heart J 110:665, 1985

281. Hiraishi S, Agata Y, Saito K et al: Interatrial
shunt flow profiles in newborn infants: a col-
our flow and pulsed Doppler echocardiographic study. Br Heart J 65:41, 1991

282. Minagoe S, Tei C, Kisanuki A et al: Noninvasive pulsed Doppler echocardiographic detection of the direction of shunt flow in patients with atrial septal defect: usefulness of
the right parasternal approach. Circulation
71:745, 1985

283. Konstantinides S, Kasper W, Geibel A et al:
Detection of left-to-right shunt in atrial septal
defect by negative contrast echocardiography: a comparison of transthoracic and transesophageal approach. Am Heart J 126:909,
1993

284. Schmidt KG, Cassidy SC, Silverman NH,
Stanger P: Doubly committed subatrial ven-

tricular septal defects: echocardiographic
featues and surgical implications. J Am Coll
Cardiol 12:1538, 1988

285. Sommer RJ, Golinko RJ, Ritter SB: Intracardiac shunting in children with ventricular
septal defect: evaluation with Doppler color
flow mapping. J Am Coll Cardiol 16:1437,
1990

286. Ludomirsky A, Tani L, Murphy DJ, Huhta
JC: Usefulness of color-flow doppler in diagnosing and in differentiating supracristal ventricular septal defect from right ventricular
outflow tract obstruction. Am J Cardiol 67:
194, 1991

287. Zotz RJ, Dohmen G, Genth S et al: Transthoracic and transesophageal echocardiography
in diagnosing ventricular septal rupture: Importance of right infarction. Coronary Artery
Dis 4:911, 1993

288. Porembka DT, Johnson DJ II, Hoit BD et al:
Penetrating cardiac trauma: a perioperative
role for transesophageal echocardiography.
Anesth Analg 77:1275, 1993

289. Jacoby SS, Gillam LD, Pandian NG, Weyman
AE: Two-dimensional and Doppler echocardiography in the evaluation of penetrating
cardiac injury. Chest 88:922, 1985

290. McIntyre RC, Moore EE, Read RR et al:
Transesophageal echocardiography in the
evaluation of a transmediastinal gunshot
wound: case report. J Trauma 36:125, 1994

291. LiMandri G, Goresnstein LA, Starr JP et al:
Use of transesophageal echocardiography in
the detection and consequences of an intracardiac bullet. Am J Emerg Med 12:105, 1994

292. Catoire P, Bonnet F, Delaunay L et al: Traumatic laceration of the ascending aorta detected by transesophageal echocardiography. Ann Emerg Med 23:356, 1994

293. Braithwaite CEM, Weiss RL, Baldino WA et
al: Multichamber gunshot wounds of the
heart. Chest 101:287, 1992

294. Skoularigis J, Essop MR, Sareli P: Usefulness
of transesophageal echocardiography in the
early diagnosis of penetrating stab wounds
to the heart. Am J Cardiol 73:407, 1994

295. Fowler NO: Pulmonary embolism. p. 283. In:
Diagnosis of Heart Disease. Springer-Verlag,
New York, 1991

296. Anderson FA Jr, Wheeler HB, Goldberg RJ
et al: A population-based perspective of the
hospital incidence and case-fatality rates of

deep vein thrombosis and pulmonary embolism. The Worcester DVT study. Arch Intern Med 151:933, 1991

297. Visner MC, Arentzen CE, O'Connor MJ et al: Alterations in left ventricular three-dimensional dynamic geometry and systolic function during acute right ventricular hypertension in the conscious dog. Circulation 67:353, 1983

298. Elliott CG: Pulmonary physiology during pulmonary embolism. Chest 101:163S, 1992

299. Come PC: Echocardiographic evaluation of pulmonary embolism and its response to therapeutic interventions. Chest 101:151S, 1992

300. Belenkie L, Dani R, Smith ER et al: Ventricular interaction during experimental acute pulmonary embolism. Circulation 78:761, 1988

301. Fitzpatrick JM, Grant JB: Effects of pulmonary vascular obstruction on right ventricular afterload. Am Rev Respir Dis 141:944, 1990

302. Dehring DJ, Arens JF: Pulmonary thromboembolism: disease recognition and patient management. Anesthesiology 73:146, 1990

303. Jardin F, Dubourg O, Gueret P et al: Quantitative two-dimensional echocardiography in massive pulmonary embolism: emphasis on ventricular interdependence and leftward septal displacement. J Am Coll Cardiol 10:1201, 1987

304. Kasper W, Meinertz T, Henkel B et al: Echocardiographic findings in patients with proved pulmonary embolism. Am Heart J 112:1284, 1986

305. Currie PJ, Seward JB, Chan KL et al: Continuous wave Doppler determination of right ventricular pressure: a simultaneous Doppler-catheterization study in 127 patients. J Am Coll Cardiol 6:750, 1985

306. Gardin JM, Burn CS, Childs WJ, Henry WL: Evaluation of blood flow velocity in the ascending aorta and main pulmonary artery of normal subjects by Doppler echocardiography. Am Heart J 107:310, 1984

307. Saada M, Catoirie P, Deleuze P et al: Diagnostic d'embolie pulmonaire grave par echocardiographie transoesophagienne. Ann Fr Anesth Reanim 9:547, 1990

308. Hunter JJ, Johnson KR, Karagianes TG et al: Detection of massive pulmonary embolus-in-transit by transesophageal echocardiography. Chest 100:1210, 1991

309. Langeron O, Goarin JP, Pansard JL et al: Massive intraoperative pulmonary embolism: diagnosis with transesophageal two-dimension echocardiography. Anesth Analg 74:148, 1992

310. Podolsky L, Manginas A, Jacobs LE et al: Superior vena caval thrombosis detected by transesophageal echocardiography. J Am Soc Echocardiogr 4:189, 1991

311. Heng Y, Shyu KG, Kuan P: Expanded indication: diagnosis of pulmonary embolism by transesophageal echocardiography. Int J Cardiol 39:91, 1993

312. Kim NH, Roldan CA, Shively BK: Pulmonary vein thrombosis. Chest 104:624, 1993

313. Pell ACH, Hughes D, Keating J et al: Brief report: fulminating fat embolism syndrome caused by paradoxical embolism through a patent foramen ovale. N Engl J Med 329:926, 1993

314. Porembka DT, Lopez A, Alspaugh JP et al: Pulmonary embolism: as diagnosed by transesophageal echocardiography. J Intensive Care Med (submitted)

315. Clements FM, de Bruin NP: Perioperative evaluation of regional wall motion by transesophageal two-dimensional echocardiography. Anesth Analg 66:249, 1987

15

Pain Management

Erin A. Sullivan
Sture G. I. Blomberg

Anesthesiologists are often consulted to manage acute surgical pain. The effective management of postoperative pain is particularly important for the cardiac surgical patient. Acute pain produces major alterations in pulmonary, cardiovascular, coagulation, gastrointestinal, and psychological function post-median sternotomy. These factors contribute to patient morbidity and mortality.

Pain sensation and its ineffective management lead to propagation of the stress response and release of stress hormones. Studies of normal volunteers infused with glucagon, cortisol, and epinephrine demonstrate an adverse synergistic effect of these three hormones on minute ventilation and the rate-pressure product.[1] It is most evident in patients during the postoperative period when increases in heart rate and minute ventilation are the normal occurrence. This increase in heart rate and minute ventilation may be harmful to patients with marginal cardiac and pulmonary function in terms of increased length of hospitalization, cost, and morbidity and mortality.

Analgesia for poststernotomy pain and the attenuation of the neurohumeral stress response may be achieved by several methods.

This chapter discusses the mechanisms of pain experienced by the cardiac surgical patient, the consequences of ineffective pain management, and alternatives for the management of postoperative sternotomy pain.

MECHANISMS OF PAIN

Poststernotomy pain syndromes are classified according to their site of origin: visceral, musculoskeletal, neurogenic, or dermal. The pain usually begins acutely and, if inadequately treated, may lead to chronic pain syndromes. Early intervention and adequate acute pain management may prevent the development of these chronic pain syndromes and enhance overall patient satisfaction and outcome.

Visceral Pain

The heart is innervated by efferent preganglionic and postganglionic sympathetic fibers, afferent sympathetic fibers, and efferent preganglionic parasympathetic fibers. Visceral pain from the heart is transmitted to the central nervous system (CNS) via the middle and inferior cervical sympathetic cardiac nerves, the thoracic cardiac sympathetic nerves (arising from the T2–T5 sympathetic ganglia), and the cardiac branches of the vagus nerve.

Caelius Aurelianus, a fifth century Roman physician, was the first to describe cardiac pain: *passio cardiaca propria*. Generally, visceral cardiac pain is described as crushing substernal or epigastric tightness that radiates to the left arm, shoulder, or neck. The etiology of the majority of cardiogenic pain is ischemia. Ischemia is caused by pathophysiologic conditions that result in coronary artery hypoperfusion (i.e., coronary artery atherosclerosis, thrombus, and coronary artery vasospasm). Endocarditis and myocarditis may also simulate the pain of cardiac ischemia.

Cardiac causalgia was described by Burch and Giles.[2] It is manifested by a constant burning and chronic substernal chest discomfort with hyperesthesia of the sternum and chest wall. Cardiac causalgia usually follows the onset of angina pectoris. Other considerations in the differential diagnosis of cardiogenic visceral pain are pains that originate from the esophagus, lungs, and aorta (aortic dissection).

Musculoskeletal Pain

Sternotomy and sternal spread during cardiac surgery commonly cause thoracic musculoskeletal pain postoperatively. The vertebrae, thorax, and surrounding soft tissue are implicated. If not adequately treated, this pain may seriously impair the patient's ability to generate an effective cough, leading to atelectasis, accumulation of secretions, and other pulmonary sequelae discussed later in this chapter.

Costochondritis

Costochondritis is usually unilateral and involves the second and third costal cartilages. It may arise from trauma to the sternum and ribs, or separation of the ribs, cartilage, and sternum, as occurs with median sternotomy.

Neurogenic Pain

Mechanical trauma resulting from sternotomy may produce a neuritis. The character of the pain is burning, lancinating, worse at night, and exacerbated by stretching the affected nerve. Fasciculations or muscle spasm, hyperesthesias, paresthesias, and dysesthesias may also be present.

Scar tissue or nerve entrapment may produce pain mediated by cutaneous receptors. The character is dull and aching, with movement-associated sharp, shooting pain exacerbated by direct pressure. This pain may radiate to areas proximal or distal to the actual scar tissue.

Prevention of Chronic Pain Syndromes

The quality of a patient's acute pain management may be an important factor for the prevention or subsequent development of chronic pain syndromes.[3,4] Studies demonstrate that patients who receive inadequate postoperative analgesia tend to have persistent pain that lasts a longer period of time than a similar group of patients who receive adequate analgesia.[5] Additionally, there appears to be a "critical time interval"[6] for providing effective acute pain management in order to reduce the incidence of delayed chronic pain sequelae.

Evidence exists to suggest that prophylactic analgesia administered preoperatively has a tendency to reduce the subsequent analgesic requirement of the patient during the postoperative period. Wang et al.[7] demonstrated that a single dose of subarachnoid morphine administered preoperatively to patients undergoing major abdominal and thoracic procedures seems to reduce the subsequent analgesic requirement during the entire hospitalization. Perhaps the attenuation of the release of algesic substances (e.g., serotonin, bradykinin, histamine, potassium, substance P, prostaglandins, and leukotrienes) by providing prophylactic analgesia preoperatively may lead to a more favorable patient outcome.[8–10]

CONSEQUENCES OF INADEQUATE POSTOPERATIVE ANALGESIA

Anesthesia and surgery alter a patient's lung volume and ventilatory pattern. Pain exacerbates these changes in pulmonary function and may contribute to a prolonged requirement for mechanical ventiltory support and an extended intensive care unit (ICU) stay.

Sternotomy incisions and intrathoracic manipulations are documented to induce a transient 50 to 70 percent reduction in the patient's vital capacity (VC)[11,12] and functional residual capacity (FRC) within 1 to 2 days after surgery. A return to baseline function occurs after 1 to 2 weeks. Residual volume increases by 13 percent, expiratory reserve volume decreases by 60 percent, and pulmonary compliance decreases by 33 percent. Tidal volume decreases by 20 percent within 24 hours after surgery and does not return to baseline values for 2 weeks. Atelectasis may result from compression of the lung,[13] pleural effusion,[14] and phrenic nerve dysfunction.[15]

The incidence of pulmonary complications increases when the postoperative FRC decreases to 60 percent of the preoperative baseline and becomes more severe as FRC decreases to 40 percent of the preoperative baseline.[16] The consequences of inadequate pulmonary function poststernotomy may be serious. An acute reduction in a patient's FRC may result in arterial hypoxemia via inadequate perfusion ($\dot{V}/\dot{Q}$ mismatch) or atelectasis (intrapulmonary shunting). Furthermore, a decrease in FRC may diminish lung compliance, leading to an increase in the work of breathing. By increasing the work of breathing, oxygen consumption increases by at least 20 percent,[17] leading to an increase in myocardial work and production of lactic acidosis.[18] Hence, acute pain may result in a reduction of tissue oxygen supply.

Finally, a VC of at least 15 ml · kg^{-1} is required to ensure effective deep breathing and coughing.[19] Inadequate deep breathing and coughing to clear pulmonary secretions and prevent atelectasis, hypoxemia, and hypercarbia is not an uncommon occurrence in the postoperative cardiac surgical patient. This is perhaps the quintessential reason that adequate early postoperative analgesia might benefit median sternotomy patients.[20]

Acute pain increases the release of catecholamines, sympathetic activity, and oxygen consumption, hence the potential disequilibrium in myocardial oxygen supply and demand. Increased myocardial oxygen demand (e.g., tachycardia, hypoxemia) increases the risk of myocardial ischemia.

Immobilization of an injured site (e.g., the legs following venous graft harvesting during coronary artery bypass graft [CABG] surgery) secondary to inadequate analgesia may cause venous pooling. Increased venous pooling in conjunction with increased platelet aggregation places the patient at risk of deep venous thrombosis and pulmonary embolism. Gastrointestinal sequelae of pain, such as gastric stasis and intestinal ileus, further complicate treatment and recovery.

The neurohumoral stress response to surgery is similar to that occurring in trauma patients.[21] In addition to the response evoked by kinins, prostaglandins, and leukotrienes,[22] there is an increase in the release of catecholamines and secretion of adrenocorticotropic hormone (ACTH) and glucagon.[23,24] Hyperglycemia, insulin resistance, gluconeogenesis, lipolysis, and protein catabolism are the end result.[25] There is supporting evidence in the literature to suggest that analgesia and sympathetic blockade may ameliorate the stress response to surgery and anesthesia.[26-30]

The quality of a patient's acute pain management may be an important factor for the prevention of subsequent development of chronic pain syndromes.[3,4] There is also evidence to support the role of inadequate acute pain management in the manifestation of "ICU psychosis."[31] Untreated pain combined with anxiety, fear, hostility, sleep deprivation, and loss of control may delay patient recovery and increase morbidity, mortality, and overall hospital cost.

POSTOPERATIVE PAIN MANAGEMENT

Goals

The primary goal of postoperative pain management is the early restoration of tissue, organ, and patient function. Surgical manipulation and tissue trauma interfere with nutrient delivery via vasoconstriction. Vasoconstriction is a consequence of pain or direct vascular injury and may result in cellular dysfunction. Sympathetic blockade can decrease pain-mediated increases in vascular resistance, thus allowing an increase in blood flow both to the skin and coronary artery grafts.[32] Regional anesthesia for pain management permits improved mobilization of the injured part.[33-36] Early mobilization helps preserve normal gastrointestinal, myofascial, and pulmonary function. Chronic myofascial pain syndromes that result from injury to the musculoskeletal structures may be minimized with early ambulation and mobilization of injured regions.

Another goal of postoperative pain management is the prevention of the adverse sequelae of pain and tissue injury. When used in high-risk patients, epidural analgesia decreases postoperative morbid events.[36-38]

How Much Analgesia Is Enough?

"In no other area of medicine has such an extravagant concern for side effects so drastically limited treatment."[39] These words epitomize the ongoing problem of inadequate postoperative analgesia.[40,41]

Weiss et al.[42] attempted to explain the basis for inadequate postoperative analgesia. Interestingly, this investigation found that 54 percent of the physicians and 74 percent of the nurses believed that their patients received adequate analgesia. However, when patients were questioned about the quality of their pain management, 41 percent complained of persistent moderate to severe pain. The explanation of these results was based on a lack of confidence in using narcotic analgesics secondary to inadequate knowledge of pharmacokinetics/pharmacodynamics; misconceptions regarding drug combinations, potential for addiction, and respiratory depression; and misconceptions regarding fictitious pain and ignorance of the variability of analgesic effect among patients. Some general misconceptions of opioid use for acute pain management are described by Mather and Phillips:[43]

1. Doses should be as small and infrequent as possible to avoid the development of addiction.
2. Doses larger than the standard do not increase pain relief and cause heavy sedation and respiratory depression.
3. Nursing and/or medical staff know when and how much pain relief each patient needs.
4. Patients requesting more pain relief than the standard are psychologically abnormal or are becoming addicted.
5. If nonopioid drugs are ordered, these should be tried in preference to opioids.
6. What is needed is a powerful nonaddictive pain reliever.

In addition to these misconceptions, one might add the following: "Immobilized, paralyzed, intubated, and mechanically ventilated patients do not hurt; analgesia renders the critically ill patient hemodynamically unstable."[44]

If one examines the actual incidence of reported complications from opioid analgesia, we find that iatrogenic dependence is rare (less than 0.1 percent) in hospitalized patients experiencing acute pain.[45] Respiratory depression secondary to opioid administration in postoperative patients has an incidence of 0.9 percent.[46] Opioids may even be used in critically ill patients to provide effective analgesia without respiratory or cardiovascular depression.[47]

Modalities of Acute Postoperative Pain Management

SYSTEMIC ANALGESIA: OPIOIDS

Opioid analgesia remains the standard to which all other modalities for treatment of poststernotomy pain are compared.[36,48–51] In order for analgesia to be effective, one should consider the route of administration, rather than the particular analgesic agent. The intramuscular route may not provide adequate analgesia in patients with poor tissue perfusion. This is often the situation in the immediate postoperative patient who arrives at the ICU slightly hypothermic and shivering. Intramuscular analgesics in this instance are erratically and unpredictably absorbed due to shunting of blood flow to the blood-rich organs (i.e., heart, brain, lung, liver, and kidneys).

The intravenous route provides immediate access to the central circulation and allows for a more rapid and predictable onset of analgesia. Intermittent intravenous doses of opioids are administered until the desired clinical effect is achieved.[52] The choice of intravenous opioid is based on the desired effect. The rapid uptake, distribution, and elimination of the synthetic opioids such as alfentanil, fentanyl, and sufentanil may be advantageous for rapidly achieving an adequate level of analgesia. However, if a longer duration of analgesia is desired, opioids such as morphine or methadone are more appropriate. The disadvantage of morphine and methadone is their delayed onset of action when compared with the more lipid-soluble agents.

Administration of the short-acting, lipid-soluble opioids by continuous intravenous infusion makes their use more practical.[53] Infusion rates are adjusted to achieve the desired clinical effect or to produce the desired plasma drug concentration. Steady-state pharmacokinetic effects are rapidly achieved with continuous intravenous infusions; superior analgesia (compared with the intermittent bolus technique) is the end result. This technique further enhances the patient-controlled analgesia method of postoperative pain management.

The major disadvantage of systemic opioid analgesics delivered by the traditional routes is that the doses required to provide effective pain relief often produce unwanted side effects: nausea, vomiting, somnolence, ileus, and respiratory depression.[54] Most studies have evaluated systemic opioids in the context of comparisons with other modes of treatment[48–50,55,56]; thus, few studies have documented the value of systemic opioids alone.

PATIENT-CONTROLLED ANALGESIA

Sechzer[56] combined the effectiveness of small intravenous bolus aliquots of opioids in achieving superior analgesia[57] with the concept of patient control, and is credited with developing patient-controlled intravenous analgesia (PCA).[58] This modality of analgesia allows the patient to self-administer predetermined aliquots of an intravenous opioid.

In theory, the patient is able to maintain steady-state therapeutic plasma levels of opioid, assuming that the appropriate drug selection, dosage, and lockout intervals are provided. This may result in decreased magnitude of pain or pain intervals, decreased anxiety, decreased analgesic requirement (total dose over time), and decreased undesired side effects (i.e., respiratory depression, oversedation).

If inappropriate doses of opioid are prescribed or lockout intervals are too lengthy, subtherapeutic levels may result and produce inadequate analgesia. Likewise, toxic drug levels may result when the less lipophilic drugs are selected in an attempt to increase the duration of the clinical effect of each aliquot. As previously stated, the onset of action of the less liphophilic opioids is longer. Since the lag time between peak levels in the plasma and CNS may be significant, and if

Table 15-1. Summary of Problems That Can Occur During Patient-Controlled Analgesia Therapy

Operator errors
  Misprogramming PCA device
  Failure to clamp or unclamp tubing
  Improperly loading syringe or cartridge
  Inability to respond to safety alarms
  Misplacing PCA pump key
Patient errors
  Failure to understand PCA therapy
  Misunderstanding PCA pump device
  Intentional analgesic abuse
Mechanical problems
  Failure to deliver on demand
  Cracked drug vials or syringes
  Defective one-way valve at Y connector
  Faulty alarm system
  Malfunctions (e.g., lock)

Abbreviation: PCA, patient-controlled analgesia.
(From White,[131] with permission.)

short lockout intervals are selected, the patient may inject a second or third dose before the first dose has achieved its maximal effect.[59,60] Recently, respiratory depression associated with PCA-controlled opioids has been reported.[61] Other problems reported during PCA therapy are depicted in Table 15-1.

Four modes of PCA are commonly described: bolus demand, bolus demand with constant infusion, infusion demand, and bolus demand with variable infusion.[62] Bolus demand and bolus demand with constant infusion pumps are currently available commercially. Although the bolus demand with constant infusion mode of PCA is lauded with excellent results,[53] more recent studies question the added benefit of continuous baseline infusion of opioids.[63]

When choosing an opioid for PCA delivery, one must consider the desired clinical effect (see previous section on intravenous opioids). Intermediate-acting agents, such as morphine, have been preferred in most clinical investigations. Shorter-acting agents (e.g., alfentanil and sufentanil) are very effective analgesics but often require a continuous infusion in order to decrease the frequency of demand boluses. Guidelines for the use of opioid analgesics in PCA modality are described by White[64] and Wolman.[44]

Regardless of the choice for postoperative analgesia, wide variations in analgesic requirements occur among patients. This may be attributed to pre-existing coping mechanisms, psychological factors, and physiologic factors (e.g., endogenous endorphin and substance P levels).[65,66] The remainder of this discussion focuses on alternatives to traditional opioid analgesic regimens.

REGIONAL ANALGESIA

Background
Regional techniques in cardiac anesthesia have no true predecessor before 1980. Prior to this time, regional techniques were used for thoracic surgery. The first documented intrathecal anesthetic for thoracic surgery was performed by Etherington-Wilson[67] in 1933. He introduced hypobaric percaine (diluted 1:1,500) intrathecally at the third lumbar interspace. The anesthetic was allowed to ascend for 40 seconds while maintaining the patient in the sitting position. The patient was subsequently placed in a slight (10 to 15-degree) Trendelenburg position for the remainder of the operation. The gradual demise in popularity of this technique occurred with the widespread adoption of endotracheal intubation and controlled respiration as standard of care for thoracic surgical procedures.

The concerns for hematoma formation following anticoagulation, alteration of hemodynamic parameters, and baroreceptor reflexes are cited as reasons for avoidance of regional anesthesia for cardiothoracic surgical patients. On the positive side, regional anesthetic techniques not only eliminate the systemic and adverse side effects of opioids but also attenuate the stress response to surgery and anesthesia. The completeness of the pain relief achieved with a few milliliters of local anesthetic coupled with the aforementioned benefits make regional anesthesia advantageous for these patients.

Table 15-2. Drugs for Intercostal Block

Drug	Duration (hr)	Concentration (%)	Dosage (mg·kg^{-1}) Plain	Dosage (mg·kg^{-1}) With Epi
Bupivacaine	8–12	0.5	2–3	2–3
Bupivacaine	6–12	0.25	2–3	2–3
Etidocaine	6–8	0.5	2–3	2–3
Tetracaine	5–9	0.10–0.15	2.0	2.0
Mepivacaine	4–8	0.5–1.0	7.0	9.0

(Adapted from Thompson and Hecker,[74] with permission.)

Several regional approaches are available for use in cardiothoracic surgical patients with median sternotomy incisions: intercostal nerve block, subarachnoid block (intrathecal), and thoracic epidural block.

Intercostal Analgesia
Intercostal nerve block is used extensively for analgesia following thoracic surgery.[68–73] Agents are administered using a variety of approaches[74]: single treatment under direct vision prior to chest closure,[69,71] single preoperative percutaneous treatment,[73] multiple percutaneous serial injections,[75,76] or continuous infusion via an indwelling intercostal catheter.[68,70,72,73]

When choosing a local anesthetic for intercostal nerve block, the following factors should be considered: total volume of solution, effective concentration of drug, total (mg) dosage of drug, volume of epinephrine to be added, and the total dosage of epinephrine. The drug should be appropriate for the block and therefore requires familiarity of effective local anesthetic doses and concentrations, as well as its recommended maximum dose. Commonly used drugs, concentrations, and acceptable drug volumes for intercostal nerve blocks are presented in Table 15-2.

A major concern with intercostal nerve block is the high degree of systemic absorption of the local anesthetic agent and subsequent toxic effect. This complication is most likely to occur when large volumes of concentrated drug are injected to provide complete motor and sensory block. Clinical studies demonstrate safe plasma levels of local anesthetics following intercostal nerve block.[49,69,77] Other potential complications from intercostal nerve block include pneumothorax and isolated hypotension.

Intrathecal and Thoracic Epidural Analgesia
Intrathecal and epidural analgesic techniques described for post-thoracotomy and post-median sternotomy pain management include intrathecal opioids, intrathecal local anesthetics combined with opioids, thoracic epidural local anesthetics, and thoracic epidural local anesthetics combined with opioids. These modalities are becoming more widely used for management of postoperative pain, given their relatively high benefit-to-risk ratio, even in the presence of systemic anticoagulation.[78–82]

Extensive reviews of these techniques, mechanisms of action, and adverse effects have been conducted.[83–85] Serious but infrequent undesired side effects of regional analgesia include unintentional high subarachnoid block, systemic toxicity secondary to local anesthetics, profound respiratory depression secondary to opioids, spinal cord or nerve root trauma, epidural hematoma formation, and infection or inflammation associated with the introduction of the catheter or needle.[86,87] Nausea, pruritis, and urinary retention may occur after the administration of epidural or intrathecal opioids.[86,87] Hypotension, temporary paralysis, urinary retention, and paresthesias may accompany epidural or intrathecal administration of local anesthetic. A low incidence of postdural puncture headache may occur with either epidural or intrathecal neuraxial blockade.

Clearly, clinical studies demonstrate that high-risk patients undergoing nonthoracic surgery benefit from epidural analgesia.[88] Preliminary studies in a canine model using thoracic epidural anesthesia demonstrated a decrease in the parameters associated with myocardial oxygen consumption, improved regional or ischemic zones of endocardial perfusion and a decrease in myocardial infarct size,[89] and a reduction in the incidence of malignant ventricular dysrhythmias.[90] Subsequent studies in humans[91] depicted improved coronary artery blood flow via selective sympathetic blockade (T1–T5) and resultant dilation of stenotic epicardial coronaries without dilating coronary arterioles. Improvement in the determinants of myocardial oxygen consumption in the absence of adversely affected coronary perfusion pressure was demonstrated using thoracic epidural anesthesia in patients with severe coronary artery disease and unstable angina.[92] Still another beneficial effect of thoracic epidural anesthesia is the improvement of global and regional ejection fractions, fewer regional wall motion abnormalities, decreased rate pressure product, and lessened ST-segment changes during exercise as evaluated by radionuclide angiography.[93] The demonstration of improved recovery time, postoperative pain relief, reduced sedation, and superior cardiac and pulmonary outcome is the conclusion of Liem et al.,[38] with the use of combined local anesthetic and opioid thoracic epidural anesthesia. This superior postoperative pain relief was also accompanied by an attenuation of the stress response (quantified by less epinephrine and cortisol release into the plasma). All the above reasons coupled with a potential reduction in the length of stay in the ICU and hospital and a decrease in overall medical cost make neuroaxial analgesia an attractive alternative to conventional pain management modalities.

Intrathecal and Thoracic Epidural Opioids

"Selective spinally mediated analgesia"[94] occurs via binding of opioids to receptors located in the spinal cord.[95,96] Specifically, opioid binding occurs to laminae II (substantia gelatinosa), III, and V of the spinal cord gray matter. These laminae are densely populated with opioid receptors.

To produce segmental analgesia, a minimum concentration of opioid in the cerebrospinal fluid (CSF) is required. Cephalad movement of hydrophilic opioids, such as morphine, occurs via CSF bulk flow.[97–99] As the opioid spreads rostrally, higher dermatomal analgesic levels are achieved.[98,100–103] Lipid-soluble opioids (e.g., fentanyl, sufentanil) tend to bind close to the site of injection and do not exhibit any significant cephalad CSF movement.[104]

Opioids may be delivered either as a single epidural or intrathecal bolus or by continuous infusion. Segmental analgesia via the intrathecal route offers advantages of faster onset of analgesia,[105] a smaller dose requirement,[106] and elimination of competition for drug absorption by epidural fat and blood vessels.[105] Commonly used dosing regimens for epidural and intrathecal opioids are listed in Tables 15-3 to 15-5.

Thoracic Epidural Local Anesthetics

Several studies[76,107–111] use thoracic epidural local anesthetics to create a circumscribed band of analgesia along a limited dermatomal distribution. In the case of median sternotomy, the desired dermatomal local anesthetic spread is from T1–T5 or T6.

Most studies in the literature describe an intermittent bolus of local anesthetic or continuous infusion of local anesthetic with concomitant administration of epidural or systemic opioids. The true efficacy of thoracic epidural local anesthesia for post-median sternotomy analgesia has yet to be elucidated.

Studies are currently ongoing at our institution to examine the effect of thoracic epi-

Table 15-3. Dosage Regimen for Intermittent Administration of Epidural Opioids

Drug	Lipid Solubility[a]	Bolus Dose	Onset (min)	Duration (hr)	Comments
Morphine	1	2–5 mg	30–60	6–24	Due to spread in cerebrospinal fluid, preferred for extensive incisions and when injection site is distant from source of nociception
Meperedine	30	50–100 mg	5–10	6–8	
Methadone	100	1–10 mg	10	6–10	May accumulate in blood with repetitive dosing
Fentanyl	800	50–100 μg	5	4–6	Not recommended when incision is extensive or injection site is distant from source of nociception
Sufentanil	1,500	10–60 μg	5	2–4	Higher doses may produce excessive sedation or ventilatory depression, presumably due to vascular uptake

[a] Octanol/pH 7.4 buffer partition coefficient relative to morphine.
(From Ferrante and VadeBoncouer,[132] with permission.)

dural anesthesia on cardiac surgical patients in terms of myocardial ischemia as well as intraoperative and postoperative analgesia. Thoracic epidural catheters are placed at the T3–T5 spinal level. An initial bolus of 2 to 3 ml of 0.5 percent bupivacaine is administered by catheter. Once the patient's level of anesthesia is determined, a continuous infusion of 0.5 percent bupivacaine is started at a rate of 2 to 5 ml · hr^{-1} and is maintained throughout the intraoperative and postoperative periods. Preliminary results are very favorable regarding postoperative pain relief, earlier ambulation times, earlier discharge from both the ICU and the hospital, and a decrease in the incidence of intraoperative and postoperative myocardial ischemia.

Combined Thoracic Epidural Local Anesthetics and Opioids
The objective of combining thoracic epidural local anesthetics and opioids is to block spinal nociceptive pathways synergistically while reducing the dose-related adverse effects of either class of agent alone. Many studies have examined the effectiveness of this technique following thoracotomy.[107, 112–118] There is also documentation in the literature of combined local anesthetic and opioid thoracic epidural anesthesia for patients undergoing CABG.[38] In this study, epidural analgesia was induced with a mixture of 0.375 percent bupivacaine plus sufentanil, 1: 200,000 (i.e., 5 μg · ml^{-1}) in an infusion dose of 0.05 ml · cm^{-1} body length. Once spread

Table 15-4. Epidural Opioid Infusions

Drug	Usual Infusion Rate (mg·hr^{-1})	Comments
Morphine	0.2–1.0	Lowest effective infusion rates should be used after a small bolus
Meperidine	10–25	Prolonged therapy may result in accumulation of normeperedine with risk of myoclonus and seizures
Fentanyl	0.03–0.01	Contribution of systemic level of analgesia may be significant

(From Ferrante and VadeBoncouer,[132] with permission.)

Table 15-5. Dosage Regimen for Subarachnoid Opioids

Drug	Dose	Onset (min)	Duration (hr)	Comments
Morphine	0.1–1.0 mg	15–30	10–30	Doses greater than 1 mg may produce an increased incidence of side effects
Meperidine	10–30 mg	5	10–30	High doses have been employed for surgical anesthesia
Fentanyl	10–50 μg	5	4–6	Higher doses will not prolong or intensify analgesia but may substantially increase side effects

(From Ferrante and VadeBoncouer,[132] with permission.)

of sensory blockade was determined, a continuous infusion of 0.125 percent bupivacaine plus sufentanil 1:1,000,000 (i.e., 1 μg · ml^{-1}) at an infusion dose of 0.05 ml · cm^{-1} body length was started. Patients maintained more stable hemodynamics both before and after cardiopulmonary bypass. They had a shorter period of recovery from the effects of anesthesia, were extubated earlier, and had superior pain relief compared with patients receiving intravenous analgesia in the postoperative period. Less release of norepinephrine occurred in the pre-bypass and bypass periods; the bypass period was also accompanied by less variability in systemic vascular resistance and less release of epinephrine. Lower levels of epinephrine and cortisol were detected in these patients postoperatively. There was no reported incidence of respiratory depression or neurologic sequelae in the thoracic epidural anesthesia group. Given the favorable results of this study, this technique clearly warrants further investigation.

Combined Intrathecal Local Anesthetics and Opioids

Our group recently examined the use of intrathecal local anesthetic plus opioid for cardiothoracic surgical patients.[119] Our protocol, a double-blind, randomized study, evaluated a series of 20 patients, 10 assigned as controls and 10 assigned as treatment. All patients received radial arterial lines, intravenous and pulmonary artery catheters that were placed prior to induction of anesthesia.

Patients received general endotracheal anesthesia consisting of fentanyl (15 to 20 μg · Kg^{-1}), midazolam (0.2 mg · kg^{-1}) and isoflurane to maintain a systolic blood pressure of less than 140 mmHg. Following induction of anesthesia, patients were placed in the lateral decubitus position, and either 3 ml of a 5 percent dextrose solution or 3 ml of active solution (100 mg lidocaine plus 1 mg preservative-free morphine in a 3-ml 5 percent dextrose solution) was administered via 25- or 26-gauge spinal needle. Patients were returned to the supine position and placed in a 15-degree Trendelenberg position for 10 minutes. The results of the study are favorable: (1) the treatment group required less isoflurane to maintain blood pressure within the specified limits; (2) no differences were noted between groups with respect to use of inotropes, vasoconstrictors, or vasodilators in the intraoperative or postoperative period; (3) emergence time was shorter in the treatment group as was time to extubation; (4) length of stay in the ICU and the hospital was shorter for patients in the treatment group; and (5) total hospital charges were lower in the treatment group. We encountered no problems with pruritis, respiratory depression, urinary retention, epidural hematoma formation, or neurologic sequelae.

In concordance with a study conducted by Yeager et al.,[37] we noted that our results still suffer from the problem of sample size. Further investigation of this type, to include a larger study sample size, is warranted.

Thoracic Epidural Adrenergic Agents

Identification of nonopioid-dependent anatomic pathways and pharmacologic receptors resulted in the investigation of nonopioid analgesics (i.e., clonidine) for management of acute postsurgical pain. Epidural adrenergic agonists have the potential for effective antinociceptive activity.[85,118] The mechanism of action is described as modulation of the endogenous postsynaptic adrenergic receptors in the dorsal horn cells.[121]

Clonidine has been sufficiently studied in animal models.[122,123] Several clinical studies demonstrate the analgesic effect of clonidine in the postoperative setting.[124–127] In theory, nonopioids do not appear to have many of the side effects of opioid analgesics (i.e., respiratory depression, urinary retention, nausea, vomiting, or pruritis). However, the nonopioids have their own side effects, such as hypotension, that tend to occur more frequently after small or medium boluses of clonidine. Larger boluses of clonidine may result in oversedation. Studies to further elucidate the benefits and risks of neuroaxial clonidine and other α_2-adrenergic agonists are ongoing.

ANTICOAGULATION AND REGIONAL ANESTHESIA

The greatest concern to the practitioner considering regional anesthesia for the cardiothoracic surgical patient is hematoma formation. To date there are insufficient conclusive outcome studies to define the safety of performing epidural or intrathecal anesthetic techniques when coagulation abnormalities exist. In order to make a rational assessment of the relevance of the risk imposed by the administration of regional anesthesia in the presence of anticoagulation, one must consider the following factors: the group of patients at risk; the incidence of the specific risk (i.e., epidural hematoma); the benefit to the patient of the technique; and the risks and benefits of alternative techniques.

Several studies document utilization of intrathecal or epidural anesthesia, either preceding or following anticoagulation.[79–82,128] No epidural hematomas or neurologic sequelae were reported. Matthews and Abrams[79] administered intrathecal morphine to 40 patients for cardiac surgery. Full anticoagulation with intravenous heparin was achieved 50 minutes after lumbar puncture. Rao and El-Etr[80] placed 4,011 spinal or epidural catheters in patients scheduled for peripheral vascular surgery. One hour after catheter placement, heparin was administered to increase the activated coagulation time to two times the baseline value. All catheters remained in place for 24 hours postoperatively. A corroborative study by Odoom and Sih[81] reported on 950 patients taking oral anticoagulants preoperatively, whose preoperative thrombotest was 19 percent (normal values reported as 70 to 130 percent). Epidural catheters were placed in these patients who were later given heparin for additional anticoagulation. El-Baz and Goldin[128] reported on continuous epidural infusion in 30 patients undergoing cardiac surgery. All patients had epidural catheters inserted 1 to 2 hours prior to administration of heparin for cardiopulmonary bypass. Liem et al.[35] describes similar results. Most recently, Horlocker et al.[129] concluded that preoperative antiplatelet therapy is not a significant risk factor for the development of neurologic dysfunction from spinal hematoma in patients receiving spinal or epidural anesthesia. This is a prospective study of 924 patients with a history of excess bruising or bleeding (12 percent of patients studied), preoperative antiplatelet therapy (39 percent of patients studied), and preoperative subcutaneous heparin administration (2 percent of patients studied). Five of 31 preoperative bleeding times were prolonged, one of 774 patients had a preoperative platelet count of less than $100,000 \cdot mm^{-3}$, 26 of 171 patients had a preoperative prothrombin time greater than normal, and 10 of 115 patients had a preoperative activated partial thromboplastin time greater than normal. Blood was noted during needle or catheter placement in 223 (22 percent) of patients, including 73 patients with frank blood in the needle or catheter. These patients did not receive further anticoagulant therapy intraoperatively, as is the usual case for cardiac surgery. Whether this would have altered the study outcome remains a matter of conjecture.

In clinical practice, the reported occurrence of neuraxial hematoma as a result of coagulation abnormalities is rare. There is a report in the Japanese literature regarding the spontaneous occurrence of an epidural hematoma around the time of cardiopulmonary bypass in a patient without instrumentation of the epidural or subarachnoid space. A review of the literature by Owens et al.[130] described 33 incidents of epidural hematoma following lumbar puncture; 70 percent of these patients had some type of hemostatic abnormality. It is impossible to determine accurately the denominator from which to calculate an accurate incidence of neuraxial hematoma. However, in a combined large series of greater than 50,000 spinal anesthetics, no epidural hematomas were noted.[130]

Cardiac surgical patients have much to gain from the use of neuraxial techniques. To reiterate, the advantages are improved pain relief, and a shorter emergence interval, and time to extubation, allowing for earlier ability to communicate with family members and practitioners, and a decreased incidence and severity of myocardial ischemia and other comorbid events.

Both patients and practitioners assume a risk of neuraxial hematoma through the incorporation of epidural or intrathecal anesthetic techniques. How high is this risk? Does this risk preclude the benefit to the patient? Only large-scale prospective studies or retrospective meta-analyses will give us the answer.

SUMMARY

Median sternotomy incisions produce acute pain that, if not adequately treated, may lead to the development of chronic pain syndromes and an increased incidence of patient morbidity and mortality. The primary goal of any acute pain management regimen is the early restoration of tissue, organ, and patient function. What is the best way to accomplish this goal? Postoperative pain can be controlled effectively in many ways. There are several considerations when selecting a modality of postoperative pain management: the experience of the practitioner and his or her familiarity with a technique; the clinical circumstances, including any contraindications to the contemplated technique or selection of medication; the appropriateness of the setting in which the therapy is to be initiated and maintained; the availability of appropriate monitors and trained personnel; patient acceptance; the ability of the technique to provide reasonable benefit to the patient in relationship to its risk; and the cost-effectiveness of the technique. Further prospective, randomized, double-blind, placebo-controlled outcome studies—particularly in patients undergoing cardiothoracic surgery—are needed to give us the final answer.

REFERENCES

1. Gil KM, Forse RA, Askanazi J et al: Energy metabolism. p. 203. In Garrow JS, Halliday D, London JL (eds): Stress, Substrate and Energy Metabolism. Libbey, London, 1985
2. Burch GE, Giles TD: Cardiac causalgia. Arch Intern Med 125:809, 1970
3. Cousins MJ, Reeve TS, Glynn CJ et al: Neurolytic lumbar sympathetic blockade: duration of denervation and relief of rest pain. Anaesth Intensive Care 7:121–35, 1979
4. Bach S, Noreng MF, Tjellden NU: Phantom limb pain in amputees during the first twelve months following limb amputation, after preoperative lumbar epidural blockade. Pain 33:297–301, 1988
5. Melzak R, Abbott FV, Zackon W et al: Pain on a surgical ward: a survey of the duration and intensity of pain and the effectiveness of medication. Pain 29:67–72, 1987
6. Cousins MJ: Pathophysiology of acute pain: immediate and prolonged effects. p. 55. In

Advances in Regional Anesthesia and Analgesia. Second International Symposium on Regional Anesthesia, 1988

7. Wang JK, Nauss LA, Thomas JE: Pain relief by intrathecally applied morphine in man. Anesthesiology 50:149–51, 1979

8. Chahl LA: Pain induced by inflammatory mediators. p. 273. In Beers RF, Basset EG (eds): Mechanisms of Pain and Analgesic Compounds. Raven Press, New York, 1979

9. Cousins MJ: Introduction to acute and chronic pain: implications for neural blockade. p. 739. In Cousins MJ, Bridenbaugh PO (eds): Neural Blockade in Clinical Anesthesia and Management of Pain. 2nd Ed. JB Lippincott, Philadelphia, 1988

10. Perl ER: Sensitization of nociceptors and its relation to sensation. p. 17. In Bonica JJ, Albe-Fessard D (eds): Advances in Pain Research and Therapy. Vol. 1. Raven Press, New York, 1976

11. Westbroo RR, Stuvs SE, Sessler AD et al: Effects of anesthesia and muscle paralysis on respiratory mechanisms in normal man. J Appl Physiol 34:81, 1973

12. Churchill E: The reduction in vital capacity following operation. Surg Gynecol Obstet 44: 483, 1927

13. Turnbull KW, Miyagishima RT, Coerein AN: Pulmonary complications and cardiopulmonary bypass: a clinical study in adults. Can Anaesth J 21:181, 1974

14. Kollel MH, Peller T, Knodel A, Cragun WH: Delayed pleuropulmonary complications following coronary artery revascularization with the internal mammary artery. Chest 94: 68, 1988

15. Wolcox P, Bailey E, Hars J et al: Phrenic nerve function and its relationship to atelectasis after coronary artery bypass surgery. Chest 93:693, 1988

16. Meyers JR, Lambeck L, O'Kane H et al: Changes in functional residual capacity of the lung after operation. Arch Surg 110:576, 1975

17. Wilson RS, Sullivan SF, Malm JR et al: The oxygen cost of breathing following anesthesia and cardiac surgery. Anesthesiology 99: 387, 1973

18. Roussos C, Macklem PT: Diaphragmatic fatigue in man. J Appl Physiol 43:189, 1977

19. Shapiro BA, Kacmarek RM, Cane RD et al: Clinical evaluation of the pulmonary system.

p. 43. In Clinical Application of Respiratory Care. 4th Ed. Mosby-Year Book Medical, Chicago, 1991

20. Craig DB: Postoperative recovery of pulmonary function. Anesth Analg 60:46, 1981

21. Jaattela A, Alho A, Avikainen V et al: Plasma catecholamines in severely injured patients: a prospective study of 45 patients with multiple injuries. Br J Surg 62:177, 1975

22. Kehlet H: The stress response to anaesthesia and surgery: release mechanisms and modifying factors. Clin Anesth 2:315, 1984

23. Gelfand RA, Matthews DE, Bier DM: Role of counterregulatory hormones in the catabolic response to stress. J Clin Invest 74:2238, 1984

24. Kehlet H, Brandt MR, Rem J: Role of neurogenic stimuli in mediating the endocrine-metabolic response to surgery. JPEN J Parenter Enteral Nutr 4:152, 1980

25. Cuthbertson DP: The metabolic response to injury and its nutritional implications: retrospect and prospect. JPEN J Parenter Enteral Nutr 3:108, 1979

26. Christenson P, Brandt MR, Rem J et al: Influence of extradural morphine on the adrenocortical and hyperglycemic response to surgery. Br J Anaesth 54:24, 1982

27. Jorgensen BC, Anderson HB, Engquist A: Influence of epidural morphine on postoperative pain, endocrine metabolic and renal responses to surgery: a controlled study. Acta Anaesthesiol Scand 26:63, 1982

28. Kehlet H, Brandt MR, Prange Hansen A et al: Effect of epidural analgesia on metabolic profiles during and after surgery. Br J Surg 66:543, 1979

29. Bromage PR, Shibata HR, Willoughby HW: Influence of prolonged epidural blockade on blood sugar and cortisol responses to operation upon the upper abdomen and thorax. Surg Gynecol Obstet 132:1051, 1971

30. Engquist A, Brandt MR, Fernandes A et al: The blocking effeect of epidural analgesia on the adrenocortical and hyperglycemic response to surgery. Acta Anaesthesiol Scand 21:330, 1977

31. McKegney FP: The intensive care syndrome: definition, treatment and prevention of a new "disease of progress." Conn Med 30:633, 1966

32. Cousins MJ, Wright CJ: Graft, muscle and skin blood flow after epidural block in vascu-

lar surgical procedures. Surg Gynecol Obstet 133:59–69, 1971

33. Pflug AE, Murphy TM, Butler SH et al: The effects of postoperative peridural analgesic on pulmonary therapy and pulmonary complications. Anesthesiology 41:8–17, 1974

34. Bridenbaugh PO: Anesthesia and influence on hospitalization time. Reg Anaesth, suppl. 7:S151–5, 1982

35. Noller DW, Gillenwater JY, Howards SS et al: Intercostal nerve block with flank incision. J Urol 117:759, 1977

36. Shulman M, Sandler AN, Bradley JW et al: Postthoracotomy pain and pulmonary function following epidural and systemic morphine. Anesthesiology 61:569–75, 1984

37. Yeager MP, Glass DD, Neff RK, Brick-Johnsen T: Epidural anesthesia and analgesia in high-risk surgical patients. Anesthesiology 66:729–36, 1987

38. Liem TH, Hasenbos MAWM, Booij LHD, Gielen MJM: Coronary artery bypass grafting using two different anesthetic techniques. Part 2. Postoperative outcome. J Cardiothorac Vasc Anesth 6:156–61, 1992

39. Angell M: The quality of mercy, editorial. N Engl J Med 306:98, 1982

40. Marks RM, Sachar EJ: Undertreatment of medical inpatients with narcotic analgesics. Ann Intern Med 78:173, 1973

41. Donovan M, Dillon P, McGuire L: Incidence and characteristics of pain in a sample of medical-surgical inpatients. Pain 6:249, 1987

42. Weiss OF, Sritwatanakul K, Alloza JL et al: Attitudes of patients, housestaff and nurses toward postoperative analgesic care. Anesth Analg 62:70, 1983

43. Mather LE, Phillips GD: Opioids and adjuvants: principles of use. p. 77. In Cousins MJ, Phillips GD (eds): Acute Pain Management. Churchill Livingstone, New York, 1986

44. Wolman RL: Patient-controlled analgesia following thoracic surgery. pp. 57–99. In Gravlee GP, Rauck RL (eds): Pain Management in Cardiothoracic Surgery. JB Lippincott, Philadelphia, 1993

45. Miller RR: Clinical effects of parenteral narcotics in hospitalized medical patients. J Clin Pharmacol 20:165, 1980

46. Miller RR: Analgesics. p. 156. In Miller RR, Greenblatt DJ (eds): Drug Effects in Hospitalized Patients. John Wiley & Sons, New York, 1976

47. Wolman RL, Luterman A: The continuous infusion of morphine sulfate for analgesia in burn patients: extending the use of an established technique, abstracted. Am Burn Assoc 20:150, 1988

48. Benzor HT, Wong HY, Belavic AM et al: A randomized, double-blind comparison of epidural fentanyl versus patient-controlled analgesia with morphine for postthoracotomy pain. Anesth Analg 76:316–22, 1993

49. Chan VWS, Chung F, Cheng DCH et al: Analgesic and pulmonary effects of continuous intercostal nerve block following thoracotomy. Can J Anaesth 38:733–9, 1991

50. Jones RM, Cashman JN, Foster JMG et al: Comparison of infusions of morphine and lysineacetyl salicylate for the relief of pain following thoracic surgery. Br J Anaesth 57:259–63, 1985

51. Salomäki TE, Laitinen JO, Nuutinen LS: A randomized, double-blind comparison of epidural versus intravenous fentanyl infusion for analgesia after thoracotomy. Anesthesiology 75:790–5, 1991

52. Churchill-Davidson HC: A Practice of Anaesthesia 4th Ed. WB Saunders, Philadelphia, 1978

53. Gourlay GK, Kowalski SR, Plummer JL et al: Fentanyl blood concentration-analgesic response relationship in the treatment of postoperative pain. Anesth Analg 67:329–37, 1988

54. Jordan C, Lehane JR, Robson PJ, Jones JG: A comparison of the respiratory effects of meptazinol, pentazocine and morphine. Br J Anaesth 51:497–502, 1979

55. Shulman M, Sandler AN, Bradley JW et al: Postthoracotomy pain and pulmonary function following epidural and systemic morphine. Anesthesiology 61:569–575, 1984

56. Salomäki TE, Laitinen JO, Nuutinen LS: A randomized, double-blind comparison of epidural versus intravenous fentanyl infusion for analgesia after thoracotomy. Anesthesiology 75:790–5, 1991

57. Roe BB: Are postoperative narcotics necessary? Arch Surg 87:912, 1963

58. Sechzer PH: Patient-controlled analgesia: a retrospective. Anesthesiology 72:735, 1990

59. Boulanger A, Choiniere M, Roy D et al: Comparison between patient controlled analgesia

and intramuscular meperidine after thoracotomy. Can J Anaesth 40:409–15, 1993

60. Lange MP, Dahn MS, Jacobs LA: Patient controlled analgesia versus intermittent analgesia dosing. Heart Lung 17:495–8, 1988

61. Etches RC: Respiratory depression associated with patient controlled analgesia: a review of eight cases. Can J Anaesth 41:125–32, 1994

62. Norman J: Terminology used in patient-controlled analgesia. p. 3. In Harmer M, Rosen M, Vickers MD (eds): Patient-Controlled Analgesia. Blackwell Scientific, Boston, 1985

63. Parker PK, Holtman NB, White PF: Patient controlled analgesia: does a concurrent opioid infusion improve pain management after surgery? JAMA 266:1947–52, 1991

64. White PF: Patient-controlled analgesia: a new approach to the management of postoperative pain. Semin Anesth 4:255–66, 1985

65. Wilson JF, Bennett RL: Coping styles, medication use and pain score score in patients using patient controlled analgesia for postoperative pain. Anesthesiology 61:A193, 1984

66. Tamsen A, Sakurada T, Wahlstrom A et al: Postoperative demand for analgesics in relation to individual levels of endorphins and substance P in cerebral spinal fluid. Pain 13:171–83, 1982

67. Etherington-Wilson W: Intrathecal nerve root block: some contributions and a new technique. Proc R Soc Med 27:323–31, 1933

68. Dryden CM, McMenemin I, Duthie DJR: Efficacy of continuous intercostal bupivacaine for pain relief after thoracotomy. Br J Anaesth 70:508–10, 1993

69. Galway JE, Caves PK, Dundee JW: Effect of intercostal nerve blockade during operation on lung function and the relief of pain following thoracotomy. Br J Anaesth 47:730–5, 1975

70. Deneauville M, Bisserier A, Regnard JF et al: Continuous intercostal analgesia with 0.5% bupivacaine after thoracotomy: a randomized study. Ann Thorac Surg 55:381–5, 1993

71. Kaplan JA, Miller ED, Gallagher EG: Postoperative analgesia ffor thoracotomy patients. Anesth Analg 54:773–7, 1975

72. Sabanathan S, Meams AJ, Bickford Smith PJ et al: Efficacy of continuous extrapleural intercostal nerve block on post-thoracotomy pain and pulmonary mechanics. Br J Surg 77:221–5, 1990

73. Swann DG, Armstrong PJ, Douglas E et al: The alkalinisation of bupivacaine for intercostal nerve blockade. Anaesthesia 46:174–6, 1991

74. Thompson GE, Hecker BR: Peripheral nerve blocks for management of thoracic surgery patients. p. 25. In Gravlee GP, Rauck RL (eds): Pain Management in Cardiothoracic Surgery. JB Lippincott, Philadelphia, 1993

75. Bergh NP, Dottori O, Lof BA et al: Effect of intercostal block on lung function after thoracotomy. Acta Anaesthesiol Scand 23:85–95, 1966

76. Asantila R, Rosenberg PH, Scheinin B: Comparison of different methods of postoperative analgesia after thoracotomy. Acta Anaesthesiol Scand 30:421–5, 1986

77. Safran D, Kuhlman G, Orhant EE et al: Continuous intercostal blockade with lidocaine after thoracic surgery: clinical and pharmacokinetic study. Anesth Analg 70:345–9, 1990

78. Williams JP, Blomberg SG: Should epidurals be used in patients who get systemic anticoagulation? Anesthesia Patient Safety Foundation News 45, 1993–4

79. Matthews ET, Abrams LD: Intrathecal morphine in open heart surgery. Lancet 2:543, 1980

80. Rao TLK, El-Etr AA: Anticoagulation following placement of epidural and subarachnoid catheters: an evaluation of neurologic sequelae. Anesthesiology 55:618–20, 1981

81. Odoom JA, Sih IL: Epidural analgesia and anticoagulant therapy: experience with one thousand cases of continuous epidurals. Anaesthesia 38:254–9, 1983

82. Waldman SD, Feldstein GS, Waldman HJ et al: Caudal administration of morphine sulfate in anticoagulated and thrombocytopenic patients. Anesth Analg 66:267–8, 1987

83. Cousins MJ, Mather LE: Intrathecal and epidural administration of opioids, review. Anesthesiology 61:276–310, 1984

84. Forrest JB: Sympathetic mechanisms in postoperative pain, editorial. Can J Anaesth 39:523–7, 1992

85. Maze M, Segal IS, Bloor BC: Clonidine and other alpha-2 adrenergic agonists: Strategies for the rational use of these novel anesthetic agents, review. J Clin Anesth 1:146–57, 1988

86. Bridenbaugh PO, Green NM: Spinal (sub-

arachnoid) neural blockade. p. 245. In Cousins MJ, Bridenbaugh PO (eds): Neural Blockade in Clinical Anesthesia and Management of Pain. JB Lippincott, Philadelphia, 1988

87. Cousins MJ, Bromage PR: Epidural neural blockade. p. 339. In Cousins MJ, Bridenbaugh PO (eds): Neural Blockade in Clinical Anesthesia and Management of Pain. JB Lippincott, Philadelphia, 1988

88. Rawal N, Sjostrand U, Christofferson E et al: Comparison of IM and epidural morphine for postoperative analgesia in the grossly obese: influence on postoperative ambulation and pulmonary function. Anesth Analg 63: 583–92, 1984

89. Davis RF, DeBoer LWV, Maroko PR: Thoracic epidural anesthesia reduces myocardial infarct size after coronary occlusion in dogs. Anesth Analg 65:711–7, 1986

90. Blomberg S, Ricksten S-E: Thoracic epidural anesthesia decreases the incidence of ventricular arrhythmias during acute myocardial ischemia in the anesthetized rat. Acta Anaesthesiol Scand 32:173–8, 1988

91. Blomberg S, Emanuelsson H, Dvist H et al: Effects of thoracic epidural anesthesia on coronary arteries and arterioles in patients with coronary artery disease. Anesthesiology 73:840–7, 1990

92. Blomberg S, Emanuelsson H, Ricksten S-E: Thoracic epidural anesthesia and central hemodynamics in patients with unstable angina pectoris. Anesth Analg 69:558–62, 1989

93. Kock M, Blomberg S, Emanuelsson H et al: Thoracic epidural anesthesia improves global and regional left ventricular function during stress-induced myocardial ischemia in patients with coronary artery disease. Anesth Analg 71:625–30, 1990

94. Cousins MJ, Mather LE, Glynn CJ et al: Selective spinal analgesia. Lancet 1:1141, 1979

95. Cousins MJ, Cherry DA, Gourlay GK: Acute and chronic pain: use of spinal opioids. p. 955. In Cousins MJ, Bridenbaugh PO (eds): Neural Blockade in Clinical Anesthesia and Management of Pain. 2nd Ed. JB Lippincott, Philadelphia, 1988

96. Yaksh TL, Noveihed R: The physiology and pharmacology of spinal opiates. Annu Rev Pharmacol Toxicol 25:443, 1975

97. Sjostrom S, Tamsen A, Perrson MP, Hartvig P: Pharmacokinetics of intrathecal morphine and meperidine in humans. Anesthesiology 67:889, 1987

98. Gourlay GK, Cherry DA, Cousins MJ: Cephalad migration of morphine in CSF following lumbar epidural administration in patients with cancer pain. Pain 23:317, 1985

99. Nordberg G: Pharmacokinetic aspects of spinal morphine analgesia. Acta Anesthesiol Scand 79:1, 1984

100. Nordberg G, Hedner T, Mellstrand T, Dahlstrom B: Pharmacokinetic aspects of epidural morphine analgesia. Anesthesiology 58:545, 1983

101. Larsen VH, Iverson AP, Christensen P et al: Postoperative pain treatment after upper abdominal surgery with epidural morphine at the thoracic or lumbar level. Acta Anaesthesiol Scand 29:566, 1985

102. Fromme GA, Steidl LJ, Danielson DR: Comparison of lumbar and thoracic epidural morphine for relief of postthoracotomy pain. Anesth Analg 64:454, 1985

103. Sullivan SP, Cherry DA: Pain from an invasive facial tumor relieved by lumbar epidural morphine. Anesth Analg 66:777, 1987

104. Mather LE: Clinical pharmacokinetics of fentanyl and its newer derivatives. Clin Pharmacokinet 8:422, 1983

105. Chauvin M, Samii K, Schermann JM et al: Plasma pharmacokinetics of morphine after IM extradural and intrathecal administration. Br J Anaesth 54:843, 1981

106. Katz J, Nelson W: Intrathecal morphine for postoperative pain relief. Reg Anesth 6:1, 1981

107. Logas WG, El-Baz N, El-Ganzouri A et al: Continuous thoracic epidural analgesia for postoperative pain relief following thoracotomy: A randomized prospective study. Anesthesiology 67:787–91, 1987

108. Matthews PJ, Govenden V: Comparison of continuous paravertebral and extradural infusions of bupivacaine for pain relief after thoracotomy. Br J Anaesth 62:204–5, 1989

109. Griffiths DPG, Diamond AW, Cameron JD: Postoperative extradural analgesia following thoracic surgery: a feasibility study. Br J Anaesth 47:48–54, 1975

110. El-Baz NM, Faber LP, Jensik RJ: Continuous epidural infusion of morphine for treatment

of pain after thoracic surgery: a new technique. Anesth Analg 63:757–64, 1984

111. James EC, Kolberg HL, Iwen GW, Gellatly TA: Epidural analgesia for postthoracotomy patients. J Thorac Cardiovasc Surg 82:898–903, 1981

112. Zwarts SJ, Hasenbos MAMW, Gielen MJM, Kho H: The effect of continuous epidural analgesia with sufentanil and bupivacaine during and after thoracic surgery on the plasma cortisol concentration and pain relief. Reg Anesth 14:183–8, 1989

113. Bigler D, Moller J, Kamp-Jensen M et al: Effect of piroxicam in addition to continuous thoracic epidural bupivacaine and morphine on postoperative pain and lung function after thoracotomy. Acta Anaesthesiol Scand 36:647–50, 1992

114. Mourisse J, Hasenbos MAWM, Gielen MJM et al: Epidural bupivacaine, sufentanil or the combination for post-thoracotomy pain. Acta Anaesthesiol Scand 36:70–4, 1992

115. George KA, Wright PMC, Chisakuta A: Continuous thoracic epidural fentanyl for post-thoracotomy pain relief: with or without bupivacaine? Anaesthesia 46:732–6, 1991

116. Harbers JBM, Hasenbos MAWM, Grot C et al: Ventilatory function and continuous high thoracic epidural administration of bupivacaine with sufentanil intravenously or epidurally: a double-blind comparison. Reg Anesth 16:65–71, 1991

117. Hasenbos MAWM, Eckhaus MN, Slappendel R, Gielen MJM: Continuous high thoracic epidural administration of bupivacaine with sufentanil or nicomorphine for postoperative pain relief after thoracic surgery. Reg Anesth 14:212–8, 1989

118. Laveaux MMD, Hasenbos MAWM, Harbers JBM, Liem T: Thoracic epidural bupivacaine plus sufentanil: High concentration/low volume versus low concentration/high volume. Reg Anesth 18:39–43, 1993

119. Hanley ES, Williams JP, Chelly J, Sweeny M et al: The effect of intrathecal morphine with lidocaine on pain relief and hemodynamics in the patient for coronary artery bypass graft. p. 254. In SCA Abstracts, Twelfth Annual Meeting, 1990

120. Tamsen A, Gordh T: Epidural clonidine produces analgesia, letter. Lancet 2:231–2, 1984

121. Howe JR, Wang IY, Yaksh TL: Selective antagonism of the antinociceptive effect on intrathecally applied alpha-adrenergic agonists by intrathecal prazosin and intrathecal yohimbine. J Pharmacol Exp Ther 224:552–8, 1983

122. Gordh T Jr, Feuk U, Norlen K: Effect of epidural clonidine on spinal cord blood flow and regional and central hemodynamics in pigs. Anesth Analg 65:1312–8, 1986

123. Eisenach J, Castro MI, Deuvan DM, Rose JC: Epidural clonidine analgesia in obstetrics: sheep studies. Anesthesiology 70:51–6, 1989

124. Rostaing S, Bonnet F, Levron JC et al: Effect of epidural clonidine on analgesia and pharmacokinetics of epidural fentanyl in the postoperative patient. Anesthesiology 75:420–5, 1991

125. Eisenach JC, Lysak SZ, Viscomi CM: Epidural clonidine analgesia following surgery: phase I. Anesthesiology 71:640–6, 1989

126. Filos KS, Goudas LC, Patroni O, Polyzou V: Hemodynamic and analgesic profile after intrathecal clonidine in humans: a dose-response study. Anesthesiology 81:591–601, 1994

127. Eisenach J, Detweiler D, Hood D: Hemodynamic and analgesic actions of epidurally administered clonidine. Anesthesiology 78:277–87, 1993

128. El-Baz N, Goldin M: Continuous epidural infusion of morphine for pain relief after cardiac operations. J Thorac Cardiovasc Surg 93:878–83, 1987

129. Horlocker TT, Wedel DJ et al: Preoperative antiplatelet therapy does not increase the risk of spinal hematoma associated with regional anesthesia. Anesth Analg 80:303–9, 1995

130. Owens EL, Kasten GW, Hessel EA: Spinal subarachnoid hematoma after lumbar puncture and heparinization: a case report, review of the literature and discussion of anesthetic implications. Anesth Analg 65:1201–7, 1986

131. White PF: Mishaps with patient-controlled analgesia. Anesthesiology 66:81–3, 1987

132. Ferrante FM, VadeBoncouer TR: Epidural and subarachnoid analgesia for thoracic surgery. p. 3. In Gravlee GP, Rauck RL (eds): Pain Management in Cardiothoracic Surgery. JB Lippincott, Philadelphia, 1993

16

Cardiovascular Pharmacology

B. V. Murthy
Ron M. Jones

The aim of this chapter is to integrate alterations in drug disposition into the typical pathophysiologic changes that occur in the perioperative cardiac patient. The pharmacokinetics and pharmacodynamics of drugs are affected by cardiovascular disease. The perioperative cardiac patient who is hypertensive and/or has valvular or ischemic heart disease (IHD) requires several medications to ameliorate symptoms. These drugs have profound effects on the cardiovascular system and produce significant implications both intraoperatively as well as in the postoperative period. An understanding of the effects of cardiopulmonary bypass (CPB) on drug disposition is important to any physician in planning strategies for the safe conduct of an anesthetic and postoperative care. A discussion of the influence of cardiac disease on pharmacology is followed by a review of the effect of CPB and surgery on drug disposition and action.

PREOPERATIVE DRUG THERAPY

The preoperative cardiac patient often requires several types of drugs, but five general categories of agents are commonly encountered: antihypertensives, antianginal drugs, drugs for management of congestive heart failure (CHF), inotropic drugs, and antidysrhythmics. Some degree of overlap exists between these categories; for example, antianginal drugs may also ameliorate the symptoms of hypertension. The pharmacologic treatment of CHF relies on the following groups of drugs: diuretics, vasodilators, and positive inotropic drugs including cardiac glycosides. Drugs used for antianginal therapy fall into three major groups: nitrates, β-blockers, and calcium antagonists. Nitrates reduce loading conditions (preload to a much greater degree than afterload) and wall tension and produce coronary vasodilation. β-blockers, in contrast, reduce heart rate (HR) and contractility and decrease myocardiol oxygen consumption (MVO_2). Calcium antagonists increase coronary blood flow (CBF) while simultaneously decreasing afterload and to some extent preload. A list of antianginal agents and their dosages is given in Table 16-6 and each are discussed in their respective sections. Calcium antagonists,[1] β-blockers,[2] and nitrates[3] all exhibit a platelet deaggregant property that is salutary in the

Table 16-1. Antihypertensive Drugs

Diuretics
  Thiazide group (e.g., bendrofluazide)
  Loop diuretics (e.g., furosemide, ethacrynic
    acid)
  Potassium sparing diuretics (e.g., spirinolac-
    tone, triameterene)
Antiadrenergic drugs
  Centrally acting (e.g., methyldopa, clonidine)
  Peripherally acting (e.g., guanethidine)
β-Blockers
  Propranolol, atenolol, metoprolol
α-Blockers
  Prazosin, doxazosin, terazosin, phentol-
    amine, phenoxybenzamine
Vasodilators
  Hydralazine, minoxidil, nitroprusside
ACE inhibitors
  Captopril, enalapril, lisinopril
Calcium antagonists
  Nifedipine, verapamil, diltiazem

Abbreviation: ACE, angiotensin-converting enzyme.

treatment of IHD. Both the drug and the disease for which it is prescribed influence the course of perioperative management.

Drug Descriptions

Hypertension is a common condition in patients undergoing cardiac surgery. Despite the incomplete understanding of the pathophysiology of essential hypertension, there has been a rapid growth in the use of pharmacologic agents for control of blood pressure. The classification of antihypertensives is outlined in Table 16-1.

Hypertension may be controlled by either a single drug or a combination of drugs that have different mechanisms of action. Antihypertensives generally act by inhibiting or modifying normal physiologic regulatory mechanisms. Hence, they may either mask or exacerbate potentially hazardous responses during the perioperative period.

DIURETIC AGENTS

Diuretics act by promoting the excretion of salt and water by blocking tubular reabsorption of chloride and sodium. The resulting

loss of fluid helps to reduce ventricular filling pressures and helps decrease wall stress and MVO_2. Loop diuretics, thiazide diuretics, and potassium-sparing diuretics (e.g., spirinolactone) are commonly used in heart failure. Diuretics also cause mild venodilation, which is complementary in the reduction of ventricular filling pressures.[4] Diuretic agents are described in Table 16-2.

Diuretics are often used in the treatment of mild to moderate hypertension. Since all classes of drugs increase urinary excretion of salt and water, there is the potential for preoperative dehydration and hypovolemia. Chronic use may also result in a variety of electrolyte disturbances including metabolic (contraction) alkalosis, hypercalcemia, hyperuricemia, and hypokalemia.

In the presence of hypokalemia the dysrhythmogenic effects of both digoxin and catecholamine sensitization to halothane may result in life-threatening dysrhythmias.[5] Potassium-sparing diuretics such as spirinolactone and triameterene are rarely primary therapy for hypertension. Spirinolactone is a competitive antagonist of aldosterone and is very effective in patients with primary hyperaldosteronism.[6] Although diuretics are the traditional choice for first-line antihypertensive therapy, evidence linking their long-term use to excess mortality resulted in a decline in primary applications.

ANTIADRENERGIC DRUGS

Antiadrenergic drugs (Table 16-3) act at different sites within the sympathetic nervous system. Drugs like reserpine and guanethidine block biogenic amines in both peripheral and central neurons. Clonidine and methyldopa reduce sympathetic outflow by a central action on the vasomotor center in the brainstem. Methyldopa reduces systemic vascular resistance (SVR) without much change in cardiac output (CO) or HR.[7] Methyldopa was commonly used in combination with a diuretic.[8] Abrupt withdrawal of clonidine may precipitate a hypertensive crisis; hence, this drug should be continued throughout the perioperative period (trans-cutaneous patch).[9]

α-Blockers

Prazosin, phentolamine, and phenoxybenza-mine all cause vasodilation by blocking the α_1-adrenergic receptor. Nonselective α-an-tagonists are rarely used currently for control of chronic hypertension. However, phentol-amine and phenoxybenzamine are still used acutely for vasodilation during the CBP pe-riod.

Prazosin decreases mean arterial pressure (MAP) and SVR without causing significant tachycardia. Cerebral and renal blood flows are well maintained. Prazosin maintains effi-cacy in the patient with hypertension associ-ated with renal insufficiency.[10] Prazosin's fa-vorable side effect profile (compared to phentolamine and phenoxybenzamine) is principally related to its postsynaptic specific-ity. Doxazosin and terazosin have properties similar to prazosin. This class of selective, postsynaptic α_1-blocker is increasingly used, as such blockers have beneficial effects on plasma lipids (unlike diuretics and β-blockers).

β-Blockers

β-Blockers competitively inhibit the effect of endogenous catecholamines at the receptor level. There are several physiologic effects. β-Blockers decrease myocardial contractility and HR.[11] β-Blockers also reduce plasma renin activity and as a result aldosterone se-cretion (for more detail on the renin-angio-tensin axis, see Ch. 9).[12] β-Blockers both de-crease MVO_2 and improve diastolic time by reducing HR, thus favorably affecting myo-cardial oxygen balance. Thus, β-blockers are also useful as antianginal agents.[13] Addition-ally, some β-blockers have potent local anes-thetic activity because of their membrane-sta-bilizing property (quinidinelike effect).[14]

Nonselective β-blockers increase broncho-motor tone and can precipitate broncho-spasm.[15] Some β-blockers have mild intrinsic sympathomimetic activity and subsequently produce less depression of CO.[16] In the dia-betic patient, β-blockers mask the symptoms of hypoglycemia, although frequent glucose assessments will mitigate this problem.[17]

Peripheral vasoconstriction due to β_2-blockade in the peripheral vasculature is often a problem in patients with peripheral vascular insufficiency. Some β-blockers are cardioselective (i.e., act predominantly on β_1-receptors in the heart) and thus have less anti-β_2 effect and cause less peripheral vaso-constriction and bronchoconstriction; such β-blockers include metoprolol, atenolol, and acebutolol.[18] Sudden withdrawal of β-block-ers can precipitate rebound adrenergic activ-ity, resulting in tachycardia, hypertension, dysrhythmias, and infarction.[19,20] β-Blockers should be continued throughout the periop-erative period unless the patient develops a new side-effect profile.[21]

CLINICAL INDICATIONS FOR β-BLOCKERS

Hypertension

Use of β-blockers is one of several strategies for initial therapy; β-blockers are particularly suitable for younger patients and those with angina pectoris. Combinations of β-blockers with diuretics, vasodilators, methyldopa, and α-blocking agents have all been used with benefit.[22]

Ischemic Heart Disease

The beneficial effect of β-blockers in IHD is in the ability of β-blockers to reduce MVO_2. They achieve this by reducing HR and de-pressing myocardial contractility. In acute myocardial infarction, early use of β-blockers reduces infarct size and decreases mortal-ity.[23,24] Although β-blockers are usually effec-tive in angina, about 20 percent of patients do not respond to any β-blocker, possibly be-cause of the unopposed α-vasoconstriction.[25] When β-blockers are withdrawn abruptly, an-gina may be exacerbated; such exacerbation usually occurs within 2 to 6 days following withdrawal.[19,20]

β-Blockers exert antianginal effects mainly by affecting myocardial oxygen balance. β-Blockers decrease MVO_2 by decreasing HR

Table 16-2. Diuretics

Generic Name	Class	Action	Factors to Watch For	Method of Administration
Bendroflumethiazide (bendrofluazide)	T	Inhibition of sodium and chloride resorption in the thick ALH and early DCT; increased potassium and HCO_3^- excretion, decreased Ca^{++} and uric acid excretion; duration of 6–12 hr	Increase in digoxin level, hemolytic anemia with methyldopa; exacerbation of hypokalemia with amphotericin; hypokalemia, adverse lipid effects, azotemia in renal insufficiency; exacerbation of gout, hyperglycemia, hypomagnesemia, hypochloremia, alkalosis, hyponatremia, hypercalcemia; contraindicated in hepatic coma	PO
Benzthiazide	T	Duration of 6–12 hr; similar to above	Similar to bendroflumethiazide	PO
Chlorthiazide	T	Duration of 6–12 hr; similar to above	Similar to bendroflumethiazide; also has a rare incidence of exfoliative dermatitis and Stevens-Johnson syndrome	IV & PO
Hydrochlorothiazide	T	Duration of 6–12 hr; similar to above	Similar to chlorthiazide	PO
Hydroflumethiazide	T	Duration of 6–12 hr; similar to above	Similar to chlorthiazide but no incidence of dermatitis	PO
Methyclothiazide	T	Duration of 24–48 hr; similar to above	Similar to chlorthiazide and hydrochlorthiazide	PO
Polythiazide	T	Duration of 24–48 hr; similar to above	Similar to chlorthiazide	PO
Trichlormethiazide	T	Duration of 24 hr, similar to above	Lichenoid dermatitis; dyspnea; similar to chlorthiazide	PO

322

Drug	Class	Mechanism	Effects	Route
Metolazone	QD	Same as above but may be more effective in patients with GFR < 20 ml·min^{-1}	Similar to thiazide group but less likely to produce hyperuricemia, hypokalemia and hypomagnesemia; different brands should not be substituted for one another (*not* same or equivalent)	PO
Quinethazone	QD	Same as above	Similar to thiazide group but is less likely to produce hypokalemia, hypomagnesemia, and uric acid retention	PO
Furosemide	L	Inhibition of sodium chloride transport at the ALH, PCT, and DCT	Can result in dramatic and rapid losses of electrolytes	PO
Ethacrynic acid	L	Same as above	Hypokalemia	PO, IV
Spironolactone	AA	Exchange of potassium for sodium at the DCT, competitive inhibitor	Hyperkalemia	PO, IV
Triamterene	AA	Same as above	Hyperkalemia	PO
Amiloride	AA	Direct effect on distal tubules	Hyperkalemia	PO
Indapamide	I	Identical to thiazide group but does not increase serum lipids	Much lower incidence of bone marrow depression	PO
Chlorthalimide	P	Similar to thiazide group	Similar to thiazide group	PO

Abbreviations: T, thiazide; GFR, glomerular filtration rate; DCT, distal convoluted tubule; ALH, ascending limb of the loop of Henle; PCT, proximal convoluted tubule; L, loop; AA, aldosterone antagonist; P, phthalimidine derivative; I, indoline.

Table 16-3. Antiadrenergic Drugs

Generic Name	Class	Action	Factors to Watch For	Method of Administration
Reserpine	ND	Depletes both central and peripheral stores of neuroamines	Orthostatic hypotension, sedation, restlessness, depression	PO
Guanethidine	ND	Same as above	Same as above	PO, IV
Methyldopa	CSI	Inhibition of central sympathetic tone and drive; requires 24 hr for full effect	Sedation, mucosal congestion, lupuslike syndrome, hemolytic anemia, thrombocytopenia	PO, IV
Clonidine	CSI	If transcutaneous form is introduced in postop period, 48 hr are required to reach steady-state level	*No* lupuslike syndromes, hemolytic anemia, or thrombocytopenia; sedation and mucosal congestion a problem; abrupt withdrawal may precipitate hypertension	PO, TTS
Propanolol	BB	Noncardioselective competitive inhibition of the β-adrenergic receptor[14,15], elimination half-life 3–6 hr	Bronchospasm, vascular insufficiency, heart block, reduction in hepatic blood flow (possibly important in patients with hepatic insufficiency); can reduce clearance of many drugs[10,13,35], potentiates the effects of Ca^{++} channel blockers, butyrophenones, hydralazine, phenothiazines, warfarin, acetominophen, disopyramide, lidocaine, ergot, prazosin, benzodiazepines; as a class BB, effects are increased by H_2-agonists, hydralazine, loop diuretics, phenothiazines, MAO inhibitors (bradycardia), propafenone, quinidine, quinolone antibiotics (ciprofloxacin)	PO, IV
Metoprolol	BB	Cardioselective inhibition; β_1 to β_2 selectivity ~30:1; better penetration into ischemic tissues[16], elimination half-life 3–4 hr	Excessive reduction in cardiac output	PO, IV
Acebutalol	BB	Cardioselective β_1 inhibition with mild ISA and MSA activity; half-life 8–12 hr; low protein binding and lipid solubility	Long half-life is possible problem in postoperative period; half-life of metabolite prolonged in renal failure; lowers total and LDL cholesterol	PO

Drug	Class	Description	Notes	Route
Atenolol	BB	Cardioselective inhibition; no ISA or MSA; half-life 6–9 hr; IV administration is 5 mg over 5 min	Long half-life[17]; half-life prolonged in renal failure (max dose 50 mg PO); does not potentiate hypoglycemia or delay recovery of blood glucose	PO, IV
Nadalol	BB	No ISA, poorly lipid soluble, 16–24 $T_{1/2\beta}$; effective half-life 6–9 hr; noncardioselective; low protein binding	If not stopped until day of surgery, can produce effects well into postoperative period; half-life increased in renal failure	PO
Esmolol	BB	Cardioselective, ultrashort duration of action; no ISA or MSA[18]; 55% protein binding; low lipid solubility	Trace amounts of methanol produced as part of enzymatic degradation	IV
Labetalol	BB, AB	Nonselective inhibition of α- and β-adrenergic receptors (ratio of 1:4 respectively); blood pressure and SVR decline concomitantly with dosage increases; stroke volume and cardiac output are minimally effected[20–23]	Hypotension; most β-blockers will increase serum lipids to one degree or another; may aggravate peripheral vascular disease; should be used with caution (if at all) in patients with cardiomyopathy; no reduction of dosage in renal failure	PO, IV
Penbutalol	BB	Nonselective inhibition of β-receptors; no MSA, mild ISA, high lipid solubility; hepatic conjugation and renal excretion; half-life 5 hr; high protein binding	Accumulation in renal failure	PO
Pindolol	BB	Nonselective β-blocker with mild MSA and marked ISA activity; moderate lipid solubility and 40% protein binding; half-life 3–4 hr; hepatic conjugation, renal excretion	Same as above, but pindolol does not significantly alter serum lipids	PO
Bisoprolol	BB	Selective β-blocker with no ISA or MSA: low lipid solubility and protein binding; half-life 9–12 hr; 50% renal excretion, 50% hepatic	Does not significantly alter serum lipids; same as BB class	PO
Betaxolol	BB	Selective β-blocker with mild MSA, no ISA, and low lipid solubility; protein binding 50% with half-life 14–22 hr; 85% hepatic, 15% renal	Same as BB class	PO
Carteolol	BB	Nonselective inhibition of β-receptors with no MSA, moderate ISA; half-life of 6 hr; 50–70% excreted unchanged in urine; low protein binding	Similar to BB group; half-life prolonged in renal failure; does not effect serum lipids	PO

(Continues)

Table 16-3. *(Continued)*

Generic Name	Class	Action	Factors to Watch For	Method of Administration
Sotalol	BB	Nonselective β-blocker with no ISA or MSA, low lipid solubility and *no* protein binding; excreted 100% renal; half-life 12 hr; useful for therapy of ventricular dysrhythmia	Bradycardia, decreased AV conduction, decreased cardiac output, hypotension; contraindicated in asthma and congenital long QT syndrome or in patients with torsade de pointes or receiving amiodarone; should be used with caution in hypokalemia and hypomagnesemia; prolonged half-life in renal failure	PO
Timolol	BB	Nonselective β-blocker; no ISA or MSA; useful in post-MI group; moderate lipid solubility and low protein binding; half-life 4 hr; 100% hepatic; prophylaxis for migraine	Same as BB group	PO
Prazosin	AB	Competitive inhibition of the α₁-adrenergic receptor at the postsyneptic receptor; does not increase heart rate or increase serum lipid levels; primarily reduces SVR	Excessive vasodilation syncope, mild orthostatic hypotension	PO
Terazosin	AB	Similar to prazosin	Same as prazosin	PO
Doxazosin	AB	Similar to prazosin	Same as prazosin	PO
Phentolamine	AB	Nonselective α-blocker	Reflex tachycardia	PO, IV
Phenoxy-benzamine	AB	Similar to phentolamine	Similar to phentolamine	PO

Abbreviations: ND, neuroamine depletion; CSI, central sympathetic inhibition; BB, β-blocker; ISA, intrinsic sympathominetic activity; AB, α-blocker; MSA, membrane-stabilizing activity; MAO, monoamine oxidase; LDL, low-density lipoprotein.

and force of contractility. Reduction in HR increases diastolic coronary flow. However, β-blockers may aggravate anginal episodes in some patients with vasospastic angina and should be used with caution.[25]

Cardiac Dysrhythmias
β-Blockers may be used in both supraventricular and ventricular dysrhythmias.[26] β-Blockers are particularly effective in dysrhythmias caused by increased circulating catecholamines (i.e., as a result of pheochromocytoma, anxiety, and exercise) or by increased sensitivity to catecholamines (thyrotoxicosis).[27] In digitalis toxicity, β-blockers may control tachydysrhythmias in the absence of a heart block.[28]

Hypertrophic Cardiomyopathy
β-Blockers reduce dynamic obstruction and decrease pressure gradients across hypertrophic subaortic stenosis by depressing the systolic function of the heart.[29] Regression of ventricular hypertrophy in cardiomyopathy may not occur but regression of ventricular hypertrophy due to hypertension can occur with β-blockers.[30]

CALCIUM ANTAGONISTS

Calcium antagonists are a heterogenous group of drugs that have similar pharmacologic actions. There are three different groups of drugs, which are described in Table 16-4.

Hemodynamic Effects
Nifedipine is a potent arterial dilator with minimal venodilating properties.[31] The intrinsic negative inotropic effect is offset to some degree by a decrease in SVR, leading to an increase in HR and CO.[32] Dihydropyridines as a class are most useful as antihypertensive agents.

Verapamil is a less potent arterial dilator than nifedipine and has predominant effects on the conduction system of the heart. Verapamil has more negative inotropic effects than nifedipine or diltiazem, especially in patients with pre-existing ventricular dysfunction.[33,34] Diltiazem causes less peripheral vasodilation than nifedipine or verapamil and produces a less negative inotropic effect when compared to verapamil.[35] There are questions regarding their long-term use in patients with coronary artery disease. The nonspecific coronary vasodilating properties may dispose those patients to coronary steal. Alternative explanations invoke reflex sympathetic activation following vasodilation with each dose (see below).

CLINICAL INDICATIONS FOR CALCIUM ANTAGONISTS

Coronary Blood Flow
Calcium antagonists are potent coronary vasodilators. Increases in CBF are seen with all calcium antagonists. Nifedipine[36] and nicardipine[37] are potent coronary vasodilators, es-

Table 16-4. Calcium Antagonists[a]

Drug	Class	Arterial[b]	Venous[b]	Negative Inotrope	CBF
Nifedipine	DHP	+ + +	+	±	+ + +
Nimodipine	DHP	+ +	+	±	+
Verapamil	PAA	+	±	+ +	+
Diltiazem	BTP	+ +	+	+	+ +
Nicardipine	DHP	+ + +	±	±	+ + +

Abbreviations: DHP, dihydropyridine derivatives; PAA, phenylalkylamines; BTP, benzothiazipines; CBF, coronary blood flow.

[a] Calcium antagonists block the slow channel in the conduction pathway and the muscle cell.

[b] Arterial and venous reflect relative activity on these beds as dose CBF. The production of possible concomitant negative inotropic effects are displayed.

4

pecially in epicardial vessels, which are prone to vasospasm. Diltiazem is effective in blocking coronary artery vasoconstriction caused by several mediators and drugs.[38,39] A recent meta-analysis in patients with known coronary artery disease has clouded this issue by noting an increase in mortality in patients treated with the short-acting forms of the dihydropyridines. The primary use of calcium antagonists as chronic anti-ischemic therapy needs further evaluation. A firm recommendation against their use in the acute postoperative period is unwarranted.

Antidysrhythmic Activity
Verapamil[40] and diltiazem[41] slow conduction velocity and prolong the effective refractory period (ERP) of the sinoatrial (SA) and atrioventricular (AV) nodes. They do not alter the ERP of atrial, ventricular, or Purkinje tissue. Verapamil is useful in the treatment of re-entrant supraventricular tachydysrhythmias (SVT). Nifedipine can enhance nodal conduction and has no antidysrhythmic properties.[42]

Antianginal Effects
The mechanism of the antianginal effect of calcium antagonists is a reduction in MVO_2 by depression of contractility and an increase in CBF by vasodilation of coronary and collateral vessels. All calcium antagonists have been proven effective in reducing angina in controlled trials.[43–45] Additionally, nifedipine[36] and nicardipine[37] have been shown to be effective in reversing coronary spasm. Combinations of nitroglycerin and calcium antagonists may be beneficial in reversing and preventing coronary spasm in variant angina.[36,46] In unstable angina, calcium antagonists have favorable effects on all three occlusive processes (i.e., vasospasm, accelerated atherosclerosis, and enhanced platelet aggregation) and are effective in relieving symptoms.[47] However, large meta-analyses demonstrate an increase in mortality with the use of the short-acting dihydropyridines (Williams JP, personal communication).[48–50]

SUMMARY
Calcium antagonists have a wide variety of clinical indications. Their use in hypertension is mainly dependent on their vasodilatory properties. They are well tolerated, do not alter exercise tolerance, and are versatile. Their wide treatment spectrum is useful in treating patients with all types of hypertension, which accounts for their rapid rise to pre-eminence in the U.S. pharmaceutical market. Recent analyses questioning their applicability in IHD may require further substantiation before firm recommendations against their use are implemented.

DIRECT VASODILATORS
When diuretics are not sufficient to control the pulmonary symptoms of CHF, the addition of vasodilators is often beneficial (Table 16-5). Vasodilators such as nitroprusside and direct smooth muscle relaxants (e.g., hydralazine)[51] cause reduction in afterload and increase CO. Nitrates (isosorbide and nitroglycerin [NTG]) and nitroprusside are also direct smooth muscle relaxants. The mechanism of action is thought to involve the release of intermediate metabolites such as nitric oxide (NO) or s-nitrosothiol, which subsequently produces smooth muscle relaxation through activation of adenylate cyclase and cyclic guanosine monophosphate (cGMP).[52]

Vasodilators are usually classified by their site of action; they range from almost pure venodilators to pure arteriolar dilators. Some drugs have mixed activity. Vasodilators that act predominantly on venous capacitance vessels (e.g., NTG) primarily reduce preload and affect CO only slightly. Those drugs acting on the arteriolar bed (e.g., hydralazine) decrease SVR and increase CO. The mixed drugs (e.g., nitroprusside) generally decrease both filling pressures and SVR with similarly mixed effects upon CO. In addition, venodilators help to redistribute pulmonary blood into the periphery, thus ameliorating pulmonary congestion.[53]

Table 16-5. Vasodilators

Generic Name	Class	Action	Factors to Watch For	Method of Administration
Hydralazine	ND	NO donor that directly relaxes vascular smooth muscle	Fluid retention, headache, reflex tachycardia, lupuslike syndrome	IV, PO
Minoxidil	ND	Similar to hydralazine	Similar to hydralazine, but no lupus-like syndrome Hypertrichosis	PO, IV

Abbreviation: ND, nitroso donor; NO, nitric oxide.

Direct vasodilators that act predominantly on the capacitance vessels (e.g., NTG) also decrease ventricular filling. These venodilators[54] not only reduce preload but thereby myocardial oxygen demand. They are useful in the treatment of congestive cardiac failure following myocardial ischemia or infarction.[55]

Hydralazine

Hydralazine, a nitroso compound, has been in use for over 30 years. It is generally administered concomitantly with a β-blocker. This is to inhibit the reflex tachycardia associated with administration of hydralazine alone. It is less commonly used in contemporary practice. Hydralazine, similar to most nitroso compounds, causes direct smooth muscle relaxation by acting as an NO donor, thereby decreasing SVR.[56] Hydralazine preferentially dilates arterioles more than veins. The major problems with hydralazine are reflex tachycardia, headache, and the appearance of a lupuslike syndrome when used in higher dosages for prolonged periods of time.[57]

Minoxidil

Minoxidil is a potent vasodilator with a mode of action similar to that of hydralazine (including the reflex increase in HR).[58] The side effects are fluid retention and hypertrichosis. Minoxidil increases sodium reabsorption in the proximal tubules and is usually combined with a diuretic to prevent fluid retention.[59]

Nitrates

NTG predominantly causes venodilation in lower doses and rapidly diminishing arteriolar dilation at higher doses.[60] NTG is a potent epicardial coronary vasodilator in both normal and diseased vessels.[61,62] The improvement in blood flow to the subendocardium is secondary to improvement in collateral flow and reductions in left ventricular end-diastolic pressure (LVEDP).[63]

Sublingual NTG (0.15 to 0.6-mg tablets) achieves blood levels adequate to cause hemodynamic changes within several minutes. The bioavailability of sublingual NTG is approximately 80 percent because this route of administration bypasses the high first-pass metabolism (90 percent) of the liver. Plasma half-life of sublingual NTG is 4 to 7 minutes.[64] NTG spray has pharmacokinetics and dynamics similar to sublingual tablets[65] (Table 16-6).

Two percent NTG ointment is readily absorbed through skin with slightly longer lasting effects. Adequate blood levels are reached within 20 to 30 minutes and the duration of action is 4 to 6 hours.[66] NTG patches contain either liquid nitroglycerin or nitroglycerin bonded on a polymer gel; in both forms NTG slowly released to the skin through a semipermeable membrane. Therapeutic blood levels are reached within 20 to 30 minutes and steady state reached after 2 hours with a maximum 24-hour duration.[67]

Intravenous NTG is available in a 5-mg ·

Table 16-6.   Antianginal Agents

Type	Action	Dose
Nitrates	Coronary vasodilation, preload reduction, mild antiplatelet effect, mild reduction in afterload; intravenous administration is preferred in critical care	*IV:* $0.1–5$ $\mu g \cdot kg^{-1} \cdot min^{-1}$ *Oral:* 5–40 mg every 6 hours *Sublingual:* 0.15–0.6 mg $\times$ 1 or 2 *Inhalational:* 0.3 ml, 1–3 inhalations *Topical:* 1–2 inches of nitropaste 6°–8° *Translingual:* 0.4-mg metered dose, 1–2 sprays *Transmucosal:* 1 mg every 3–5 hr *Transdermal:* 0.1–0.6 mg for 12 hr every day
Dipyridamole	Antithrombotic effect; FDA has announced plans to withdraw approval for long-term therapy of angina	*Oral:* 25–75 mg TID
β-Blockers	Reduction in myocardial oxygen consumption, decrease in heart rate	See Table 16-3
Calcium antagonists	Coronary vasodilation, afterload reduction	See Table 16-4

ml^{-1} solution of 70 percent alcohol. Therapeutic blood levels are achieved within minutes but marked systemic hypotension can occur.[68] Dose is adjusted according to the volume status of the patient and titrated to the desired effect. The infusion is started usually at 5 to 10 $\mu g \cdot min^{-1}$ initially and doses up to 75 to 150 $\mu g \cdot min^{-1}$ may be needed. The offset of effects is rapid (2 to 5 min) after discontinuation.

Furosemide

Intravenous furosemide, apart from producing diuresis, also causes mild venodilation. Boluses of furosemide or an intravenous infusion of furosemide are especially valuable in patients who are on diuretics preoperatively as well as in patients with renal dysfunction.[69,70]

ANGIOTENSIN-CONVERTING ENZYME INHIBITORS

The renin-angiotensin system (RAS) is involved in many types of hypertension and is currently the center of attention in the control of blood pressure. Angiotensin-converting enzyme (ACE) inhibitors produce a competitive inhibition that prevents the release of angiotensin II, thus preventing secretion of aldosterone. The antihypertensive effect, however, is more complex, as the RAS is widely distributed in the body and is present in tissue as well as plasma (Fig. 16-1). It appears that a part of the antihypertensive influence is related to an increase in vasodilatory bradykinin, the breakdown of which is enhanced by angiotensin II. (For further discussion of the RAS, see Ch. 9).

Since the introduction of the first orally available drug, captopril, ACE inhibitors rapidly became mainstay therapy in many clinical situations, including hypertension and CHF. Their increasing popularity is associated with the fact that they appear to reverse some of the long-term cardiac changes associated with hypertension and CHF. However, sporadic anecdotal reports of renal failure occurring after surgery in patients taking ACE inhibitors prompted some authorities to advocate stopping them preoperatively and substituting other drugs such as calcium antagonists. This practice has not found wide acceptance in the United States.

All ACE inhibitors are used orally in lowering blood pressure in essential hyperten-

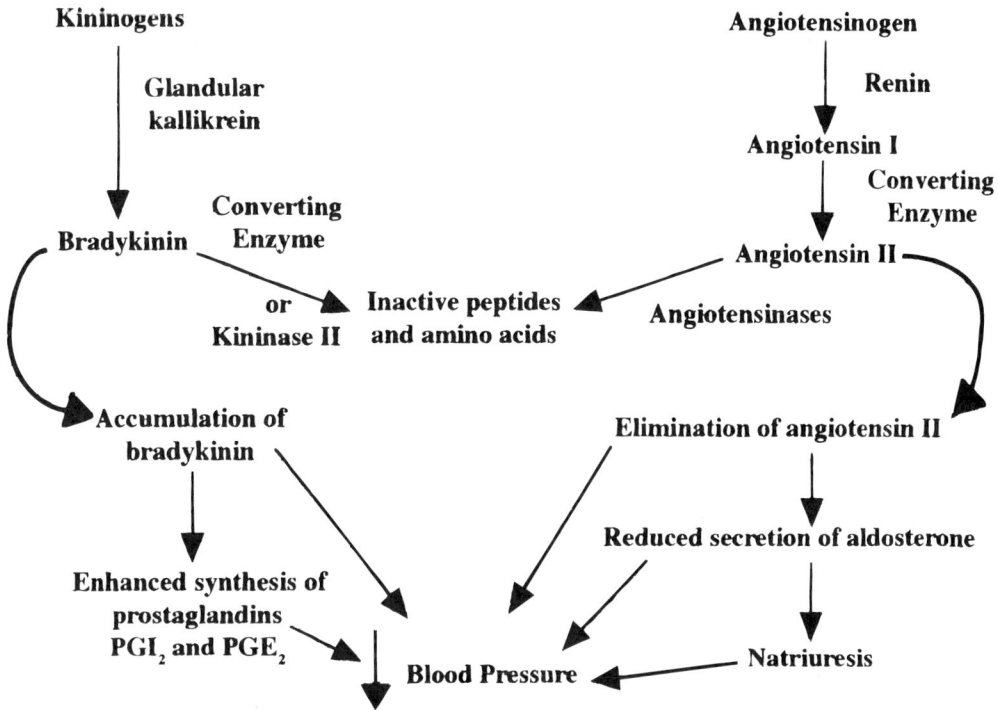

Fig. 16-1. Location of active enzyme systems inhibited by angiotensin-converting enzyme (ACE) inhibitors. ACE inhibitors produce a reduction of blood pressure through both a decrease in the action of angiotensin (natriuresis and vasodilation) as well as an increase in the action of bradykinin (increased production of vasodilatory prostaglandins (PGEs) and direct vasodilation from bradykinin).

sion.[71] They are characterized hemodynamically by a decrease in blood pressure secondary to a decrease in SVR with little effect on CO. Plasma renin activity increases significantly because of negative feedback. There is also a marked decrease in aldosterone secretion. ACE inhibitors may also act directly on the vascular smooth muscle to produce vasodilation.[72] Enalaprilat is the only intravenous formulation available (Table 16-7).

INOTROPIC AGENTS

Catecholamines activate β_1-receptors in the myocardium and increase intracellular cyclic adenosine monophosphate (cAMP). This second messenger in turn increases intracellular calcium. Phosphodiesterase (PDE) inhibitors eliminate the catalysis of cAMP by inhibiting the isoenzyme III of PDE, thereby increasing intracellular cAMP independent of β-receptor activation. Digoxin increases intracellular calcium by inhibiting sodium- and potassium-activated adenosine triphosphatase (Na$^+$, k$^+$-ATPase) and exchanging intracellular sodium for extracellular calcium. Increasing intracellular calcium during systole is the final common pathway for all inotropic drugs.[73] Catecholamines and PDE inhibitors individually or in combination are commonly used to augment myocardial contractility in the intensive care period.

Cardiac Glycosides

Although cardiac glycosides have been in use for a long time, it is now well recognized that afterload reduction is the most beneficial pharmacologic maneuver in CHF (i.e., by helping to lower the impedance to ejection of the failing myocardium).

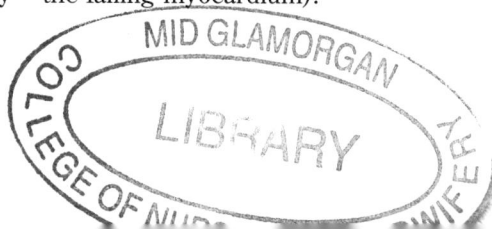

Table 16-7. Angiotensin-Converting Enzyme Inhibitors

Generic Name	Class	Action	Factors to Watch For	Method of Administration
Captopril	ACEI	Competative inhibition of the enzyme-converting angiotensinogen to aniotensin; may have direct smooth muscle relaxant properties; poorly understood	Angioedema, proteinuria, glomerulonephritis; marked first dose effect with CHF and renovascular hypertension	PO
Enalapril	ACEI	Same as captopril; however, enalapril is a prodrug and must be converted to its active congener enalaprilat	Similar to captopril but with less marked effects	PO, IV
Lisinopil	ACEI	Longer acting compound similar to captopril; may have mild negative inotropic activity	Same as above	PO

Abbreviation: ACEI, angiotensin-converting enzyme inhibitor; CHF, congestive heart failure.

Cardiac glycosides are no longer extensively used in the management of failing contractility, although when such failure is associated with atrial fibrillation, cardiac glycosides are useful in reducing the rate of ventricular response.[74,75] Digoxin remains the most commonly used glycoside. Digoxin has a positive inotropic action by competitive inhibition of membrane-bound Na^+, K^+-ATPase, producing high intracellular levels of sodium. The intracellular sodium is exchanged for extracellular calcium. High intracellular calcium levels allow increased binding of the contractile proteins actin and myosin, thus enhancing the force of myocardial contraction.[76]

Digoxin also has important effects on the conduction tissue. Digoxin delays conduction through both the AV node and Purkinje system.[77] The duration of the action potential is shortened. Digoxin also has a vagotonic effect, thus reducing the atrial refractory period but prolonging the refractory period of the AV node. These effects lead to a reduction in the ventricular rate in atrial fibrillation. Automaticity in Purkinje cells is enhanced; in digoxin toxicity this can lead to a variety of dysrhythmias that are potentiated by hypokalemia.

Pharmacokinetics Digoxin is absorbed well orally with a bioavailability of approximately 85 percent and has a large volume of distribution. It is highly protein bound, giving rise to potential drug interactions. Approximately 90 percent of digoxin is excreted unchanged in the urine with an elimination half-life of 36 hours.[78] Digoxin has a narrow therapeutic ratio. Therapeutic plasma levels of digoxin are 0.5 to 2 ng · ml^{-1} and toxicity appears at 2.5 ng · ml^{-1} or greater. Digoxin levels should be monitored carefully in both acute and chronic administration and the doses should be reduced in renal insufficiency.[79] Concomitant administration of quinidine,[80] amiodarone,[81] or verapamil[82] increase serum digoxin concentrations.

Adrenergic Agonists

Adrenergic agonists commonly used in the perioperative period are epinephrine, norepinephrine, dopamine, dobutamine, and isoproterenol (see Table 16-9).

Epinephrine Epinephrine is an endogenous catecholamine synthesized and excreted by the adrenal medulla. It is a potent activator of α- and β-receptors released during the sympathetic response. At low intravenous infusion rates (less than .03 $\mu g \cdot kg^{-1} \cdot min^{-1}$) β effects predominate. In middle dosage ranges (.03 to .15 $\mu g \cdot kg^{-1} \cdot min^{-1}$) both α and β effects predominate. Epinephrine preferentially dilates skeletal muscle via β-receptor stimulation, while constricting splanchnic, renal, and cutaneous vessels. In lower doses epinephrine is a potent bronchodilator, and nebulized preparations are used for reactive airway disease as well as bronchospasm associated with anaphylaxis. Epinephrine is useful perioperatively in certain cardiac surgery patients who may benefit from its positive inotropic and chronotropic effects, as well as its direct vasoconstricting actions. However, because of the chronotropic effects, it may be detrimental to the patient with cardiogenic shock or ongoing ischemia. Because epinephrine is dysrhythmogenic, this drug should be used cautiously in patients recieving those potent inhalational agents that sensitize the myocardium to its effects (e.g., halodane).

Norepinephrine Norepinephrine is the chemical precursor of epinephrine. It is released by postganglionic nerves in the adrenergic sympathetic system. Norepinephrine is a potent α- and β_1- agonist with weak effects on β_2-receptors. Intravenous infusion produces elevations in systolic and diastolic arterial pressure mediated by peripheral vasoconstriction. Its direct chronotropic effects are mitigated by the compensatory vagal response to increased arterial pressure, and thus HR remains relatively stable with an increase in SV. Deleterious effects of norepinephrine include splanchnic and renal vasoconstriction, as well as coronary artery vasoconstriction. In the patient with unstable angina or ongoing ischemia, norepinephrine may worsen oxygen delivery to the myocardium while increasing myocardial work load via elevated afterload and preload. However, recent reports indicate that lower infusion rates of norepinephrine may produce better oxygen delivery/consumption profiles. An additional complication related to its use is local tissue necrosis when peripheral infiltration occurs.

Dopamine Dopamine is the chemical precursor of norepinephrine and epinephrine. It is present in the adrenal medulla, sympathetic postganglionic neurons, and central nervous system. Dopamine stimulates α-, β-, and dopaminergic receptors. At low levels (1 to 5 $\mu g \cdot kg \cdot min^{-1}$) renal, splanchnic, and coronary vasodilation occur, mediated through dopamine-1 receptors. At this dosage range β effects also predominate, producing positive inotropic and chronotropic effects as well as peripheral vasodilation. Additionally, dopamine stimulates norepinephrine release in the middle dosage ranges. At higher dosage ranges (7 to 10 $\mu g \cdot kg^{-1} \cdot min^{-1}$) α effects become more pronounced. Infusion rates greater than 10 $\mu g \cdot kg^{-1} min^{-1}$ produce predominantly α stimulation, which presumably negates the vasodilation derived from dopaminergic receptor activation. Because dopamine administration produces increases in glomerular filtration and renal blood flow, it has been widely used in patients with renal dysfunction, multisystem organ failure, and shock.

In a study of patients with renal insufficiency, however, dopamine-induced increases in glomerular filtration rate and renal flow were much less pronounced than in normal patients.[83] Furthermore, there has been no clear documentation of improvement in outcome of renal function after dopamine administration. Finally, dopamine crosses readily into the pituitary and suppresses the release of prolactin, leutinizing, and growth hormones.[84]

Dobutamine Dobutamine is a synthetic inotrope structurally related to dopamine and isoproterenol. Dobutamine has a greater affinity for β_1- than β_2-receptors. It has very weak α-stimulating properties, and virtually no dopaminergic activity. Dobutamine has potent inotropic effects on the heart. However, it has less chronotropic effect than isoproterenol. Thus, it increases inotropic state with minimal changes on HR or peripheral vascular resistance. Dobutamine increases SV and CO in patients with CHF or ongoing myocardial ischemia. Additionally, dobutamine inhibits hypoxic pulmonary vasoconstriction and produces some direct pulmonary vasodilation, making it a useful drug in patients with right ventricular dysfunction or elevated pulmonary artery pressures. Tachydysrhythmias can occur with dobutamine administration, especially in the higher dose ranges (greater than 10 to 15 $\mu g \cdot kg^{-1} \cdot min^{-1}$).

Isoproterenol Isoproterenol is a potent β-agonist with virtually no α effects. Through β_1 effects, isoproterenol increases cardiac contractility and rate. Through β_2 effects, isoproterenol lowers SVR and pulmonary vascular resistance. Because of its pronounced chronotropic effect, isoproterenol is primarily used to increase HR in patients with bradysrhythmias or heart block. It is less useful in patients with CHF or shock, due to its peripheral vasodilatory actions, which may lower arterial pressure. Additionally, tachydysrhythmias frequently occur with administration of this drug. Because it markedly increases the inotropic and chronotropic state, thus increasing myocardial oxygen requirements, it is not appropriate in patients with myocardial ischemia. Via β_2 stimulation, isoproterenol produces bronchodilation, making it useful in patients with reactive airway disease and concomitant cardiovascular disease.

Phosphodiesterase Inhibitors
PDE inhibitors inhibit the breakdown of cAMP, thereby causing accumulation of cAMP. Amrinone, milrinone, and enoximone all cause positive inotropic action coupled with peripheral vasodilation (inodilators).[85,86] However, their beneficial effects with long-term use are unclear. They are useful in short-term therapy in critically ill patients who do not respond to standard therapy. A major drawback to their use is an increase in platelet activation and consumption. This frequently results in a dose-related decrease in platelet count, but rarely necessitates platelet transfusion. This side effect is especially troublesome when PDE inhibitors are used in combination with mechanical circulatory support.

Pharmacokinetics in Cardiac Disease
PATHOPHYSIOLOGIC CONSIDERATIONS
The pharmacodynamics and pharmacokinetics of most drugs are characterized in healthy volunteers or during the stable phase of a disease in patients. Changes in drug disposition and action occur in pathophysiologic states such as CHF and in the critically ill. CHF may be regarded as the prototypical heart disease in which there are specific pathophysiologic changes with important pharmacologic implications. A discussion of these changes will serve to define important principles in understanding strategies of therapy in the perioperative cardiac patient.

In CHF, CO is reduced. Compensatory mechanisms induce increased sympathetic activity, resulting in chronically high sympathetic tone and elevated circulating catecholamine concentrations. The renin-angiotensin aldosterone system is activated, leading to vasoconstriction and sodium and water retention.

As CHF progresses, the myocardial catecholamine stores are depleted. Sympathetic nerve endings in the heart fail to synthesize, store, and release catecholamines. β-Receptors exhibit a decreased response to catecholamines (down-regulation) in CHF and in patients given prolonged infusions of catecholamines.[87]

Clinically, these changes lead to decreased

perfusion of kidney, liver, and gut, resulting in altered uptake, distribution, and elimination of drugs. In addition to the reduction in renal blood flow, intrarenal redistribution of blood flow from the outer cortex to medulla occurs in CHF, with further impairment of drug clearance.[88] In addition, in CHF right heart pressure is elevated, which causes hepatic and gastrointestinal congestion leading to alterations in drug disposition.[89] These factors alter pharmacokinetics of drugs in CHF to a varying extent depending on the type of the drug and mode of elimination.[90]

PHARMACOKINETIC CONSIDERATIONS

Absorption

Most drug absorption from the intestinal tract takes place in the upper jejunum. Reduced gastric emptying alters drug delivery into the upper small intestine and thus alters the rate of absorption of drugs like furosemide, bumetanide and digoxin. In addition, gut edema may decrease absorption of drugs in CHF.[91] Absorption from muscle depends on the physicochemical properties of the drug and muscle blood flow. Muscle blood flow is decreased in severe heart failure and absorption of drugs is impaired.[92,93]

Distribution

Some proportion of orally administered drugs is metabolized, both in the gut mucosa and in the liver, and such drugs may not reach the systemic circulation (reduced bioavailability). The clearance of drugs with a high hepatic extraction ratio (e.g., organic nitrates, morphine, prazosin, and hydralazine) depends on hepatic perfusion.[94] Hence, higher concentrations of these drugs can be expected in CHF due to reduced hepatic perfusion. The apparent V_d is a theoretical volume of plasma into which a drug is distributed to achieve the measured plasma concentration. V_d thus helps to define appropriate loading dose. The V_d of several drugs (e.g., lidocaine) is reduced in heart failure and loading doses may need to be appropriately reduced.[95]

Clearance and Excretion

The clearance of a drug is the volume of plasma cleared of the drug per unit time. Some water soluble drugs are excreted unchanged in urine but most drugs are lipid soluble and are metabolized in the liver to water soluble compounds before being excreted by the kidneys. In CHF there is a reduction of hepatic blood flow and venous congestion. Hepatic venous congestion can impair microsomal function and affect drugs with low extraction (e.g., warfarin).[96] The renal clearance is the net result of filtration and active secretion or reabsorption in the tubules. Glomerular filtration is usually reduced in heart failure and elimination of renally cleared drugs is impaired. For many drugs the decrease in clearance is associated with a reduced V_d such that the elimination half-life may not be very different from that in a healthy subject.[97] Because hepatic blood flow and enzyme activity are affected more than renal function in heart failure, drug toxicity is more likely to occur with drugs that are metabolized in the liver than with those that are eliminated solely by the kidneys.[95]

DRUG-SPECIFIC ALTERATIONS

Lidocaine

Lidocaine, a class I antidysrhythmic drug, has a high hepatic extraction ratio and is rapidly metobolized in the liver. Thus, the clearance is flow dependent. When CO is decreased, its clearance is reduced due to decreased hepatic blood flow. Thomson and colleagues[97] also reported that the V_d at steady state (V_{dSS}) and clearance are reduced in patients with CHF, and plasma drug concentrations were found to be in an inverse relationship with the cardiac index.[97] Thus, is it is advisable to decrease both the loading dose as well as infusion of lidocaine in patients with a reduced cardiac index. Lidocaine concentrations are also found to be increased in myocardial infarction with a decrease in clearance regardless of cardiac index. This is attributed to an increase in acute phase proteins, especially α_1-acid glycoprotein, with a consequent increase in lidocaine protein binding leading to a decrease in V_d.[98]

Procainamide

Procainamide produces higher blood levels than normal when given in standard doses in patients with CHF. About one-half the administered dose is exececreted unchanged in urine and the remainder is metabolized prior to excretion. One of the metabolites, N-acetylprocainamide, has antidysrhythmic activity and will accumulate in conditions of renal impairment. Koch-Weser and Klein[99] demonstrated that steady state concentrations were higher during renal impairment. They also reported that the V_d of procainamide was decreased in patients with CHF compared with healthy subjects. As a result, higher drug levels are expected in patients with a low cardiac index, and loading doses should be reduced appropriately in such patients.[100]

Digoxin

Digoxin absorption is slower and peak concentrations are lower in patients with CHF compared with healthy subjects.[101,102] Digoxin has an extensive V_d and most of the dose is excreted unchanged in urine. Digoxin is susceptible to the renal effects of CHF. With a narrow therapeutic index, it is mandatory to monitor digoxin levels since renal clearance is lower in patients with CHF.[103] However, the dose of digoxin should be reduced only in the presence of renal impairment, as there is little evidence that heart failure per se alters the elimination half-life or clearance of digoxin.[102]

Nitrates

Nitrates are vasodilators commonly used in heart failure (both acute heart failure and CHF), ischemic heart disease, and for blood pressure control perioperatively. Some patients exhibit lower total clearance of NTG in CHF. However, they do not show toxic levels when titrated closely to hemodynamic end points.[104] Variations in bioavailability with the transdermal route of administration of NTG has been observed in CHF.[105] NTG has a short duration of action with a half-life of 1.9 minutes. Acute tolerance can be a major problem with NTG. The pharmacokinetics of the longer acting nitrates, isosorbide mononitrate and dinitrate, appear to be unaltered in the presence of CHF, hepatic disease,[106] or during digestion.[106]

The hemodynamic effects of NTG have been extensively reviewed in patients with acute and chronic CHF.[53,107,108] It has predominant affect on large veins and a lesser affect on arteries.[109] In patients with CHF, there are consistent decreases in pulmonary arterial pressure (PAP), pulmonary capillary wedge pressure (PCWP), central venous pressure (CVP), and pulmonary vascular resistance (PVR). NTG also causes mild pulmonary arterial vasodilation.

Hydralazine

Hydralazine is mainly metabolized in the liver by acetylation, the degree of which appears to be genetically determined. Some individuals are rapid acetylators compared with others. The bioavailability of the orally administered drug is less in rapid acetylators.[110] In patients with CHF, oral absorption is not affected but elimination half-life is increased.[111] Impaired hepatic metabolism in CHF may reduce hydralazine acetylation. Interindividual variability upon oral dosage is observed and oral doses are higher due to low bioavailability in rapid acetylators. Clearance after intravenous administration appears to be similar to that in healthy subjects.[111]

Diuretics

Diuretics and sodium restriction serve to activate the RAS and increase afterload. Reduced peak plasma concentrations and delayed peak concentrations are observed with furosemide in patients with CHF.[112] Absorption, however, is unaffected. The diuretic response appears to be blunted and may be due to the reduced delivery of the drug to the renal tubules in CHF.[112] Bumetinide shows similar altered pharmacokinetics in CHF.[113]

Phosphodiesterase Inhibitors
PDE inhibitors are drugs that inhibit phosphodiesterase isoenzyme III, the enzyme that catalyses the breakdown of cAMP in cardiac and smooth muscle. The clinical effects are an increase in myocardial contractility and marked peripheral vasodilation. The clearance of amrinone ranges from 0.28 to 0.42 L $\cdot$ hr^{-1} $\cdot$ kg^{-1} in healthy individuals but in CHF it is decreased to 0.12 to 0.15 L $\cdot$ hr^{-1} $\cdot$ kg^{-1}, resulting in a prolonged elimination half-life. The infusion rate should be monitored closely and adjusted according to hemodynamic response. Milrinone clearance is also decreased and the elimination half-life prolonged.[110] Dosages of both milrinone and amrinone should be titrated closely to hemodynamic responses in CHF. Chronic use of amrinone and milrinone in CHF has been associated with increased mortality and at present they are used mainly in the postoperative period for myocardial insufficiency.[114]

Angiotensin-Converting Enzyme Inhibitors
One of the compensatory mechanisms in cardiac failure is activation of the renin-angiotensin-aldosterone system. Angiotensin II produces vasoconstriction, thereby maintaining systemic blood pressure. It also stimulates aldosterone secretion, leading to sodium and water retention (see Ch. 9).

Although vasoconstriction may lead to reduced organ blood flow and renal hypoperfusion, vasoconstriction of postglomerular capillaries helps to restore renal perfusion and keep it above the threshold of autoregulation.[115] The intrarenal actions of angiotensin II help to adjust intraglomerular pressure in order to maintain glomerular filtration.

Blockade of the RAS in severe heart failure may therefore interfere critically with the homeostatic mechanisms of renal excretion.[116] Hence, the beneficial effect of unloading the heart by reducing SVR and improving renal plasma flow are balanced by a potentially harmful effect of unloading the kidney by preferentially reducing the outflow resistance of the glomerulus. However, the development of functional renal insufficiency is unlikely and is a rare cause for withdrawal of ACE inhibitors when the following precautions are taken during chronic drug therapy:[117]

1. The initial dose of ACE inhibitor has to be reduced with increasing severity of heart failure.
2. The concomitant administration of inhibitors of prostaglandin synthesis (e.g., nonsteroidal anti-inflammatory drugs) appears to be associated with a high risk of renal impairment.

Captopril Changes in the pharmacokinetics of captopril in heart failure are related to secondary renal dysfunction. Deterioration in renal function may occur during chronic therapy due to the attenuation of angiotensin-II–mediated vasoconstriction of the efferent glomerular arterioles that maintain glomerular filtration.[118]

Enalapril The bioavailability of enalaprilat (the active metabolite produced from enalapril) is reduced in CHF due to a reduction in the rate of absorption and decreased hydrolysis. Peak plasma concentrations and the onset of clinical effect therefore tend to be delayed.[119] Both enalapril and enalaprilat are excreted primarily in the urine, and plasma concentrations tend to be higher in the presence of renal impairment.

Lisinopril Lisinopril is the lysine analog of enalaprilat, the active metabolite of enalapril. It is active after oral administration and does not require biotransformation to induce pharmacologic effects. Compared with healthy volunteers, absorption in patients with heart failure is reduced,[120] but plasma concentrations are higher, suggesting a reduced V_d. As a result, the onset of action is delayed, but more prolonged.[121]

CARDIOPULMONARY BYPASS AND PHARMACOKINETICS

The institution of CPB is accompanied by profound physiologic changes that have important pharmacokinetic implications. Changes in blood pressure leading to alterations in regional blood flow, hemodilution, and hypothermia all contribute to alterations in the pharmacokinetics of drugs. Studies of the pharmacokinetics of drugs during CPB are difficult both to undertake and evaluate. Many attempts at pharmacokinetic evaluation and modeling assumed a consistent steady state for the period of the study. However, there are continuous changes, both during and after bypass surgery, due to the release of vasoactive endogenous substances (see Ch. 5), fluctuation of the metabolic state, changes in temperature, and so on.

If a substance is given by intravenous bolus or as an intravenous infusion that is discontinued either during or shortly after bypass surgery, observations over a period several times longer than the half-life of the substance are needed to measure the distribution and elimination parameters correctly. Pharmacokinetic studies usually use time-averaged values over a period of study.[122] For statistical accuracy, the study period should be at least twice the duration of the longest half-life estimated; it is difficult to estimate clearance of drugs on bypass, most of whose elimination half-lives far exceed that of the average bypass duration.[123]

Physiologic Considerations

CBP is accompanied by profound physiologic changes apart from those induced by surgery and anesthesia that may alter the pharmacokinetics of many drugs.[124] Drug distribution can be altered by both hemodilution and a decrease in protein binding. Elimination kinetics are also altered secondary to changes in hepatic and renal function during CPB (Table 16-8).

Metabolism of drugs is depressed in general. In the case of neuromuscular blockers, hypothermia prolongs the action, probably by a decrease in local acetylcholine synthesis as well as by reduced clearance due to decreased RBF.[125]

Pharmacokinetic implications of using pulsatile versus nonpulsatile flow during CPB are unclear. Hynynen and colleagues[126] demonstrated no significant alterations in thiopental pharmacokinetics using pulsatile or nonpulsatile flow during CPB.

Table 16-8. Pharmacokinetic Changes During Cardiopulmonary Bypass

Parameter	Pathophysiologic Change	Effects on Pharmacokinetics
Absorption	Hypotension and regional perfusion changes	Reduced oral or intramuscular absorption
Distribution	Pulmonary sequestration Decreased pulmonary blood flow Hypotension; altered regional perfusion Hemodilution; dilution of binding proteins Postoperative increase in α_1-AG; increase in postoperative protein binding	Decreased volume of distribution Decreased pulmonary drug distribution Decreased volume of distribution Increased volume of distribution Decreased volume of distribution
Elimination	Decreased hepatic blood flow Hypothermia Hypotension; decreased renal blood flow	Decreased clearance of drugs Decreased hepatic metabolism Decreased renal clearance

Abbreviations: α_1-AG, α_1-acid glycoprotein.

CHANGES IN BLOOD PRESSURE

Changes in blood pressure lead to alterations in regional blood flow distribution and decreased perfusion of organ systems. There is indirect evidence to suggest a decrease of blood flow to nonvital organs such as skeletal muscle.[127] A decrease in hepatic blood flow as measured by the clearance of indocyanine green has been reported.[128] The administration of vasoactive substances further alters regional blood flow (e.g., an increase in hepatic blood flow occurs with isoproterenol or glucagon and a decrease with β-adrenergic blockers[129]).

HEMODILUTION

Hemodilution has pronounced effects on drug levels. The addition of the CPB pump priming solution results in an increase in V_d and a decrease in plasma protein binding with an increase in free drug fraction. This will initially lower drug concentrations. This decrease is soon corrected by redistribution from tissues to serum. The results will depend on the characteristics of the drug. For drugs with a high initial V_d, the drug concentrations after re-equilibration will be only slightly lower than those before hemodilution. The degree of plasma protein binding alters such that for drugs that are highly protein bound the decreased concentration of binding proteins will lead to an increase in the fraction of unbound drug. This will favor distribution of drug from plasma to tissues and lead to decreased concentration of the drug.

Heparin decreases the protein binding of many drugs to an unknown extent through an increase in nonesterified fatty acids. In the immediate postoperative period, there is an increase in the synthesis of acute phase proteins (e.g., α_1-acid glycoprotein), which leads to increased binding of basic drugs such as lidocaine, propranolol, disopyramide, and fentanyl.[130]

HUMORAL RESPONSES

CPB induces a marked physiologic stress response leading to release of vasoactive intermediates. Hypothermia, hemodilution, and nonpulsatile flow all result in the release of catecholamines, insulin, prostaglandins, and renin. Up to a 200 percent increase in plasma norepinephrine and a 1,500 percent increase in plasma epinephrine were recorded during CPB.[131] Epinephrine levels peak during rewarming[132] and both epinephrine and norepinephrine continue to increase into the postbypass period.[133] (For a more complete discussion, see Ch. 5.)

Hyperglycemia commonly occurs during CPB. This is probably the result of several factors: increased glycogenolysis secondary to increased catecholamine levels; decreased insulin response due to hypothermia; reduced glucose transport and uptake; and binding of insulin to the extracorporeal circuit.[134] Although there is a possibility of greater metabolic derangement and neurologic injury with hyperglycemia, Metz and Keats[135] found no significant difference in outcome with varying blood glucose levels during CPB.

The acute phase reaction is a homeostatic response of the organism to injury and inflammation.[136] Changes occur in the concentrations of various plasma protein fractions with pharmacokinetic implications. The plasma concentrations of α_1-acid glycoprotein rise two- to fivefold and albumin and transferrin concentrations decrease in acute phase response to surgery. The rise in α_1-acid glycoprotein leads to an increased binding of basic drugs such as amide local anesthetics,[137] disopyramide, fentanyl, and propranolol.

HYPOTHERMIA

Hypothermia can itself influence drug distribution and metabolism. Hepatic enzymatic activity is depressed during hypothermia. In addition, there is marked intrahepatic redistribution of blood flow with development of intrahepatic shunting. Hypothermia also affects renal function. GFR is decreased by 65 percent at 25°C in dogs[138] and there is evidence that drug clearance is decreased similarly during hypothermia.[139]

ORGAN BLOOD FLOW

The elimination of drugs can be influenced by several changes occurring during and after CPB. The elimination of drugs that are cleared by the lungs either by local metabolism or exhalation can be expected to be altered. Renal clearance is altered by the accompanying circulatory changes of CPB. The glomerular filtration of a drug normally depends on the degree of protein binding and is usually flow independent. Tubular secretion is flow dependent and tubular reabsorption is likely to be affected by changes in pH and filtrate volume. However, because of the impairment of the metabolic state of the kidney due to hypoperfusion and hypothermia, such a change is not always found in the elimination kinetics of drugs.[140] Many drugs are metabolized in the liver before being eliminated. The determinants of hepatic clearance are blood flow, drug protein binding, and the activity of hepatic enzyme systems. Hepatic flow decreases during CPB. Protein binding can decrease during the CPB due to hemodilution, as already discussed. However, postoperatively, due to an increase in α_1-acid glycoprotein, increased binding of basic drugs is also possible. Intrinsic enzyme system activity is difficult to measure in the context of CPB, but a depression of the enzyme systems is expected due to hypothermia and hypoperfusion.[130]

After institution of CPB, pulmonary blood flow is reduced markedly and is confined to bronchial vessels only. This isolation of the pulmonary circulation produces some changes in disposition of certain basic drugs such as lidocaine, imipramine, propranolol, and fentanyl that distribute into lung significantly.[141] On restoration of pulmonary circulation at the end of CPB, washout of this accumulated drug may increase the plasma concentration briefly. Pharmacokinetic changes during cardiopulmonary bypass are summarized in Table 16-8.

CARDIOPULMONARY BYPASS APPARATUS

Some drugs are absorbed by the CPB apparatus. NTG, fentanyl, and thiopental have all been shown to be absorbed by the CPB apparatus. This leads to an additional decrease in the final drug concentrations while on CPB, not commensurate with hemodilution alone.[142]

Pharmacokinetics of Some Individual Drugs During Cardiopulmonary Bypass

PHARMACOKINETIC CONSIDERATIONS

Absorption
Theoretically, the absorption of oral and intramuscular drugs will be altered during CPB. However, as most intraoperative drugs are administered intravenously, other routes of administration will not be discussed further here.

Distribution
The distribution kinetics of most drugs are altered during CPB by several mechanisms. Changes in blood pressure and regional blood flow, hemodilution, pulmonary sequestration, hypothermia, altered protein binding, and sequestration by the CPB apparatus all lead to alterations in drug disposition.

BENZODIAZEPINES

Aaltonen and colleagues[143] reported that the total serum concentrations of lorazepam and of its conjugates decreased abruptly after initiation of the CPB. An increase in the serum concentrations of lorazepam following CPB has been reported; this was possibly due to redistribution of the drug from tissues. The elimination half-life after CPB was not different from that of healthy volunteers. As with midazolam, a decrease in concentration at the start of CPB and an increase at the termination of CPB has been reported.[144] After CPB, the elimination half-life was found to be prolonged compared with studies in healthy subjects.

LIDOCAINE

Holley and colleagues[137] have studied lidocaine pharmacokinetics before and after CPB using patients as their own control. No changes were found in either clearance, V_d, or elimination half-life after a bolus dose of 100 mg lidocaine when compared to the preoperative state 15 minutes after start of CPB or one day postoperatively.[137] These findings suggest that whatever changes that occur during CPB are quickly reversed after CPB.

These authors also gave intravenous bolus injections of lidocaine three and seven days after surgery. Lidocaine clearance was decreased by 42 percent and V_d was reduced by 40 percent three days after surgery. Seven days after surgery the pharmacokinetic parameters returned to normal. The kinetic changes on the third day were coincident with a 46 percent decrease in lidocaine free fraction because of an increased protein binding due to an increase in the levels of α_1-acid glycoprotein of up to 200 percent. The reductions in clearance and V_d produce higher lidocaine levels in these patients recovering from cardiac surgery; however, toxicity may not occur because of the decrease in the free fraction of lidocaine.

The assessment of therapeutic efficacy in relation to drug levels must be made cautiously during this period because of alterations in protein binding. Morrel and Harrison[145] observed an increase in V_d of lidocaine without change in clearance, leading to an increase in elimination half-life. The changes in distribution are explained by hemodilution and decreased protein binding. On this basis the authors recommend a larger than normal loading dose.

DIGOXIN

In contemporary practice, digoxin is less commonly used in the preoperative preparation of patients undergoing cardiac surgery. However, it is often used in the immediate postoperative period for the prophylactic treatment of supraventricular dysrhythmias.[146,147] Digoxin has low protein binding,

a large V_d, and is excreted predominantly unchanged in the urine. Digoxin concentrations decrease significantly on initiation of CPB due to hemodilution. Digoxin protein binding is too low to affect V_d in this context.[148-150] Digoxin concentrations remain low during the procedure and for several hours thereafter. Morrison and Killip[149] found that approximately 13 hours following the onset of CPB, serum digoxin concentrations rebounded in some patients, the mechanism of which is not fully understood. Digoxin levels before and immediately after CPB in patients on chronic digoxin therapy are therefore generally similar. This may be due to the long elimination half-life and low protein binding of digoxin. However, clearance may be reduced commensurate with any reduction in creatinine clearance. These data suggest that perioperative supplementation of digoxin is probably unnecessary for patients on chronic therapy, and monitoring of drug levels is important in the early postoperative period until renal function returns to normal.

INTRAVENOUS ANESTHETICS

Thiopental

Nancheria and colleagues[151] studied thiopental pharmacokinetics after a bolus of 6 mg · kg^{-1} given after CPB was initiated and cardioplegia given. The V_d of the central compartment was similar to the values reported in healthy volunteers but the total clearance and metabolism were significantly impaired, possibly by hypothermia.[151] Morgan and colleagues[152] administered thiopental by an exponentially decreasing infusion to achieve a relatively constant plasma concentration. Concentrations were maintained until the onset of CPB, whereupon the total thiopental concentration decreased abruptly by 50 percent.[152] They also found that the unbound fraction nearly doubled due to hemodilution. Thus, although the total drug levels decreased markedly with the onset of CPB, free drug levels were more constant. Whereas the debate continues on the virtues of pulsatile flow during CPB, no differences in pharmacokinetic parameters of thiopental were found in patients undergoing CPB with pulsatile or nonpulsatile flows.

Methohexital

The pharmacokinetic profile of methohexital was found to be similar to that of thiopental.[153] Concentrations of methohexital, which is slightly less protein bound (73 percent) compared with thiopental (84 percent), decreased on initiation of bypass with a gradual recovery during CPB. The investigators observed a strong correlation between the albumin concentrations and the degree of plasma protein binding for both methohexital and thiopental.

Etomidate

Etomidate pharmacokinetics during CPB were studied after a bolus injection followed by a continuous infusion.[154] A marked decrease in etomidate concentration was observed after the onset of CPB. The concentration increased again during the procedure, possibly due to hypothermia-induced inhibition of metabolism. Concentrations of etomidate decreased again during rewarming, possibly due to increased metabolism. The observed increase in concentration again in the post-CPB period was explained by the authors as release from the bypass apparatus, although there are no confirmed reports of etomidate sequestration during CPB.

Propofol

Propofol has been used for induction of anesthesia and also as an infusion during the bypass period.[155-157] Propofol infusion in combination with fentanyl was used to predict plateau concentrations before bypass. The onset of CPB resulted in a decrease in propofol concentration as a result of hemodilution. Propofol concentration recovered rapidly, probably due to hypothermia and hepatic hypoperfusion during CPB. Laycock and Alston,[157] using propofol infusions during CPB, found a reduction in SVR and systemic VO_2, possibly indicating impaired tissue perfusion.

INHALATIONAL ANAESTHETICS

Isoflurane

Inhalational drugs are often used during CPB via the pump oxygenator to maintain anesthesia. With the implications of continued myocardial depression by inhalational drugs in the postoperative period in the background, Henderson and colleagues[158] studied the washin and washout of isoflurane during CPB with hypothermia. Initially, blood concentrations increased rapidly followed by a slower but steady increase such that a steady state was not attained during the period of CPB (40 minutes). After the isoflurane was discontinued, blood concentrations rapidly decreased to 50 percent of maximal values within 2 minutes. This was followed by a slower terminal elimination such that by 15 minutes the concentration had fallen to 75 percent of maximum. The authors opined that up to 2 percent isoflurane can be administered during CPB to maintain anesthesia and the enhanced washout will facilitate a rapid decrease in concentration to 0.5 percent at the termination of CPB. Thomson and colleagues[159] reported that isoflurane and desflurane in equipotent doses appear to have similar hemodynamic effects during CPB, although systemic hypotension was found to be slightly more common with desflurane.

MUSCLE RELAXANTS

Nondepolarizing muscle relaxants have a small V_D and low clearance values. In general, concentrations of nondepolarizing muscle relaxant were found to be higher during CPB despite hemodilution. This may be due to decreased drug clearance and a reduction in distribution due to hypoperfusion. Isolation of the pulmonary circulation (into which these drugs accumulate in appreciable amounts) may be one of the contributing factors.[160]

Protein binding of tubocurarine is markedly decreased as a result of hemodilution. This results in an increase in free fraction relative to the increase in total concentration. A decrease in renal clearance and hepatic clearance could also contribute to the increase in concentration of tubocurarine during CPB.[161] Atracurium infusion requirements needed to maintain a 92 to 95 percent block of initial twitch height during CPB are reduced compared with pre-CPB levels.[162] Pancuronium concentrations decrease on initiation of CPB, probably due to hemodilution, and remain relatively constant during bypass until rewarming.[163] Thus, the dosage requirements of nondepolarizing relaxants, such as pancuronium, atracurium, and vecuronium, are uniformly decreased during CPB.[162–164]

VASODILATORS

Nitroglycerin

The influence of CPB on NTG clearance was studied by Dasta and colleagues[165,166] in patients receiving an infusion of NTG. They found a 20 percent increase in the clearance of NTG; however, due to the interindividual variability in the pharmacokinetics of the drug, it is difficult to draw conclusions from this finding.[167] NTG is also absorbed by the bypass apparatus (primarily the polyurethane defoaming sponge in the bubble oxygenator). This observation is in keeping with the absorption of the drug by certain plastics.[143]

Sodium Nitroprusside

Sodium nitroprusside (SNP) is metabolized by a nonenzymatic reaction in the red blood cells to yield cyanide ions. Cyanide ions are detoxified by the enzymatic addition of sulfur to yield thiocyanate. Thiocyanate is excreted via the kidney with a half-life of about 4 to 7 days. During hypothermic CPB, nonenzymatic release of the cyanide ion from SNP is not affected but the enzyme detoxification is delayed[168] because hypothermia inhibits the enzymatic detoxification. The red blood cell cyanide concentration during hypothermia reached a mean concentration of about 0.55 $\mu g \cdot ml^{-1}$, which decreased rapidly on rewarming. Hence, the possibility of cyanide toxicity following the use of large doses of SNP in hypothermic patients must be considered.

β-BLOCKERS

Plachetka and colleagues[169] reported that propranolol concentrations decreased on initiation of CPB and remained low throughout the procedure. There was a sudden increase in the concentration at the end of the procedure that remained elevated for up to 4 hours after bypass. This was attributed by the authors to washout from the lungs. The authors concluded that hypothermia, via its inhibition of hepatic metabolism of propranolol, leads to a marked increase in propranolol concentrations offset only by hemodilution.

Wood and coworkers[170] reported a doubling of the unbound fraction of propranolol after heparinization—an effect reversed following protamine administration. This effect is thought to be due to an increase in free fatty acid concentration produced by heparin, which decreases protein binding of propranolol. Due to the highly protein-bound nature of propranolol (90 to 95 percent), this effect is very likely. The degree of difference in the changes of propranolol concentration observed in these studies may also reflect high interindividual variation.

In summary, it appears that propranolol concentrations decrease upon initiation of bypass with a relative rise in free fraction. Hypothermia induces an inhibition of hepatic metabolism, then leads to an increase in plasma concentrations during the procedure, followed by a rise upon termination of bypass due to pulmonary washout. The clinical advantages of chronic propranolol therapy in the perioperative management of dysrhythmias and hemodynamic stability are established. The effect of CPB on propranolol pharmacokinetics does not appear to be a major problem.

ANTIBIOTICS

Cephalosporins

Antibiotic prophylaxis during cardiac surgery is common and cephalosporins are commonly used for this purpose. Miller and colleagues[171] have studied the pharmacokinetics of cefazolin. They reported a decrease in concentration at the initiation of CPB, followed by a plateau or a slow increase during the course of CPB. Renal clearance of cefazolin did not show deterioration during bypass surgery. Cephalothin is metabolized by the liver and eliminated by the kidney.[172] The effects of CPB on cephalothin appeared to be similar to those of cefazolin. Sato and coworkers[173] reported that the elimination half-life of cephalothin was significantly prolonged both during and after bypass surgery. It would appear from the pharmacokinetic profile of cephalosporins that although there is a decline in concentration soon after initiation of bypass, the concentration regains a plateau phase, and final elimination may by slightly prolonged. On balance, the dosage requirements are probably no different from that in noncardiac surgery.

OPIOIDS

The influence of CPB on the pharmacokinetics of opioids is well characterized.[174,175] Fentanyl, which is a lipid-soluble drug with high hepatic extraction and protein binding of 80 percent, has received the most attention. Fentanyl concentrations decrease abruptly on initiation of bypass, usually by 30 to 50 percent. This is attributed variously to hemodilution and an increased V_d. Concentrations did not change for much of the duration of bypass without supplemental dosing; this suggests a reduced clearance, probably due to hypothermia. When fentanyl is administered at a rate calculated to produce constant levels, serum fentanyl concentrations increase during bypass, suggesting either reduced hepatic clearance or impaired peripheral drug redistribution.

Bently and colleagues[176] have reported a rise in fentanyl levels on termination of CPB, possibly due to washout of fentanyl from the lungs. Koska and coworkers[177] demonstrated a prolonged elimination half-life after the bypass period, possibly related to reduced hepatic clearance. Koren and colleagues[178] reported the decrease in fentanyl concentrations on institution of bypass was not commensurate with the degree of hemo-

dilution. Also in an in vitro study they demonstrated that fentanyl was absorbed by the CPB apparatus (mainly by the membrane oxygenator).[179]

Thus, it would appear that initially, fentanyl concentrations decrease due both to hemodilution and absorption onto the bypass apparatus. At the end of bypass, an increase in fentanyl concentration occurs due to washout from the lungs. The clearance and post-CPB elimination half-life are prolonged due to hypothermia-induced hepatic hypoperfusion.

The elimination of alfentanil after CPB is also prolonged (elimination half-life of 195 minutes versus 72 minutes). The difference is attributed to an increase in V_d.[180] Alfentanil concentrations decrease after the onset of CPB by approximately 50 percent.[180] This occurs predominantly with the bound fraction due to dilution of the binding protein to which alfentanil binds (α_1-acid glycoprotein). Hug and colleagues[181] also reported a prolonged elimination half-life for alfentanil after bypass due to an increase in V_d. No change in clearance was reported.[181]

THE POSTOPERATIVE PERIOD

The postoperative period of the cardiac surgical patient is a critical period with intricate hemodynamic implications. However, it is in many respects similar to that of any patient undergoing a major operation with similar neuroendocrine and stress responses to surgery. The use of CPB imposes additional metabolic stress and neurohumeral and biochemical changes.

Physiologic Changes

The initial response to surgical trauma is an increase in the circulating concentration of catabolic hormones such as catecholamines, glucagon, and cortisol and a concomitant decrease in plasma concentration of the anabolic hormones insulin and testosterone.[182] Plasma cortisol concentrations are rapidly elevated in response to surgical simulation.[183] The increase in cortisol concentration leads to hyperglycemia, protein breakdown, salt and water retention, and potassium loss. The concentrations of growth hormone[184] and glucagon[185] are increased by a wide variety of surgical procedures.

Insulin concentrations are decreased during surgery and in the immediate postoperative period despite coexisting hyperglycemia. The relationship of insulin and glucagon secretions in the postoperative period is complex. Allison[186] suggested that the supression of insulin secretion is primarily a result of the predominance of α-adrenergic activity.

SALT AND WATER RETENTION

Sodium and water retention and potassium loss are among the most constant features of the body's response to surgery.[187] Plasma antidiuretic hormone (ADH) and renin and aldosterone are increased during surgery and contribute to sodium and water retention.[188]

SURGICAL STRESS RESPONSE

Some aspects of the stress response to operative trauma may be modified by anesthetic agents and techniques.[189,190] A reduction of endocrine and metabolic responses may be achieved by afferent neural blockade with local anesthetics (epidural or spinal block)[191] or by inhibition of the hypothalamus with large doses of opioids. The latter method is commonly employed in cardiac surgical patients as both morphine, 4 mg $\cdot$ kg^{-1}, and fentanyl, 75 μg $\cdot$ kg^{-1}, inhibit hormonal and metabolic responses to cardiac surgery.[192,193]

Pharmacologic Implications

NONSPECIFIC ALTERATIONS

Cardiovascular surgery imposes major pathophysiologic changes in the human organism. Fluid, electrolyte and acid base changes, hemodynamic instability, and hypothermia all influence postoperative pharmacodynamics and pharmacokinetics. In addition, the acute phase proteins secreted during stress response alter the pharmacokinetics of many pharmacologic agents.

In the days following surgery, alterations occur in plasma protein fractions (a so-called acute phase response), notably, an increase in α_1-acid glycoprotein levels and a decrease in albumin concentrations.[136] The increase in α_1-acid glycoprotein levels leads to an increased binding of basic drugs such as amide local anesthetics, disopyramide, fentanyl, and propranolol.[136,195,196]

Preoperative drug therapy and alterations in pharmacokinetics during CPB and surgery, have implications in the postoperative period. Profound β-blockade may exert residual bradycardia or produce myocardial depression after cardiac surgery. Alternatively, withdrawal of β-blockers before surgery may lead to withdrawal hypersensitivity, tachycardia, and dysrhythmias.[19,20] Continuing the administration of β-blocker through cardiac surgery results in more stable intraoperative hemodynamics and offers considerable protection from rhythm disturbances.[21]

The use of amiodarone prior to CPB often results in a trio of unwanted side effects: an atropine-resistant bradycardia, peripheral vasodilation, and myocardial depression. In the postoperative period the myocardium is unresponsive to inotropic agents.

Calcium antagonists should be continued throughout the perioperative period to ensure stable hemodynamics.[195] However, caution should be exercised in the administration of verapamil to patients with left ventricular dysfunction since myocardial depression can occur, especially when used in combination with β-blockers.[196,197] The myocardial depressant effect of calcium antagonists is potentiated by inhalational anaesthetic agents.[198,199]

Digoxin has a long elimination half-life and a large V$_d$. Hence, drug levels are not altered markedly by CPB. Patients on digoxin receive close monitoring of serum levels as the concomitant use of some drugs (e.g., quinidine, amiodarone, and verapamil) can compete for protein binding with a subsequent elevation of serum digoxin levels.

In patients with renal insufficiency, the clearance of ACE inhibitors may decrease and renal impairment can worsen.[116] Calcium antagonists have additive antihypertensive effects with ACE inhibitors but significant pharmacokinetic interactions between these two groups of drugs are unlikely. Inhibition of drug metabolism by cimetidine will impair the elimination of warfarin, diazepam, propranolol, and lidocaine.[200]

Cholinesterase activity is reduced at the onset of CPB and remains depressed for several days postoperatively.[201] This has interesting pharmacokinetic implications for mivacurium, a nondepolarizing muscle relaxant hydrolized by cholinesterase. The effects of other nondepolarizing muscle relaxants are potentiated by diuretics, calcium antagonists, and aminoglysides.[202-204]

SPECIFIC PROBLEMS

Hypertension

Postoperative hypertension following cardiac surgery occurs for several reasons. Endogenous catecholamines, increased plasma renin activity, and angiotensin II all lead to hypertension. Hypothermia, pain, and anxiety all cause increases in SVR. Postoperative hypertension leads to an increase in myocardial oxygen demand, ischemia, and increased bleeding, and poses a possible risk of cerebrovascular accident. Increased SVR due to hypothermia and depressed CO leads to decreased organ perfusion and metabolic acidosis. In such situations vasodilator therapy is beneficial.

NTG and SNP are the most commonly used vasodilators in the postoperative period.

Nitroglycerin

NTG is the most commonly used venodilator in the postoperative cardiac patient. In doses of 5 to 10 $\mu g \cdot min^{-1}$ it causes coronary vasodilation, decreases preload by venodilation, and decreases afterload by arteriolar dilation in the hypothermic postoperative patient.[205] Tolerance is observed with chronic use and

wide individual variability is noted. Doses as high as 50 to 150 $\mu g \cdot min^{-1}$ may be required to achieve the desired effect in "tolerant" individuals.[206]

Sodium Nitroprusside

SNP is a potent arteriolar dilator with some venodilating properties. The hemodynamic effects of SNP are reduction in SVR and systemic blood pressure and significant increase in CO and SV along with decreases in PAP, PCWP, CVP, and PVR. The onset and offset are rapid after intravenous infusion. During an infusion, reflex baroceptor activity causes tachycardia. Rebound hypertension may occur after withdrawal of the drug due to residual activation of the RAS. For this reason it is best to use SNP principally as an acute control agent. As soon as control of hypertension is achieved, a long-acting agent should supplant the use of SNP. In no case should the use of SNP exceed 4 hours.[205]

Low Cardiac Output

Vasodilators in Postoperative Low Output Syndrome   Both NTG and SNP have been used to improve hemodynamics in postoperative low syndrome. Kaplan and colleagues[205] showed that both drugs are useful in CHF following bypass surgery. NTG decreases filling pressures more than SNP but both drugs improve overall hemodynamics. Stinson and coworkers[207] demonstrated significantly greater improvement in CO with SNP than with NTG in the postoperative low output syndrome. Vasodilators are often beneficial for children with the postoperative low output syndrome; cardiogenic shock due to ruptured ventricular septum following myocardial infarction; and therapy in regurgitant valvular heart disease.[208] (For a more complete discussion of afterload reduction, see Ch. 7.)

In mitral and aortic regurgitation, vasodilators decrease the regurgitant fraction and improve the forward fraction.[209] NTG, SNP, and phentolamine are also useful for decreasing pulmonary hypertension in patients undergoing surgery for mitral stenosis. Thus, vasodilators, used alone or in combination with ino-

Table 16-9.   Positive Inotropic Drugs and Dosages

	Bolus Dose	Infusion	Predominant Receptor Action		
			α	β	DA
Epinephrine	2–16 μg	2–10 μg·min^{-1}	+ + +	+ + +	—
Norepinephrine	2–16 μg	2–16 μg·min^{-1}	+ + + +	+ +	—
Dopamine	NA	2–25 μg·kg·min^{-1}	+ +	+ + +	+ +
Dobutamine	NA	2–20 μg·kg^{-1}·min^{-1}	+	+ + +	—
Dopexamine	NA	0.5–4 μg·kg^{-1}·min^{-1}	—	+ +	+ +
Isoproterenol	2–16 μg	1–5 μg·min^{-1}	—	+ + +	

tropes, are useful in postoperative low cardiac output syndrome following coronary artery bypass grafting or valvular heart surgery. In patients requiring mechanical circulatory support, vasodilators are occasionally beneficial.[210]

Positive Inotropic Drugs

After optimal preload and afterload conditions are achieved, preservation or augmentation of myocardial contractility is addressed by pharmacotherapy. Often pharmacologic intervention is required to improve myocardial contractility. In addition to positive inotropic drugs, it is important to ensure normal or near normal cardiac rhythm, since dysrhythmias decrease myocardial performance. A list of inotropic drugs and their usual doses is given in Table 16-9.

Inotrope and Vasodilator Combination

In patients with postoperative left ventricular failure, a combination of inotropic and vasodilator drugs is often more effective than either group used alone (see Ch. 7). The inotropic drugs increase myocardial contractility whereas vasodilators help to increase SV by decreasing afterload. Both groups of drugs decrease elevated filling pressures and maintain and augment CO and organ perfusion while decreasing SVR and PVR. Various combinations of inotropes and vasodilators have been used with benefit.

Pulmonary Hypertension

  Nitric Oxide NO is an endothelium-derived relaxing factor (EDRF).[211] It produces its actions through a reversible binding of the heme moiety of guanylyl cyclase, stimulating the production of cyclic guanosine monophosphate (cGMP), which causes vasodilation of the vascular smooth muscle.[212] It is widely distributed in the body and appears to be an important messenger in the immune, neurologic, and cardiovascular systems. Although it is an endogenous substance, it is now known that nitrosodilators including organic nitrates and nitroprusside act by producing NO.[213]

Inhaled NO is a selective pulmonary vasodilator and reverses hypoxic pulmonary vasoconstriction. The use of inhaled NO is presently being evaluated in several clinical conditions.[214] NO has been used in the treatment of idiopathic pulmonary hypertension[215] and pulmonary hypertension due to congenital heart disease in the newborn.[214] It has also been useful in pulmonary hypertension associated with severe adult respiratory distress syndrome.[216]

It is possible that halogenated anesthetics may attenuate NO-dependent vascular smooth muscle relaxation by competing with NO for binding sites on the enzyme guanylyl cyclase.[217] NO readily reacts with high concentrations of inspired oxygen to form toxic nitrogen dioxide. NO may also play a role in the control of coronary vascular tone and blood flow and postischemic reperfusion.[218] In the presence of atherosclerosis, NO-dependent relaxation is altered in humans. Untreated hypertension[219] and diabetes[220] are known to have an altered response to NO-mediated relaxation.

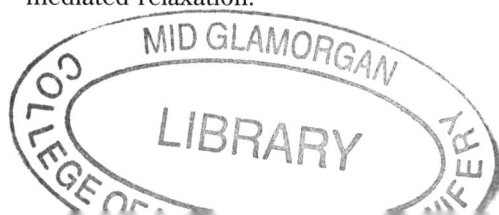

Thus, NO is an interesting substance with potential implications in the physiology and pathology of cardiopulmonary disorders. Further controlled trials are needed to evaluate the safety and benefit of NO therapy.[221]

SUMMARY

The pharmacokinetics of many perioperative drugs undergo alterations during cardiac surgery with cardiopulmonary bypass. Some of these are hemodynamically induced (altered perfusion of organs), some iatrogenic (hemodilution, hypothermia), and some metabolic (altered protein binding). In general, for drugs with very long half-lives and high V_d, of the changes are minimal. Concurrent hemodynamic status influences drug metabolism and elimination and successful hemodynamic management in the postoperative period results in predictable outcome both in pharmacologic and clinical terms.

REFERENCES

1. Kiyomoto A, Sasaki Y, Odawara A et al: Inhibition of platelet aggregation by diltiazem. Comparison with verapamil and nifedipine and inhibitory potensies of diltazem metabolites. Circ Res 52:1–115, 1983
2. Frishman WH, Christodoulou J, Weksler B et al: Abrupt propranolol withdrawal in angina pectoris: effects on platelet aggregation and exercise tolerance. Am Heart J 95:169, 1978
3. Diodati J, Theroux P, Latour JG et al: Effects of nitroglycerin at theraputic doses on platelet aggregation in unstable angina pectoris and acute myocardial infarction. Am J Cardiol 66:683, 1990
4. Dikshit K, Vyden JK, Forrester JS et al: Renal and extrarenal effects of furosemide in congestive heart failure after myocardial infarction. N Engl J Med 288:1087, 1973
5. Stewart DE, Ikram H, Espiner EA et al: Arrhythmigenic potential of diuretic induced hypokalaemia in patients with mild hypertension and ischaemic heart disease. Br Heart J 54:290, 1985
6. Johnston LC, Greible HG: Treatment of hypertensive disease with diuretics. V: Spirinolactone, an aldosterone antagonist. Arch Intern Med 119:225, 1967
7. Fouad FM, Nakashima Y, Tarazi R et al: Reversal of left ventricular hypertrophy in hypertensive patients treated with methyldopa: lack of association with blood pressure control. Am J Cardiol 49:795, 1982
8. Gilman AF, Goodman LS, Rall TW et al: The Pharmacological Basis of Therapeutics. 7th Ed. p. 789. Macmillan, New York, 1985
9. Bruce DL, Croley TF, Lee JS: Preoperative clonidine withdrawal syndrome. Anesthesiology 51:90, 1979
10. Mancia G, Ferrari A, Gegorini L et al: Effect of prazosin on automatic control of circulation in essential hypertension. Hypertension 2:700, 1980
11. Lund-Johansen P: Haemodynamic changes at rest and during exercise in long-term beta-blockade therapy of essential hypertension. Acta Med Scand 195:117, 1974
12. Morgan TO, Roberts R, Carney SL et al: Beta-adrenergic receptor blocking drugs, hypertension and plasma renin. Br J Clin Pharmacol 2:159, 1975
13. Royster RL: Anti-ischemic drug therapy. p. 88. In Kaplan JA (ed): Cardiac Anaesthesia. 3rd Ed. WB Saunders, Philadelphia, 1993
14. Nies AS, Shand DG: Clinical pharmacology of propranolol. Circulation 52:6, 1975
15. Decalmer PBS, Chatterjee SS, Cruickshank JM et al: Beta-blockers and asthma. Br Heart J 40:184, 1978
16. Svendsen TL, Hartling OJ, Jrap-Jensen J et al: Adrenergic beta receptor blockade: hemodynamic importance of intrinsic sympathomimetic activity at rest. Clin Pharmacol Ther 29:711, 1981
17. Ryan JR, LaCorte W, Jain A et al: Hypertension in hypoglycemic diabetics treated with beta adrenergic antagonists. Hypertension 7:443, 1985
18. Breckenridge A: Which beta blocker? Br Med J 286:1085, 1983
19. Egstrup K: Transient myocardial ischemia after abrupt withdrawal of antianginal therapy in chronic stable angina. Ann J Cardiol 61:1219, 1988
20. Pantano JA, Lee YC: Abrupt propranolol withdrawl and myocardial contractility. A study

of effects in normal man. Arch Int Med 136: 867, 1976

21. Wechsler AS: Assessment of prospectively randomised patients receiving propranolol therapy before coronary bypass operation. Ann Thorac Surg 30:128, 1980

22. Chruchill-Davidson HC: Anaesthesia and cardiac disease. p. 469. In: A Practice of Anaesthesia. Lloyd-Luke (Medical Books) Ltd., London, 1984

23. Peter T, Norris RM, Clarke ED et al: Reduction of enzyme levels of propranolol after acute myocardial infarction. Circulation 57: 1091, 1978

24. Beta-blocker Heart Attack Trial Research Group: A randomized trial of propranolol in patients with acute myocardial infarction. I. Mortality results. JAMA 247:1707, 1982

25. Kern MJ, Ganz P, Howitz JD et al: Potentiation of coronary vasoconstriction by beta-blockade in patients with coronary artery disease. Circulation 67:1178, 1983

26. Silverman NA, Wright R, Levitsky S: Efficacy of low dose propranolol in preventing postoperative supraventricular arrhythmias: a prospective randomized study. Ann Surg 196: 194, 1982

27. Feely J, Penden N: Use of beta-adrenoceptor blocking drugs in hyperthyroidism. Drugs 27:425, 1984

28. Braunwald E: Heart failure. p. 1360. In Petersdorf RG, Raymond D (eds): Harrison's Principles of Internal Medicine. 10th Ed. McGraw Hill, New York, 1983

29. Swan DA, Bell B, Oakley CM et al: Analysis of symptomatic course and prognosis and treatment of hypertrophic obstructive cardiomyopathy. Br Heart J 33:671, 1971

30. Hachamovitch R, Sonnenblick EH, Strom JA et al: Left ventricular hypertrophy in hypertension and the effects of antihypertensive drug therapy. Curr Probl Cardiol 13:375, 1988

31. Robinson BF, Dobbs RJ, Kelsey CR: Effects of nifedipine on resistant vessels, arteries and veins in man. Br J Clin Pharmacol 10: 433, 1980

32. Serruys PW, Brower RW, Ten Katen JH et al: Regional wall motion from radioopaque markers after intravenous and intracoronary injections of nifedipine. Circulation 63:584, 1981

33. Singh BN, Roche AHG: Effects of intravenous verapamil on hemodynamics in patients with heart disease. Am Heart J 94:593, 1977

34. Chew CYC, Hecht HS, Collett JT et al: Influence of severity of ventricular dysfunction on hemodynamic responses to intravenously administered verapamil in ischemic heart disease. Ann J Cardiol 47:917, 1981

35. Josephson MA, Hopkins J, Singh BN: Hemodynamic and metabolic effects of diltiazem during coronary sinus pacing with particular reference to left ventricular ejection fraction. Am J Cardiol 55:286, 1985

36. Schwartz JS, Bache RJ: Combined effects of calcium antagonists and nitroglycerin on large coronary artery diameter. Am Heart J 115:964, 1988

37. Turlapaty P, Wary R, Kaplan JA: Nicardipine, a new intravenous calcium antagonist. A review of its pharmacology, pharmacokinetics and perioperative applications. J Cardiothorac Anesth 3:344, 1989

38. Brolon BG, Bolson EL, Dodge HT: Dynamic mechanisms in human coronary stenosis. Circulation 70:917, 1984

39. Sato O, Ohashi M, Metz MZ et al: Inhibitory effect of a calcium antagonist (diltiazem) on aortic and coronary contractions in rabbits. J Mol Cell Cardiol 14:741, 1982

40. Wellens HJJ, TanSL, Bar FWH et al: Effect of verapamil studied by programmed electrical stimulation of the heart in patients with paroxysmal re-entrant supraventricular tachycardia. Br Heart J 39:1058, 1977

41. Sugimoto T, Ishikawa T, Kaseno K et al: Electrophysiologic effects of diltiazem, a calcium antagonist, in patients with impaired sinus or atrio-ventricular node function. Angiology 31:700, 1980

42. Rowland E, Evans T, Krikler D: Effect of nifedipine on atrioventricular conduction as compared with verapamil. Intracardiac electrophysiological study. Br Heart J 42:124, 1979

43. Moskowitz RM, Piccini PA, Nacarelli GV et al: Nifedipine therapy for stable angina pectoris: preliminary results of effects on angina frequency and treadmill exercise response. Am J Cardiol 44:811, 1979

44. Strauss WE, Mcintyre KM, Parisi AR et al: Safety and efficacy of diltiazem hydrochloride for the treatment of stable angina pecto-

ris: report of a cooperative clinical trial. Am J Cardiol 49:560, 1982

45. Pine MB, Citron PD, Bailly DJ et al: Verapamil versus placebo in relieving stable angina pectoris. Circulation, suppl. 1. 65:17, 1982

46. Johnson SM, Mauritson DR, Willerson JT et al: A controlled trial of verapamil in Prinzmetal's varient angina. N Engl J Med 304:862, 1981

47. McCall D, Walsh RA, Frohlich ED et al: Calcium entry blocking drugs: mechanisms of action, experimental studies and clinical uses. Cur Probl Cardiol 10:1, 1985

48. Ruzicka M, Leenen F: Relevance of intermittent increases in sympathetic activity for adverse outcome on short-acting calcium antagonists. In pp. 2819–25. Larugh JH, Brenner BM (eds): Hypertension: Pathophysiology, Diagnosis, and Management, 2nd Ed. Raven Press, New York, 1995

49. McClellan K: Unexpected results from MIDAS in atherosclerosis. Summary of results presented at the 15th Scientific Meeting of the International Society of Hypertension in Melbourne, Australia, March 1994. Inpharma Wkly 932:4, 1994

50. Psaty B, Heckbert S, Koepsell T et al: The risk of myocardial infarction associated with antihypertensive drug therapies. JAMA 274: 620–5, 1995

51. Smucker ML, Samford CF, Lipscomb KM: Effects of hydralazine on pressure-volume and stress-volume relations in congestive heart failure to secondary to idiopathic dilated cardiomyopathy. Am J Cardiol 56:690, 1985

52. Abrams J: Pharmacology of nitroglycerin and long acting nitrates. Am J Cardiol 56:12A, 1985

53. Miller RR, Vismara L, Williams DO et al: Pharmacological mechanism for left ventricular unloading and clinical congestive heart failure: differential effects of nitroprusside, phentolamine and nitroglycerin on cardiac function in the peripheral circulation. Circ Res 39:127, 1976

54. Taylor WR, Forrester JS, Magnsson P et al: Hemodynamic effects of nitroglycerine ointment in congestive heart failure. Am J Cardiol 38:469, 1976

55. Chatterjee K, Rouleau JL: Hemodynamic and metabolic effects of vasodilators, nitrates, hydralazine, prazosin and captopril in chronic ischemic heart failure. Acta Med Scand, Suppl. 651. 210:295, 1981

56. Ablad B: A study of the mechanism of the hemodynamic effects of hydralazine in man. Acta Pharmacol Toxicol suppl. 1. 20:1, 1963

57. Perry HM: Late toxicity to hydralazine resembling systemic lupus erythematosus or rheumatoid arthritis. Ann J Med 54:58, 1973

58. Pettinger WA: Minoxidil and the treatment of severe hypertension. N Engl J Med 303: 922, 1980

59. Zins GR: Alterations in renal function during vasodilator therapy. p. 165. In Wesson LG, Faneli GM (eds): Recent Advances in Renal Physiology and Pharmacology. University Park Press, Baltimore, 1974

60. Imhof PR, Ott B, Frankhauser P et al: Difference in nitroglycerin dose-response in the venous and arterial beds. Eur J Clin Pharmacol 18:455, 1980

61. Abrams J: Hemodynamic effects of nitroglycerin in pulmonary hypertension. Ann Intern Med 99:9, 1983

62. Brown G, Bolson E, Peterson RB et al: The mechanisms of nitroglycerin action. Stenosis vasodilatation as a major component of drug response. Circulation 64:1089, 1981

63. Moir TW: Subendocardial distribution of coronary blood flow and the effect of antianginal drugs. Circ Res. 30:621, 1972

64. Armstrong PW, Armstrong JA, Marks GS: Blood levels after sublingual nitroglycerin. Circulation. 59:585, 1979

65. Parker JO, Vankoughnett KA, Farrel B: Nitroglycerin lingual spray: clinical efficacy and dose-response relation. Amn J Cardiol 57:1, 1986

66. Reichek N, Goldstein RE, Redwood DR et al: Sustained effects of nitroglycerin treatment in patients with angina pectoris. Circulation 50:348, 1974

67. Chien YW: Pharmaceutical considerations of transdermal nitroglycerin delivery: the various approaches. Am Heart J 108:207, 1984

68. DePace NL, Herling IM, Kotler MN et al: Intravenous nitroglycerin for rest angina: potential pathophysiologic mechanisms of action. Arch Intern Med 142:1806, 1982

69. Krasna MJ, Scott GE, Scholz PM et al: Postoperative enhancement of urinary output in

patients with acute renal failure using continuous furosemide therapy. Chest 89:294, 1986

70. Lerman BB, Belardinelli L: Cardiac electrophysiology of adenosine, basic and clinical concepts. Circulation 83:1499, 1991

71. Williams GH: Converting enzyme inhibitors in the treatment of hypertension. N Engl J Med. 319:1517, 1988

72. Antonaccio MJ: Angiotensin converting enzyme inhibitors. Annu Rev Pharmacol Toxicol 22:57, 1982

73. Braunwald E, Colucci WS: Evaluating the efficacy of new inotropic agents. J Am Coll Cardiol 3:1570, 1984

74. Parmley WW, Smith TW, Pitt B: Should digoxin be the drug of first choice after diuretics in chronic congestive heart failure? Am Coll Cardiol 12:265, 1988

75. Kulick DL, Rahimtoola SH: Current role of digitalis therapy in patients with congestive heart failure. JAMA 265:2995, 1991

76. Smith TW: Digitalis: mechanism of action and clinical use. N Engl J Med 318:358, 1988

77. Rosen MR, Wit AL, Hoffman BF: Electrophysiology and pharmacology of cardiac arrhythmias. IV. Cardiac antiarrhythmic and toxic effects of digitalis. Am Heart J 89:391, 1975

78. Doherty JE, Hall WH, Murphy ML et al: New information regarding digitalis metabolism. Chest 59:433, 1971

79. Doherty JE, Perkins WH, Wilson MC: Studies with titrated digoxin in renal failure. Am J Med 37:536, 1964

80. Doering W: Digoxin-quinidine interaction. N Engl J Med 301:400, 1979

81. Zipes DP, Prystowsky EN, Heger JJ: Amiodarone: electrophysiologic actions and clinical effects. J Am Coll Cardiol 3:1057, 1984

82. Pederson KE, Dorph-Pederson A, Hvidt S et al: Digoxin-verapamil interaction. Clin Pharmacol Ther 30:311, 1981

83. Smit AJ: Dopamine in chronic renal failure. Am J Hypertens 3:755–75, 1990

84. Chrousos, G.: The hypothalamic-pituitary-adrenal axis and immune-mediated inflammation. N Engl J Med 332:1351–62, 1995

85. Rutman HI, LeJemtel TH, Sonnenblick EH: New cardiotonic agents: implications for patients with heart failure and ischemic heart disease. J Cardiothorac Anesth 1:59, 1987

86. Benotti RJ, Grossman W, Braunwald E et al: Effects of amrinone on myocardial energy metabolism and hemodynamics in patients with severe congestive heart failure due to coronary artery disease. Circulation 62:28, 1980

87. Brodde O-E: Pathophysiology of the beta-adrenoceptor system in chronic heart failure: consequences of treatment with agonist, partial agonist or antagonist. Eur Heart J, suppl. F. 12:54, 1991

88. Kilcoyne MM, Schmidt DH, Cannon PJ: Intrarenal blood flow in congestive heart failure. Circulation 47:786, 1973

89. Bodenham A, Shelly MP, Rarrk GR: The altered pharmacokinetics and pharmacodynamics of drugs commanly used in clinically ill patients. Clin Pharmacokinet 14:347, 1988

90. Benowitz NL, Meister W: Pharmacokinetics in patients with cardiac failure. Clin Pharmacokinet 1:389, 1976

91. Beskowitz D, Droll MN, Likoff W: Malabsorption as a complication of congestive heart failure. Am J Cardiol 11:43, 1963

92. Greenblatt DJ, Koch-Weser J: Intramuscular injection of drugs. N Engl J Med 295:542, 1976

93. Jonkman JHG, von Bork LE, de Zeenw RA, Orie NGM: Bioavailability after intramuscular injection. Lancet 1:693, 1976

94. Sherlock S: Disease of the Liver and Biliary System. Ed. Mosby-Year Book, St. Louis, 1985

95. Woosley RL: Pharmacokinetics and pharmacodynamics of antiarrhythmic agents in patients with congestive heart failure. Am Heart J 114:1280, 1987

96. Hepner GW, Vessel ES, Tantum KR: Reduced drug elimination in congestive heart failure. Studies using aminopyrine as a model drug. Am J Med 65:271, 1978

97. Thomson PD, Melmon KL, Richardson JA et al: Lidocaine pharmacokinetics in advanced heart failure, liver disease and renal failure in humans. Ann Intern Med 78:499, 1973

98. Prescott LF, Adjepon-Yamoah KK, Talbott RG. Impaired lignocaine metabolism in patient with myocardial infarction and cardiac failure. Br Med J 1:939, 1976

99. Koch-Weser J, Klien SW: Procainamide dosage schedules, plasma concentrations and clinical effects. JAMA 215:1454, 1971

100. Gibson TP, Matusik EJ, Briggs WA: N-acetyl

procainamide levels in patients with end-stage renal failure. Clin Pharmacol Ther 19: 206, 1976

101. Korhonen UR, Jonnela AJ, Pakarinem AJ, Pentilainen PJ, Takkunen JT: Pharmacokinetic of digoxin in patients with acute MI. Am J Cardiol 44:1190–4, 1979

102. Ohnhans EE, Vozeh S, Nuesch E: Absorption of digoxin in severe right heart failure. Eur J Clin Pharmacol 15:11–120, 1979

103. Naafs MAB, Vander Hoek C, Van Guin S et al: Decreased renal clearance of digoxin in chronic congestive heart failure. Eur J Clin Pharmacol 29:249, 1985

104. Armstrong PW, Armstrong SA, Marks GS: Pharmacokinetic hemodynamic studies of intravenous nitroglycerin in congestive heart failure. Circulation 62:160, 1980

105. Armstrong PW, Armstrong JA, Mark GS: Pharmacokinetic hemodynamic studies of nitroglycerin ointment in congestive heart failure. Am J Cardiol 46:670, 1980

106. Parker JO: Nitrate therapy in stable angina pectoris. N Engl J Med 316:1635, 1987

107. Lavine SJ, Campbell CA, Held AC et al: Effect of nitroglycerin induced reduction of left ventricular filling pressure on diastolic filling in acute dilated heart failure. J Am Coll Cardiol 14:233, 1989

108. Natarajan D, Khurana TR, Kamade V et al: Sustained hemodynamic effects with theraputic doses of intravenous nitroglycerine in congestive heart failure. Am J Cardiol 62:319, 1988

109. Miller RR, Fennel WH, Yong JB et al: Differential systemic arterial and venous action and consequent cardiac effects of vasodilator drugs. Prog Cardiovasc Dis 24:353, 1982

110. Shammas FV, Dickstein K: Clinical pharmacokinetics in heart failure: an updated review. Clin Pharmacokinet 15:94, 1988

111. Crawford MH, Ludden TM, Kennedy GT: Determinants of systemic availability of oral hydrallazine in heart failure. Clin Pharmacol Ther 38:538, 1985

112. Brater DC, Day B, Beudette A, Anderson S: Bemutanide and furosemide in heart failure. Kidney Int 26:183, 1984

113. Vasko MR, Brown-Cartwright D, Knochel PA et al: Furosemide absorption altered in decompensated congestive heart failure. Ann Intern Med 102:314, 1985

114. Packer M, Carven JR, Rodihesser RJ et al: Effect of oral milrinone on mortality in severe chronic heart failure. N Engl J Med 325:1468, 1991

115. Curtiss C, Cohn JN, Vrobel T, Fransiosa JA: Role of the renin-angiotensin system in systemic vasoconstriction of congestive heart failure. Circulation 58:763, 1978

116. Dietz R, Nagel F, Osterziel KJ: Angiotensin-converting enzyme inhibitors and renal function in heart failure. Am J Cardiol 70:119C, 1992

117. Dzau VJ, Packer M, Lilly LS et al: Prostaglandins in severe congestive heart failure. Relation to activation of the renin-angiotensin system and hyponatremia. N Engl J Med 310: 347, 1984

118. Packer M, Lee WH, Kessler PD: Preservation of glomerular filtration rate in human heart failure by activation of the renin-angiotensin system. Circulation 74:766, 1986

119. Dickstein K, Till AE, Aarsland T et al: The pharmacokinetics of enalapril in hospitalised patients with congestive heart failure. Br J Clin Pharmacol 23:403, 1987

120. Beerman B, Jungren IL, Cocchetto D et al: Lisinopril steady-state kinetics in healthy subjects. J Clin Pharmacol 25:471, 1985

121. Dickstein K: Hemodynamic, hormonal and pharmacokinetic aspects of treatment with lisinopril in congestive heart failure. J Cardiovasc Pharmacol, Suppl. 3. 9:73, 1987

122. Runciman WB, Ilsley AH, Mather LE et al: A sheep preparation for studying interactions between blood flow and drug disposition. I: Physiological profile. Br J Anaesth 6:1015, 1984

123. Wood M: Pharmacokinetics and principles of drug infusions in cardiac patients. In Kaplan JA (ed): Cardiac Anesthesia. 3rd Edition WB Saunders, Philadelphia, 1993

124. Nimmo WS, Peacock JE: Effect of surgery and anaesthesia on pharmacokinetics and pharmacodynamics. Br Med Bull 44:286, 1988

125. Ham J, Miller RD, Benet LJ et al: Pharmacokinetics and pharmacodynamics of d-tubocurarine during hypothermia in cat. Anesthesiology 49:324, 1978

126. Hynynen M, Olkkola KT, Naveri E et al: Thiopentone pharmacokinetics during cardiopulmonary bypass with a nonpulsatie or pul-

satile flow. Acta Anesthesiol Scand 33:554, 1989

127. Stanley TH: Arterial blood pressure and deltoid muscle gas tension during cardiopulmonary bypass in man. Can Anaesth Soc J 25: 286, 1987

128. Koska AJ, Romagnoli A, Kramer WG: Effect of cardiopulmonary bypass on fentanyl distribution and elimination. Clin Pharm Ther 29: 100, 1981

129. Pentel P, Benowitz N: Pharmacokinetic and pharmacodynamic considerations in drug therapy of cardiac emergencies. Clinic Pharmacokinet 9:29, 1984

130. Buyleart WA, Herregods LL, Mortier EP, Bogaert MG: Cardiopulmonary bypass and the pharmacokinetics of drugs: an update. Clin Pharmacokinet 17:10, 1989

131. Riplogle R, Levy M, Dewall RA, Lillehei RC: Catecholamine and serotonin response to cardiopulmonary bypass. J Thorac Cardiovasc Surg 44:638, 1962

132. Reves JG, Karp RB, Buttner EE et al: Neuronal and adrenomedullary catecholamine release in response to cardiopulmonary bypass in man. Circulation 66:49, 1982

133. Philbin DM, Levine FH, Kono K et al: Attenuation of the stress response to cardiopulmonary bypass by addition of pulsatile flow. Circulation 64:808, 1981

134. Swain JA: Endocrine responses to cardiopulmonery bypass. In Uttley JR (ed): Pathophysiology of Cardiopulmonery Bypass. Williams & Wilkins, Baltimore, 1983

135. Metz S, Keats AS: Benefits of a glucose containing priming solution for cardiopulmonary bypass. Anesth Analg 72:428, 1991

136. Geneva M, Omann, Hinshaw DB: Inflamation. In Greenfield LJ (ed): Surgery: Scientific Principles and Practice. JB Lippincott, Philadelphia, 1993

137. Holley FO, Ponganis KV, Stanski DR: Effects of cardiac surgery with cardiopulmonary bypass on lidocaine disposition. Clin Pharmacol Ther 35:617, 1984

138. Boylan JW, Hong SK: Regulation of renal function in hypothermia. Am J Physiol 211: 1371, 1966

139. Davis FM, Perimalazhagan KN, Harris EA: Thermal balance during cardiopulmonery bypass with moderate hypothermia in man. Br J Anaesth 49:1127, 1977

140. Miller KW, McCoy HG, Chan KKH et al: Effect of cardiopulmonary bypass on cefazoline disposition. Clin Pharmacol Ther 27:551, 1980

141. Roth RA, Wiersma DA: Role of the lung in total body clearance of circulating drugs. Clin Pharmacokinetic 4:355, 1979

142. Hall R: The pharmacokinetic behaviours of opioids administered during cardiac surgery. Can J Anesth 38:747, 1991

143. Aaltonen L, Kanto J, Arola M et al: Effect of age and cardiopulmonary bypass on the pharmacokinetics of lorazepam. Acta Pharmacol Toxicol 51:126, 1982

144. Kanto J, Himberg JJ, Heikkila H et al: Midazolam kinetics before, during and after cardiopulmonary bypass surgery. Int J Clin Pharmacol Res 2:123, 1985

145. Morrel DF, Harrison GG: Lidocaine kinetics during cardiopulmonary bypass. Br J Anaesth 55:1173, 1983

146. Roffman JA, Fieldman A: Digoxin and propranolol in the prophylaxis of supraventricular tachydysrhythmias after coronary bypass surgery. Ann Thorac Surg 31:496, 1981

147. Cski JF, Schatzlein MH, King RD: Immediate postoperative digitalization in the prophylaxis of supraventricular arrhythmias following coronary artery bypass. J Thorac Cardiovasc Surg 81:419, 1981

148. Krasula RW, Hastreiter AR, Levitsky S et al: Serum, atrial, and urinary digoxin levels during cardiopulmonary bypass in children. Circulation 49:1047, 1974

149. Morrison J, Killip T: Serum digitalis and arrhythmia in patients undergoing cardiopulmonary bypass. Circulation 47:341, 1973

150. Coltart DJ, Chamberlain DA, Howard MR et al: Effect of cardiopulmonary bypass on plasma digoxin concentrations. Br Heart J 33:334, 1971

151. Nancheria AR, Narang PK, Kim YD et al: Sodium thiopental kinetics during cardiopulmonary bypass. Anesth Analg 65:S111, 1986

152. Morgan DJ, Crankshaw DP, Prideaux PR et al: Thiopentone levels during cardiopulmonary bypass. Anaesthesia 41:4, 1986

153. Bjorksten AR, Crankshaw DP, Morgan DJ, Prideaux PR: The effects of cardiopulmonary bypass on plasma concentrations and protein binding of methohexital and thiopental. J Cardiothorac Vasc Anesth 2:281, 1988

154. Oduro A, Tomlinson AA, Davies GK: The use of etomidate infusions during anaesthesia for cardiopulmonary bypass. Anaesthesia 38S: 66, 1983

155. Massey NJA, Sherry KM, Oldroyd S, Peacock JE: Pharmacokinetics of an infusion of propofol during cardiac surgery. Br J Anaesth 65:475, 1990

156. Russell GN, Wright EL, Fox MA et al: Propofol-fentanyl anaesthesia for coronary artery surgery and cardiopulmonary bypass. Anaesthesia 44:205, 1989

157. Laycock GJA, Alston RP: Propofol and hypothermic cardiopulmonary bypass: vasodilation and enhanced metabolic protection? Anaesthesia 47:382, 1992

158. Henderson JM, Nathan HJ, Lalande M et al: Washin and washout of isoflurane during cardiopulmonary bypass. Can J Anaesth 35:587, 1988

159. Thomson IR, Bowering JB, Hudson RJ et al: A comparison of desflurane and isoflurane in patients undergoing coronary artery surgery. Anesthesiology 75:776, 1991

160. Walker JS, Brown KF, Shanks CA: Alcuronium kinetics in patients undergoing cardiopulmonary bypass surgery. Br J Clin Pharmacol 15:237, 1983

161. Walker JS, Shanks CA, Brown KF: Altered d-tubocurarine disposition during cardiopulmonary bypass surgery. Clin Pharmacol Ther 35:686, 1984

162. Flynn PJ, Hughes R, Walton B: Use of atracurium in cardiac surgery involving cardiopulmonary bypass with induced hypothermia. Br J Anaesth 56:967, 1984

163. d'Hollander AA, Duvaldestin P, Henzel D et al: Variations in pancuronium requirement, plasma concentration, and urinary excretion induced by cardiopulmonary bypass with hypothermia. Anesthesiology 58:505, 1983

164. Buzello W, Schulermann D, Schindler M, Spinner G: Hypothermic cardiopulmonary bypass and neuromuscular blockade by pancuronium and vecuronium. Anesthesiology 62:201, 1985

165. Dasta JF, Jacobi J, Wu LS et al: Loss of nitroglycerin to cardiopulmonary bypass apparatus. Crit Care Med 11:50, 1983

166. Dasta JF, Webber RJ, Wu LS et al: Influence of cardiopulmonary bypass on nitroglycerin clearance. J Clin Pharmacol 26:165, 1986

167. Bogaert MG: Clinical pharmacokinetics of glyceryl trinitrate following the use of systemic and topical preparations. Clin Pharmacokinet 12:1, 1987

168. Moore RA, Geller EA, Gallagher JD, Clark DL: Effect of hypothermic cardiopulmonary bypass on nitroprusside metabolism. Clin Pharmacol Ther 37:680, 1985

169. Plachetka JR, Salomon NW, Copeland JG: Plasma propranolol before, during and after cardiopulmonary bypass. Clin Pharmacol Ther 30:745, 1981

170. Wood M, Shand DG, Wood AJJ: Propranolol binding in plasma during cardiopulmonary bypass. Anesthesiology 51:512, 1979

171. Miller KW, McCoy HG, Chan KKH et al: Effect of cardiopulmonary bypass on cefazolin disposition. Clin Pharmacol Ther 27:550, 1980

172. Miller KW, Chan KKH, McCoy HG et al: Cephalothin kinetics before, during and after cardiopulmonary bypass surgery. Clin Pharmacol Ther 265:55, 1979

173. Sato Y, Kanazawa H, Okazaki H et al: A comparison of the penetration characteristics of latamoxef and cephalothin into right atrial appendage and pericardial fluid of adult patient undergoing open-heart surgery. J Antibiot (Tokyo) 37:678, 1984

174. Lunn JK, Stanley TH, Eisele J et al: High dose fentanyl anesthesia for coronary artery surgery: plasma fentanyl concentrations and influence of nitrous oxide on cardiovascular responses. Anesth Analg 58:390, 1979

175. Bovill JG, Sebel PS: Pharmacokinetics of high-dose fentanyl. Br J Anaesth 52:795, 1980

176. Bentley JB, Conahan TJ, Cork RC: Fentanyl sequestration in lung during cardiopulmonary bypass. Clin Pharmacol Ther 34:703, 1983

177. Koska AJ, Romagnoli A, Kramer WG: Effect of cardiopulmonary bypass on fentanyl distribution and elimination. Clin Pharmacol Ther 29:100, 1981

178. Koren G, Crean P, Klein J et al: Sequestration of fentanyl by the cardiopulmonary bypass (CPBP). Eur J Clin Pharmacol 27:51, 1984

179. Rosen DA, Rosen KR, Davidson B et al: Absorption of fentanyl by the membrane oxygenator. Anesthesiology 63:A281, 1985

180. Kumar K, Crankshaw DP, Morgan DJ, Beemer GH: The effect of cardiopulmonary

bypass on plasma protein binding of alfentanil. Eur J Clin Pharmacol 35:47, 1988

181. Hug CC, De Lange S, Burn AGL: Alfentanil pharmacokinetics in patients before and after cardiopulmonary bypass (CPB), Anesth Analg 62:266, 1983

182. Traynor C, Hali GM: Endocrine and metabolic changes during surgery: anaesthesia implications. Br J Anaesth 53:153, 1981

183. Lush D, Thorpe JN, Richardson DJ, Bower DJ: The effect of epidural analgesia on the adrenocortical response to surgery. Br J Anaesth 44:1169, 1972

184. Cartensen H, Terner N, Thoren L, Wide L: Testosterone, leutinising hormone and growth hormone in blood following surgical trauma. Acta Chir Scand 138:1, 1972

185. Russel RCG, Walker CJ, Bloom SR: Hyperglucagonaemia in surgical patient. Br Med J 1:10, 1975

186. Allison SP: Changes in insulin secretion during open-heart surgery. Br J Anaesth 43:138, 1971

187. Oyama T: Endocrine responses to anaesthetic agents. Br J Anaesth 45:276, 1973

188. Robertson D, Michaelis AM: Effect of anesthesia and surgery on plasma renin activity in man. J Clin Endocrinol Metab 34:831, 1972

189. Engquist A, Blichert-Toft M, Flgaard K et al: Inhibition of aldosterone response to surgery by saline administration. Br J Surg 65:224, 1978

190. Hall GM: The anaesthetic modification of the endocrine and metabolic response to surgery. Ann R Coll Surg Engl 67:25, 1985

191. Kehlet H, Brandt MR, Hansen AP, Alberti KG: Effect of epidural analgesia on metabolic profiles during and after surgery. Br J Surg 66:543, 1979

192. George JM, Reier E, Lanese RR, Rower JM: Morphine anesthesia blocks cortisol and growth hormone response to stress in humans. J Clin Endocrinol Metab 38:736, 1974

193. Stanley TH, Berman L, Green O et al: Plasmacatecholamine and cortisol responses to fentanyl-oxygen anesthesia for coronary-artery operations. Anesthesiology 53:250, 1980

194. Rouleau J-L, Warnica JW, Burgess JH: Prazosin and congestive heart failure: short and long term therapy. Am J Med 71:147, 1981

195. Casson WR, Jones RM, Parson RS: Nifedipine and cardiopulmonary bypass: post bypass management after continuation or withdrawl of therapy. Anaesthesia 39:1197, 1984

196. Jenkins LC, Scoates PJ: Anaesthetic implications of calcium channel blockers. Can Anaesth Soc J 32:436, 1985

197. Packer M, Meller J, Media N et al: Hemodynamic consequences of combined beta-adrenergic and slow calcium channel blockade in man. Circulation 65:660, 1982

198. Kapur PA, Bloor BC, Flacke WE and Olewine SK: Comparison of CVS responses to verapamil during enflurane, isoflurane or halothane anesthesia in dog. Anesthesiology 61:156, 1984

199. Maze M, Mason DM, Kates RE: Verapamil decreases MAC for halothane in dogs. Anesthesiology 59:327, 1983

200. Feely J, Wilkinson GR, Wood AJJ: Reduction of liver blood flow and propranolol metabolism by cimetidine. N Engl J Med 304:692, 1981

201. Shearer EH, Russel GN: The effect of cardiopulmonary bypass on cholinesterase activity. Anesthesiology 48:293, 1993

202. Miller RD, Sohn YJ, Matteo RS: Enhancement of d-tubocurane neuromuscular blockade by diuretics in man. Anesthesiology 45:442, 1976

203. Anderson KA, Marshall RJ: Interactions between calcium entry blockers and vecuronium bromide in anesthetised cats. Br J Anaesth 57:775, 1985

204. McIndewar IC, Marshall RJ: Interactions between the neuromuscular blocking drug ORG NC 45 and some anaesthetic, analgesic and antimicrobial agents. Br J Anaesth 53:785, 1981

205. Kaplan JA, Finlayson DC, Woodward S: Vasodilator therapy after cardiac surgery: a review of the efficacy and toxicity of nitroglycerin and nitroprusside. Can Anaesth Soc J 27:253, 1980

206. Dupius J, Lalonde G, Lebean R et al: Sustained beneficial effect of a seventy-two hour intravenous infusion of nitroglycerin in patients with severe chronic congestive heart failure. Am Heart J 120:625, 1990

207. Stinson EB, Holloway EL, Derby G et al: Comparative hemodynamic responses to chlorpromazine, nitroprusside, nitroglycerin and trimelaphan immediately after open heart operations. Circulation 51:126, 1975

208. Greenberg BH, Rahimtoola SH: Vasodilator treatment for valvular heart disease. JAMA 246:269, 1981

209. Greenbaum DA, Dillon JC, Felgenbaum H: The effect of nitroglycerin upon pulmonary and left arterial pressures in patients with mitral stenosis. Am Heart J 91:156, 1976

210. Strum JT, Furhaman TM, Igo SR et al: Efficiency of nitroprusside treatment in the postcardiotomy low output syndrome needing intra-aortic balloon pump. J Thorac Cardiovasc Surg 78:254, 1974

211. Palmer RMJ, Ferrige AG, Moncada S: Nitric oxide release accounts for the biological activity of endothelium-derived relaxing factor. Nature 327:524, 1987

212. Moncada S, Palmer RMS, Higgs EA: Nitric oxide: physiology, pathophysiology and pharmacology. Pharmacol Rev 43:109, 1991

213. Harrison DG, Bates JN: The nitrovasodilators. New ideas about old drugs. Circulation 87:1461, 1993

214. Tibbalis J: Clinical applications of gaseous nitric oxide. Anaesth Intensive Care 21:866, 1993

215. Kinsella JP, Toews WH, Henry D, Abman SH: Selective and sustained pulmonary vaso- dilatation with inhalational nitric oxide therapy in a child with idiopatric pulmonary hypertension. J Pediatr 122:803, 1993

216. Rosaint R, Falke KJ, Lopez F et al: Inhaled nitric oxide for adult respiratory distress syndrome. N Engl J Med 328:399, 1993

217. Hart JL, Jing M, Bina S et al: Effects of halothane on EDRF/cGMP mediated vascular smooth muscle relaxations. Anesthesiology 79:323, 1993

218. Siegfried MR, Carey MAXL, Lefer AM: Beneficial effects of SPM-5185 a cystine-containing NO donor in myocardial ischemia–reperfusion. Am J Physiol 263:H771, 1992

219. Panza JA, Cassino PR, Kilcoyn CM, Quyymi AA: Role of endothelium-derived nitric oxide in the abnormal endothelium-dependant vascular relaxation of patients with essential hypertension. Circulation 87:1468, 1993

220. Calver A, Collier J, Vallance P: Inhibition and stimulation of nitric oxide synthesis in the human forearm arterial bed of patients with insulin-dependent diabetes. J Clin Invest 90:2548, 1992

221. Foubert L, Fleming B, Latimer R et al: Safety guidelines for use of nitric oxide. Lancet 399:1615, 1992

17

Mechanical Circulatory Support

Howard I. Chait
John P. Williams

WHY DO WE NEED MECHANICAL CIRCULATORY SUPPORT SYSTEMS?

Mechanical support is a lot like marriage: it is not to be entered into reservedly or unadvisedly. Although there are compelling physiologic reasons for selecting a mechanical over a pharmacologic form of circulatory support, from the patient's perspective the summary risk is similar. For this reason it is best to discuss the need for and use of a mechanical circulatory support system (MCSS) with the patient *before* surgery. There is mounting evidence that patients favor such "advance directives." Most physicians are loath to discuss the use of tools such as MCSS with patients. Physicians, when asked a similar question regarding their personal medical care, however, responded that they favor the use of advance directives.[1]

This chapter should serve as a starting point for anyone interested in the use of MCSS. It is not intended to serve as an exhaustive review of the literature or the final word in the technical description and utilization of every type of MCSS. This chapter does provide the reader with a general survey of MCSS from a clinical perspective, reviews the need and utilization criteria for MCSS, briefly reviews the outcome data available from a variety of devices, and finally reviews the contraindications to utilization. The reading list available at the end of this chapter provides a good source for the detail omitted because of space constraints.

Goals of Therapy

The reasons that favor MCSS in preference to pharmacologic support are primarily physiologic. These physiologic reasons are divisible into two broad categories: the deleterious effects of pharmacologic support, and the ameliorative effects of mechanical circulatory support.

DELETERIOUS EFFECTS OF PHARMACOLOGIC SUPPORT

The precise myocardial response of a patient to pharmacologic intervention is difficult if not impossible to predict. The appearance of untoward side effects is the result of a variety of problems, including pre-existing organ dysfunction (renal, hepatic, or pulmonary insufficiency), pre-existing alterations in organ blood flow (renal, carotid, vertebral, or coronary arterial stenosis), alterations in metabolism (chronic myocardial ischemia), and alterations in receptor density, expression and function, and the maximum dosage of the agent to name just a few.[2]

Drugs such as isoproterenol or norepinephrine, when used in the nonfailing myocardium, can unfavorably alter the myocardial supply/demand ratio and aggravate or initiate an ischemic event. Yet these agents can re-establish a normal supply-demand relationship when administered to the failing myocardium.[3] The best one can hope to accomplish is to initiate therapy to eliminate or amend the physiologic derangement present and to choose pharmacologic agents based on the effects they produce in a population of normal humans or an animal model. This approach requires one to wait for a complication to occur, rather than anticipating a change and averting a negative outcome.

Besides the routine complications that attend the use of catecholamines (either natural or synthetic) and other positive inotropic agents, high levels of the sympathomimetic amines can produce necrotic changes in the myocardium.[4,5] Endogenous sympathetic release during stressful events in humans may also result in myocardial necrosis.[6] Alterations in serum electrolytes (sodium, potassium, magnesium, zinc, and calcium)[7-10] and the stress hormones (insulin, glucocorticoids, and thyroid)[2,11] are capable of exacerbating the deleterious effects of both natural and synthetic catecholamines. All these changes can occur during or following the onset of cardiopulmonary bypass.

Table 17-1 describes the type of agent and most common reasons for eliminating therapy with that agent. Many of the recently introduced synthetic amines (e.g., dobutamine), and bypyridines (e.g., amrinone) are less likely to produce myocardial necrosis than are the naturally occurring sympathomimetics.[12-15] Enoximone, the most recently developed of the bypyridines, was touted as a "pharmacologic" bridge to transplant.[16]

Table 17-1. Comparative Analysis of Positive Inotropic Agents

Agent	Family	Drawback
Isoproterenol	Catecholamine (synthetic)	Tachycardia, coronary steal, dysrhythmogenic, excessive vasodilation
Epinephrine	C (natural)	Tachycardia, excessive vasoconstriction, decrease in splanchnic blood flow and renal blood flow, dysrhythmogenic
Norepinephrine	C (natural)	Severe reduction in renal and splanchnic flow, excessive vasoconstriction
Dopamine	C (natural)	Tachycardia, dysrhythmias, vasoconstriction
Dobutamine	C (synthetic)	Tachycardia, dysrhythmias
Digitalis	Glycoside	Dysrhythmias, excessive AV nodal blockade, long half-life
Amrinone	PDE-III$_i$	Excessive vasodilation, increased AV nodal conduction velocity, thrombocytopenia, dysrhythmias
Milrinone	PDE-III$_i$ (15 times potency of amrinone)	Similar to amrinone
Enoximone	PDE-III$_i$	Similar to amrinone

Abbreviation: PDE-III$_i$, phosphodiesterase-III inhibitor.

However, a more recent prospective evaluation found pharmacologic support with enoximone adequate in only 65 percent of 201 patients.[17] Unfortunately, no pharmacologic agent is capable of sustaining myocardial function or prolonging life over a period of months, as several clinical trials have recently demonstrated.[18-23] The prolongation of life is the specific purview of MCSS. In all clinical trials to date, no agent is capable of prolonging life in chronic utilization.

AMELIORATIVE EFFECTS OF MCSS

Unlike any of the pharmacologic agents, MCSS provides the failing myocardium with an opportunity for repair in addition to providing the body a stable metabolic transport system. It is not clear how pathologic conditions lead to an acute or chronic loss of myocardial contractile function. However, the most common acute, reversible, contractile defect is myocardial "stunning."[24] A period of ischemia (usually greater than 15 minutes at normothermia) that is of insufficient duration to produce necrotic changes reliably reproduces the "stunning" phenomena. Of the numerous mechanistic postulates available, one of the more significant is a loss of nucleotide (energy) precursors from the cell. Replacement of these precursors is not complete for days after a brief period of warm ischemia.[25,26]

Further abnormalities that may contribute to the depression in function that follows a "stunning" type of myocardial insult include interstitial and intra- or intercellular edema. Water regulation and oncotic pressure are under tight regulation in the myocardium. Small changes in total water content can result in large changes in myocardial compliance and function.[27,28] MCSS may not only provide a stable period that allows for resolution of this edematous state, but may also accelerate this process by avoiding increases in central venous pressure. Increases in central venous pressure (CVP), which typically occur with myocardial failure, lead to an increase in myocardial lymphatic outflow pressure. This increase in myocardial lymphatic outflow pressure will reduce the rate of egress of interstitial edema fluid.[29]

The intra-aortic balloon pump (IABP) and the ventricular assist device (VAD) MCSS are capable of reducing infarct size in animal models.[30-34] In the IABP-MCSS, human studies generally document an increase in coronary blood flow; however, most of these patients are hypotensive at the initiation of MCSS support.[35-40] In animals, the IABP and VAD improve the ratio of epicardial to endocardial blood flow in peri-infarct zones.[30,36,40]

In the setting of chronic ischemia and myocardial failure, the MCSS produces a decompressed heart requiring minimal energy expenditure, while it continues to provide forward flow to the remainder of the body.[33,41,42] In both animal and human subjects, MCSS achieves this reduction in the metabolic and oxygen demands of the myocardium primarily through a decline in wall tension. Both left ventricular intracavitary pressures (peak systolic and end-diastolic) decrease following the institution of MCSS.[43,44] Both IABP and VAD MCSS provide the clinician with the unique opportunity to augment cardiac output while simultaneously decreasing total myocardial energy expenditure.

Background and Significance

In 1985 the working group on MCSS conducted a population-based study in Minnesota to estimate the need for MCSS. That study projected an annual eligibility of 17,000 to 35,000 candidates in the United States.[45] These projections, however, do not include patients who could benefit from temporary support with the anticipated return of native cardiac function. Approximately 250,000 to 300,000 people undergo cardiac surgery each year.[46] About 3 to 6 percent of these patients will require MCSS after surgery.[47,48] This adds an additional 10,000 to 18,000 patients each year who will require some form of temporary MCSS.

The most recent estimates for the utilization of MCSS are from the Institute of Medicine (IOM). The study group that examined the future of the artificial heart program, reported an annual estimate of 10,000 to 20,000 patients requiring a total artificial heart (TAH) and 25,000 to 60,000 patients requiring a VAD. However, these investigators noted that as the population aged, and if a successful device became available, the total number of implants could reach 200,000 by the year 2020.[49] These estimates rely solely on mortality statistics from patients aged 35 to 75 years, with coronary artery disease. If the mortality statistics expanded to include patients aged 25 to 85, as well as those succumbing to congestive heart failure, worldwide utilization could exceed 500,000 patients by the year 2020.

Finally, if the eventual market cost of a TAH is $100,000 (in 1991 dollars), and the cost of a VAD is $50,000, the increase in health care costs for the device alone would be $5 billion per year. The above financial implications and the extensive commitment of medical resources require the need to assess the appropriateness and applicability of MCSS.

SOCIAL AND ETHICAL CONCERNS

No other medical issues (with the obvious exceptions of organ transplantation and fetal tissue utilization) engender as many social and ethical dilemmas as MCSS. An estimated development cost for the TAH (1963 to 1992) is $270 million.[50] This enormous expenditure plus the yearly estimated costs of $10 million prompted Claude Lenfant, director of the National Heart, Lung, and Blood Institute (NHLBI), to suspend funding of the TAH program in 1988. An industrial and public outcry, restored funding; but, with the caveat that the IOM initiate a re-evaluation of the TAH's costs and benefits.[51] Subsequently, this IOM committee, chaired by John R. Hogness, recommended a continuation of current funding but concluded that projected costs would be greater and the benefits lower than for any

medical procedure now in use. The estimated cost per quality-adjusted-life-year gained is $105,000, which is substantially lower than other health care technologies (for a comparison of selected health care technologies see Appendix 17-1). The committee also made acceptance of the report contingent on the following proposals: (1) completion of clinical trials on the VAD, (2) collection of data regarding the quality of the hardware and psychological and social issues accompanying the widespread utilization of the TAH and (3) a re-evaluation in 1994 following an assessment of data collection; before continuation of funding.[51]

Finally, the planning committee that set up the aforementioned IOM panel also made several basic recommendations regarding patient involvement. First, an examination of human costs to the patient and family is necessary; especially a propos the long-term use of MCSS. Second, patient selection and clinical trial conduct should *follow* the development of detailed criteria for these procedures. Third, close monitoring of the trials by all parties involved (NHLBI, FDA, contractors, grantees, and the local IRB) is mandatory. Fourth, the patient, surrogate decision makers and the patient's primary care physicians must receive adequately illuminating, incremental information.[51] Finally, in those centers where the possibility of anticipated utilization of MCSS exists, all patients and families must receive basic information concerning MCSS. This should avoid last-minute confusion regarding patients' wishes.[51] A durable power of attorney further provides for compliance with advance directives.

Many social and ethical concerns remain. For further discussions and explanations of the many dilemmas raised by MCSS. The reader is referred to "The Artificial Heart: Prototypes, Policies, and Patients," edited by J. R. Hogness and M. Van Antwerp.

HISTORY

There were several early attempts to mimic the circulatory effects of the heart.[52–65] All these early attempts at circulatory support

Table 17-2.   Level of Federal Funding, 1966–1991[a]

Year	66	70	74	78	82	86	91
Expenditures	18	34	34	28	18	16	15

[a] All expenditures are in millions of dollars, approximated, and adjusted to reflect costs in 1991 dollars.[51]

were in animals. Application of a mechanical circulatory device in humans occurred late in the twentieth century.[66–68]

The modern history of MCSS is a direct result of the rise in popularity and safety of cardiac surgery. However, it would be a gross misstatement to ascribe the forces that initiated this sojourn to "market pressure" alone. Without the drive, ambition, and prescience of a number of pioneers' there would be no MCSS. This section should give the reader some perspective on the fiscal and chronologic resources expended to bring us to the present.

Table 17-2 compares the level of federal funding from 1966 through 1991. What is not represented in this table is the number of grants supported for each year. The first year of federal support was 1964 and awarded $581,000 in six contracts. For the fiscal year ending 1991, projected expenditures are approximately $15.5 Million, which supports six research and development (R&D) grants for the TAH, two for thermal power, and 23 others. The trend in funding, however, is downward. The year for maximum federal support was 1974 with the dollar total (adjusted to 1991) peaking around $34 million.

From 1964 to 1969, the approach for MCSS development research was through systems engineering, since developing a MCSS seemed similar in scope to the space program. This approach changed in 1969 to focus on an integrated device. This decision followed, in part, the first successful use of such a design in humans by Denton Cooley, although the integration of numerous considerations (biocompatibility, power source and the prevention of infection and thromboembolism to name a few) was proving to be a more formidable obstacle than previously projected.

The termination of the nuclear powered MCSS in early 1974 required a redirection of many man-hours of labor; however, an interim assessment panel strongly advised against its use. Further recommendations by this panel urged the continuation of efforts to develop a left ventricular assist device (LVAD) as well as the TAH. The acceptance of this advice would have implications reaching into 1990. Then, in 1984 and 1985, two successful bridge-to-transplant operations occur with the use of pneumatically powered LVADs: one in Stanford, and one at the Texas Heart Institute.

Late in 1981, the Food and Drug Administration (FDA) approved a request from the University of Utah for an investigational device exemption (IDE). This would culminate in the first long-term human implantation in Dr. Barney Clark later in 1982. The survival time was 112 days, but this limited success results in four further implantations (including one in Sweden), all with similarly positive results. Then, in 1988, the recommendations of the Working Group (convened to discuss the results of these first human implants) result in funding for four further R&D contracts to produce a TAH. Five months later, funding was suspended coincident with the publication by Devries and his group of the results of the first four Jarvik-7 implants; however, the primary reason given for this action was an inability to fund both the TAH and LVAD programs. The LVAD program appeared closer to producing a viable product.

Late in 1990, the FDA withdrew Symbion's IDE. After 186 implants worldwide, the production of the device halted. Later in the same year, the NHLBI funded contracts with the University of Pittsburgh and St. Louis University for a joint clinical trial of 20 Novacor LVADs.

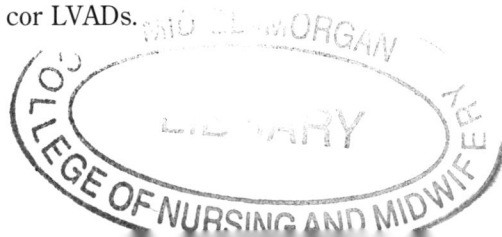

As of late 1995, approximately 293 TAH implants, 1,384 LVADs, 196 right VADs, and 1,000 biventricular VADs had been inserted worldwide. Of these insertions, 1,721 patients weaned from their support and approximately 1,452 left the hospital.[69,70] (Fasnacht A, ABIOMED Cardiovascular, Inc., Danvers, MA, and Olsen DB, Salt Lake City, personal communications). These are impressive figures, as all these patients would have died in hospitals less than 15 years ago. The appropriate use of these devices and patient selection is the focus of the next sections of this chapter.

DEVICE DESCRIPTIONS

The devices and systems available for open utilization include roller pumps (Fig. 17-1),

IABPs (Fig. 17-2), centrifugal pumps (Fig. 17-3), and the ABIOMED BVS-5000 (Fig. 17-4). The specific features of these devices are summarized in Table 17-3. Those devices available under experimental protocols include the Hemopump (Fig. 17-5), the Novacor (Fig. 17-6), the Thermedics (Fig. 17-7), the Nimbus (Fig. 17-8) the Utah, the Penn State Thoratec (Fig. 17-9), and the Penn State Rollerscrew. The specific features of these systems are summarized in Table 17-4. Appendix 17-2 lists the manufacturers' addresses of many of these devices.

CONTRAINDICATIONS TO MCSS

There are at least three categories into which the contraindications to the use of MCSS can be ascribed. These categories are

Table 17-3.   Summary of Specific Features of Devices Available for Open Utilization

Device	Roller Pump	IABP	Centrifugal Pump	ABIOMED BVS-5000
Blood pump	D/C brushless motor	Helium-filled balloon	Centrifugal force	Pneumatic drive, dual chamber, blood pumps with two trileaflet polyurethane valves each
Power supply	A/C with transformer and battery	A/C with transformer and battery	A/C with transformer and battery	A/C with transformer and battery
Insertion sites (outflow)	Femoral artery, aorta	Femoral artery, aorta, subclavian	Femoral artery, aorta	Aorta or main pulmonary artery
Insertion sites (inflow)	Right atrium vena cavae, femoral vein		Right atrium, vena cavae, femoral vein	Right atrium or left atrium
Position of device	Extracorporeal	Extracorporeal	Extracorporeal	Extracorporeal
Vol. of displacement (stroke volume)	5–25 ml per revolution	Depends on size of balloon (20, 40, 50, 60)	40–80 ml	70–80 ml
Flow characteristics	Nonpulsatile, pseudopulsatile	Pulsatile	Nonpulsatile	Pulsatile
Figure No.	17-1	17-2A–F	17-3A,B	17-4A–C
Ref. No.	30, 69, 71–77	78–81	82	Fasnacht A, (personal communication)

Abbreviations: IABP, intra-aortic balloon pump; D/C, direct current; A/C, alternating current; CO, cardiac output.

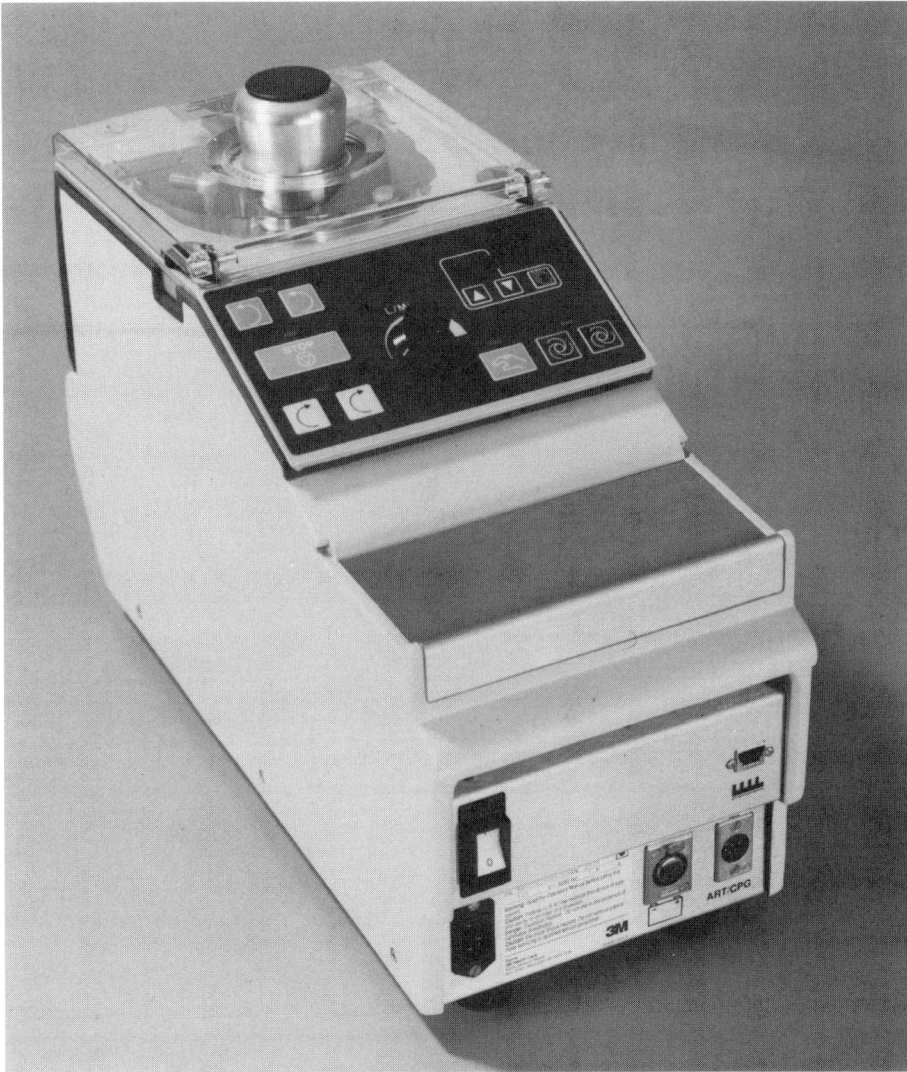

Fig. 17-1. Roller pump console pump head and controls.

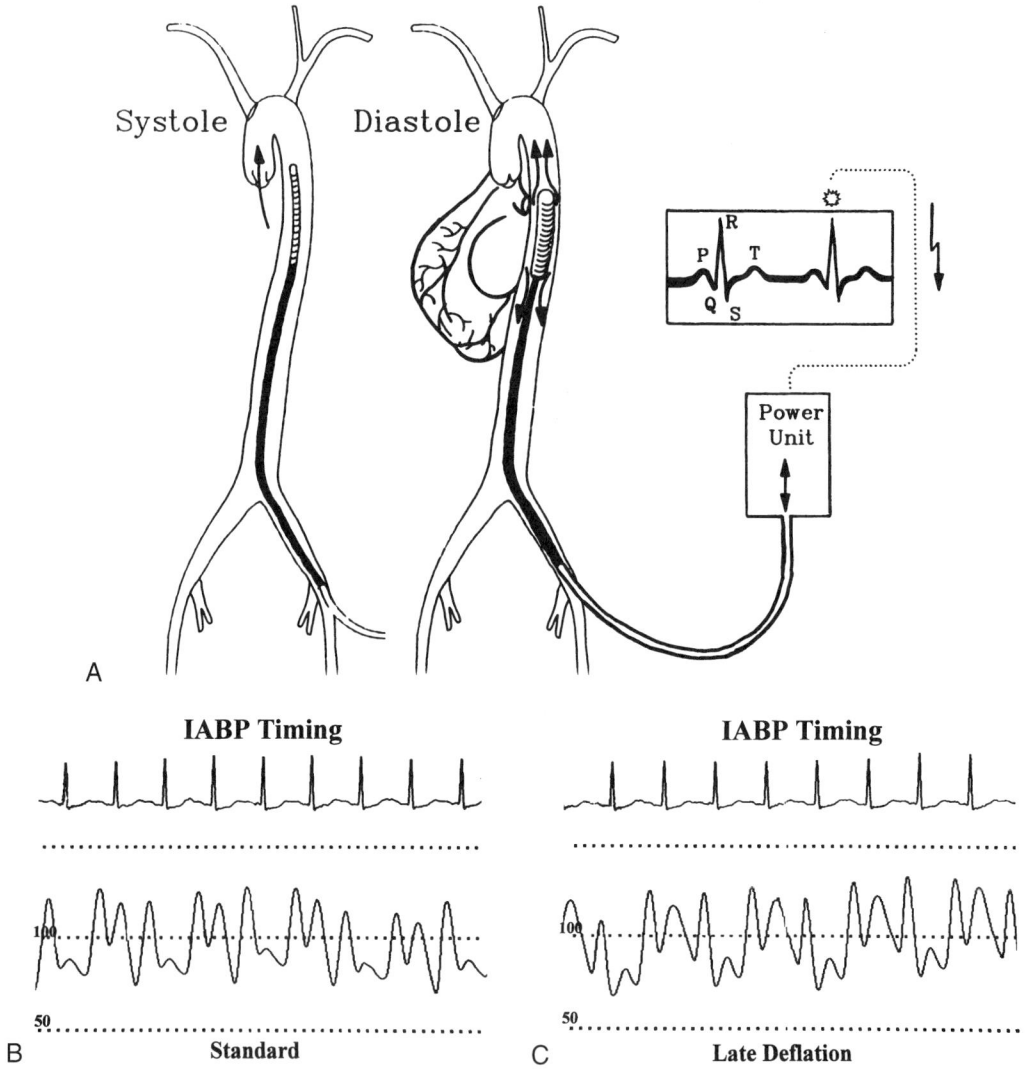

Fig. 17-2. (A) Schematic of the intra-aortic balloon pump (IABP) during systole and asystole. **(B)** Normal timing and functioning in the 1:2 mode. **(B)** Normal timing and function in the 1:2 mode. **(C)** Late deflation in the 1:2 mode. (*Figure continues.*)

IABP Timing

IABP Timing

D **Early Deflation**

E **Early Inflation**

IABP Timing

F **Late Inflation**

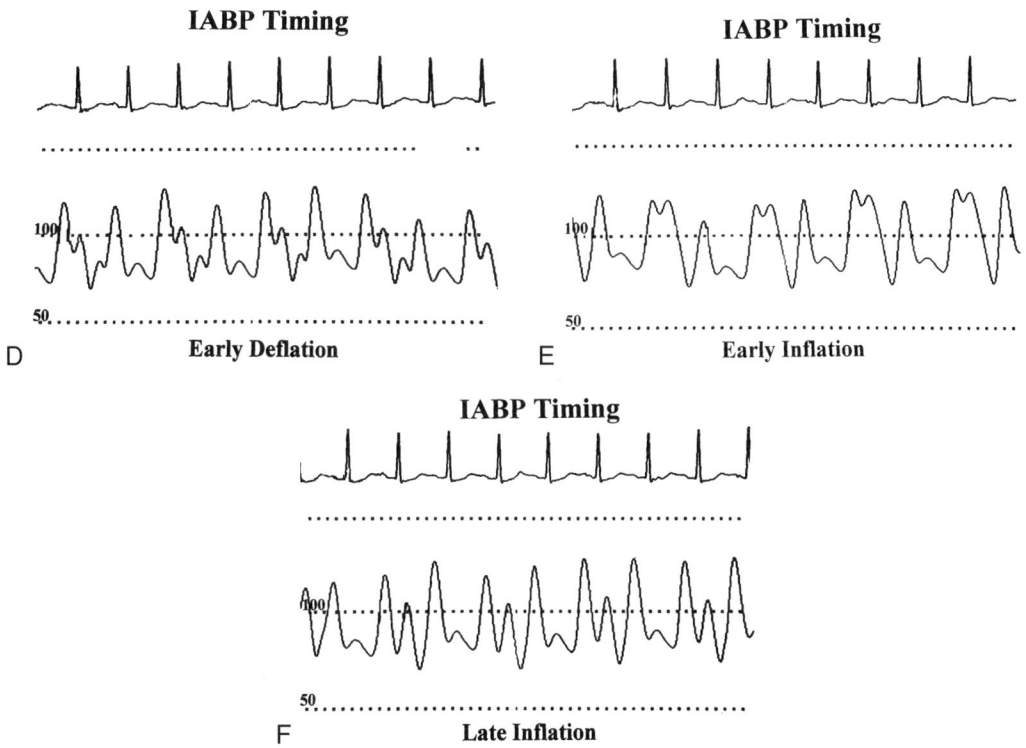

Fig. 17-2 (*Continued*). **(D)** Early deflation in the 1:2 mode. **(E)** Early inflation in the 1:2 mode. **(F)** Late inflation in the 1:2 mode.

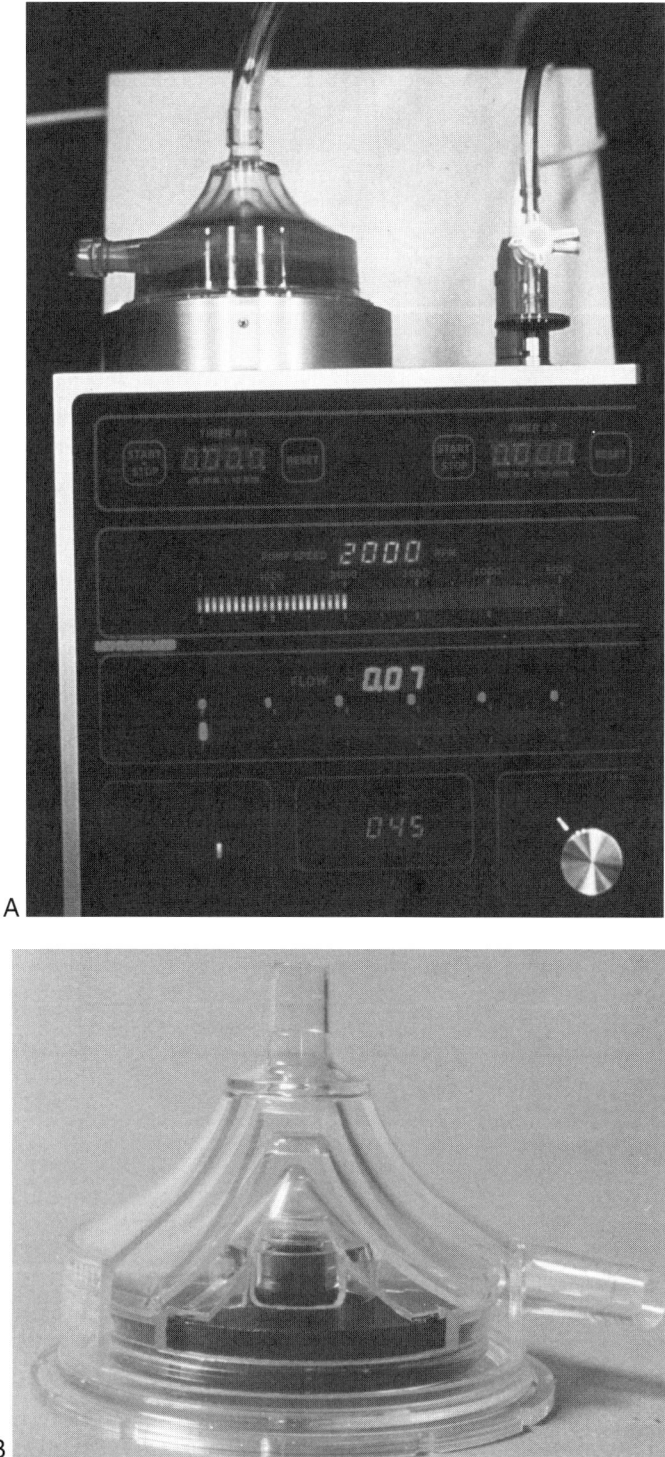

Fig. 17-3. (A) Centrifugal pump drive console. **(B)** Constrained vortex produced by the internal cones.

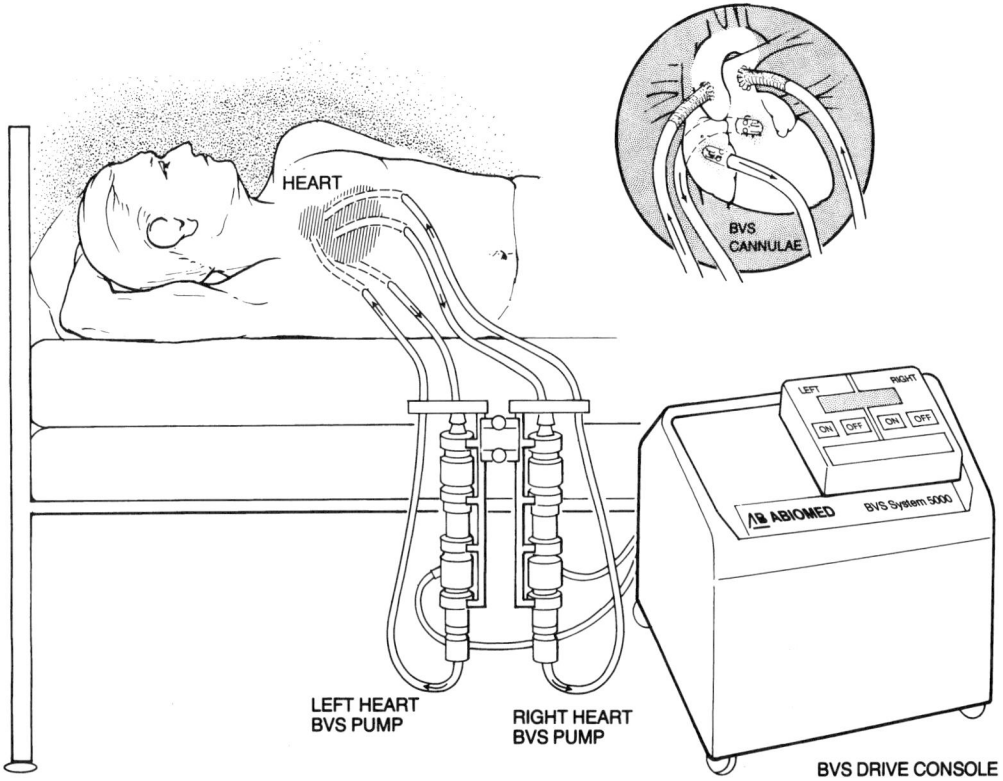

Fig. 17-4. Diagram of suggested placement of the BVS-5000 in a patient with biventricular failure. Actual placement may vary secondary to anatomic constraints. The pump is constructed as a plastic tube filled with two polymer chambers. The left and right BVS pumps are identical in construction. Each pump is configured with a passively filled, upper "atrial" chamber and a lower, actively emptied "ventricular" chamber (the lines running from the console to the pumps lead to the "ventricular" housing and chamber). During diastole, air is actively exhausted from around the "ventricular" chamber, thus allowing the "atrial" chamber to passively empty into the "ventricular" chamber. Bioprosthetic valves maintain unidirectional flow from "atrial" to "ventricular" chambers and on to the pulmonary or systemic circulations. Once the "ventricular" chamber fills, air is injected into the plastic housing around the polymer chamber, this action compresses the chamber and results in the ejection of blood. The "atrial" chamber then fills passively in preparation for the next cycle.

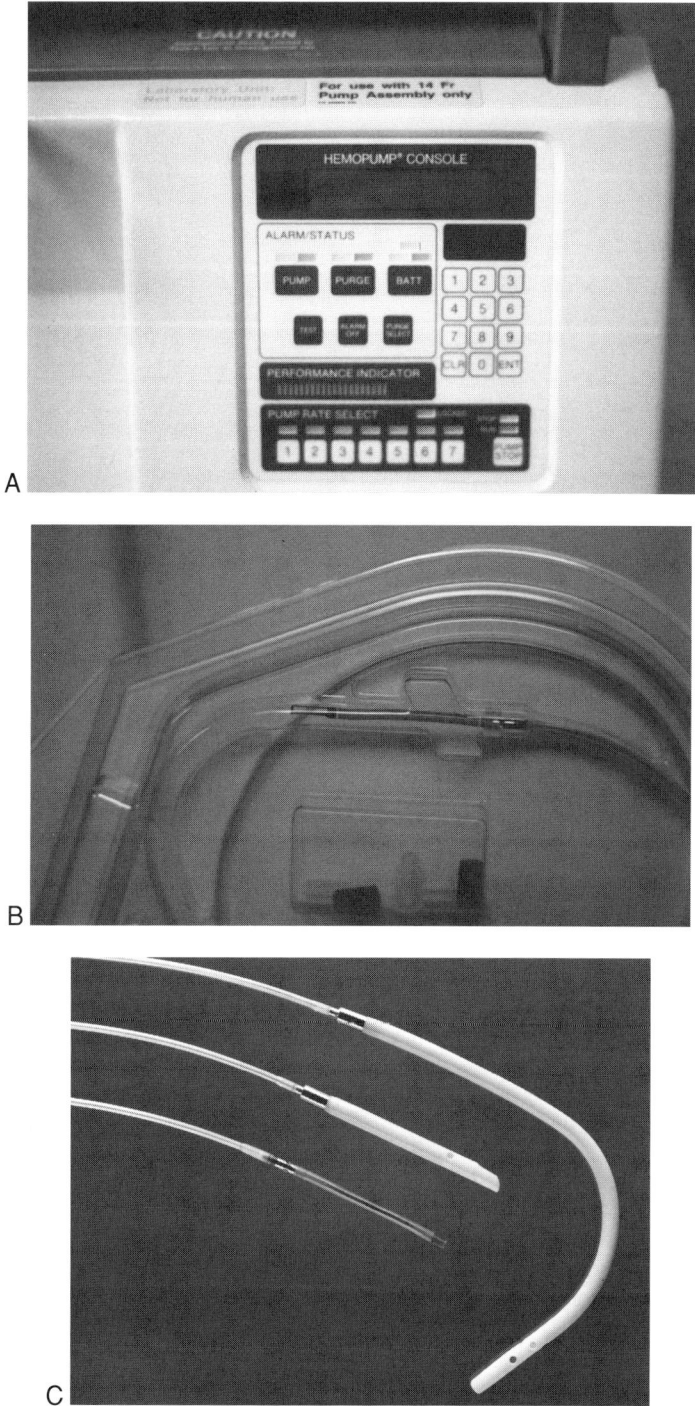

Fig. 17-5. Hemopump. **(A)** Console. **(B)** Tip of the Hemopump that resides within the left ventricle. **(C)** Three available tip sizes (Fig. B courtesy of Johnson & Johnson Intervention Systems, Rancho Cordova, CA; Fig. C from Phillips,[168] with permission.)

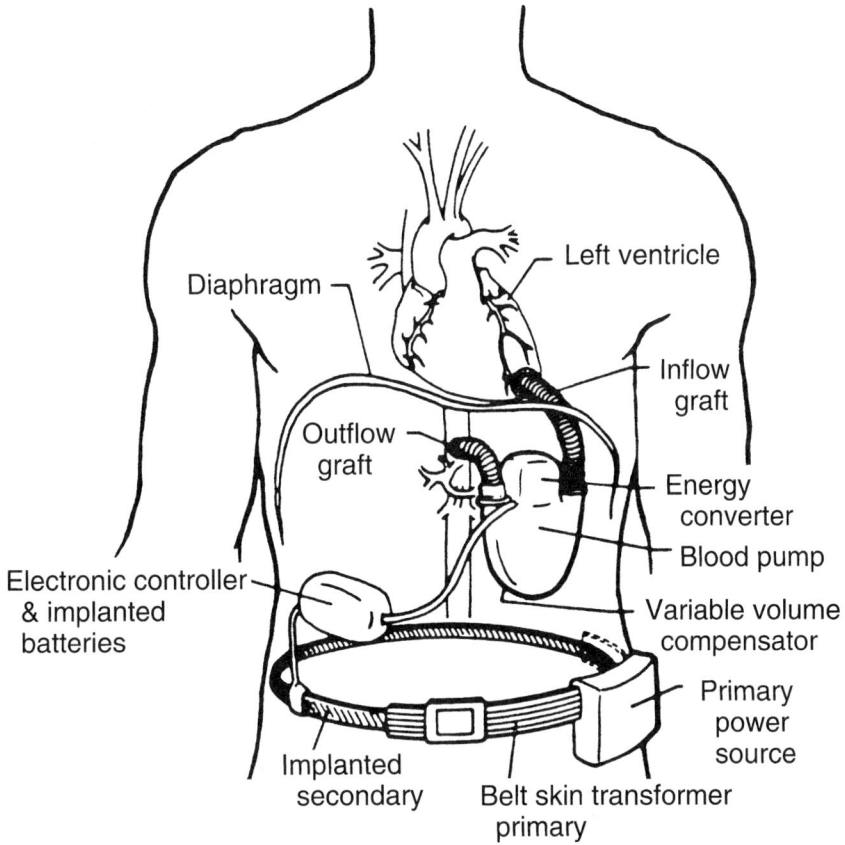

Fig. 17-6. Novacor left ventricular assist device. **(A)** Anatomic location. (*Figure continues.*)

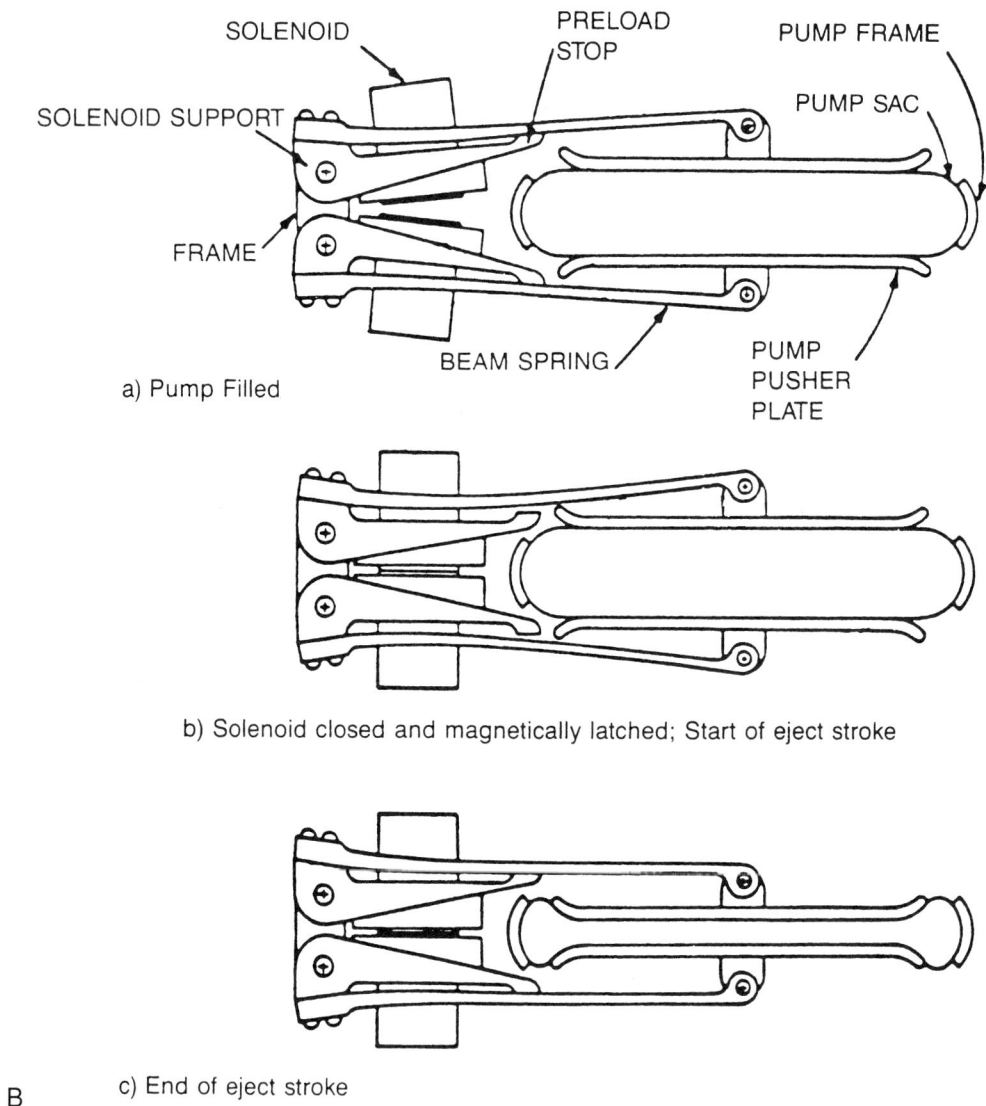

a) Pump Filled

b) Solenoid closed and magnetically latched; Start of eject stroke

B

c) End of eject stroke

Fig. 17-6 (*Continued*). (**B**) Energy converter operation. (From Altieri et al.,[86] with permission.)

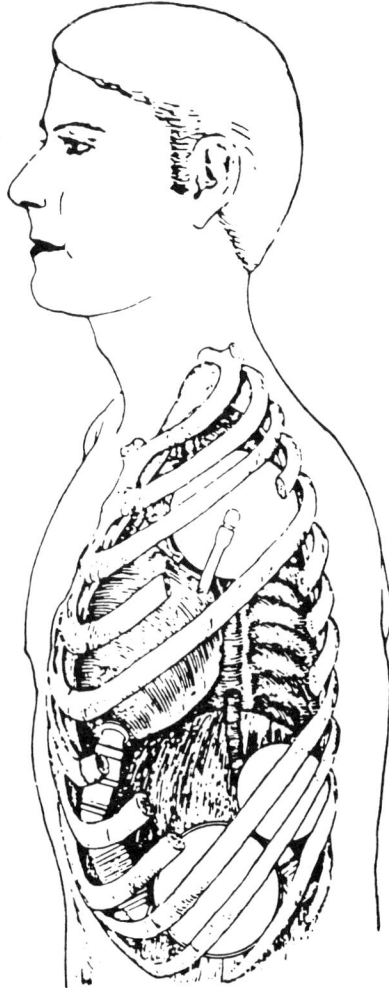

A

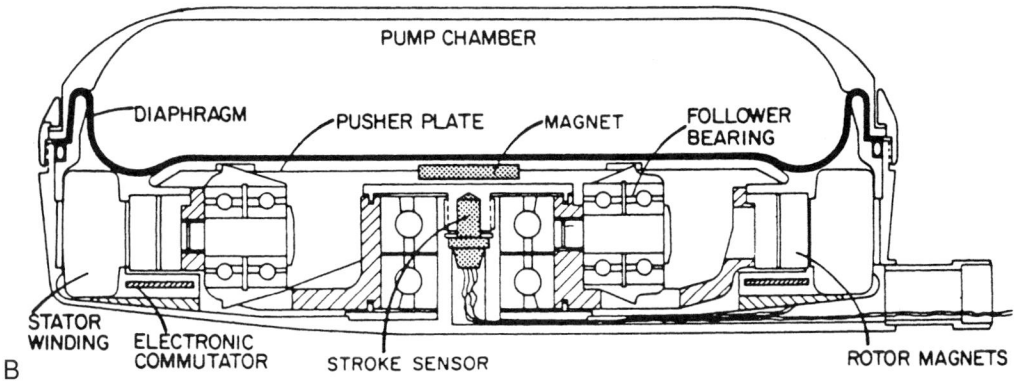

B

Fig. 17-7. Thermedics left ventricular assist device. **(A)** Anatomic location. The device implantation now occurs in the left upper to mid-upper abdomen. **(B)** Blood/pump energy converter assembly. In the pneumatic version the motor assembly is replaced by a pneumatic sac. (*Figure continues.*)

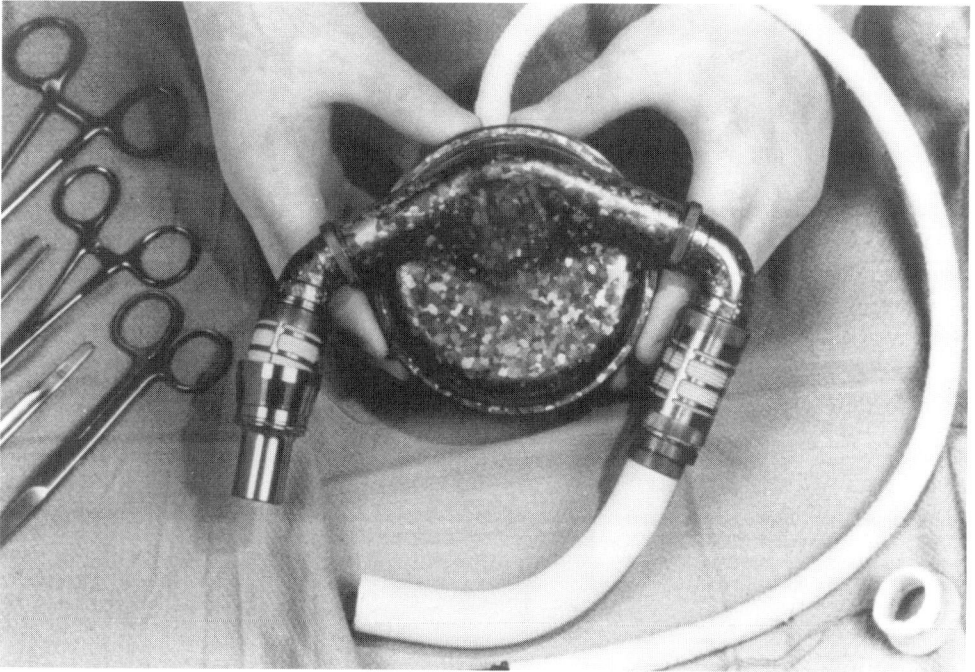

Fig. 17-7 (*Continued*). (**C**) Device prior to insertion. (Fig. C from Szycher et al.,[169] with permission.)

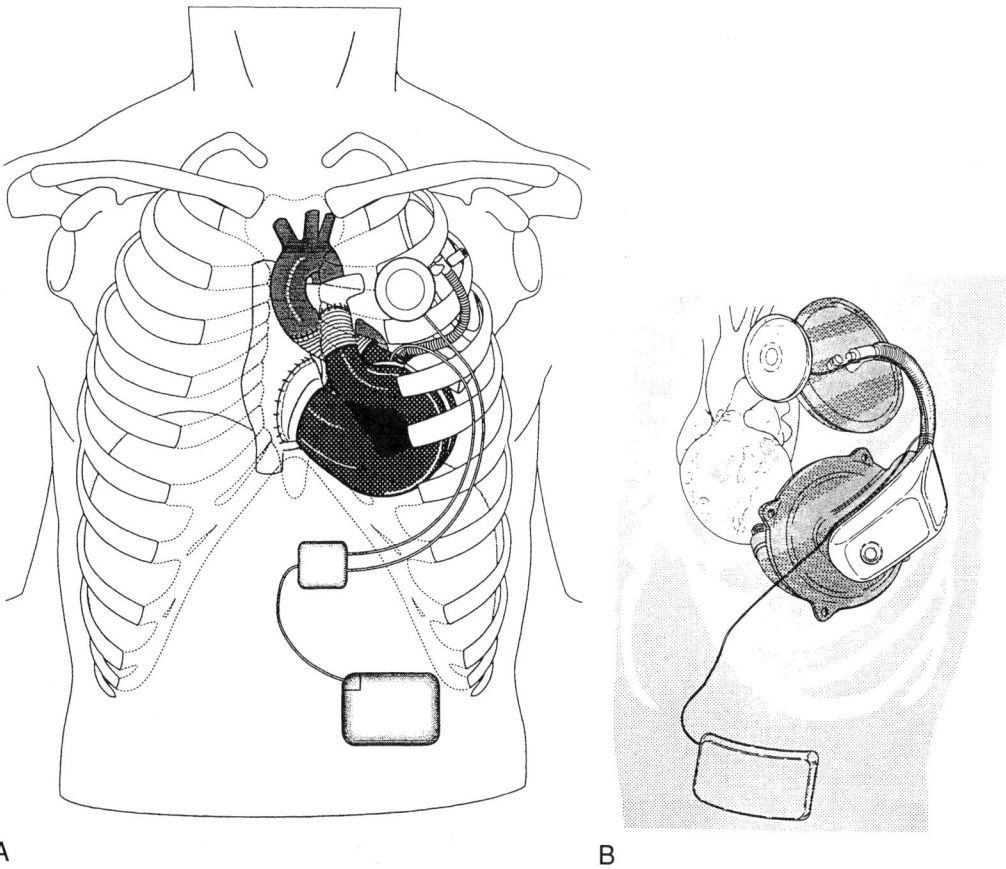

Fig. 17-8. Nimbus devices. **(A)** Anatomic location of the Nimbus CCF device. **(B)** Anatomic location of ET4 total artificial heart. (Fig. A courtesy of CCF-Nimbus Inc., Rancho Cordova, CA; Fig. B from Altieri et al.,[86] with permission.)

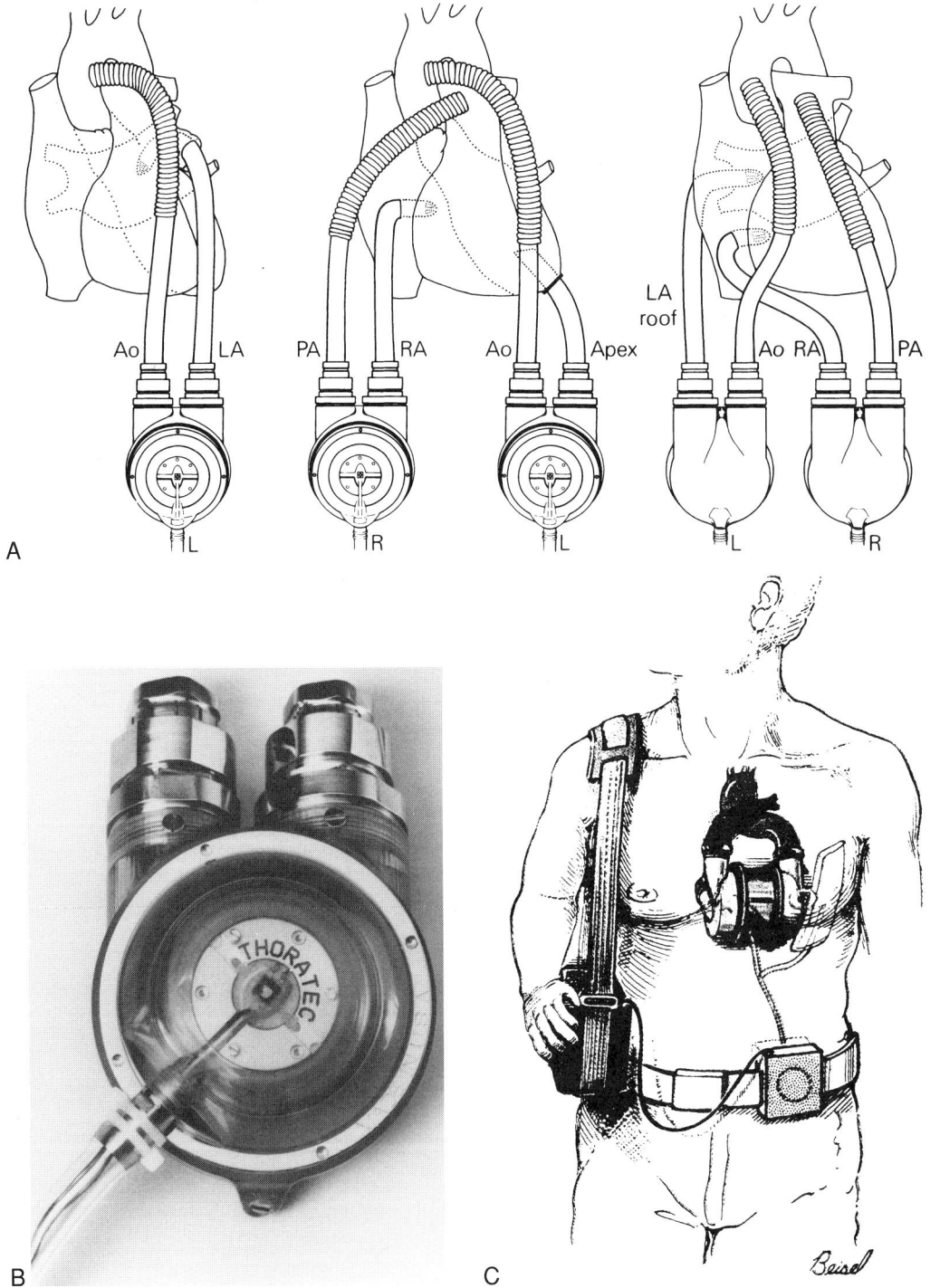

Fig. 17-9. Various placements for the Thoratec device. **(A)** Left ventricular placement. **(B)** Biventricular placement with the draining left ventricular cannula in the left ventricle and **(C)** in a left atrial position. (Courtesy of Thoratec Laboratories Corp., Berkeley, CA.)

Table 17-4. Devices Available on Experimental Protocol

Device	Hemopump	Novacor	Thermedics	Nimbus	Utah	Penn State Thoratec	Penn State Rollerscrew	ABIOMED TAH
Pump mechanism	Centrifugal (axial flow)	Dual spring-loaded pusher plate compression of containment vessel	Single pusher plate, flexing flexing surface onto rigid containment vessel	Double-acting hydraulic cylinder driving dual pusher plates	Biomer pump sac, externalize pneumatic controller	Flexing membrane compresses blood containment vessel	Roller screw attached to pusher plates alternately pumping left and right sides	Toroidal blood pump attached to a centrifugal hydraulic fluid pump
Power supply	Axial flow rotor	Solenoid conversion of electrical energy	Pneumatic or electrical	Electrical	Pneumatic	Pneumatic	Electric motor	Electric motor
Insertion sites (outflow)	Femoral	Aorta (asc or desc)	Aorta (asc or desc) porcine valve	Aorta or pulmonary artery	Aorta or pulmonary artery	Aorta or pulmonary artery	Aorta or pulmonary artery	Aorta or pulmonary artery
Insertion sites (inflow)	Reside in LV	LV apex	LV apex porcine valve recession	RA, LA	RA, LA	RA, LA	RA, LA	RA, LA
Position of device		Left upper quadrant	Upper abdomen/ left chest	Mediastinal	Mediastinal	Paracorporeal	Mediastinal	Mediastinal
Volume of displacement/ flow	3 L·m^{-1}	64–67 ml	83 ml	53 ml	80 ml	65 ml	—	—
Variable volume control	Yes	Yes	Yes	Yes	No	No	Yes	No
Flow characteristics	Nonpulsatile	Pulsatile	Pulsatile	Pulsatile	Pulsatile	Pulsatile	Pulsatile	Pulsatile
Figure No.	17-5A,B	17-6A,B	17-7A–C	17-8A,B	—	17-9A–C	—	—
Ref. No.		85, 86		24, 75, 87, 88	86, 89	90, 91	92–95	96

Abbreviations: asc, ascending; desc, descending; RA, right atrium; LA, left atrium.

Table 17-5. Contraindications to Using MCSS

Scenario	Device	Contraindication
Post-cardiotomy failure	Percutaneous IABP	Severe femoral atherosclerosis Aortic regurgitation Descending thoracic aneurysm Tenuous aortic suture line Forward stroke volume <20 ml
	VAD	Age Pulmonary hypertension Psychogenic instability Active drug abuse Uncontrollable hemorrhage Active endocarditis Pre-existing organ dysfunction Metastatic carcinoma
Bridge to transplant	VAD	Age Small size Active infection Established organ dysfunction (pulmonary, renal, neurologic hepatic, or rheologic) Metastatic carcinoma Psychogenic instability Active drug abuse Severe diabetes Severe peripheral vascular disease

Abbreviations: IABP, intra-aortic balloon pump; VAD, ventricular assist device.

physiologic, psychological, and anatomic. Of these three, the last contains the only absolute contraindications to the use of MCSS, but, anatomic contraindications are rarely a problem in the adult population. Table 17-5 presents a complete outline of these categories, but, the applicability (i.e., relative strength of the contraindication) within each of these categories to a patient is described in the sections below.

Physiologic

There are at least three further subdivisions that describe the physiologic reasons for avoiding or not progressing to a MCSS: effect on vital organ function, pre-existing organ dysfunction, and rheologic (coagulation and hemolytic) disorders.

VITAL ORGAN PERFUSION

There is general agreement that all the LVADs improve vital organ perfusion and function, as compared to the immediate pre-

implant condition.[97-103] Little is known about the dynamics of vital organ blood flow in the MCSS recipient. Studies in dogs in hemorrhagic shock reflect an improvement in splanchnic perfusion during IABP assist.[104] Presumably this ameliorative effect occurs with all forms of MCSS and may account for the improvement in organ function often noticed following implantation (see the following section).

Several examinations of ventilatory interactions with the Jarvik device are also available.[105-107] In both animals and humans, the hyperpnea associated with exercise appears unrelated to cardiac output per se. However, in animals, a reduction in cardiac output during exercise leads to a rise in both ventilation and lactate levels and a drop in oxygen consumption. The ventilatory response occurs is related to pH and pCO_2, and the fall in oxygen consumption follows the reduction in oxygen delivery.

Phasic events during respiration with an

artificial heart in place mimic normal cardio-respiratory interactions but occur for very different reasons. The normal respiratory variation in cardiac output is secondary to an augmentation of right ventricular preload during inspiration, which reduces left ventricular preload (ventricular interdependence). Inspiration also increases left ventricular afterload when the blood leaves the intrathoracic aorta to enter the extrathoracic arterial tree. This increase in afterload summates with the former decrease in preload to produce the normal respiratory variation.

With the Jarvik device in place, the ventricles are exposed to atmospheric pressure; thus, changes in intrathoracic pressure are not transferred to the ventricular chambers. Furthermore, the ventricles are functionally independent, with little direct interaction. During inspiration, intrathoracic pressure decreases and both right and left ventricular afterload decrease. Left ventricular filling decreases, but there is no net change in right ventricular volume. The end result of these changes is an increase in right ventricular stroke volume, with a simultaneous decrease on the left.[102] As the Jarvik device is usually set in the "complete fill to incomplete empty" mode on the right and the "incomplete fill to complete empty" mode on the left, the effect of ventilation is rarely noticeable in the right ventricle.

Further investigations are necessary, however. Other designs of TAH will not respond to vascular resistance changes in a similar fashion.[108]

PRE-EXISTING ORGAN DYSFUNCTION

There are no hard and fast rules regarding the degree of organ dysfunction that prohibits the use of MCSS. In general, two or more failing organ systems or irreversible neurologic injury constitute sufficient damage to preclude MCSS. Many institutions consider age greater than 60 years to be a relative contraindication to bridging. If advanced age and single organ dysfunction

exist in concert, this will often result in exclusion from bridging support.

A recent article from the German Heart Institute is indicative of the present problems involved in excluding patients for bridging based on pre-existing organ dysfunction. Thirty-four patients were supported for a mean duration of 19.2 days. Neurologic impairment was present in 21 patients prior to implant, but 16 patients recovered during support and 14 were transplanted. Renal dysfunction as characterized by oliguria for greater than 6 hours or creatinine greater than 1.5 mg percent was present in 18 patients (2 on dialysis). Fourteen patients responded to implant and 13 were transplanted. Fourteen patients also demonstrated liver dysfunction with SGOT and SGPT levels in excess of 100 U/L. Twelve patients recovered completely and 11 were transplanted. Their conclusion was that no preimplant data could accurately predict irreversible organ damage.

Other investigators also note this inability to distinguish with certainty which patients will respond positively to implant: they tend to err on the side of excessive implantation. In a second report from the French group at la Pitié in Paris, not only was the differentiation of positive responders impossible, as assessed by the presence of preoperative hepatic or renal dysfunction, but the absolute level of dysfunction was not indicative of eventual organ recovery.[109] In their experience, the single criterion that seems to predict poor outcome reliably is the presence of immunosuppression with or without systemic sepsis.[88,97,98,103]

The presence of a pulmonary infection per se does not reliably predict poor outcome. However, this caveat may be somewhat device-specific as those investigators who utilize the Jarvik-7 generally report a higher incidence of mediastinitis. This may be secondary to the large amount of unfilled space in the mediastinum into which blood and serum can pool and become a culture medium.[110,111]

RHEOLOGIC ABNORMALITIES

Two of the most common contraindications as well as complications surrounding the use of a MCSS are bleeding and thromboembolism. Their status as "malefactorum primum" remains unchanged over the 30-year course of modern mechanical support. In the most recent Combined Registry report, bleeding, ventricular failure, and renal failure are the most important univariate predictors of failure to transplant.[69a,69b] Many of these authors suggest the rate of thromboembolism is related to infection. In animals the relationship of sepsis and thromboembolism is positive in more than 70 percent of cases.[112] Thus, a diligent search for all sources of infection and/or sepsis must precede the decision to implant.

The role of renal dysfunction is equally important secondary to the decrease in platelet function. Dialysis can correct these defects to an extent; however, the reversal is not permanent. This partial inhibition is more important to the TAH recipient than to the VAD recipient. The TAH device requires cardiopulmonary bypass (CPB) for placement. Once CPB is initiated, platelet counts fall to 50 percent of normal. Plasma levels of both platelet factor 4 (PF4) and β-thromboglobulin rise, indicative of α-granule release. Fibrinogen receptors decline in these platelets, and the platelets demonstrate a reduced sensitivity to soluble platelet agonists.[113–115] Thus, it is not surprising that bleeding is a very common complication following implantation, but the implication for anesthesiologists is to assess coagulation with as wide a selection of assays as possible (prothrombin time [PT], partial thromboplastin time [PTT], fibrinogen, fibrin split products, PF4, and bleeding time). It is also necessary to ensure an adequate supply of coagulation factors for the post-CPB period.

Once the immediate post-CPB period is past, attention is directed to decreasing thromboembolic complications. A number of strategies are available, but there is no technique that is 100 percent successful. Iloprost, a stable analogue of prostacyclin, is available for experimental use in humans. Currently, the major use for Iloprost is to inhibit platelet function in those patients with heparin-induced thrombocytopenia during CPB. Iloprost does have the significant disadvantage of inducing hypotension during administration.[116] Other experimental agents available to inhibit platelet aggregation (OKY-046, a thromboxane A_2 synthetase inhibitor) and protease activation (nafamostat mesilate, or FUT-175, is a specific, reversible inhibitor of kallikrein, thrombin and plasmin) are being tested in animals and humans in Japan.[117]

Finally, good evidence exists that measures of blood viscosity and red cell fragility are predictive of thrombotic episodes. In patients with LVADs in place, increases in fibrinogen, whole blood viscosity, and red cell rigidity preceded thrombotic episodes. If these same measures were available preimplantation, efforts could be directed to improving these measures and, it is hoped, to decreasing the incidence of neurologic thrombotic episodes.[113,118]

Although thromboembolic episodes are the leading cause of neurologic morbidity in the use of the TAH,[119] it is far from clear what the ideal antithrombotic protocol is. Table 17-6 compares the neurologic versus anticoagulation protocol results from the first 100 patients who received a Jarvik-7 device. Nine patients of the group suffered a neurologic event: three patients were receiving heparin alone, four received heparin and dipyridamole, one received nothing, and one received heparin, dipyridamole, and aspirin.

Anatomic Contraindications

Anatomic contraindications to the use of MCSS are divided into two categories: IABP and VAD/TAH. The anatomic contraindications for the IABP invariably involve atherosclerotic changes in the femoral or iliac arteries and abdominal or descending thoracic aorta. Severe atherosclerotic disease will

Table 17-6. Neurologic Versus Anticoagulation Protocol Results From the First 100 Recipients of the Jarvik-7 Device

Type of Anticoagulation	Total Number in Group	Neurologic Event[a]
None	8	1 (12.5)
Heparin	12	3 (25)
Heparin/Dipyridamole	36	4 (11)
Heparin/Dipyridamole/ASA	35	1 (3)

[a] Numbers in parentheses reflect the percentage of the respective group.

either make cannulation of the selected vessel impossible or will not allow passage of the guidewire or sheath. Other areas of cannulation are available (i.e., the axillary artery or a transthoracic placement), but outcome does not appear to be as gratifying with these alternative approaches. Other anatomic lesions that preclude the use of the IABP include aortic regurgitation or a tenuous aortic suture line. In the former case, institution of IABP support will lead to a massive increase in the regurgitant fraction and will rapidly precipitate left ventricular failure. In the latter, the increase in the diastolic pressure during balloon inflation will place additional stress on an already friable aorta. In this type of patient, it is best to proceed directly to the use of a VAD.

Pure right ventricular failure is a relative contraindication to the use of the IABP. Although the IABP provides diastolic augmentation and increases diastolic coronary blood flow in an ischemic setting, the nonhypertrophied right ventricle relies on both systole and diastole for the provision of nutrient flow. Thus, in the setting of a recent right ventricular infarct, diastolic flow will be increased at the expense of systolic flow. In the hypertrophied or chronic pressure-overloaded ventricle, the relationship of coronary blood flow to systole and diastole resembles that of the left ventricle. In this scenario, the IABP may be more useful. It is important to remember that whenever the use of the IABP is contemplated, there must be forward flow of at least 20 ml · beat^{-1}. Flow below this will result in insufficient augmentation and eventual failure.

Anatomic constraints on the use of VADs and the TAH are easily understood. The primary issue is space in the thorax to accommodate the inflow, pump, outflow, and drive lines (either pneumatic or electric). The specific contraindications that preclude the use of a VAD include a VSD following a perforating septal myocardial infarction, thrombotic material in the diseased heart, and severe valvular dysfunction.[96] In the presence of the above factors, the better choice may be the TAH. Unfortunately, this option does not presently exist in the United States.

There are no internal devices currently in clinical trial that will function in the pediatric age range. Thus, size of the thorax remains a constraining factor, but it is applicable in only the rare patient. Paracorporeal (i.e., 3M Sarns Pulsatile and Pierce-Donachy VADs) and extracorporeal (i.e., BioMedicus and 3M Sarns) require only sufficient space to place cannula for inflow and outflow. The Jarvik device, which was originally manufactured in two stroke volumes (70 or 100), required an assessment of both the anteroposterior (AP) diameter (the so-called DT 10) and total surface area. In those patients with surface areas of greater than 2 m^2 the 100 model was preferred, although many institutions had abandoned this criteria prior to removal of the device from the market. The use of the 70 model appeared adequate in almost all clinical trials. The DT 10 (AP diameter at the level of the 10th thoracic vertebrae) determined lateral versus medial placement of the device. Medial placement increased the risk of IVC and right atrial compression, while lateral placement increased the incidence of pulmonary infection.[103]

Psychological

The psychological contraindications for the use of MCSS are essentially those of heart transplantation.[120] The application of these criteria must be tempered by the expectation of the result. If the patient is to be supported as a bridge to transplant, the criteria are rigidly applied; if, however, the patient is supported with the expectation of return of native cardiac function, these criteria are interpreted with greater latitude. Neither space nor time is available to examine this issue in detail, and the reader is referred to the reference above for a complete discussion of the psychological impact of MCSS.

PHARMACOLOGIC INTERACTIONS

Inotropic and Vasoactive Agents

Although many of the patients receiving a MCSS are also receiving pharmacologic support, few data are available in the literature to quantify objectively which agent is used or when. If univentricular support is initiated, the need for inotropic support for the remaining ventricle is usually mandatory. The choice of agent reflects institutional orientation. At many institutions, the older catecholamine agents, epinephrine and isoproterenol, predominate; at other institutions, the more recent agents dopamine and dobutamine, or various combinations of these agents, are used. The most common agent used in European reports at present is enoximone (a phosphodiesterase III inhibitor). While some investigators consider this drug a pharmacologic bridge to transplant,[121] other investigators remain skeptical. In a prospective study of 24 patients referred to the Berlin Heart Institute, 15 stabilized on enoximone therapy, but the remainder failed to respond and required urgent MCSS placement.

Despite the paucity of data available to make a decision concerning the choice of agent for these patients, some data are available regarding their effects in the patient with a TAH. Table 17-7 represents the hemodynamic results of stepped infusions of both inotropic and vasodilating compounds.[122] The drugs were administered to a patient with a Jarvik 7-70 device, approximately 7 days after implantation. The settings for the device were as follows: systolic duration of 50 percent, with a device rate of 100, and left and right drive pressures of 170 and 35 mmHg, respectively. The infusions were administered through a left internal jugular venous catheter, and dosages increased at 15-minute intervals. One hour elapsed between drug changes. All pressures were measured directly, and cardiac output was measured from the COMDU driver unit previously calibrated by the Fick method.

Both epinephrine and dopamine caused dose-dependent decreases in systemic vascular pressure (SVR) and mean arterial pressure (MAP). Epinephrine at the highest dose studied ($75 \text{ ng} \cdot \text{kg}^{-1} \cdot \text{min}^{-1}$) resulted in a reversal of this trend, but this increase did not return the parameters to baseline. Both dopamine and epinephrine cause dose-dependent increases in P-rate. Little change was noted in pulmonary vascular resistance (PVR) with either drug.

Nitroprusside resulted in dose-dependent decreases in MAP, SVR, mean pulmonary arterial pressure [MPAP], and PVR. Accompanying the decrease in PVR and MPAP was a 35 percent decrease in PaO_2 and a 25 percent increase in the systemic A-VO_2 difference. Nitroglycerin produced the most interesting results of this group. Both MAP and SVR exhibited an increase with administration. Although there was a reversal of this trend in the MAP, it did not return MAP to baseline levels. There was also a slight rise in both CVP and left atrial pressure (LAP) as the dosage increased, which returned to baseline at the highest dosage studied ($2 \text{ mg} \cdot \text{kg}^{-1} \cdot \text{min}^{-1}$). The changes produced by nitroglyc-

Table 17-7. Hemodynamic Results of Stepped Infusions of Ionotropic and Vasodilating Compounds

Drug and Dosage	Hemodynamic Results						
	CO	MAP	SVR	LAP	CVP	PVR	P-rate
Dopamine (mg·kg^{-1}·min^{-1})							
BL	5.5	100	17	7.5	7.5	2.5	105
2.5	6.0	80	12.5	9.0	7.0	2.5	106
5.0	6.0	80	13	8.0	7.0	2.0	110
7.5	6.1	78	12	8.0	7.0	2.5	115
Epinephrine (ng·kg^{-1}·min^{-1})							
BL	5.5	107	17.5	7	7	2.5	92
25	5.8	92	14.5	8	9	2.1	102
50	6.0	78	12	8	7	2.2	103
75	6.0	85	13	9	9	2.0	107
Nitroglycerin (mg·kg^{-1}·min^{-1})							
BL	5.1	80	14	7	7	2	92
0.5	5.2	91	15.1	9	9	2.2	94
1.0	5.5	95	15	8	8	2.1	93
2.0	5.1	84	14.9	7	6	2	92
Nitroprusside (mg·kg^{-1}·min^{-1})							
BL	5.5	95	16	8	8	2.6	90
0.5	5.3	90	16	8	7.5	2.1	93
1.0	5.2	80	14	8	8	1.9	93
2.0	5.1	72	13.5	7	7	1.6	91

Abbreviations: BL, baseline; CO, cardiac output (expressed in L·min^{-1}); SVR, systemic vascular resistance (expressed in Wood units); PVR, pulmonary vascular resistance (expressed in Wood units); P-rate, rate of remnant atrium (expressed in beats·min^{-1}); MAP, mean arterial pressure (expressed in mmHg); LAP, left atrial pressure (expressed in mmHg); CVP, central venous pressure (expressed in mmHg).

erin may be related to the relative capacitance of the venous and arterial systems. It is conceivable that in the normal heart (which is far more sensitive to changes in venous resistance than arterial resistance) the predominate effect is one of a reduction in venous pressure with little change in cardiac output. In the Jarvik heart (operating at equal systole and diastole), the influence of this change in venous resistance is less and, in fact, a slight increase in arterial compliance predominates.[108] Furthermore, alteration of the design characteristics of the TAH (or in this specific device) would also change the response to these (and presumably other) alterations in circulatory physiology. Much more work remains to be done to elucidate the interactions of these agents with the artificial heart and to integrate this into normal human circulatory physiology.

Anticoagulation

As is abundantly clear from the preceding section, there is no widely accepted protocol for anticoagulation in the patient on MCSS. It is also imperative to know which type of

Table 17-8. Anticoagulation Recommendations

Device	Anticoagulation Recommendations
BioMedicus/3M Sarns	Maintain ACT 150–200
ABIOMED BVS-5000	Maintain ACT 200
Thermo Cardiosystems LVAD	ASA and DP; ± DEX
Thoratec/Pierce-Donachy VAD	ASA and DP; ± DEX
HEMOPUMP	Maintain ACT 150–200; DEX
Novactor LVAD	ASA and DP; ± DEX
Scimed ECMO	Maintain ACT 400

Abbreviations: BVS, biventricular support; LVAD, left ventricular assist device; ECMO, extracorporeal membrane oxygenation; DEX, dextran; DP, dipyridamole; ASA, aspirin; ACT, activated clotting time.

device is in use. The pneumatic group seems to require a less rigid anticoagulation protocol than the roller-pump or ECMO groups, but not as low as some of the electrically actuated devices. Table 17-8 is a composite of recommendations from the literature and device manufacturers.[110,111,113,123,124] The types of agents used to achieve "anticoagulation" are not all inhibitory of the intrinsic or extrinsic systems; some are inhibitors of platelet degranulation, activation, or adhesion.

Monitoring of the various parameters of coagulation is an absolute necessity. At most institutions, the basic coagulatory measures suffice: PT, activated partial thromboplastin time (APTT) fibrinogen, fibrin degradation products, activated clotting time (ACT), platelet count, and bleeding time. In other institutions however, the repertoire is expanded to include reptilase time, whole blood and Raby's tranference tests, thromboelastography, platelet aggregation, plasma and serum antithrombin III levels, fibrinopeptide A levels (α_2-antiplasmin levels), PF4, and β-thromboglobulin. Unfortunately, little work other than the study previously cited in the rheologic contraindications section examined a method to predict thrombotic complications; hence goal-directed therapy is impossible. Thus, there remains no widely accepted means of providing anticoagulation in this group of patients.

Anesthetic Considerations

There are no clinical data to substantiate many of the theoretical alterations mentioned in this section. The rate of uptake of anesthetics is inversely related to the cardiac output. As the level of anesthetic increases and results in a depression of the cardiac output, the rate of anesthetic uptake is subsequently increased. In the patient with a TAH or biventricular support system, this is not possible. In the patient with an LVAD, this remains a possibility. Thus, there is an anesthetic implication for not only the type of device selected but also the extent of support.

The peripheral vascular effects of two inhalation anesthetics are available in the literature. Halothane and isoflurane were recently compared in five patients following implantation of a Jarvik-7 device. Most importantly (relative to the previous discussion about the effects of vascular resistance), the Jarvik-7 device was set to operate in a preload-independent mode, thus, cardiac output was held constant. The patients received two concentrations of the anesthetic agents, 1 (0.75 percent for halothane and 1.25 percent for isoflurane) and 1.5 (1.125 percent for halothane and 1.875 percent for isoflurane) MAC. The anesthetics were administered 6 to 24 hours apart, and all measurements were made after a stable end-tidal concentration was reached. Table 17-9 represents the hemodynamic changes described.

Table 17-9. Hemodynamic Effects of Halothane and Isoflurane

Agent and Dose	CI	MAP	SVRI	LAP	MPAP	PVRI	CVP
Halothane							
C	2.9	100	27	14	22	3.6	15
1	2.8	77	22	10	19	3.6	14
1.5	2.8	66	18	11	17	2.6	13
Isoflurane							
C	2.8	102	30	11	19	3.2	16
1	2.6	65	20	6	14	3.5	12
1.5	2.8	48	13	6	14	2.9	11

Abbreviations: CI, cardiac index (expressed in $L \cdot min^{-1} \cdot m^{-2}$); C, control (recorded immediately prior to the anesthetic); SVRI, systemic vascular resistance (expressed in Wood units·m^{-2}); MAP, mean arterial pressure; MPAP, mean pulmonary artery pressure (expressed in mmHg); PVRI, pulmonary vascular resistance (expressed in Wood units·m^{-2}); CVP, central venous pressure.

Briefly, both isoflurane and halothane produced significant reductions in both SVR and MAP. Halothane resulted in an approximately 30 percent fall in both parameters, while isoflurane resulted in an approximately 50 percent decrease. MPAP, CVP, and LAP all fell with increasing concentrations of the inhalation agents with no difference between the agents. Shunt fraction, serum catecholamine concentration, and PaO_2 did not change with administration of either agent.[125] The authors of this study believed that the hemodynamic stability of halothane in this group of patients was superior to isoflurane. However, the issue of recurrent anesthetic exposure in this group (who are at high risk of liver dysfunction) was not addressed. Undoubtedly, the most common anesthetic administered for placement of MCSS is opiate based.

Other areas of interest that are not available in the literature include alterations in pharmacokinetics and dynamics of drug effect, both orally and parenterally; alterations in the respiratory effects of the inhalation agents; alterations in baroreceptor function; and alterations in venous and systemic compliance, to name just a few. The field is rich with the possibility of application to later human clinical trials or to the understanding the interaction of many complex human physiologic responses.

MONITORING
Heart and Whole Body
NONINVASIVE TECHNIQUES

For those patients in whom the return of native cardiac function is anticipated, there are a range of possible monitoring modalities. The simplest to use and obtain is ultrasonography. Although conventional transthoracic ultrasonography has limited application in this group of patient (because of "shadowing" or "masking" of structures underlying the prosthetic device), transesophageal ultrasound (TEE) examination is very helpful. TEE, ventricular anatomy, loading conditions (filling volumes), wall motion, and valvular integrity can all be easily visualized and monitored on a daily basis. This may require the administration of daily anesthetics if the patient is extubated but is well worth the effort on a cost/benefit basis.

Gated radionuclide scans represent the second common method of following ventricular function after implantation.[126-128] These devices are not as portable as the TEE but do allow for unrestricted visualization of all areas of the myocardium. Their use on a daily basis is restricted, however, as each examination requires exposure to a fixed radiation dose. Thus, these tests are best used on a weekly, rather than daily, basis or for only those patients in whom there is concern that the device may be contributing to a difficult or protracted weaning process. Previous work suggests that those patients with an ejection fraction of greater than 35 percent will wean and survive to discharge.

Two other types of scans are available at some institutions: positron emission tomography (PET) and single photon emission computed tomography (SPECT). None has the utility and portability of the TEE or gated nuclide scans just mentioned. The section Devices discusses the use of the cardiac output monitoring and diagnostic unit (COMDU) for tracking cardiac output and device flows; however, the issue of assessing patient flow requirements is covered next.

INVASIVE

Almost all discussions of adequacy of device flow depend on a preselected normal figure that varies by device and institution. This ranges from a low of 90 ml $\cdot$ min^{-1} $\cdot$ kg^{-1} (proposed by the Cleveland group) to a high of 175 ml $\cdot$ min^{-1} $\cdot$ kg^{-1} (proposed by the Baylor group) with the Berlin group in the middle at 120. The goal of most of these devices, with the exception of the IABP and ECMO, is to provide adequate systemic perfusion and to keep LAP as low as possible. The latter is done in an effort to avoid pulmonary edema and pulmonary hypertension. Thus, much of the engineering of these devices is exemplified in the manner in which they deal with increases in venous (either systemic for a right-sided or pulmonary for a left-sided device) pressures. Most of the TAH and VAD devices rely on the inverse relationship between $S\bar{v}O_2$ and right atrial pressure as the control mechanism for increasing pump flows (i.e., as $S\bar{v}O_2$ declines right atrial pressure increases). The devices are not perfect, however, and inflow restriction is a common problem with many, rendering this relationship questionable.

The body deals not only with systemic flow-pressure relationships, but also with oxygen transport. As such, any given flow may be insufficient to meet total oxygen demands either because oxygen utilization is increased (e.g., fever, thyrotoxicosis, malignant hyperthermia, shivering) or because oxygen delivery is impaired (e.g., decrease in hemoglobin, left-shifted oxyhemoglobin dissociation curve, decrease in PaO_2, carbon monoxide poisoning).

Recently, the group at Baylor suggested that the more appropriate measure of pump adequacy is ml $\cdot$ min^{-1} $\cdot$ kg^{-1} of O_2. When these investigators applied this measure to pump flows, they found good agreement with all the various levels of flow just described; the only change was the level of hemoglobin: from 15 g percent to 10 to 7.5 g percent. Furthermore, they demonstrated that exercising their animals (goats) at varying levels of oxygen delivery resulted in rapid but inversely proportional changes in blood lactate levels. Unfortunately, they did not adjust oxygen tension, only pump flows.[129]

As the most common complications surrounding the use of MCSS are bleeding, infection, and renal failure (all of which negatively impact oxygen delivery), it seems that $S\bar{v}O_2$ is a very important measure in this group of patients. Other important measures for adequacy of whole body perfusion include lactate and pyruvate levels, pH, and $P\bar{v}O_2$. In those patients with drastic left shifts in the oxyhemoglobin dissociation curve, $P\bar{v}O_2$ is more important than $S\bar{v}O_2$. The reason for the change in position is as the P_{50} value moves to the left (a leftward shifted curve) greater amounts of oxygen are bound to hemoglobin below a PO_2 of 20 mmHg. Functionally, the body cannot derive oxygen from the blood below this PO_2 because the gradient from erythrocyte to tissue is too low. Although our current means of obtaining these data are invasive, the Baylor group are considering incorporating a sensor for $S\bar{v}O_2$ monitoring in their device.

Other invasive measures are available to assess myocardial thickening directly. A recent study compared several measures of global function against a superficially implanted but extractable wall motion crystal.[130] The crystal accurately reflected changes in wall motion when compared to TEE but did not reliably track measures of global contractility (dP/dt-40 or dP/dt_{max} and cardiac output). Not examined in this abstract but of great importance for use in the postcardiotomy patient would be the predictive value of sequential changes (better or worse) in the thickening fraction. It is likely that this tool would allow one to monitor the return (or absence thereof) of native cardiac function more accurately. Furthermore, it would save the need for either TEE or MUGA scans as screening examinations. Weaning could proceed more smoothly and "on-line" if a minimum level of thickening were established for each patient.

Routine monitors of global perfusion (PA catheters with or without $S\bar{v}O_2$, RVEF, or CCO) monitoring may be of benefit during the acute postoperative period and for the postcardiotomy patient. However, during bridge to transplant use, the fewer indwelling lines (to decrease the incidence of sepsis) the better. Ideally, all measures should be noninvasive.

Other Vital Organs

CEREBRAL

The best monitor of adequate cerebral blood flow (CBF) and function is a patient capable of responding to a questioner. This makes the first rule regarding the care of these patients simple: try to limit their anesthetic periods to the minimum time necessary to complete a procedure. Frequently, however, this is not possible and other methods of assessing CBF and function are necessary.

There are several methods to measure CBF; only a representative sample are covered here. Four major techniques are available to estimate CBF; these methods also apply to all the other organs that are discussed later: Doppler interrogation of blood flow velocity, dilutional tracer effects (e.g., Kety-Schmidt, Fick, thermodilution, indocya-

nine green dye [ICG]), computed tomography [CT], magnetic resonance imaging [MRI], relative radioactivity distribution (e.g., PET, SPECT, Xenon), and oxygen-mediated measures (e.g., near-infrared spectroscopy).

Most of these are not applicable to the patient on MCSS because of a requirement for the patient to physically transport to the location of the device. In the acute postoperative setting this is not feasible. For the longer-term bridge to transplant, this may not present as great a problem. The second major stumbling block is the presence of magnetic materials in all the devices, thus rendering the MRI scan useless. Perhaps the most useful for bedside monitoring are the techniques that are portable and relatively easy to use: near-infrared spectroscopy, Doppler interrogation, and dilutional tracer effects—primarily continuous jugular venous thermodilution and the Kety-Schmidt technique using N_2O.

Knowing the CBF is only part of the answer, however, and some measure of cerebral activity must accompany these measures. Thus, a combination of the near-infrared spectroscopy or electrical activity monitor (e.g., electroencephalography [EEG]), compressed spectral array, spectral edge detection scheme, evoked potentials and a measure of flow are probably the best monitors in the absence of a conscious patient. Studies during long-term support with the PET or SPECT scan would prove very helpful in learning more about the normal human response to TAH or nonpulsatile perfusion.

RENAL

The measurement of renal blood flow (RBF) and function is also a complex issue. Although the same four basic methods apply to this measure, the ability of the kidney to concentrate, secrete, and absorb agents at a variety of levels complicates any measure of RBF, glomerular filtration (GFR), filtration fraction (FF), or renal plasma flow. This section focuses on some easily portable methods for estimating renal clearance. The best method for estimating RBF, GFR, and FF is use of the clearance of inulin and hippurate.[131] Unfortunately, this method is time, labor, and resource intensive. This makes it a less than ideal method for routine use in an intensive care unit (ICU). The other common method for estimating GFR and RBF uses radionuclides.[132] Despite numerous theoretical problems in calculating RBF and GFR, the use of radionuclides for the noninvasive evaluation of renal function is readily available and acceptable. However, similar to inulin and hippurate measurements, this method is labor, time, and resource intensive for producing accurate and reproducible results.

A common method for estimating GFR is the use of serum and urinary concentrations of creatinine. GFR can be obtained by either following serial evaluations of serum creatinine or measuring urinary excretion of creatinine.[133] Although this measure suffices for routine clincal care, numerous errors contribute to its unfavorable status as a tool for clinical research.[134] Recently, a new method became available for daily estimations of GFR. This method, which requires the use of iodinated contrast, compares favorably (r = 0.86) to inulin and radionuclide (r = 0.89) clearance. It does not require the administration of radioactive tracers or the use of timed urinary collections. The length of time required to process each sample is about 10 minutes. It does, however, require the purchase of a special device to measure the iodine concentration in the serum.[135] This appears to be an ideal method to follow GFR and when combined with other routine measures of renal competence (concentrating, secretory, and resorbtive functions) allows for a more detailed picture of renal function.

HEPATIC

Measurement of hepatic blood flow is slightly more complex than the two organ systems previously mentioned. The liver is provided with both an arterial and venous (portal) source of inflow. Although both invasive and noninvasive methods are available to estimate hepatic blood flow, only the noninvasive methods are covered here.[136]

Two basic methods are used to estimate hepatic blood flow: clearance of dyes or tracers and inert gas washout. Continuous infusions of indocyanine green dye (ICG), bromosulfthalein (BSP), or galactose will all provide reasonable estimates of hepatic blood flow, but all require placement of a hepatic venous catheter to ensure their accuracy. A significant disdvantage of the continuous infusion technique with ICG is the poor extraction and back diffusion that occurs in inverse proportion to the health of the liver. Single bolus techniques with either BSP or ICG offer the advantages of speed, precision, and reproducibility but still require the placement of hepatic venous catheters for accuracy.

Radioactive colloids are also available to estimate hepatic blood flow. Unfortunately, as noted in both the previous sections, this requires repeated radiation exposure for the patient. It is possible that a single dose of ^{99m}Tc-pertechnetate could suffice to measure both hepatic and renal blood flow simultaneously; however, this would require close supervision and superb timing to ensure the accuracy of both measures. It is unlikely that more than a few centers are capable of this kind of reproducible accuracy and effort.

Finally, the inert gas washout technique provides an inhalational measure of estimated hepatic blood flow. Similar to the radioactive colloid measure, however, it requires repeated radiation exposure for repeated assessments. Furthermore, if the constituency of the liver is altered by drugs or disease, the partition coefficient will change and the subsequent assumptions regarding blood flow are altered unpredictably. Background radioactivity from the lung can also interfere with the liver washout counting.

Devices

INTRA-AORTIC BALLOON PUMP

The IABPs that are currently available do the majority of the device monitoring themselves. The common problems that result in

Table 17-10. IABP Alarm Messages and Their Probable Causes[a]

Alarm Message	Probable Causes
Loss of trigger source	
ECG	QRS signal insufficient (<120 mV)
Arterial pressure	Arterial pressure signal insufficient rhythm, or deflation set too late
V-pace	AV pace mode active, normal QRS detected, or no pacer spike
AV pace	No A *and* V spike, AV interval inappropriate (<50 or >250 msec), or heart rate >110 beats·min^{-1}
Internal	Detection of R-wave
High-pressure alarm	
Catheter	Kink in tubing or unwrapped IABP
Drive	Pressure in balloon *system* is elevated or vacuum level is decreased
Gas escape	
Disconnect	IABP tubing disconnected
Rapid gas loss	Rupture of IABP or tubing
Slow gas loss	Leak in tubing, connector or IABP

Abbreviations: IABP, intra-arterial balloon pump; ECG, electrocardiogram.

[a] Although there are differences between manufacturers regarding the display of these alarm conditions, the essential cause and remedy are similar.

visible alarms on the console are loss of augmentation, loss of trigger source, high-pressure alarm, and gas escape. Loss of trigger source, high-pressure alarms, and gas escape alarms will suspend balloon function. The primary causes of these alarms are listed in Table 17-10.

The low augmentation alarm is user adjustable in most systems and will not cause a suspension of pumping if activated. In most cases, the remedies for these problems are obvious. Any of the loss of trigger source alarms should result in a search beginning at the patient and continuing to the device for a functional discontinuity. If no disconnection is found, a search for alternative trigger sources is made. If a different trigger source is used, timing must be re-examined (see the section Device Descriptions for timing discussion).

The high-pressure alarms are also self explanatory and result in a similar patient to device systems check. If no physical obstruction is found in the catheter, failure of the IABP to deploy is the cause. In general, this latter high-pressure alarm, and all gas escape alarms, result in discontinuation of IABP support and necessitate removal of the catheter. If blood is noted in the IABP catheter at any

time, a leak must be suspected and the IABP catheter removed. Condensation in the IABP catheter can result in abnormal function but is easily remedied by briefly operating the IABP pump while disconnected from the patient and catheter.

VENTRICULAR ASSIST DEVICES AND TOTAL ARTIFICIAL HEART

The most common method for noninvasively monitoring pneumatic ventricular function has been the COMDU. Although recent studies suggest that the COMDU produced as much as a negative 16 percent error,[137] these errors were systematically investigated and reduced to a more tolerable 0.1 percent (range of 4.8 to −3.65 percent). The set of hemodynamic conditions that produced the largest aberration was low preload (3 mmHg), high afterload (135 mmHg), and high heart rate (150 mmHg). None of these was an uncommon value for postoperative implant patients.

The COMDU functions by integrating the TAH pneumatic outflow over a measured pressure difference and relating this integral to the systolic and diastolic periods. When blood moves into the pneumatic ventricle, the blood/air diaphragm is displaced and air is sent through the exhaust line of the diver to the COMDU. Once diastole is triggered from the driver, the COMDU analyzes the exhaust flow for 1.2 seconds or until systole is triggered, whichever is shorter. The volume of blood ejected is then derived from a linear calibration constant and multiplied by the frequency of pumping to produce a cardiac output. The cause of the aberrations noted above appears secondary to a discrepancy between fill volume and stroke volume. As afterload increases, the rate of ejection decreases (although this parameter can be independently set; increasing dP/dt increases the degree of hemolysis) and the relative duration of the monitoring period for the COMDU increases. If the monitoring period is increased, the errors relative to the monitoring period increase. These monitoring period errors will also increase with increases in heart rate, decreases in preload, and increases in afterload. Presumbably, future algorithms for the COMDU will avoid some of these errors with a resultant improvement in accuracy.

Another recent enhancement of the pneumatically driven ventricles includes noninvasive assessment of pulmonary artery pressure. Although the description of the technique is available only in abstract form at the present, once published this should give the clinician another method of following the pulmonary artery pressure. This method does not appear to be influenced by alterations in fill volume, as it was tested in a mock circulation with fill volumes from 30 to 60 ml with an r value of greater than 0.92.[138]

UTILIZATION CRITERIA

Postoperative Cardiac Failure

While it is easiest to examine only a physiologic paradigm, the decision to implement MCSS in a patient is a distillation of several important criteria, and a constellation of considerations is the rule. Very broadly, these criteria divide into physiologic, psychologi-

Table 17-11.   Criteria for Implementation of MCSS[a]

Cardiac index <2.0 L·min^{-1}·m^{-2}
Systemic vascular resistance $>2,100$ dynes ·sec^{-1}·cm^{-5}
Left atrial pressure >18 mmHg
Urine output <20 ml·hr^{-1}

[a] These criteria are assessed during the administration of maximal dosages of inotropes and in the absence of gross metabolic derangements.

cal, and ethical issues. Most institutions have elected to assign patients by only the physiologic criteria listed in Table 17-11;[47] however, both the patient's and family's wishes can and should modify this approach. The inclusion of third-party payers, in this already complex formula, will occur in the not-so-distant future. The simplest answer for the assessment of psychological issues may be to use any of the currently available heart transplant evaluations. The criteria for the Stanford experience are readily available in the literature.[120]

INFLUENCE OF TIME OF ONSET

Feelings of inadequacy, guilt, or shame on the part of both the surgeon and anesthesiologist generally accompany the use of MCSS in the immediate postoperative period. As the need for postoperative support is usually unanticipated, the family is often in a state of grief, shock, and turmoil. The patient is no longer able to make decisions for himself. If the delicate interplay between physician and patient is to be the final arbiter, it can only occur if the patient knows that the option of MCSS is available before it is needed. During highly stressful periods, advance directives avoid the indiscreetly prepared and often regrettable choices made by dubious surrogate decision makers.

The influence of personal feelings of ineptitude is less likely the less proximate the time of onset of cardiac failure is to the time of surgery. The patient may also be able to participate to a greater degree than in the immediate postanesthetic period. Similar to the patient awaiting heart transplantation, the family has the psychological advantage of a slower transition into the MCSS period. None of these factors demotes or mitigates in any way the need for a thorough discussion of MCSS before surgery.

The longer the interval between the discontinuance of CPB and the initiation of MCSS, the less likely is the chance of survival. This emphasizes the importance of utilizing predetermined criteria to initiate MCSS support.[39,139,140]

HIERARCHIC TRANSITION AND DIRECTED SUPPORT

Generally, the first MCSS applied is the IABP. This is a minimally invasive, easily controlled, and widely available form of MCSS. The device does not need FDA clearance for its use, and the institution of support occurs expeditiously. This ease of use makes consideration of IABP application a much less feared option than previously. The ease of applicability also contributes to a lack of appreciation of the IABP as a form of MCSS.

Although this device provides primarily a left-sided assist, the amelioration of left ventricular failure will often improve a marginally functioning right ventricle. This may be true even in the patient with relatively pure right-sided failure secondary to pulmonary hypertension. The right ventricle takes on many of the characteristics of the left ventricle secondary to the large increase in ventricular wall thickness. The alteration in wall thickness also alters the coronary flow pattern and transmural distribution, making the right ventricle much more dependent on diastolic coronary blood flow.[141] For a description of the IABP as well as its salutary physiologic effects, see below.

The use of more invasive, less easily controlled, and much more intensive devices supplants the IABP when the patient fails to meet the physiologic criteria outlined in Table 17-11 or biventricular failure supervenes. This step represents a logarithmic escalation in level of care and responsibility, however. The option of more aggressive

MCSS should only occur after a thorough discussion with the patient and family.

It is worth mentioning that although many institutions adopt this type of graduated approach to MCSS, there is evidence that a more aggressive approach would yield a greater likelihood of survival.[119,142] It is unlikely that many institutions will be able to adopt this approach primarily for a lack of man power. One device that does rival the IABP for ease of use but still requires a surgical intervention for placement is the Hemopump.[74,143–145] A detailed description of this new approach to MCSS is available in the section Device Descriptions, but it shows great promise as a device that may supplant the use of the IABP.

OUTCOME ASSESSMENTS

Intra-aortic Balloon Pump
No well-controlled clinical trials of the sequential use of IABP and VADs exist. All the available data involve the use of either one or the other device. The most recent results from the combined registry for the clinical use of mechanical ventricular assist devices following postcardiotomy cardiogenic shock do not include IABP insertion in any of the categories.[146] Approximately 30,000 IABP insertions occur each year for both medical and surgical indications. Approximately 300,000 implantations have occurred since the inception of the device.[147]

Table 17-12 displays the results from four large trials of the IABP. The most recent is almost 10 years old, however, and as such may not be representative of recent results. Table 17-12 includes results from both nonsurgical and surgical placements. There is no intent to compare these two categories, but it is instructive to examine the differences in outcome of these two groups. The best survival in all three series occurred in the patient with limited permanent loss of myocardium. Restriction of IABP application to those patients with limited permanent myocardial loss (those in whom "stunning" is the primary reason for ventricular failure following

Table 17-12. Outcome Assessment of IABPs Based on Four Large Trials

Area of Utilization	Investigators			
	Bolooki (N)	Beckman (N)	McEnany (N)	Pennington (N)
Medical				
Acute MI	17	3	NA	NA
Unstable angina	5	4	22	22[a]
Cardiogenic shock	101	32	145	33[a]
	Overall survival about 40%			
Surgical				
Preoperative insertion	88	91	146	55
Postoperative insertion	206	80	225	323
	Overall survival about 60%			

[a] Patients went on to surgery; survival statistics are represented with the surgical group.

an ischemic insult) implies that one is able to assess the loss of myocardium rapidly, efficiently, and accurately.[148] Prior experience demonstrates that IABP support is sufficient in more than 70 percent of patients presenting with postcardiotomy myocardial failure.[47,48]

VENTRICULAR ASSIST DEVICE

The use of ventricular bypass techniques, either uni- or biventricular in origin, following postcardiotomy procedures is relatively rare. The Combined Registry reported approximately 1,300 patients (about 0.1 percent of all cardiac procedures performed) during the past 10 years.[149,149a] The Combined Registry for the clinical use of mechanical ventricular assist devices is an organization formed in 1985 and consists of approximately 70 centers, with more being added each year. Fourty-four of these centers are in the United States and 26 are outside. The peak year for the use of VADs was 1987, with approximately 100 to 110 implants. Each year since has shown a decline in their use.

An early comparison of mortality rates among the three types of devices used for postcardiotomy support revealed a marked difference. The roller and centrifugal devices were associated with statistically higher survival rates (32 percent and 25 percent, respectively) when compared to the pneumatic group (16 percent).[150] Through the subsequent 6 years, the experience with pneumatic ventricles has increased, and this situation is no longer true. However, the roller pump and centrifugal devices are both more available and familiar in use than the currently available pneumatic device, although experience with the ABIOMED BVS-5000 is growing. Finally, the roller pump and centrifugal groups represent the only devices that are currently capable of support in children.[151]

Table 17-13 displays the number of implants for selected years, from 1980 to 1991. Also included is an approximation of the total cardiac procedures performed during each of

Table 17-13. Number of Implants and Cardiac Procedures Performed Between 1980 and 1991[a]

Year of Use	No. of Implants	Yearly Cardiac Procedures
1980	25	196,000
1984	50	308,000
1987	138	584,000
1990	109	595,000

[a] All figures are approximate and are based on the information provided to the Combined Registry[69, 69b] and the reported rates of discharge for disease states. (Bureau of Vital Statistics).

Table 17-14. Types and Placements of Implants and Survival

Type of Placement	No. of Procedures	Percentage Weaned	Percentage Discharged
Univentricular	615	48.9	27.3
Right	121	38.8	25.6
Left	494	51.4	27.7
Biventricular	350	37.7	19.7
Total	965	44.9	~27

those years. Table 17-14 gives a breakdown of the types and placements of these implants, as well as a percentage survival for each of those categories. Although a cursory review of these data would suggest that the use of VADs to support the failing circulation is of little benefit, two important points are not included in these data.

Before the advent of MCSS, predicted mortality would approach 90 to 100 percent for the vast majority of these patients. Second, patients who reach hospital discharge have a 2-year actuarial survival of 82 percent. Finally, the quality of life for discharged patients is relatively unimpaired; 86 percent function at a New York Heart Association (NYHA) level II or better.[149a]

In a recent review of the Registry Data,[69b,123] a significantly decreased incidence of bleeding was noted in the pneumatic group compared to the centrifugal group (32 percent versus 45 percent), although bleeding did not discriminate between survivors and nonsurvivors. Among the complications that did discriminate between survivors and nonsurvivors was renal failure, biventricular failure, and respiratory failure. (For a more complete description of the complications associated with VAD support postcardiotomy, see the section, Complications, below.) There remains no difference in the rate of weaning or discharge with regard to type of device used (pneumatic, 43 percent and 21 percent, respectively; centrifugal, 45 percent and 26 percent, respectively).

Although these data demonstrate a statistically worse outcome if the mode of support chosen is biventricular assist device (BVAD), this is presumably a reflection of the severity of insult to the myocardium, not a direct reflection of the problems of biventricular support. Support for this contention is available from work in animals. In a group of 10 goats that underwent a standard anoxic myocardial insult, the presence of biventricular support added the following benefits: better systemic perfusion, lower right atrial pressures, lower right ventricular workloads, and decreased right ventricular distension. Other investigators report that the use of hybrid devices (see the section, Bridge to Transplant, below) decreases the survival rate in bridge to transplant candidates and that phenomenon could be present in these results as well.

HEMOPUMP

The Medtronic HEMOPUMP is not included in these results. In a review of the first 53 patients to meet criteria for placement, 41 underwent successful implantation. The majority of insertion failures were an inability to traverse the iliac or aortic bifurcations, although in two patients the device did not negotiate the arch. Of the 41 patients implanted, 35 percent were weaned and 30 percent were 30-day survivors. Complications of support included bleeding and arterial injury in those patients with difficult passage of the device.[152] A further refinement of the device is currently undergoing clinical trials in Europe. This refinement will shrink the size of the device to 14 Fr (see the Device Description section).

Novacor

The Novacor device is rarely used for post-cardiotomy support. As of January 1992, the total number of patients supported was nine, with only one patient surviving the weaning process. That patient was a long-term survivor at 39 months post-device removal. The longest period of support was 216 hours, with a mean duration of support of 39 hours.

ABIOMED

To date, the ABIOMED BVS–5000 device was implanted in approximately 1,200 patients. Two hundred centers worldwide are currently involved in clinical trials. The mean duration of support is 6.2 days, with a maximum of 62 days. Biventricular support (BVS) is the most common mode (60 percent of cases) of operation. The primary intended use for this device is postcardiotomy support, although it is effective as a bridge to transplant. (Fasnacht A: ABIOMED Cardiovascular, Inc., Danvers, MA, personal communication).

Bridge to Transplant

PATIENT SELECTION

The criteria to initiate MCSS in the bridge-to-transplant patient remain ambiguous. From a physiologic perspective, criteria similar to those outlined for the acute use of MCSS are also applicable in this scenario. Ethical and psychological issues are easier to address in these patients primarily because their disease process is chronic in nature. This allows for an accommodation period during which patients can gain further comprehension of MCSS and of how its use will effect their lives. There is some disagreement on the applicability of MCSS, once secondary organ dysfunction appears.[69,96,153,154] However, in other recent studies, pre-existing organ dysfunction (if secondary to chronic cardiac failure) or advanced age does not necessarily prohibit the utilization of MCSS.[17,155,155a] The progression of the patient to transplantation is dependent on the resolution of the chronic organ dysfunction.

Table 17-15. Contraindications to Bridging

Age > ? 60 yrs	Pulmonary
"Irreversible" organ	hypertension
damage	Sepsis
Severe Atherosclerosis	Illicit or legal drug
Psychogenic instability	abuse
Small size	Severe diabetes
	Metastatic carcinoma

(Data from Refs. 92, 100, 119, 148, and 151.)

Table 17-15 lists contraindications to heart transplant bridging.

TYPE OF DEVICE

Early results with the three main types of assist devices—centrifugal, pneumatic, and electric—were not dramatically different.[69a,69b,76,77,114,146,149a] The Novacor LVAD is the first electrically activated device to seek an FDA IDE for the clinical setting; however, the Thermo Cardiosystems Heartmate is the first device to receive premarket approval (PMA) as a bridge to transplant. With regard to duration of implantation, the current trend is for the pneumatically activated devices to have the longest duration (51.3 days, in a range of 0 to 344), the electric group second (45.8 days, in a range of 0 to 370) and the centrifugal group the shortest duration (8.1 in a range of 1 to 29 days).

The type of device used for bridging also affects the rate of hospital discharge significantly. The rate of hospital discharge following transplantation varies from a high of 87.4 percent for the univentricular support (i.e., LVAD) group to 69.5 percent for the paracorporeal BVS group to 49.6 percent for the TAH. Furthermore, the combination of two different types of devices (pneumatic or electric combined with centrifugal—60 percent and 50 percent, respectively) resulted in a worse rate of discharge compared to the exclusive use of either pneumatic or centrifugal devices (71.8 percent and 64.7 percent, respectively).

PORTABILITY

The ease with which a device can be transported to or from a particular patient's locale is an important determinant of utilization. If a device demands the commitment of large amounts of chronologic, personnel, and fiscal resources, it is less likely to become a viable option. As the portability of the device improves, the amount of time required to prepare for utilization decreases. As the amount of preparatory time decreases, the areas in which the device is available increase. As the areas available for use increase, the experience with the device improves. As the experience with the device improves, the results (outcome) also improve. As the outcome from utilization improves, the device is more widely sought as an option. Furthermore, the more frugal the device is with personnel resources (i.e., less complex), the more likely its use in a variety of institutions and settings. Thus, the need for a portable (i.e., simple and reliable) form of MCSS is important to an institution.

But what about the patient? Included in the above discussion is an implicit assumption that the patient is to remain in one area of a hospital. If the device sees use in the bridge-to-transplant candidate, the patient's abilities to walk, talk, and interact with the outside world become of paramount concern. In an ideal device, drive lines would not tether the patient to a chair or console. The movement of the patient would not impair the function of the device. This last criterion is the most important from a functional point of view. If walking or sitting with the device in place is inhibited, a variety of problems ensue.

The least of these physiologically, although not psychologically, is the loss of the patient's ability to interact with his environment. The greatest problem is the loss of erect posture. This inevitably leads to muscle wasting, protein catabolism, and the loss of the normal pathway to clear secretions. Although these changes do not ineluctably result in complications, the likelihood of their occurrence is increased. However, for almost all successful device implantations, the patient is more mobile and alert than while moribund and ill with NYHA class IV failure.

DURATION OF SUPPORT

Although there was an initial tendency to initiate shorter duration support with the centrifugal group of devices, this is no longer true.[76,77,114,146] All types of devices are currently used for the patient requiring a bridge to transplant. Selection of the device is generally based on institutional bias and not upon objective evidence. The selection of a device for bridge-to-transplant use based on chronologic criteria is very difficult. This is due to the unpredictable availability of donor organs.

The recent assessment of MCSS by the NHLBI divided the devices into two categories: those devices used for less than or more than 180 days.[50] Using these criteria, the types of devices available are described in Table 17-16. The outcomes from these devices are described in the following section.

OUTCOME STUDIES

The broadest source of information is the Combined Registry, although other sources of information are used in this section.[17,70,153,156–159] Since many of these devices are not widely available, little time will be spent on describing their outcomes in detail. There are, however, expanded descriptions of outcome for devices whose utilization exceeds 50 patients worldwide.

General Overview

The overall use of MCSS for bridging is declining from the peak year of 1988. About 25 percent of the 476 patients reported to the Combined Registry had isolated left ventricular support, 34 percent had paracorporeal biventricular support, and about 40 percent underwent total artificial heart replacement (all pneumatic). Four patients underwent isolated right ventricular support but only one survived to transplant and discharge. If this latter group is ignored (because of small sample size), rates for transplantation were equal, regardless of device type; however, the rates of hospital discharge were significantly better for the isolated left ventricular support group.

Table 17-16.   MCSS Devices Classified by Length of Use

Devices Available for Less Than 180 Days	Devices Available for More Than 180 Days

Pneumatic artificial hearts
  Penn State Heart/3M Sarns
  Symbion/Utah Heart/CardioWest
  Nimbus/Cleveland Clinic
  University of Perkinje, Czechoslovakia
  Tokyo Heart
	Temporary assist devices
	  Penn State/3M
	  Nimbus
	  Novacor
	  Thermedics
	  Europe—various centers
	  Japan—various centers

Pulsatile ventricular assist devices
  ABIOMED BVS-5000
  Novacor
  Pierce/Donachy—Thoratec
  Thermedics Heartmate
  Electrocath
	Permanent total artificial hearts
	  ABIOMED/Texas Heart Institute
	  Penn State Heart/3M
	  University of Utah
	  Nimbus/Cleveland Clinic

Constant flow devices
  BioMedicus/Biopump
  3M Sarns
  Medtronic HEMOPUMP	

The total days of support for those patients who were transplanted and discharged (217 of the 476) ranged from 0 to 370, with an average of 24.3. The worst performance was the pneumatic TAH group (these results are all prior to the disbanding of Symbion and do not reflect the more recent results of the CardioWest organization). For all transplanted patients in this group, the percentage discharged was 49.6. Of the isolated left ventricular support group who survived to transplant, 87.4 percent were discharged. This result is not significantly different from the survival following orthotopic heart transplantation alone. The rate of discharge following transplantation for the BVS group was 69.5 percent. This was significantly less than the isolated LVAD group but is significantly greater than the pneumatic TAH group.

The average duration of support following LVAD placement was 30.6 days, with a range of 0 to 370. There was a significantly shorter duration of support for those patients (n = 26) undergoing centrifugal LVAD placement (6.1 mean, range 0 to 29 days). There was no significant difference between the electric and pneumatic groups with respect to duration of support (mean of 48.1 versus 31.9 days, respectively). The rates of discharge following transplantation were not significantly different between the three groups (C, 80.0 percent; E, 92.6 percent; P, 92.1 percent). The use of either pneumatic or electrical devices combined with centrifugal devices (n = 22) resulted in significantly poorer outcomes (overall 40 percent survived to transplant and of those 56 percent survived to discharge).

Selected Device Outcomes

Pneumatic Total Artificial Heart (Jarvik-7) As of 1995, there were 247 implants worldwide with the vast majority of this experience coming from the Jarvik-7 series (more than 82 percent). Approximately 69 percent of these patients were transplanted and 34 percent ultimately discharged (47 percent of those transplanted). At present, the Symbion Corporation is disbanded, but the Jarvik device reverted to the University of Utah. The Universities of Utah and Arizona are currently working together under the name "CardioWest" and regained their IDE in January of 1993.

Pneumatic Thoratec Device As of 1995, 367 of these devices were implanted. Approximately 63.4 percent of the 367 patients were transplanted, and 85 percent of those were discharged. The device was utilized as an LVAD in 34.9 percent of these patients and in a biventricular configuration in the remainder (Olsen DB, Salt Lake City, personal communication). Mean duration of support was 8.5 days, with a maximum of 74 days. Overall mortality was not affected by duration of pump support. Principal reasons for non-transplantation were bleeding and multiorgan failure.

Novacor Device There are 358 patients as of November, 1995; 61.2 percent transplanted and 91.1 percent of those were discharged. Multiorgan failure and stroke accounted for the majority of the reasons for not transplanting. There were 11 operative deaths included in the 42 patients who were not transplanted. Mean duration of support is 45 days, with a range of 1 to 370 days. Approximately 19 percent of patients required concomitant right ventricular support. Of this subgroup, about 28 percent were successfully transplanted. In those patients not transplanted there were six operative deaths.

Thermo Cardiosystems (Thermedics) Heart Mate 1000 As of late 1995, 502 patients were treated at 90 centers around the world. Mean duration of support is 102 days, with a range of 15 to 324 days. Approximately 65.5 percent of this group survived to transplantation, and 89 percent of the transplanted group were discharged. Twenty-seven of the bridging patients were also included in a comparison of renal and hepatic function following either transplantation alone or bridging.[155a] Although there were no differences between the groups at 30 days, hepatic function (bilirubin levels) was significantly better in the LVAD group at 60 days postprocedure. The average time required to return to normal levels was about 40 days. Renal function during LVAD support was also improved compared to the transplant group; however, this was ascribed to the effect of the immunosuppressive regimen[159] in the latter. Both blood urea nitrogen and creatinine (38 mg · dl^{-1} and 1.7 mg · dl^{-1} respectively) declined

following implantation and were within normal limits at the time of transplantation.

Finally, the quality of life was compared through the use of the NYHA classification. All 27 patients in the bridging group were class III (4) or IV (23) prior to implantation. Following either implantation or transplantation, all patients improved by at least two classifications with the majority (greater than 90 percent) residing in the class I category.

Intra-aortic Balloon Pump Little recent work is available on the use of IABP as a bridge to transplant. In a 1987 report,[160] five patients were supported for a mean duration of 6.2 days (range 1 to 15); 80 percent of patients were transplanted and 75 percent of those survived to discharge. In a second report from 1989,[161] eight patients were supported for 1.5 to 27 days; 88 percent of these patients were transplanted and 57 percent of that group (n = 4) survived to discharge.

Penn State University Roller Screw Electrically Driven Total Artificial Heart
The device has been implanted in animals with encouraging long-term results. With the electric motor and the pump implanted and the supply externally, two animals had the device in place for 222 and 205 days, respectively. These results were obtained in an electric motor device in which a cam-type to rectilinear motion translator was used: Subsequent modifications to the roller screw mechanism have had good results. Six calves were instrumented, the longest survival time being 131 days. These animals were able to eat, drink, and perform moderate exercise with the power pack and the device functioning automatically.[92] Three humans have received a similar device with one surviving to transplantation (Olsen DB, Salt Lake City, personal communication).

COMPLICATIONS

Intra-aortic Balloon Pump
The incidence of complications with the IABP is directly related to the degree of preexisting myocardial dysfunction, patient size, duration of support, and perhaps the type of

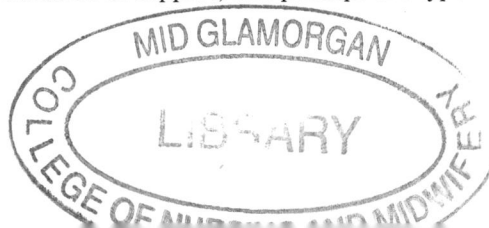

placement (i.e., surgical versus percutaneous). At least 20 studies report complications following IABP insertion from 1973 through 1992.[162] These studies encompass more than 4,000 patients. Prior to publication of the 1992 study, the most commonly reported type of complication was vascular (e.g., thrombosis of an extremity, ischemia, paraplegia, embolization), which occurred at an average rate of approximately 16 percent. Following publication of this study, a new variable, delirium, was added, which occurred in approximately 34 percent of patients. Unfortunately, this group of investigators did not report an incidence of delirium in similar patients not requiring IABP support, thus making any firm conclusions regarding the relationship of this complication to placement difficult.

Table 17-17 is a distillation of the complication rates from the 20 studies mentioned previously. In descending order of incidence, they are delirium (34 percent), vascular (15.8 percent),[163] renal failure (5.1 percent), sepsis (3.4 percent), bleeding (3.2 percent), aortic dissection (2.0 percent), cerebral infarction (1.4 percent), and mesenteric infarction (1.1 percent). Not all investigators reported all of these complications, however. The second column of Table 17-17 lists the number of investigators who reported the complication. This can be used as a rough measure of the

Table 17-17. Incidence of Complications Associated With IABP

Complication	Incidence (%)	Report Rate[a]
Delirium	34	1
Vascular	15.8	20
Renal	5.1	6
Sepsis	3.4	19
Bleeding	3.2	16
Dissection	2.0	15
Cerebral infarction	1.4	10
Mesenteric infarction	1.1	9

Abbreviations: IABP, intra-aortic balloon pump.
[a] Number of investigators who reported the respective complications.

reliablity of the incidence measure (i.e., the greater the number of investigators reporting a particular complication, the better the estimate of its incidence). However, because the definitions for many of these complications vary, it is not possible to make strict comparisons without a more detailed analysis (i.e., a meta-analysis). Although it is not addressed in Table 17-17, the risk factors associated with these morbidities were very similar across the groups.

Of note, in many if not all of the studies reported here, female gender is associated with an increase in both mortality and morbidity; however, the body size of the patients is neither recorded nor compared in many of these studies. A similar conclusion was promulgated by the original CASS study, until the data were re-evaluated in light of patient body size (in square meters). It then became apparant that the risk factor was not, in fact, gender, but rather size. It is for this reason that many investigators have chosen to replace gender with patient size in this section as well. This application of the CASS data may be premature but is, in our opinion, justified.

Ventricular Assist Device

In their 1990 report, the Combined Registry described complications in 448 patients following the use of MCSS related only to postcardiotomy cardiogenic shock (as opposed to its use for bridge to transplant). These results are not very different from those reported following the use of IABPs, although the mortality rates are higher (see the section on VAD outcome). The average length of support was 3.3 days (range 0 to 39) and did not differ with regard to type of device, type of support (LVAD, RVAD, or BVAD) or outcome (weaned, expired, or discharged). Table 17-18 lists complications ranked from highest to lowest incidence. Many patients had more than one complication. Also included in Table 17-18 is a list of the multivariate discriminators that predicted the ability to wean, or, once weaned, discharge patients.

The five most common complications fol-

Table 17-18. Ranking of Complications Associated With Ventricular Assist Devices

Complication	Incidence (%)	Predict Wean	Predict Discharge
Bleeding	45	N	N
Renal failure	38	N	Y[a]
Biventricular failure	32	Y[a]	N
Respiratory failure	22	N	N
Thromboembolism	16	N	N
Infection	15	Y[a]	N
Low cardiac output	14	Y[a]	Y[a]
Neurologic injury	13.5	N	N
Perioperative infarct	13	N	N
Coagulopathy	8	N	Y[a]
Hemolysis	7	N	N
Flow obstruction	5	Y[a]	N
Patent foramen ovale	2	N	N
Mechanical failure	1	N	N

[a] Negative influence on selected outcome.
(Data from Miller et al.[146])

lowing postcardiotomy support were bleeding, renal failure, biventricular failure, respiratory failure, and thromboembolism. The incidence of biventricular failure was significantly higher in those patients not weaning (41 percent versus 22 percent). Although this may seem superficially obvious, many physicians elect to support only the left ventricle, believing that the right ventricle is a pure conduit and not an important pumping chamber. These data would indicate otherwise. Other investigators also notice improved outcomes in animals when BVS is intiated soon after injury.[164] The BVAD group maintained better outputs and lower right atrial pressures than those in the LVAD group, as well as an improvement in mortality.

Although the incidence of renal failure did not discriminate between those patients weaning and not weaning, it did discriminate between those patients being discharged after weaning (57 percent in those patients expiring after weaning versus 15 percent for those discharged).

A more recent examination of this Registry revealed similar findings with a few exceptions. The seven most common complications (in descending order of incidence) are now bleeding (41 percent), renal failure (30 percent), biventricular failure (23 percent), respiratory failure (18 percent), infection (13 percent), neurologic injury (13 percent), and thromboembolism (7 percent). There remains no difference in the rate of weaning or discharge with regard to type of device used (see the section, Selected Device Outcomes, above). There is a difference with regard to postoperative bleeding between two devices. The incidence of bleeding in the pneumatic group is 32 percent, while in the centrifugal group it is 45 percent. Renal failure (14 percent versus 38 percent), biventricular failure (12 percent versus 31 percent), and respiratory failure (12 percent versus 21 percent) are currently the discriminators for survival versus nonsurvival when the groups are combined.[123]

Two of the pneumatic devices, the ABIOMED and Thoratec, have been inserted in enough patients to generate data regarding their individual incidence of complications. The ABIOMED device has been inserted in approximately 1,200 patients for postcardiotomy support. The most common adverse

Table 17-19. Complications of MCSS[a]

Complication	Type of Support		
	Univentricular (%)	Biventricular (%)	TAH (%)
Bleeding	*32.6	*45	*47.2
Ventricular failure	*15.0	*11.9	*8.1
Renal failure	*13.4	*26.3	*28.5
Respiratory failure	8.6	16.3	*23.6
Infection	24.6	30.0	*34.2
Perioperative MI	*1.6	0	1.6
Thrombus/embolus	*19.8	15.0	15.5
Neurologic injury	*8.0	*8.1	10.6

[a] Those complications with asterisks preceding their percentage occurrence were univariate predictors of not receiving a transplant within their respective device category (e.g., univentricular, TAH).

event has been bleeding requiring reoperation. The incidence of thromboembolic complications and device failure has been zero. Data regarding the incidence of respiratory and renal failure, neurologic events, and perioperative infarction are not available (Fasnacht A, Danvers, MA, personal communication).

The Thoratec device has been inserted in approximately 367 patients. The incidence and type of complication are very similar to those reported in Table 17-18. The most common problem was biventricular failure (65 percent). Furthermore, the rate of survival was significantly influenced by the use of MCSS for biventricular failure. Six of 16 patients supported biventricularly survived to discharge, while only one of eight patients who underwent solely left-sided support survived.

Bridge to Transplant
In general, complications following the use of MCSS are similar in character to those following postcardiotomy support. Table 17-19 lists complications reported to the Combined Registry up to June 1995.[69b] All the complications listed in Table 17-19 are univariate predictors of not receiving a transplant and many of the patients suffered from more than one complication. A total of 181 patients are reported from a pool of 584. Thus, the overall rate of complications is about 31 percent.

The incidence of complications among the different devices does vary slightly. Most notably, the incidence of poor pumping (ventricular failure) was only 8 percent with the TAH but was a problem in 12 to 15 percent of patients in the other two groups (univentricular and biventricular support). Conversely, the incidence of respiratory failure with the TAH was 24 percent, while univentricular and biventricular devices averaged about one-half that rate. When comparing these statistics, it is important to remember that there has been a moratorium on the use of the TAH device since 1991. Thus, direct comparisons are no longer as meaningful. Current results with the CardioWest device suggest little difference in overall complication rates. In a series of 53 patients entered since January 1993, 68 percent of patients were transplanted and 94 percent of those survived (Olsen DB, Salt Lake City, personal communication).

However, a general impression continues to be that patient demographics supercede device characteristics with regard to the incidence of complications. It is this impression that drives the search for more and better ways of delineating presupport survivors (i.e., improved patient selection).

REFERENCES

1. Wallace J: Most physicians with a critical illness would choose to have their own treatment withheld. Anesthesiol News 1991

2. Merin RG: Autonomic nervous system pharmacology. p. 471. In Miller RD (ed): Anesthesia, Churchill Livingstone, New York, 1990

3. Mueller H, Ayres SM, Gregory JJ et al: Hemodynamics, coronary blood flow, and myocardial metabolism in coronary shock; response to norepinephrine and isoproterenol. J Clin Invest 49:1885–1902, 1970

4. Lehr D, Krukowski M, Chau R: Acute myocardial injury produced by sympathomimetic amines. Isr J Med Sci 5:519–24, 1969

5. Balazs T, Bloom S: Cardiotoxicity of adrenergic bronchodilator and vasodilating antihypertensive drugs. p. 199. In Van Stee EW (ed): Cardiovascular Toxicology. Raven Press, New York, 1982

6. Rockhold RW: Cardiotoxicity of naturally occurring catecholamines. p. 347. In Baskin SI (ed): Principles of Cardiac Toxicology. CRC Press, Boca Raton, FL, 1991

7. Rona G: Catecholamine cardiotoxicity, editorial review. J Mol Cell Cardiol 17:291–306, 1985

8. Vormann J, Fischer G, Classen HG, Thoni H: Influence of decreased and increased magnesium supply on the cardiotoxic effects of epinephrine in rats. Arzneimitteforschun, 33:205–10, 1983

9. Selye H, Bajusz E: Stress and cardiac infarcts. Angiology 10:412–20, 1959

10. Selye H: Genesis and prevention of cardiopathies: Part III. Hormonal, neural, neuroendocrine, and miscellaneous mechanisms. Ann NY Acad Sci 156:195–206, 1969

11. Selye H, Bajusz E: Conditioning by corticoids for the production of cardiac lesions with noradrenaline. Acta Endocrinol 30:183–7, 1959

12. Keogh B, Priddy R, Morgan C, Gillbe C: Comparative study of the effects of enoximone and dobutamine in patients with impaired left ventricular function undergoing cardiac surgery. Cardiology, suppl 3. 77:58–61, 1990

13. Dage RC, Okerholm RA: Pharmacology and pharmacokinetics of enoximone. Cardiology, suppl 3. 77:2–13, 1990

14. Gage J, Rutman H, Lucido D, LeJemtel TH: Additive effects of dobutamine and amrinone on myocardial contractility and ventricular performance in patients with severe heart failure. Circulation 74:367–73, 1986

15. Sundram P, Reddy HK, McElroy PA et al: Myocardial energetics and efficiency in patients with idiopathic cardiomyopathy: response to dobutamine and amrinone. Am Heart J 119:891–8, 1990

16. Loisance DY: Mechanical bridge to cardiac transplantation, editorial. Int J Artif Organs 14:269, 1991

17. Schiessler A, Warnecke H, Friedel N et al: Clinical use of the Berlin Biventricular Assist Device as a bridge to transplantation. ASAIO Trans 36:M706–8, 1990

18. Packer M, Carver JR, Rodeheffer RJ et al: Effect of oral milrinone on mortality in severe chronic heart failure. The PROMISE Study Research Group [see comments]. N Engl J Med 325:1468–75, 1991

19. DiBianco R, Shabetai R, Kostuk W et al: A comparison of oral milrinone, digoxin, and their combination in the treatment of patients with chronic heart failure [see comments]. N Engl J Med 320:677–83, 1989

20. Uretsky BF, Jessup M, Konstam MA et al: Multicenter trial of oral enoximone in patients with moderate to moderately severe congestive heart failure. Lack of benefit compared with placebo. Enoximone Multicenter Trial Group [see comments]. Circulation 82:774–80, 1990

21. Szycher M, Gernes CD, Sherman C: Thermedics' approach to ventricular support systems. J Biomater Appl 1:39–105, 1986

22. Yusef S, Teo K: Inotropic agents increase mortality in patients with congestive heart failure. Circulation, suppl III. 82:III-673, 1990

23. Dies F, Krell MJ, Whitlow P et al: Intermittent dobutamine in ambulatory outpatients with chronic cardiac failure. Circulation, suppl 2. 74:II-38, 1986

24. Bregman D, Kaskel P: Advances in percutaneous intra-aortic balloon pumping. Crit Care Clin 2:221–36, 1986

25. Reimer KA, Hill ML, Jennings RB: Prolonged depletion of ATP and of the adenine nucleotide pool due to delayed resynthesis of adenine nucleotides following reversible myocardial ischemic injury in dogs. J Mol Cell Cardiol 13:229–39, 1981

26. Kloner RA, DeBoer LWV, Darsee JR et al: Prolonged abnormalities of myocardium salvaged by reperfusion. Am J Physiol 241:H591–9, 1981

27. Foglia RP, Steed DL, Manganaro AJ, Buck-

berg GD: Iatrogenic myocardial edema with crystalloid primes: effects on left ventricular compliance performance, and perfusion. Surg Forum 29:312–5, 1978

28. Laine GA, Allen SJ: Left ventricular myocardial edema. Lymph flow, interstitial fibrosis, and cardiac function. Circ Res 68:1713–21, 1991

29. Williams JP: Myocardial lymphatics and cardiac function. p. 37. In Stanley TH, Sperry RJ (eds). Anesthesiology and the Heart. Kluwer Academic, Dordrecht, 1990

30. Pennock JL, Pae WE, Pierce WS, Waldhausen JA: Reduction of myocardial infarct size: comparison between left atrial and left ventricular bypass. Circulation 59:275–9, 1979

31. Dennis C, Carlens E, Senning A et al: Clinical use of a cannula for left heart bypass without thoracotomy: experimental protection against fibrillation by left heart bypass. Ann Surg 156:623–37, 1962

32. Sugg WL, Webb WR, Ecker RR: Reduction of extent of myocardial infarction by counterpulsation. Ann Thorac Surg 7:310–6, 1969

33. Laks H, Ott RA, Standeven JW et al: The effect of left atrial-to-aortic assistance on infarct size. Circulation, suppl 2. 56:II-38–II-43, 1977

34. Maroko PR, Bernstein EF, Libby P et al: Effects of intraaortic balloon counterpulsation on the severity of myocardial ischemic injury following acute coronary occlusion. Circulation XLV:1150–9, 1972

35. Williams DO, Korr KS, Gewirtz H, Most AS: The effect of intraaortic balloon counterpulsation on regional myocardial blood flow and oxygen consumption in the presence of coronary artery stenosis in patients with unstable angina. Circulation 66:593–6, 1982

36. Gewirtz H, Ohley W, Williams DO et al: Effect of intraaortic balloon counterpulsation on regional myocardial blood flow and oxygen consumption in the presence of coronary artery stenosis: Observations in an awake animal model. Am J Cardiol 50:829–36, 1982

37. Fuchs RM, Brin KP, Brinker JA et al: Augmentation of regional coronary blood flow by intra-aortic balloon counterpulsation in patients with unstable angina. Circulation 68: 117–23, 1983

38. Jett GK, Dengle SK, Barnett PA et al: Intraaortic balloon counterpulsation: its influ-

ence alone and combined with various pharmacological agents on regional myocardial blood flow during experimental acute coronary occlusion. Ann Thorac Surg 31:144–54, 1981

39. DeWood MA, Notske RN, Hensley GR et al: Intraaortic balloon counterpulsation with and without reperfusion for myocardial infarction shock. Circulation 61:1105–12, 1980

40. Shaw J, Taylor DR, Pitt B: Effects of intraaortic balloon counterpulsation on regional coronary blood flow in experimental myocardial infarction. Am J Cardiol 34:552–6, 1974

41. Nasu M, Shinkai M, Fujiwara H et al: Recovery of end-stage organ dysfunction by circulatory assist. ASAIO Trans 37:M345–7, 1991

42. Pennock JL, Pierce WS, Waldhausen JA: Quantitative evaluation of left ventricular bypass in reducing myocardial ischemia. Surgery 79:523–33, 1976

43. Bavaria JE, Furukawa S, Kreiner G et al: Effect of circulatory assist devices on stunned myocardium. Ann Thorac Surg 49:123–8, 1990

44. Spotnitz HM, Covell JW, Ross J, Braunwald E: Left ventricular mechanics and oxygen consumption during arterial counterpulsation. Am J Physiol 217:1352–8, 1969

45. Pennington DG, Swartz MT: Management: by circulatory assist devices. Cardiol Clin 7: 195–204, 1989

46. Anonymous: Vital and Health Statistics. Detailed diagnoses and procedures, National Hospital Discharge Survey, 1987. Vital and Health Statistics, Series 13: Data from the National Health Survey No. 100:5, 1989

47. Norman JC, Cooley DA, Igo SR et al: Prognostic indices for survival during postcardiotomy intra-aortic balloon pumping. J Thorac Cardiovasc Surg 74:709–20, 1977

48. McEnany MT, Kay HR, Buckley MJ et al: Clinical experience with intraaortic balloon pump support in 728 patients. Circulation, suppl I. 58:I-124–32, 1978

49. Funk M: Epidemiology of end-stage heart disease. Appendix D. p. 251. In Hogness JR, Van Antwerp M (eds): The Artificial Heart. Prototypes, Policies and Patients. National Academy Press, Washington DC, 1991

50. Anonymous: The Artificial Heart. Prototypes, Policies and Patients. National Academy Press, Washington, DC, 1991

51. Annas GJ: The health care proxy and the living will. N Engl J Med 324:1210–3, 1991

52. LeGallois M: Experiments on the principle of life. p. 130. M Thomas, Philadelphia, Translated by NC & JG Nancrede. 1813

53. Jacobi C: Ein Beitrag zur Technik der kunstichen Durchblutung uberlebender organe. Arch Exp Pathol Pharm 36:330–48, 1895

54. Brodie TC: The perfusion of surviving organs. J Physiol (Lond) 29:266–75, 1903

55. Embley EH, Martin CJ: The action of anaesthetic quantities of chloroform upon the blood vessels of the bowel and kidney; with an account of an artificial circulation apparatus. J Physiol (Lond) 29:266–75, 1905

56. Hooker DR: A study of the isolated kidney. The influence of pulse pressure upon renal function. Am J Physiol (Lond) 27:24–44, 1910

57. Richards AN, Drinker CK: An apparatus for the perfusion of isolated organs. J Pharmacol Exp Ther 7:467–83, 1915

58. Dixon WE: A simple perfusion apparatus. J Physiol (Lond) 56:xl–xlii, 1922

59. Dale HH, Schuster EHJ: A double perfusion-pump. J Physiol (Lond) 64:356–64, 1928

60. Gibbs OS: An artificial heart. J Pharmacol Exp Ther 38:197–215, 1930

61. Van Allen CM: A pump for clinical and laboratory purposes which employs the milking principle. JAMA 98:1805–6, 1932

62. Gibbs OS: An artificial heart for dogs. J Pharmacol Exp Ther 49:181–6, 1933

63. Barcroft H: Observations on the pumping action of the heart. J Physiol (Lond) 78:186–95, 1933

64. Gibbon JH: Artificial maintenance of circulation during experimental occlusion of pulmonary artery. Arch Surg 34:1105–31, 1937

65. Gibbon JH: The maintenance of life during experimental occlusion of the pulmonary artery followed by survival. Surg Gynecol Obstet 69:602–14, 1939

66. Cooley DA, Liotta D, Hallman GL et al: Orthotopic cardiac prosthesis for two-staged cardiac replacement. Am J Cardiol 24:723–30, 1969

67. Norman JC, Cooley DA, Kahan BD et al: Total support of the circulation of a patient with post-cardiotomy stone-heart syndrome by a partial artificial heart (ALVAD) for 5 days followed by heart and kidney transplantation. Lancet 1:1125–7, 1978

68. De Vries WC, Anderson JL, Joyce LD et al: Clinical use of the total artificial heart. N Engl J Med 310:273–8, 1984

69. Oaks TE, Pae WE Jr, Miller CA, Pierce WS: Combined Registry for the Clinical Use of Mechanical Ventricular Assist Pumps and the Total Artificial Heart in Conjunction with Heart Transplantation: Fifth Official Report—1990. J Heart Lung Transplant 10:621–5, 1991

69a. Pae WE Jr. Miller CA, Matthew Y, Pierce WS: Ventricular assist devices for postcardiotomy cardiogenic shock. J Thorac Cardiovasc Surg 104:541–53, 1992

69b. Mehta AM, Aufiero TX, Pae WE Jr et al: Combined registry for the clinical use of mechanical ventricular assist pumps and the total artificial heart in conjunction with heart transplantation: sixth official report—1994. J Heart Lung Transplant 14:585–93, 1995

70. Joyce LD, Johnson KE, Cabrol C et al: Nine year experience with the clinical use of total artificial hearts as cardiac support devices. ASAIO Trans 34:703–7, 1988

71. Rose DM, Connolly M, Cunningham JN Jr, Spencer FC: Technique and results with a roller pump left and right heart assist device. Ann Thorac Surg 47:124–9, 1989

72. Litwak RS, Koffsky RM, Jurado RA et al: Use of a left heart assist device after intracardiac surgery: technique and clinical experience. Ann Thorac Surg 21:191–202, 1976

73. Rose DM, Colvin SB, Culliford AT et al: Long-term survival with partial left heart bypass following perioperative myocardial infarction and shock. J Thorac Cardiovasc Surg 83:483–92, 1982

74. Frazier OH, Nakatani T, Duncan JM et al: Clinical experience with the Hemopump. ASAIO Trans 35:604–6, 1989

75. Abou-Awdi NL: Thermo cardiosystems left ventricular assist device as a bridge to cardiac transplant. AACN Clin Issues Crit Care Nurs 2:545–51, 1991

76. Miller CA, Pae WE Jr, Pierce WS: Combined Registry for the Clinical Use of Mechanical Ventricular Assist Pumps and the Total Artificial Heart in conjunction with heart transplantation: fourth official report—1989. J Heart Transplant 9:453–8, 1990

77. Pae WE Jr, Miller CA, Pierce WS: Combined registry for the clinical use of mechanical

ventricular assist pumps and the total artificial heart: third official report—1988. J Heart Transplant 8:277–80, 1989

78. Moulopoulos SD, Topaz S, Kolff WJ: Diastolic balloon pumping (with carbon dioxide) in the aorta. A mechanical assistance to the failing circulation. Am Heart J 63:669–75, 1962

79. Topaz SR: How the balloon pump was conceived. A personal reminiscence. Cardiovasc Dis 4:422–7, 1977

80. McBride LR, Miller LW, Naunheim KS, Pennington DG: Axillary artery insertion of an intraaortic balloon pump. Ann Thorac Surg 48:874–5, 1989

81. Mertlich GB, Quaal SJ, Borgmeier PR, DeVries KL: Effect of increased intra-aortic balloon pressure on catheter volume: relationship to changing altitudes. Crit Care Med 20:297–303, 1992

82. Noon GP, Sekela ME, Glueck J et al: Comparison of delphin and biomedicus pumps. Trans Am Soc Artif Intern Organs 36:M616–9, 1990

83. Zapol WM, Snider MT, Hill JD et al: Extracorporeal membrane oxygenation in severe acute respiratory failure. A randomized prospective study. JAMA 242:2193–6, 1979

84. Zwischenberger JB, Cilley RE, Hirschl RB et al: Life-threatening intrathoracic complications during treatment with extracorporeal membrane oxygenation. J Pediatr Surg 23:599–604, 1988

85. Shinn JA: Novacor left ventricular assist system. AACN Clin Issues Crit Care Nurs 2:575–86, 1991

86. Altieri FD, Watson JT, Taylor KD: Mechanical support for the failing heart. J Biomater Appl 1:106–56, 1986

87. Dasse KA, Chipman SE, Sherman CN et al: Clinical experience with textured blood contacting surfaces in ventricular assist devices. Trans Am Soc Artif Intern Organs 33:418–25, 1987

88. Griffith BP, Kormos RL, Hardesty RL et al: The artificial heart:infection-related morbidity and its effect on transplantation. Ann Thorac Surg 45:409–14, 1988

89. Himley SC, Butler KC, Massiello A et al: Development of the E4T electrohydraulic total artificial heart. ASAIO Trans 36:M234–7, 1990

90. Pennington DG, Kanter KR, McBride LR et al: Seven years' experience with the Pierce-Donachy ventricular assist device. J Thorac Cardiovasc Surg 96:901–11, 1988

91. Rosenberg G, Snyder AJ, Landis DL et al: An electric motor-driven total artificial heart: seven months survival in the calf. Trans Am Soc Artif Intern Organs 30:69–74, 1984

92. Davis PK, Pae WE Jr, Pierce WS: Toward an implantable artificial heart. Experimental and clinical experience at the Pennsylvania State University. Invest Radiol 24:81–7, 1989

93. Wisman CB, Rosenberg G, Weiss WJ et al: The development and successful application of an intrathoracic compliance chamber for the implantable electric motor-driven ventricular assist pump. Surg Forum 34:253, 1983

94. Kaan GL, Noyez L, Vincent JG et al: Management of postcardiotomy cardiogenic shock with a new pulsatile ventricular assist device. Initial clinical results. ASAIO Trans 37:559–63, 1991

95. Snyder AJ, Rosenberg G, Landis DL et al: Indirect estimation of circulatory pressures for control of on electric motor-driven total artificial heart. p. 87. In Langrana NA (ed) Advances in Bioengineering: American Society of Mechanical Engineering, New York, 1985

96. Rokitansky A, Wolner E: Total artificial heart and assist devices as a bridge to transplantation. Int J Artif Organs 12:77–84, 1989

97. Friedel N, Viazis P, Schiessler A et al: Patient selection for mechanical circulatory support as a bridge to cardiac transplantation. Int J Artif Organs 14:276–9, 1991

98. Moritz A, Rokitansky A, Trubel W et al: Timing for implantation and transplantation in mechanical bridge to transplantation. Int J Artif Organs 14:270–5, 1991

99. Reedy JE, Swartz MT, Termuhlen DF et al: Bridge to heart transplantation: importance of patient selection. J Heart Transplant 9:473–80; discussion, 1990

100. Solis E, Leger P, Muneretto C et al: Clinical application and patient selection in the use of a total artificial heart as a bridge for transplantation. Eur J Cardiothorac Surg 2:65–71, 1988

101. Schiedermayer DL, Shapiro RS: The artificial heart as a bridge to transplant: ethical and

legal issues at the bedside. J Heart Transplant 8:471–3, 1989
102. Farrar DJ, Hill JD, Gray LA Jr et al: Heterotopic prosthetic ventricles as a bridge to cardiac transplantation. A multicenter study in 29 patients. N Engl J Med 318:333–40, 1988
103. Muneretto C, Solis E, Pavie A et al: Total artificial heart: survival and complications. Ann Thorac Surg 47:151–7, 1989
104. Landreneau RJ, Horton JW, Cochran RP: Splanchnic blood flow response to intraaortic balloon pump assist of hemorrhagic shock. J Surg Res 51:281–7, 1991
105. Huszczuk A, Whipp BJ, Adams TD et al: Ventilatory control during exercise in calves with artificial hearts [see comments]. J Appl Physiol 68:2604–11, 1990
106. Robotham JL, Mays JB, Williams MA, DeVries WC: Cardiorespiratory interactions in patients with an artificial heart. Anesthesiology 73:599–609, 1990
107. Marconi C, Grassi B, Meyer M et al: Ventilatory and gas exchange kinetics in a human recipient of a Jarvik-7 total artificial heart [letter; comment]. J Appl Physiol 70:1406–7, 1991
108. Sharp MK, Olsen DB: Sensitivity of the artificial heart to changes in vascular resistance. ASAIO Trans 36:805–10, 1990
109. Kawaguchi AT, Gandjbahch I, Pavie A et al: Liver and kidney function in patients undergoing mechanical circulatory support with Jarvik-7 artificial heart as a bridge to transplantation. J Heart Transplant 9:631–7, 1990
110. Joyce LD, Johnson KE, Toninato CJ et al: Results of the first 100 patients who received Symbion Total Artificial Hearts as a bridge to cardiac transplantation. Circulation 80: III192–201, 1989
111. Griffith BP: Interim use of the Jarvik-7 artificial heart: lessons learned at Presbyterian–University Hospital of Pittsburgh. Ann Thorac Surg 47:158–66, 1989
112. Hastings WL, Aaron JL, Deneris J et al: A retrospective study of nine calves surviving five months of the pneumatic total artificial heart. Trans Am Soc Artif Intern Organs 27: 71–5, 1981
113. Borovetz HS, Kormos RL, Griffith BP, Hung TC: Clinical utilization of the artificial heart. Crit Rev Biomed Eng 17:179–201, 1989
114. Pae WE Jr, Pierce WS: Combined registry for the clinical use of mechanical ventricular assist pumps and the total artificial heart: second official report—1987. J Heart Transplant 8:1–4, 1989
115. Addonizio VP: Platelet function in cardiopulmonary bypass and artificial organs. Hematol Oncol Clin North Am 4:145–55, 1990
116. Cottrell ED, Kappa JR, Stenach N et al: Temporary inhibition of platelet function with iloprost (ZK36374) preserves canine platelets during extracorporeal membrane oxygenation. J Thorac Cardiovasc Surg 96:535–41, 1988
117. Takahama T, Kanai F, Hiraishi M et al: Combined administration of protease inhibitor and thromboxane A2 synthetase inhibitor for anticoagulation of a left ventricular assist device. ASAIO Trans 36:M141–4, 1990
118. Hung TC, Borovetz HS, Kormos RL et al: Artificial heart. Hemorrheology and transient ischemic attacks. ASAIO Trans 36:M132–5, 1990
119. Vlahakes GJ, Turley K, Hoffman JIE: The pathophysiology of failure in acute right ventricular hypertension: hemodynamic and biochemical correlations. Circulation 63:87–95, 1981
120. Christopherson LK: Heart transplants. Hastings Cent Rep 12:18–21, 1982
121. Loisance D, Dubois Rande JL, Deleuze PH et al: Pharmacological bridge to cardiac transplantation. Eur J Cardiothorac Surg 3: 196–202, 1989
122. Liska J, Brodin LA, Koul B: Hemodynamic effects of epinephrine, dopamine, nitroglycerin, and nitroprusside in a patient with a total artificial heart (TAH). Anesthesiology 72:757–60, 1990
123. Pennington DG, Swartz MT: Temporary circulatory support in patients with postcardiotomy cardiogenic shock. Cardiac Surg State of the Art Rev 5:373–92, 1991
124. Bolman RM, Cox JL, Marshall W et al: Circulatory support with a centrifugal pump as a bridge to cardiac transplantation. Ann Thorac Surg 47:108–12, 1989
125. Rouby JJ, Leger P, Andreev A et al: Peripheral vascular effects of halothane and isoflurane in humans with an artificial heart. Anesthesiology 72:462–9, 1990
126. Sweet SE, Sussman HA, Ryan TJ et al: Se-

quential radionuclide imaging during paracorporeal left ventricular support. Chest 78: 423–8, 1980

127. Taylor A Jr, Milton W, Christian PE et al: The role of nuclear imaging in the management of the first total artificial heart recipient. Clin Nucl Med 10:427–31, 1985

128. Moritz A, Napoli CA, Feiglin D et al: Radionuclide assessment of the natural heart ejection fraction before and after LVAD implantation. Int J Artif Organs 12:41–6, 1989

129. Takatani S, Noda H, Takano H, Akutsu T: Continuous in-line monitoring of oxygen delivery to control artificial heart output. Artif Organs 14:458–65, 1990

130. Williams JP, Brooks M, Chelly J et al: Do changes in myocardial wall-thickening fractions reflect changes in global functions? Anesthesiology 73:A162, 1990

131. Brenner BM, Dworkin LD, Ichikawa I: Glomerular ultrafiltration. p. 124. In Brenner BM, Rector FG (eds): The Kidney. WB Saunders, Philadelphia 1986

132. Peters AM: Quantification of renal haemodynamics with radionuclides. Eur J Nucl Med 18:274–86, 1991

133. Kampmann JP, Hansen JM: Glomerular filtration rate and creatinine clearance. Br J Clin Pharmacol 12:7–14, 1981

134. Bauer JH, Brooks CS, Burch RN: Clinical appraisal of creatinine clearance as a measurement of glomerular filtration rate. Am J Kidney Dis 2:337–46, 1982

135. Lewis R, Kerr N, Van Buren C et al: Comparative evaluation of urographic contrast media, inulin, and 99mTc-DTPA clearance methods for determination of glomerular filtration rate in clinical transplantation. Transplantation 48:790–6, 1989

136. Johnson DJ, Muhlbacher R, Wilmore DW: Current research review. Measurement of hepatic blood flow. J Surg Res 39:470–81, 1985

137. Shaw WJ, Pantalos GM, Everett S, Olsen DB: Factors influencing the accuracy of the cardiac output monitoring and diagnostic unit for pneumatic artificial hearts. ASAIO Trans 36:M264–8, 1990

138. Vonesh MJ, Cork RC, Mylrea KC: A noninvasive method of estimating mean pulmonary artery pressure in the pneumatic total artificial heart. J Clin Monit 7:294–303, 1991

139. Bolooki H, Williams W, Thurer RJ et al: Clinical and hemodynamic criteria for use of the intra-aortic balloon pump in patients requiring cardiac surgery. J Thorac Cardiovasc Surg 72:756–68, 1976

140. Golding LAR, Loop FD, Peter M et al: Late survival following use of intraaortic balloon pump in revascularization operations. Ann Thorac Surg 30:48–51, 1980

141. Foex P: Evaluating the right ventricle. p. 13. In Stanley TH, Sperry RJ (eds): Anesthesiology and the Heart. Kluwer Academic, Dordrecht, 1990

142. Mickleborough LL, Rebeyka I, Wilson GJ, Gray G, Desrosiers A: Comparison of left ventricular assist and intra-aortic balloon counterpulsation during early reperfusion after ischemic arrest of the heart. J Thorac Cardiovasc Surg 93:597–608, 1987

143. Duncan JM, Frazier OH, Radovancevic B, Velebit V: Implantation techniques for the Hemopump. Ann Thorac Surg 48:733–5, 1989

144. Merhige ME, Smalling RW, Cassidy D et al: Effect of the hemopump left ventricular assist device on regional myocardial perfusion and function. Reduction of ischemia during coronary occlusion. Circulation 80: III158–66, 1989

145. Frazier OH, Wampler RK, Duncan JM et al: First human use of the Hemopump, a catheter-mounted ventricular assist device. Ann Thorac Surg 49:299–304, 1990

146. Miller CA, Pae WE Jr, Pierce WS: Combined registry for the clinical use of mechanical ventricular assist devices. Postcardiotomy cardiogenic shock. ASAIO Trans 36:43–6, 1990

147. Veasy LG, Webster HF, McGough EC: Intra-aortic balloon pumping: adaptation for pediatric use. Crit Care Clin 2:237–49, 1986

148. Ballantyne CM, Verani MS, Short D et al: Delayed recovery of severely "stunned" myocardium with the support of a left ventricular assist device after coronary artery bypass graft surgery. J Am Coll Cardiol 10:710–2, 1987

149. Rosenberg G: Technological opportunities and barriers in the development of mechanical circulatory support systems. p. 211. In Hogness Jr, Van Antwerp M (eds): The Artificial Heart. Prototypes, Policies and Patients.

(eds): National Academy Press, Washington, DC, 1991

149a. Pae WE Jr: Ventricular assist devices and total artificial hearts: a combined registry experience. Ann Thorac Surg 55:295–8, 1993

150. Pliam MB: Temporary left heart assist for open heart surgery patients: clinical experience from a Community Hospital and review of the literature. Minn Med 69:341–52, 1986

151. Drinkwater DC, Laks H: Clinical experience with centrifugal pump ventricular support at UCLA Medical Center. ASAIO Trans 34: 505–8, 1988

152. Wampler RK: Investigational trials of the hemopump. Temporary cardiac assist with an axial pump system. Edited by Flameng W. New York, Springer-Verlag, 1991, pp 39–46

153. Hill JD: Bridging to cardiac transplantation. Ann Thorac Surg 47:167–71, 1989

154. Magovern GJ, Golding LA, Oyer PE, Cabrol C: Circulatory support 1988. Weaning and bridging. Ann Thorac Surg 47:102–7, 1989

155. Wareing TH, Kouchoukos NT: Postcardiotomy mechanical circulatory support in the elderly. Ann Thorac Surg 51:443–7, 1991

155a. Dasse KA, Frazier OH, Lesniak JM et al: Clinical responses to ventricular assistance versus transplantation in a series of bridge to transplant patients. ASAIO J 38:M622–6, 1992

156. Davis PK, Rosenberg G, Snyder AJ, Pierce WS: Current status of permanent total artificial hearts. Ann Thorac Surg 47:172–8, 1989

157. Rokitansky A, Laczkovics A, Prodinger A et al: The new small Viennese total artificial heart: experimental and first clinical experiences. Artif Organs 15:129–35, 1991

158. Lammermeier D, Frazier OH, Igo SR, Cooley DA: Total artificial hearts and ventricular assist devices as bridges to heart transplantation. Tex Med 84:56–60, 1988

159. Lewis RM, Van Buren CT, Radovancevic B et al: Impact of long-term cyclosporine immunosuppressive therapy on native kidneys versus renal allografts: serial renal function in heart and kidney transplant recipients. J Heart Lung Transplant 10(1 pt 1):63–70, 1991

160. Bolman RM, Spray TL, Cox JL et al: Heart transplantation in patients requiring preoperative mechanical support. J Heart Transplant 6:273–280, 1987

161. Oaks TE, Wisman CB, Pae WE et al: Results of mechanical circulatory assistance before heart transplantation. J Heart Transplant 8: 113–5, 1989

162. Sanders KM, Stern TA, O'Gara PT et al: Medical and neuropsychiatric complications associated with use of the intraaortic balloon pump. J Intensive Care Med 7:154–64, 1992

163. Perler BA, McCabe CJ, Abbott WM, Buckley MJ: Vascular complications of intra-aortic balloon counterpulsation. Arch Surg 118: 957–62, 1983

164. Nakatani T, Takano H, Noda H et al: Prerequisites to salvage profound biventricular failure patients with ventricular assist devices. Int J Artif Organs 12:234–41, 1989

165. Kankaanpaa J: Cost-effectiveness of liver transplantations—how to apply the results in resource allocation. Prev Med 19:700–4, 1990

166. Valenzuela TD, Criss EA, Spaite D et al: Cost-effectiveness analysis of paramedic emergency medical services in the treatment of prehospital cardiopulmonary arrest. Ann Emerg Med 19:1407–11, 1990

167. Kelley MD: Hypercholesterolemia: the cost of treatment in perspective. South Med J 83: 1421–5, 1990

168. Phillips SJ: Hemopump support for the failing heart. ASAIO Trans 36:2M629–32, 1990

169. Szycher M, Clay W, Gernes D, Sherman C: Thermedics approach to ventricular support systems. J Biomater Appl 1:39–105, 1986

Appendix 17-1

Cost per Quality Adjusted Life-Year of Selected Health Care Options

Health Care Option	Cost per Quality Adjusted Life Year
Medical therapy for hypercholesterolemia with	
Diet	$-$2,536
Oat bran 1.5 cups · day^{-1}	$20,448
Fish oil 25 g · day^{-1}	$77,534
Gemfibrozil 600 mg bid	$108,826
Coronary care units for	
High-risk patients	$69,900
Low-risk patients	$294,400
Coronary angioplasty for	
Severe angina	$12,700
Mild angina	$102,400
Coronary artery bypass surgery for	
Left main disease	$6.900
Mild angina, poor LV function	$9,500
3-vessel disease	$143,800
Mild angina, good LV function	
3-vessel disease	
Mild angina, 1-vessel disease	$899,300
Surgical repair of congenital heart disease	
Ventricular septal defect	NA
Tetralogy of Fallot	NA
Hypoplastic left heart	NA
Transplantation of	
Lung	NA
Liver	$45,000
Heart	$32,000
Total artificial heart	$105,000

(Data abstracted from refs. 50, 165–167.)

Appendix 17-2

Manufacturers of Devices

Intra-aortic balloon pump
Aries Medical
Division of St. Judes Medical
12 Elizabeth Drive
Chelmsford, MA 01824
(508) 250-8020

Datascope Corporation
14 Phillips Parkway
Montvale, NJ 07645
(800) 288-2121

Arrow International
(formerly Kontron Instrument)
3000 Bernville Road
Reading, PA 19605

Mansfield Scientific
135 Forbes Boulevard
Mansfield, MA 02048
(800) 842-0996

Centrifugal pump
BioMedicus-Medtronics
9600 West 76th Street
Eden Prairie, MN 55344
(612) 944-7784

3M Health Care
6200 Jackson Road
Ann Arbor, MI 48103
(800) 521-2818

Roller pump
Cobe Laboratories
Cardiovascular Division
14401 West 65th Way
Arvada, CO 80004-3599
(800) 525-2623

Polystan
Vital Core
Division of Columbia Vital Systems
100 East Chestnut
Westmont, IL 60559
(800) 874-8358

3M Health Care
6200 Jackson Road
Ann Arbor, MI 48103
(800) 521-2818

Sorin Biomedical
Cardiopulmonary Marketing
17600 Gillette Avenue
P.O. Box 19503
Irvine, CA 92713-9503
(800) 854-3683

Paracorporeal ventricular assist device
BVS-5000
ABIOMED
33 Cherryhill Drive
Danvers, MA 01923
(508) 777-5410

Thoratec (AKA-Pierce-Donachy)
2023 Eighth Street
Berkeley, CA 94710
(510) 841-1213

Corporeal ventricular assist device
Thermo Cardiosystems, Inc.
Subsidiary of Thermedics
P.O. Box 2999
Woburn, MA 01888-2697
(617) 932-8668

HEMOPUMP
Medtronic DLP
Hemodynamics Division
620 Watson, SW
P.O. Box 409
Grand Rapids, MI 49501-0409

Novacor
Division of Baxter Healthcare Corporation
7799 Pardee Lane
Oakland, CA 94621
(510) 568-8338

407

TAH
ABIOMED
33 Cherryhill Drive
Danvers, MA 01923
(508) 777-5410

E4T-2
Nimbus Corporation
2945 Kilgore Road
Rancho Cordova, CA 95670
(916) 852-2833

Pennsylvania State University
Hershey Medical Center
P.O. Box 850
Hershey, PA 17033
(717) 534-8521

EH-TAH & Utah-100
University of Utah
Artificial Heart Research Laboratory
Institute for Biomedical Engineering
803 North 300 West
Salt Lake City, UT 84103-1414
(801) 581-6991

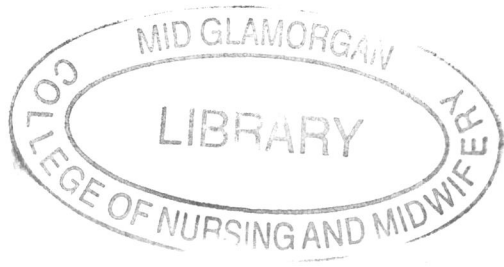

Index

Page numbers followed by f indicate figures; those followed by t indicate tables.

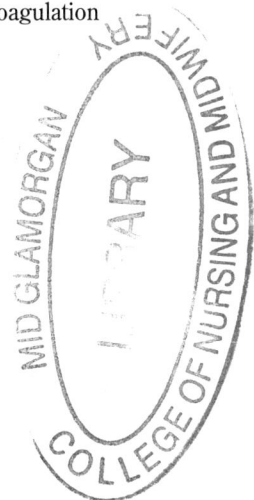

neurologic assessment in
   after full recovery, 236
   in immediate postoperative period, 227,
      234–236, 235t
   open vs. closed ventricular procedures in, 227
   risk factors for, 225–227, 225t
   summary of, 236
   with ventricular assist devices, 397, 397t
Neurotoxicity, of cyclosporine, 71–72
Nicardipine
   antianginal effects of, 328
   in cardiopulmonary bypass
      interaction with endothelin, 162
      renal effects of, 162
   classification of, 327f
   coronary vasodilation with, 327–328
Nifedipine
   antianginal effects of, 328
   classification of, 327f
   coronary vasodilation with, 327–328
   hemodynamic effects of, 327
Nimbus mechanical circulatory support device
   anatomic location of, 373f
   features of, 375t
Nimodipine, 327f
Nitrates
   mode of action, 328, 329–330, 330t
   pharmacokinetic alterations, in heart disease,
      336
Nitric oxide, inhaled
   for pulmonary hypertension, 347–348
   for right ventricular failure, 127, 134, 135f
Nitroglycerin
   absorption by CPB apparatus, 340
   action of, 329–330, 330t
   interaction with mechanical circulatory sup-
      port devices, 380–381, 381t
   pharmacokinetics, during CPB, 343
   postoperative
      dosage of, 346
      for hemodynamic management, 141
      for low cardiac output syndrome, 346
Nitroprusside
   interaction with mechanical circulatory sup-
      port devices, 380, 381t
   pharmacokinetics, during CPB, 343
   postoperative
      dosage of, 346
      for hemodynamic management, 140–141
      for low cardiac output syndrome, 346
   preoperative therapy with, 328
Norepinephrine
   adverse effects of, 358, 358t
   for cardiomyopathy, 60
   perioperative use of, 333

postoperative
   dosage of, 347t
   for hemodynamic management, 140
   transforming growth factor stimulation by, 31
   for ventricular hypertrophy, 29
Nosocomial infection. *See under* Infections
Novacor ventricular assist device
   anatomic location of, 369f
   energy converter operation of, 370f
   features of, 375t
   outcome assessment of, 392, 395
Nutritional support. *See also* Malnutrition
   in cardiac surgery, 149–150
   in mechanical ventilation, 117

O

Obliterative cardiomyopathy. *See* Restrictive-
   obliterative cardiomyopathy
OKT3. *See* AntiCD-3 monoclonal antibody
   (OKT3)
OKT4-LEU-3a monoclonal antibody, 76t
OKT8-LEU-2 monoclonal antibody, 76t
OKY-045, 378
Oncogenes. *See also* Proto-oncogenes
   activation of, in ventricular hypertrophy,
      30–31
   in ventricular pressure overload, 30–31
Ophthalmologic complications of CABG surgery,
   224
Opiate antagonists, 235
Opioid analgesia. *See also* specific agents
   combined with
      intrathecal local anesthetics, 310
      local thoracic epidural analgesia, 309–310
   misconceptions about, 304
   pharmacokinetics, during CPB, 344
   for postoperative stress response, 345
   systemic, 305
   thoracic epidural, 308, 309t–310t
Organ failure, multiple. *See* Multiorgan failure
Outcome assessment, for MCSS
   as bridge to transplant, 393–395
   in postoperative cardiac failure, 389–392,
      390t–391t
Oxacillin, 202
Oximetry, cerebral, 232–233
Oxygen
   concentration of, in weaning process, 111
   systemic delivery of
      monitoring of, in mechanical circulatory sup-
         port, 384
      PEEP ventilation interference with, 105
      postoperative management of, 124

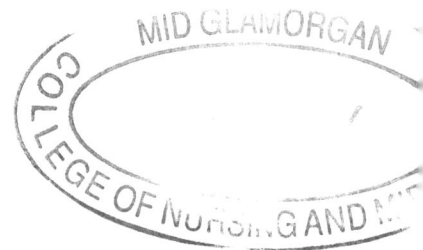